# PROGRESS IN CLINICAL AND BIOLOGICAL RESEARCH

## RECENT TITLES

Please contact the publisher for information about previous titles in this series.

# ADVANCES IN NEUROBLASTOMA RESEARCH 2

# Advances in Neuroblastoma Research 2

Proceedings of the Fourth Symposium on Advances in Neuroblastoma
Research Held in Philadelphia, Pennsylvania, May 14–16, 1987

Editors

**Audrey E. Evans**
The Children's Hospital of Philadelphia
Philadelphia

**Giulio J. D'Angio**
The Children's Hospital of Philadelphia
Philadelphia

**Alfred G. Knudson**
Fox Chase Cancer Research Center
University of Pennsylvania
Philadelphia

**Robert C. Seeger**
The Jonsson Comprehensive Cancer Center
UCLA School of Medicine
Los Angeles

ALAN R. LISS, INC. • NEW YORK

**Address all Inquiries to the Publisher**
**Alan R. Liss, Inc., 41 East 11th Street, New York, NY 10003**

**While the authors, editors, and publisher believe that drug selection and dosage and the specifications and usage of equipment and devices, as set forth in this book, are in accord with current recommendations and practice at the time of publication, they accept no legal responsibility for any errors or omissions, and make no warranty, express or implied, with respect to material contained herein. In view of ongoing research, equipment modifications, changes in governmental regulations and the constant flow of information relating to drug therapy, drug reactions and the use of equipment and devices, the reader is urged to review and evaluate the information provided in the package insert or instructions for each drug, piece of equipment or device for, among other things, any changes in the instructions or indications of dosage or usage and for added warnings and precautions.**

**Library of Congress Cataloging-in-Publication Data**

Symposium on Advances in Neuroblastoma Research
   (4th  :  1987  :  Philadelphia, Pa.)
   Advances in neuroblastoma research 2.

   (Progress in clinical and biological research  ;
271)
   Includes bibliographies and index.
   1. Neuroblastoma—Congresses.  2. Cancer cells—
Congresses.  3. Oncogenes—Congresses.  I. Evans,
Audrey E., 1925-  .  II. Title.  III. Series:
Progress in clinical and biological research  ; v.  271.
[DNLM: 1. Bone Marrow—transplantation—congresses.
2. Cell Transformation, Neoplastic—congresses.
3. Iodine Radioisotopes—therapeutic use—congresses.
4. Iodobenzenes—therapeutic use—congresses.
5. Neuroblastoma—therapy—congresses. 6. Oncogenes—congresses.  W, 1 PR668E v. 271  /  QZ 380 S989 1987a]
RC280.N4S95  1987     618.92'9948     88–843
ISBN 0-8451-5121-5

# Contents

## ONCOGENES

# DIFFERENTIATION AND CELL BIOLOGY

## [131]I-META-IODOBENZYLGUANIDINE THERAPY

# Contributors

**Chizuru Abe-Nakagawa,** Department of Molecular Biology, Toho University School of Medicine, Tokyo 143, Japan **[121]**

**H. Ando,** Japan **[525]**

**Bernard Aubert,** Department of Physics, INSERM U66, Institut Gustave-Roussy, 94805 Villejuif Cedex, France **[655]**

**Ann Barrett,** Glasgow Institute of Radiotherapeutics and Oncology, Glasgow G31 4PG, Scotland **[509]**

**Chantal Bayle,** Department of Hematology, Institut Gustave-Roussy, Villejuif, France **[689]**

**A. Bernard,** Institut G. Roussy, Villejuif, France **[225]**

**J.L. Bernard,** Department of Pediatric Oncology, Hôpital d'Enfants de la Timone, 13385 Marseille Cedex 5, France **[583]**

**F. Berthold,** Department of Pediatrics, University of Köln, 5000 Köln, Federal Republic of Germany **[669]**

**June L. Biedler,** Cell Biology Program and Laboratory of Cellular and Biochemical Genetics, Memorial Sloan-Kettering Cancer Center, New York, NY 10021 and Walker Laboratory, Rye, NY 10580 **[103,265,277,449]**

**P. Biron,** Centre Léon Bérard, 69373 Lyon, France **[225]**

**Robert L. Bjork,** Department of Pediatrics and the Jonsson Comprehensive Cancer Center, UCLA School of Medicine, Los Angeles, CA 90024 **[41]**

**Joseph B. Bolen,** Pediatric Branch, Laboratory of Tumor Virus Biology, Division of Cancer Etiology, National Cancer Institute, National Institutes of Health, Bethesda, MD 20892 **[185]**

**Bruce Bostrom,** Divisions of Clinical Pharmacology and Pediatric Oncology, Departments of Pediatrics and Pharmacology, University of Minnesota Medical School, Minneapolis, MN 55455 **[557]**

**Eric Bouffet,** Department of Pediatric Oncology, Centre Leon Berard, 69373 Lyon, France **[573]**

**J.F. Bouvier,** Department of Nuclear Medicine, Centre Leon Berard, 69373 Lyon Cedex 08, France **[707]**

**Jennifer P. Boyd,** Department of Pediatrics, University of Pennsylvania Medical School, Philadelphia, PA 19104 **[353]**

**V. Breant,** Laboratoire Hospitalo-Universitaire-U 278, Faculté de Pharmacie, 13385 Marseille Cedex 5, France **[583]**

**Garrett M. Brodeur,** Departments of Pediatrics and Genetics, Washington University School of Medicine, St. Louis, MO 63110 **[3,41,57,91,291,509]**

The numbers in brackets are the opening page numbers of the contributors' articles.

xiii

**Maud Brunat-Mentigny,** Department of Pediatric Oncology, Centre Leon Berard, 69373 Lyon, France **[573,707]**

**Jean M. Caillaud,** Department of Pathology, Institut Gustave-Roussy, 94805 Villejuif Cedex, France **[689]**

**J.P. Cano,** Laboratoire Hospitalo-Universitaire-U 278, Faculté de Pharmacie, 13385 Marseille Cedex 5, France **[583]**

**Christian Carrie,** Department of Pediatric Oncology, Centre Leon Berard, 69373 Lyon, France **[573]**

**A. Casalaro,** Pediatric Oncology Research Laboratory, G. Gaslini Research Children's Hospital, 16148 Genoa, Italy **[437]**

**J. Casper,** University of Wisconsin, Milwaukee, WI and the Pediatric Oncology Group, St. Louis, MO **[215]**

**Robert P. Castleberry,** University of Alabama, Birmingham, AL 35233 **[509]**

**Andrea O. Cavazzana,** Laboratory of Pathology, National Cancer Institute, National Institutes of Health, Bethesda, MD 20184 **[463,475,487]**

**Lorraine Cazenave,** Pediatric Branch, National Cancer Institute, National Institutes of Health, Bethesda, MD 20892 **[185]**

**Tien-ding Chang,** Laboratory of Cellular and Biochemical Genetics, Memorial Sloan-Kettering Cancer Center, New York, NY 10021 **[265]**

**M. Charbit,** Laboratoire Hospitalo-Universitaire-U 278, Faculté de Pharmacie, 13385 Marseille Cedex 5, France **[583]**

**P. Chauvot,** Department of Nuclear Medicine, Centre Leon Berard, 69373 Lyon Cedex 08, France **[707]**

**Nai-Kong V. Cheung,** Departments of Pediatrics, Radiology, Pathology, and Medicine, Case Western Reserve University, Cleveland, OH 44106 and Department of Pediatrics, Memorial Sloan-Kettering Cancer Center, New York, NY 10021 **[237,249,595,619]**

**Valentina Ciccarone,** Laboratory of Neurobiology, Department of Biological Sciences, Fordham University, Bronx, NY 10458 **[277]**

**C. Cirillo,** Pediatric Oncology Research Laboratory, G. Gaslini Research Children's Hospital, 16148 Genoa, Italy **[437]**

**J. Clarke,** Imperial Cancer Research Fund, Oncology Laboratory, Institute of Child Health, London, England **[605,643]**

**Peter Coccia,** Departments of Pediatrics and Medicine, Case Western Reserve University, Cleveland, OH 44106 and Memorial Sloan-Kettering Cancer Center, New York, NY 10021 **[237]**

**V. Combaret,** Centre Léon Bérard, 69373 Lyon, France **[225]**

**Mark J. Cooper,** Pediatric Branch, National Cancer Institue, National Institutes of Health, Bethesda, MD 20892 **[175]**

**Sabine Coornaert,** ORIS-I-CEA, 91190 France **[655,689]**

**P. Cornaglia-Ferraris,** Pediatric Oncology Research Laboratory, G. Gaslini Research Children's Hospital, 16148 Genoa, Italy **[437]**

**Dominique Couanet,** Department of Radiology, Institut Gustave-Roussy, 94805 Villejuif Cedex, France **[547,689]**

**Giulio D'Angio,** Children's Hospital of Philadelphia, Philadelphia, PA 19145 **[509]**

**Bruno De Bernardi,** Instituto Giannina Gaslini, 16148 Genova, Italy **[509]**

**J. de Kraker,** Department of Pediatric Oncology, Emma Kinderziekenhuis, 1018 HJ Amsterdam, The Netherlands **[679]**

**Ludvik Donner,** Laboratory of Pathology, National Cancer Institute, National Institutes of Health, Bethesda, MD 20184 **[291]**

**R. Dopfer,** Department of Pediatrics, University of Tübingen, 7400 Tübingen, Federal Republic of Germany **[669]**

**F. Ducrettet,** Department of Nuclear Medicine, Centre Leon Berard, 69373 Lyon Cedex 08, France **[707]**

**Reggie E. Duerst,** Department of Pediatrics, University of Rochester Medical Center, Rochester, NY 14642 **[249]**

**G. Elsom,** Imperial Cancer Research Fund, Oncology Laboratory, Institute of Child Health, London, England **[605]**

**Noriko Esumi,** Department of Pediatrics, Kyoto Prefectural University of Medicine, Kyoto 602, Japan **[327]**

**Audrey E. Evans,** Division of Oncology, Children's Hospital of Philadelphia, Philadelphia, PA 19104 **[175,509]**

**Anne Farge,** Department of Pediatric Oncology, Centre Leon Berard, 69373 Lyon, France **[573]**

**Marie C. Favrot,** Centre Léon Bérard, 69373 Lyon, France **[225,509]**

**Stephen A. Feig,** Department of Pediatrics and the Jonsson Comprehensive Cancer Center, UCLA School of Medicine, Los Angeles, CA 90024 **[203]**

**U. Feine,** Department of Nuclear Medicine, University of Tübingen, 7400 Tübingen, Federal Republic of Germany **[669]**

**Donald W. Fink,** Department of Pharmacology, Division of Clinical Pharmacology, University of Minnesota, Minneapolis, MN 55455 **[317]**

**Chin-to Fong,** Department of Pediatrics, Washington University School of Medicine, St. Louis, MO 63110 **[3]**

**Christopher S. Foster,** Joseph Stokes, Jr. Research Institute, and the Department of Pediatrics, University of Pennsylvania Medical School, Philadelphia, PA 19104 **[421]**

**Christopher N. Frantz,** Department of Pediatrics, University of Rochester Medical Center, Rochester, NY 14642 **[249]**

**Arnold I. Freeman,** Roswell Park Memorial Institute, Buffalo, NY **[509]**

**J. A. Garson,** ICRF Oncology Laboratory, ICH, London, England **[151]**

**Adrian P. Gee,** Department of Pediatrics Hematology/Oncology, University of Florida, Gainesville, FL 32610 and the Pediatric Oncology Group, St. Louis, MO **[215]**

**Jean-Claude Gentet,** Department of Pediatric Oncology, Hôpital d'Enfants de la Timone, 13385 Marseille Cedex 5, France **[573,583]**

**Anne Geoffray,** Department of Radiology, Institut Gustave-Roussy, 94805 Villejuif Cedex, France **[547]**

**V. Gerein,** Department of Pediatric Oncology, Children's Hospital of the University, 6000 Frankfurt, Federal Republic of Germany **[669]**

**Stanley Gerson,** Departments of Pediatrics and Medicine, Case Western Reserve University, Cleveland, OH 44106 and Memorial Sloan-Kettering Cancer Center, New York, NY 10021 **[237]**

**Fred Gilbert,** Department of Pediatrics, Division of Medical Genetics, Mt. Sinai School of Medicine, New York, NY 10029 **[17]**

**Mary Catherine Glick,** Department of Pediatrics, University of Pennsylvania Medical School, Philadelphia, PA 19104 **[353,421]**

**I. Gordon,** The Hospital for Sick Children, London, England **[605,643]**

**M. Graham,** Johns Hopkins University, Baltimore, MD, and The Pediatric Oncology Group, St. Louis, MO **[215]**

**John Graham-Pole,** Department of Pediatrics Hematology/Oncology, University of Florida, Gainesville, FL 32610 and the Pediatric Oncology Group, St. Louis, MO **[215]**

**Mark Greene,** Department of Pathology and Laboratory Medicine, University of Pennsylvania School of Medicine, Philadelphia, PA 19104 **[165]**

**Rogers Griffith,** Department of Pathology, Washington University School of Medicine, St. Louis, MO 63110 **[3]**

**Samuel Gross,** Department of Pediatrics Hematology/Oncology, University of Florida, Gainesville, FL 32610 and the Pediatric Oncology Group, St. Louis, MO **[215]**

**Fadhel Guermazi,** Department of Nuclear Medicine, Institut Gustave-Roussy, Villejuif, France **[689]**

**Gerald Haase,** Children's Hospital of Denver, Denver, CO 80218 **[509]**

**Y. Hanawa,** Japan **[525]**

**J. Happ,** Department of Radiology, University of Frankfurt, 6000 Frankfurt, Federal Republic of Germany **[669]**

**Richard Harris,** Department of Pediatrics, University of Cincinnati College of Medicine, Cincinnati, OH 45229 **[203]**

**Olivier Hartmann,** Department of Pédiatric Oncology, Institut Gustave-Roussy, 94805 Villejuif Cedex, France **[509,547,655,689]**

**W. Harvey,** Brooke Army Medical Center, San Antonio, TX and The Pediatric Oncology Group, St. Louis, MO **[215]**

**F. Ann Hayes,** Department of Hematology-Oncology, St. Jude Children's Research Hospital, Memphis, TN 38101 **[3,509]**

**Lee J. Helman,** Pediatric Branch, National Cancer Institute, National Institutes of Health, Bethesda, MD 20892 **[175]**

**Lawrence Helson,** Clinical and Medical Affairs Department, ICI Americas, and Stewart Pharmaceuticals, Wilmington, DE 19897 **[175,291,509]**

**Shigeyoshi Hibi,** Department of Pediatrics, Kyoto Prefectural University of Medicine, Kyoto 602, Japan **[327]**

**Ken Higashi,** Department of Biochemistry, University of Occupational and Environmental Health, Kitakyushu 807, Japan **[31]**

**Tamaki Hino,** Department of Pediatrics, Kyoto Perfectural University of Medicine, Kyoto 602, Japan **[337]**

**C.A. Hoefnagel,** Department of Nuclear Medicine, The Netherlands Cancer Institute, 1066 CX Amsterdam, The Netherlands **[679]**

**G. Hör,** Department of Radiology, University of Frankfurt, 6000 Frankfurt, Federal Republic of Germany **[669]**

**Yoshihiro Horii,** Department of Pediatrics, Kyoto Prefectural University of Medicine, Kyoto 602, Japan **[337]**

**Keiichi Ikeda,** Department of Pediatric Surgery, Faculty of Medicine, Kyushu University 60, Fukuoka 812, Japan **[31]**

**Naohiko Ikegaki,** Department of Human Genetics, University of Pennsylvania School of Medicine, Philadelphia, PA 19104 **[133]**

**Shinsaku Imashuku,** Department of Pediatrics, Children's Research Hospital, Kyoto Prefectural University of Medicine, Kyoto 602, Japan **[327]**

**Y. Ishiguro,** Japan **[525]**

**Mark A. Israel,** Pediatric Branch, National Cancer Institute, National Institutes of Health, Bethesda, MD 20892 **[175,185]**

**H. Jürgens,** Department of Pediatrics, University of Düsseldorf, 4000 Düsseldorf, Federal Republic of Germany **[669]**

**Naotoshi Kanda,** Department of Anatomy, Tokyo Women's Medical College, Tokyo 162, Japan **[121]**

**M. Kaneko,** Japan **[525]**

**N. Kapoor,** The Pediatric Oncology Group, St. Louis, MO **[215]**

**Kanefusa Kato,** Department of Biochemistry, Institute for Developmental Research, Aichi Prefectural Colony, Kasugai 480-03, Japan **[327]**

**John T. Kemshead,** Imperial Cancer Research Fund, Oncology Laboratory, Institute of Child Health, London, England **[151,337,395,509,535,605,643]**

**Roger H. Kennett,** Department of Human Genetics, University of Pennsylvania School of Medicine, Philadelphia, PA 19104 **[133]**

**Takanobu Kikuchi,** Department of Molecular Biology, Toho University School of Medicine, Tokyo 143, Japan **[121]**

**Th. Klingebiel,** Department of Pediatric Oncology, Children's Hospital of the University, 7400 Tübingen, Federal Republic of Germany **[669]**

**P. Koch,** Montreal Children's Hospital, Montreal, Quebec, Canada, and the Pediatric Oncology Group, St. Louis, MO **[215]**

**R. Koide,** Japan **[525]**

**B. Kornhuber,** Department of Pediatrics, University of Frankfurt, 6000 Frankfurt, Federal Republic of Germany **[669]**

**Bernard Kremens,** Department of Pediatric Oncology, Centre Leon Berard, 69373 Lyon, France **[573]**

**Gundula LaBadie,** Department of Pediatrics, Division of Medical Genetics, Mt. Sinai School of Medicine, New York, NY 10029 **[17]**

**B.E. Lahneche,** Department of Nuclear Medicine, Centre Léon Bérard, 69373 Lyon Cedex 08, France **[707]**

**Faustina LaLatta,** Department of Pediatrics, Division of Medical Genetics, Mt. Sinai School of Medicine, New York, NY 10029 **[17]**

**Fritz Lampert,** Leiter der Kinder-Poliklinik der Justus Liebig-Universitat, Giessen, Federal Republic of Germany **[509]**

**Lois A. Lampson,** Children's Cancer Research Center, Children's Hospital of Philadelphia, Philadelphia, PA 19104; present address: Center for Neurological Diseases, Brigham and Women's Hospital, Boston, MA 02115 **[409]**

**L.S. Lashford,** Imperial Cancer Research Fund, Oncology Laboratory, Institute of Child Health, and The Hospital for Sick Children, London, England **[605,643]**

**Yuk M. Law,** Department of Pediatrics and the Jonsson Comprehensive Cancer Center, UCLA School of Medicine, Los Angeles, CA 90024 **[91]**

**Hillard Lazarus,** Departments of Pediatrics and Medicine, Case Western Reserve University, Cleveland, OH 44106 and Memorial Sloan-Kettering Cancer Center, New York, NY 10021 **[237]**

**Jérôme G. Leclère,** Department of Nuclear Medicine, Institut Gustave-Roussy, 94805 Villejuif Cedex, France **[547,689]**

**Jean Lemerle,** Department of Pediatrics, Institut Gustave-Roussy, 94805 Villejuif Cedex, France **[655,689]**

**Carl Lenarsky,** Department of Pediatrics and the Jonsson Comprehensive Cancer Center, UCLA School of Medicine, Los Angeles, CA 90024 **[203]**

**Jean D. Lumbroso,** Department of Nuclear Medicine, Institut Gustave-Roussy, 94805 Villejuif Cedex, France **[547,655,689]**

**John L. Magnani,** Laboratory of Structural Biology, NIDDK, National Institutes of Health, Bethesda, MD 20184 **[487]**

**Henry C. Maguire, Jr.,** Department of Pathology and Laboratory Medicine, University of Pennsylvania School of Medicine, Philadelphia, PA 19104 **[165]**

**N. Maïassi,** Department of Nuclear Medicine, Centre Leon Berard, 69373 Lyon Cedex 08, France **[707]**

**M. Majoor,** Werkgroep Kindertumoren and Department of Nuclear Medicine, the Netherlands Cancer Institute, Emma Kinderziekenhuis, 1018 HJ Amsterdam, The Netherlands **[679]**

**Takafumi Matsumura,** Department of Pediatrics, Kyoto Prefectural University of Medicine, Kyoto 602, Japan **[337,395,525]**

**F. Maul,** Department of Radiology, University of Frankfurt, 6000 Frankfurt, Federal Republic of Germany **[669]**

**Bernard M. Mechler,** Institute of Genetics, Johannes Gutenberg University, D-6500 Mainz, Federal Republic of Germany **[377]**

**M. Edward Medof,** Department of Pediatrics, Memorial Sloan-Kettering Cancer Center, New York, NY 10021 and Departments of Pediatrics and Pathology, Case Western Reserve University, Cleveland, OH 44106 **[619]**

**Peter W. Melera,** Molecular Biology Program, Memorial Sloan-Kettering Cancer Center, Walker Laboratory, Rye, NY 10580 **[71,103]**

**A. Melodia,** Pediatric Oncology Research Laboratory, G. Gaslini Research Children's Hospital, 16148 Genoa, Italy **[437]**

**N. Mendenhall,** University of Florida, Gainesville, FL and the Pediatric Oncology Group, St. Louis, MO **[215]**

**Louis Merlin,** ORIS-I-CEA, 91190 France **[655]**

**Marian B. Meyers,** Laboratory of Cellular and Biochemical Genetics, Memorial Sloan-Kettering Cancer Center, New York, NY 10021 **[277,449]**

**Fathia Meziane,** Department of Pediatric Oncology, Centre Leon Berard, 69373 Lyon, France **[573]**

**Richard W. Michitsch,** Molecular and Cell Biology Programs, Memorial Sloan-Kettering Cancer Center, New York, NY 10021 **[103]**

**Floro D. Miraldi,** Departments of Pediatrics and Radiology, Case Western Reserve University, Cleveland, OH 44106 **[595]**

**Bernard L. Mirkin,** Divisions of Clinical Pharmacology and Pediatric Oncology, Departments of Pediatrics and Pharmacology, University of Minnesota Medical School, Minneapolis, MN 55455 **[317,557]**

**J. Miser,** Department of Pediatrics, Mayo Clinic, Rochester, MN **[487]**

**Kate T. Montgomery,** Molecular Biology Program, Memorial Sloan-Kettering Cancer Center, Walker Laboratory, Rye, NY 10580; present address: Department of Molecular Pharmacology, Albert Einstein College of Medicine, Bronx, NY 10461 **[71]**

**J. Morisset,** Institut G. Roussy, Villejuif, France **[225]**

**Michon Morita,** Department of Pediatrics, Washington University School of Medicine, St. Louis, MO 63110 **[3]**

**Thomas J. Moss,** Department of Pediatrics and the Jonsson Comprehensive Cancer Center, UCLA School of Medicine, Los Angeles, CA 90024 **[41,91,203]**

**David Munn,** Department of Pediatrics, Memorial Sloan-Kettering Cancer Center, New York, NY 10021 and Departments of Pediatrics and Pathology, Case Western Reserve University, Cleveland, OH 44106 **[619]**

**N. Nagahara,** Japan **[525]**

**Akira Nakagawara,** Department of Pediatric Surgery, Faculty of Medicine, Kyushu University 60, Fukuoka 812, Japan **[31]**

**N. Nakata,** Japan **[525]**

**Samuel Navarro,** Laboratory of Pathology, National Cancer Institute, National Institutes of Health, Bethesda, MD 20184 **[463,475]**

**Robert W. Newburgh,** Office of Naval Research, Arlington, VA 22217 **[307]**

**D. Niethammer,** Department of Pediatrics, University of Tübingen, 7400 Tübingen, Federal Republic of Germany **[669]**

**Jacques Ninane,** Cliniques St. Luc, Brussels B-1200, Belgium **[509]**

**K. Nishihira,** Japan **[525]**

**Rosa Noguera,** Laboratory of Pathology, National Cancer Institute, National Institutes of Health, Bethesda, MD 20184 **[463]**

**D. Norris,** Cleveland Clinic, Cleveland, OH, and The Pediatric Oncology Group, St. Louis, MO **[215]**

**Daniel T. O'Connor,** Division of Nephrology-Hypertension, VA Medical Center, San Diego, CA 92161 **[175]**

**Robert F. O'Dea,** Departments of Pediatrics and Pharmacology, Division of Clinical Pharmacology, University of Minnesota, Minneapolis, MN 55455 **[317]**

**I. Okabe,** Japan **[525]**

**Masaaki Okada,** Eisai Co. Ltd., Tokyo 112, Japan **[337]**

**Claude Parmentier,** Department of Nuclear Medicine, Institut Gustave-Roussy, 94805 Villejuif Cedex, France **[655,689]**

**Thierry Philip,** Department of Pediatric Oncology, Centre Léon Bérard, 69373 Lyon, France **[225,509,573,583,707]**

**T. Pick,** Cook Children's Hospital, Ft. Worth, TX, and The Pediatric Oncology Group, St. Louis, MO **[215]**

**Katarina Polakova,** Department of Human Genetics, University of Pennsylvania School of Medicine, Philadelphia, PA 19104, and Cancer Research Institute, Slovak Academy of Science, 81232 Bratislava, Czechoslovakia **[133]**

**M. Ponzoni,** Pediatric Oncology Research Laboratory, G. Gaslini Research Children's Hospital, 16148 Genoa, Italy **[437]**

**V.R. Potluri,** Department of Pediatrics, Division of Medical Genetics, Mt. Sinai School of Medicine, New York, NY 10029 **[17]**

**Laura Prince,** Department of Biomedical Science, Drexel University, Philadelphia, PA 19104 **[133]**

**Jon Pritchard,** The Hospital for Sick Children, London WC1N 3JH, England **[509,643]**

**Yvon Rabarison,** U66 INSERM, Villejuif, France **[689]**

**Norma Ramsay,** Department of Pediatrics, University of Minnesota School of Medicine, Minneapolis, MN 55455 **[203]**

**C. Raybaud,** Department of Pediatric Oncology, Hôpital d'Enfant de la Timone, 13385 Marseille Cedex 5, France **[583]**

**Sylvia A. Rayner,** Department of Pediatrics and the Jonsson Comprehensive Cancer Center, UCLA School of Medicine, Los Angeles, CA 90024 **[57]**

**C. Patrick Reynolds,** Department of Pediatrics and the Jonsson Comprehensive Cancer Center, UCLA School of Medicine, Los Angeles, CA 90024 **[57,203,291,307,463,475]**

**Marcel Ricard,** Department of Physics, INSERM U66, Institut Gustave-Roussy, 94805 Villejuif Cedex, France **[655]**

**Robert A. Ross,** Laboratory of Neurobiology, Department of Biological Sciences, Fordham University, Bronx, NY 10458 **[265,277,487]**

**Daniel H. Ryan,** Department of Pediatrics, University of Rochester Medical Center, Rochester, NY 14642 **[249]**

**Ulla Saarinen,** Departments of Pediatrics and Medicine, Case Western Reserve University, Cleveland, OH 44106 and Memorial Sloan-Kettering Cancer Center, New York, NY 10021 **[237]**

**Tohru Saida,** Department of Pediatrics, Kyoto Prefectural University of Medicine, Kyoto 602, Japan **[395]**

**N. Sasaki,** Japan **[525]**

**Harland Sather,** Children's Cancer Study Group, Pasadena, CA 91101 **[203]**

**Tadashi Sawada,** Department of Pediatrics, Kyoto Prefectural University of Medicine, Kyoto 602, Japan **[337,395,525]**

**Martin Schlumberger,** Department of Nuclear Medicine, Institut Gustave-Roussy, 94805 Villejuif Cedex, France **[655]**

**D. Schwabe,** Department of Pediatric Oncology, Children's Hospital of the University, 6000 Frankfurt, Federal Republic of Germany **[669]**

**Robert C. Seeger,** Department of Pediatrics and the Jonsson Comprehensive Cancer Center, UCLA School of Medicine, Los Angeles, CA 90024 **[3,41,57,91,203,291,475,509]**

**Michael Selch,** Department of Radiation Oncology and the Jonsson Comprehensive Cancer Center, UCLA School of Medicine, Los Angeles, CA 90024 **[203]**

**P. Sheppard,** Cambridge Research Biochemistry, Harston, Cambridge, England **[151]**

**Hiroyuki Shimatake,** Department of Molecular Biology, Toho University School of Medicine, Tokyo 143, Japan **[121]**

**Erica Sibinga,** Department of Pathology and Laboratory Medicine, University of Pennsylvania School of Medicine, Philadelphia, PA 19104 **[165]**

**Stuart Siegel,** Children's Hospital of Los Angeles, Los Angeles, CA 90027 **[509]**

**Dennis J. Slamon,** Department of Medicine and the Jonsson Comprehensive Cancer Center, UCLA School of Medicine, Los Angeles, CA 90024 **[41,57,91,475]**

**Ide E. Smith,** Oklahoma Children's Hospital, Oklahoma City, OK 73126 **[509]**

**Lawrence Sousa,** Amgen, Inc., Thousand Oaks, CA and Children's Cancer Study Group, Pasadena, CA 91101 **[41]**

**Barbara A. Spengler,** Laboratory of Cellular and Biochemical Genetics, Memorial Sloan-Kettering Cancer Center, New York, NY 10021 **[265,277]**

**Jerry Stein,** Department of Pediatrics and Medicine, Case Western Reserve University, Cleveland, OH 44106 and Memorial Sloane-Kettering Cancer Center, New York, NY 10021 **[237]**

**Sarah Strandjord,** Department of Pediatrics and Medicine, Case Western Reserve University, Cleveland, OH 44106 and Memorial Sloan-Kettering Cancer Center, New York, NY 10021 **[237]**

**Tohru Sugimoto,** Children's Research Hospital and the Department of Pediatrics, Kyoto Prefectural University of Medicine, Kyoto 602, Japan **[337,395,525]**

**Yoshikazu Suzuki,** Eisai Co. Ltd., Tokyo 112, Japan **[337]**

**Sudha Swamy,** Pediatric Branch, National Cancer Institute, National Institutes of Health, Bethesda, MD 20892 **[175]**

**Osamu Tagaya,** Eisai Co. Ltd., Tokyo 112, Japan **[337]**

**T. Takeda,** Japan **[525]**

**Carol J. Thiele,** Pediatric Branch, National Cancer Institute, National Institutes of Health, Bethesda, MD 20892 **[185]**

**P. Thomas,** Brooke Army Medical Center, San Antonio, TX and The Pediatric Oncology Group, St. Louis, MO **[215]**

**Mary M. Tomayko,** Department of Pediatrics and the Jonsson Comprehensive Cancer Center, UCLA School of Medicine, Los Angeles, CA 90024 **[57,291,307]**

**J. Treuner,** Department of Pediatric Oncology, Children's Hospital of the University, 7400 Tübingen, Federal Republic of Germany **[669]**

**Timothy J. Triche,** Laboratory of Pathology, National Cancer Institute, National Institutes of Health, Bethesda, MD 20184 **[291,307,463,475,487]**

**Kwei-Lan Tsao,** Department of Pediatrics, Division of Medical Genetics, Mt. Sinai School of Medicine, New York, NY 10029 **[17]**

**Yoshiaki Tsuchida,** Department of Surgery, National Children's Hospital, Tokyo 154, Japan **[121]**

**Tohru Tsuda,** Department of Biochemistry, University of Occupational and Environmental Health, Kitakyushu 807, Japan **[31]**

**Kentaro Tsunamoto,** Department of Pediatrics, Kyoto Prefectural University of Medicine, Kyoto 602, Japan **[327]**

**A. Tunoda,** Japan **[525]**

**J. van den Berghe,** Mothercare Unit, ICH, London, England **[151]**

**P.A. Voûte,** Werkgroep Kindertumoren, Emma Kinderziekenhuis, and the Department of Nuclear Medicine, The Netherlands Cancer Institute, NL-1018 HJ Amsterdam, The Netherlands **[509,679]**

**Daniel Von Hoff,** Departments of Pediatrics and Medicine, Case Western Reserve University, Cleveland, OH 44106 and Memorial Sloan-Kettering Cancer Center, New York, NY 10021 **[237]**

**Randal Wada,** Department of Pediatrics and the Jonsson Comprehensive Cancer Center, UCLA School of Medicine, Los Angeles, CA 90024 **[41,57]**

**Phyllis Warkentin,** Departments of Pediatrics and Medicine, Case Western Reserve University, Cleveland, OH 44106 and Memorial Sloan-Kettering Cancer Center, New York, NY 10021 **[237]**

**David Weiner,** Department of Pathology and Laboratory Medicine, University of Pennsylvania School of Medicine, Philadelphia, PA 19104 **[165]**

**John Wells,** Department of Medicine and the Jonsson Comprehensive Cancer Center, UCLA School of Medicine, Los Angeles, CA 90024 **[203]**

**David C. Wilbur,** Department of Pediatrics, University of Rochester Medical Center, Rochester, NY 14642 **[249]**

**Ling Xu,** Department of Pediatrics, Division of Medical Genetics, Mt. Sinai School of Medicine, New York, NY 10029 **[17]**

**K. Yamamoto,** Japan **[525]**

**T. Yazawa,** Japan **[525]**

**Jean-Michel Zucker,** Institut Curie, Paris, France **[573,583]**

# Preface

This volume contains papers presented at the Fourth Symposium on Neuroblastoma Research held at The Children's Hospital of Philadelphia in May 1987. The preface to the previous volume noted an explosion in the basic research in human neuroblastoma starting at the beginning of this decade. At this fourth meeting, the number of people attending and the number of abstracts submitted (83) were similar to the 1984 meeting, but there was an increase in the depth of research, and larger numbers of papers reported results of molecular biological research.

The discussions, which occupied almost half of the total conference time, have been summarized by the chairperson of each session and are included after each group of papers dealing with a given topic.

The first day of the conference was devoted to studies of oncogenes, the second to cell biology and differentiation, and the third to innovative therapies. There were enough reports related to $^{131}$I-meta-iodobenzylguanidine ($^{131}$I-MIBG) to fill an entire afternoon. One evening during the conference was devoted to clinical studies of bone marrow transplantation for primary treatment of patients with neuroblastoma and for treatment of patients in relapse. Two international reports were presented during the clinical session, one devoted to a proposed international staging system for neuroblastoma (with response criteria) and another to a multi-center blind study on the reactivity of a panel of monoclonal antibodies on neuroblastoma and other small round-cell tumors of childhood.

The first six papers published here and two related discussion periods were devoted to amplification of N-*myc* and its biological characteristics. Two papers reported neuroblastoma cell lines that expressed only one copy of the N-*myc* oncogene. In a second session devoted to molecular genetics, N-*myc* protein expression was characterized, and one paper reported the immunologic characteristics of the N-*myc* protein as measured by monoclonal antibodies. The session included a paper on the *neu*-oncogene, originally discovered in rats and now studied in human neuroblastoma. Another participant reported alterations in gene expression during retinoic acid induced differentiation.

The papers in the second section of this volume are devoted to differentiation and various aspects of cell biology. Several papers address the changes in various characteristics of the cells after differentiation, including expression of different proteins such as intermediate filament and fibronectin, S-100 protein induced by 5-bromo-2-deoxyuridine. One paper addresses neuronal differentiation by synthetic polyprenoic acid and in situ modulation of murine neuroblastoma nerve growth factor.

In a major invited lecture, Dr. Bernard M. Mechler reported his and Elizabeth Gateff's extraordinary studies on the neuroblastoma genes in *Drosophila* and the hereditary expression of tumor development by gene transfer.

Monoclonal antibodies were used in several studies to determine various changes in the expression of the cell membrane. One presentation provided comparison of the membrane phenotypes of neuroblastoma cells with fetal neuroblasts, and another demonstrated the significance of the absence of HLA-A, B, and C expression in neuroblastoma cells and other related cell lines.

The clinical sessions involved both diagnostic and therapeutic studies. As mentioned earlier, a proposal for a new staging system, including the studies necessary to confirm response to treatment, was discussed at length. There was general agreement to try the new staging system, but conference participants disagreed about which studies would be necessary for confirmation. The European group feels that [131]I-MIBG provides the most effective means of detecting small amounts of neuroblastoma, but it was pointed out that this nuclide study is not commonly available in the United States. The Japanese group presented data on mass screening of neuroblastoma in infancy, and this program was discussed with great interest. The session also included an interesting radiographic study of bone marrow metastasis detected by magnetic resonance imaging.

The papers that address recent advances in therapy fall mainly into two groups dealing with [131]I-MIBG and bone marrow transplantation. It is striking that there are only two papers on chemotherapy—carboplatin and very-high-dose cisplatin—which points up the fact that there have not been many recent advances in chemotherapy regimens. The six papers on [131]I-MIBG are all from Europe and report single institution or collaborative studies that show the effectiveness of this radiolabeled metabolic compound. However, the therapeutic response seems to be short-lived. Perhaps the next series of studies will be related to use of this compound earlier in the course of disease.

Papers reporting results of bone marrow transplantation had larger numbers and more uniform patients than the series reported at the previous meeting. It appears that the inclusion of superlethal chemotherapy and irradiation during first remission has led to larger numbers of long-term survivors. The improvement in results between transplantation after recurrence or in first remission of neuroblastoma are not as impressive as for acute myeloid leukemias, where long-term survival improved from 25% to 60%. Three papers addressed the therapeutic use of monoclonal antibodies, both conjugated to 131 iodine and unconjugated. These are essentially phase I/II studies that include significant responses in a small number of patients. The group working in London pointed out some problems in using monoclonal antibodies against human tumors, particularly the very small uptake in the tumor and the large uptake in the reticuloendothelial system, particularly the liver. The results using the unlabeled GD2-specific monoclonal antibody seem to be a little more hopeful.

This volume will be of primary interest to the basic scientist working in the field of neuroblastoma, although the studies on mechanisms of transformation and cellular control would be of value to anyone working in the area of cancer cell biology. The reports on tumor markers and therapy will be of use to the clinician, who needs to improve the treatment of neuroblastoma, which historically has not been very successful.

**Audrey E. Evans**
**Philadelphia, Pennsylvania**
**February 1988**

# Acknowledgments

The organizers of the conference wish to express their gratitude for the generous support from the following companies:

Adria Laboratories
Bristol Myers
The Childrens Cancer Research Foundation
The Seligson Foundation

The organizers and conference participants would also like to acknowledge the patience and efforts of Lila Philson, whose hard work in planning the conference and in assembling the papers for this volume have, in large measure, led to its success.

# ONCOGENES

Advances in Neuroblastoma Research 2, pages 3–15
© 1988 Alan R. Liss, Inc.

# MOLECULAR ANALYSIS AND CLINICAL SIGNIFICANCE OF N-MYC AMPLIFICATION AND CHROMOSOME 1P MONOSOMY IN HUMAN NEUROBLASTOMAS.

Garrett M. Brodeur, Chin-to Fong, Michon Morita, Rogers Griffith, F. Ann Hayes, Robert C. Seeger.

Department of Pediatrics (GMB; CTF; MM) and Pathology (RG), Washington University School of Medicine, St. Louis, Missouri 63110; Department of Hematology-Oncology (FAH), St. Jude Children's Research Hospital, Memphis, Tennessee 38101; Department of Pediatrics (RCS), UCLA School of Medicine, Los Angeles, California 90024; Pediatric Oncology Group, St. Louis, Missouri; Children's Cancer Study Group, Los Angeles, California.

## INTRODUCTION

Cytogenetic analysis of human cancer cells has suggested genetic mechanisms of malignant trans-formation or progression (Brodeur, 1986; Brodeur, 1987). The most common forms of cytogenetic rearrangement include deletions, translocations and cytogenetic manifestations of gene amplification. The former represents loss of DNA from the karyotype and may indicate the site of suppressor or regulatory genes that prevent uncontrolled growth or promote differentiation. The latter two cytogenetic rearrangements have been associated with mechanisms of oncogene activation in some cases and may result in unregulated expression or overexpression of a particular oncogene.

We are conducting a cytogenetic and molecular analysis of neuroblastoma cells from primary tumor tissue and cell lines. This analysis has identified mechanisms of oncogenesis as well as the probable location of genes involved in tumori-genesis. What follows is the progress we have made in examining these cytogenetic rearrangements at the molecular level to more precisely define the genes involved in the tranformation or progression of neuroblastoma.

## CHROMOSOME 1P MONOSOMY

We first described partial monosomy for the short arm of chromosome 1 as the most characteristic cytogenetic abnormality in human neuroblastomas (Brodeur, et al, 1975; Brodeur, et al, 1977). Partial 1p monosomy is found in 70-80% of primary tumors and cell lines (Brodeur, et al; 1981; Brodeur, et al, 1982; Biedler, et al, 1980; Gilbert, et al, 1982; Gilbert, et al, 1984). Cytogenetic analysis of neuroblastomas reveals that 70% (23/33) of primary tumors and 85% (22/26) of established cell lines have deletions or rearrangements of the short arm of chromosome 1 (Table 1), resulting in partial 1p monosomy (Figure 1). However, most neuroblastomas that have been karyotyped come from patients with advanced stages of disease (III and IV, or C and D), so it is not clear if these findings are representative of all neuroblastomas (Franke, et al, 1986a; Franke, et al, 1986b; Kaneko, et al, 1987; Brodeur, unpublished observations).

Table 1.  SELECTED CHROMOSOME ABNORMALITIES IN HUMAN NEUROBLASTOMAS

| Tissue Source | Del 1p* | DMs* | HSRs* |
|---|---|---|---|
| Primary Tumors | 23/33 | 14/33 | 2/33 |
| Cell Lines | 22/26 | 14/26 | 14/26 |
| Total | 45/59 | 28/59 | 16/59 |

*Del 1p = deletion of short arm of chromosome 1; DMs = double minutes; HSRs = homogeneously staining regions.

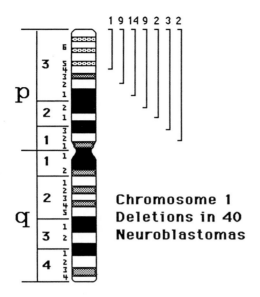

Chromosome 1
Deletions in 40
Neuroblastomas

Figure 1. Diagram of deletions of the short arm of chromosome 1 seen in 40 neuroblastoma cell lines and primary tumors. The brackets show the region deleted, and the numbers above the brackets show the number of tumors or cell lines with the corresponding deletion.

The chromosome 1 deletion is analogous to the 13q14 chromosome deletion in retinoblastomas, or the deletion of 11p13 in Wilms tumors (Knudson, et al, 1976; Francke, 1976; Francke, et al, 1977; Riccardi, et al, 1978). Although constitutional deletions of the respective chromosomes have been identified in the latter two tumors, no chromosome deletion syndrome has been identified as yet that predisposes to the development of neuroblastoma (Moorhead, et al, 1980; Brodeur, 1982). Since there have not been any descriptions of 1p deletion syndromes, it is likely that deletions large enough to be visible with the light microscope are incompatible with life (i.e., embryonic lethal mutations are expressed).

The three tumors described above and some other tumors have in common a loss of tumor DNA from a particular chromosome that is specific for each type of tumor. These genetic lesions are thought to represent the loss of regulatory or suppressor genes, whose absence may play a role in malignant transformation. In some cases, the tumor karyotypes do not show gross chromosomal deletions. Instead, molecular analysis with restriction fragment length polymorphisms (RFLP's) has revealed submicroscopic mutations, mitotic recombination, or loss of heterozygosity (LOH) involving the implicated chromosome (Cavenee, et al, 1983; Cavenee, et al, 1986; Dryja, et al, 1984; Hansen, et al, 1985; Koufos, et al, 1985; Murphree and Benedict, 1984). Molecular approaches to identify the gene that is consistently deleted in retinoblastoma have led to the cloning of the putative retinoblastoma gene (Friend, et al, 1986; Lee, et al, 1987; Fung, et al, 1987). Similar approaches are being applied to the cloning of the Wilms tumor predisposition gene on chromosome 11, as well as the localization of a number of other putative tumor loci.

In order to more precisely define the region that is consistently deleted in neuroblastomas, and to determine if deletions occurred in tumors that could not be karyotyped, we are taking a molecular approach to mapping the chromosome 1 deletion in these tumors (Fong, et al, 1987). This approach should lead to the localization, identification and characterization of the putative neuroblastoma (Nb) gene on the short arm of chromosome 1. We are using RFLP analysis with DNA probes that map to the short arm of chromosome 1 to look for LOH and to more precisely define the region that is consistently deleted to a chromosome band or subband. Initially, we decided to evaluate DNA probes that had already been mapped to chromosome 1 (or regionally mapped along the chromosome), and about which there was already RFLP information.

We have already obtained preliminary information on pairs of somatic and tumor DNAs from 45 individual patients with the following probes: alpha-fucosidase (FUCA) (1p34); L-*myc* (1p32); alpha-amylase (1p22); antithrombin-III (ATIII) (1q23); renin (1q23-25); and a random DNA marker that maps to chromosome 1 (L1.22) (Human Gene Mapping 8, 1985). Of the DNA pairs analyzed to date, 40 are informative: 18 at only one locus, 11 at two loci, 8 at three loci, and 3 at four loci. Overall, 34/40 show no LOH for chromosome 1, 2/40 show LOH at the only informative locus (FUCA—1p34), and 4 show LOH at 1p32-1p34 but do not show LOH with proximal short arm and long arm probes.

These latter results are consistent with either deletion of the distal short arm (at or between between 1p32 and 1p34) in these cases, or mitotic recombination, with resulting partial homozygosity for the distal short arm (Fong, et al, 1987). Thus, LOH for the entire chromosome rarely if ever occurs in neuroblastomas, perhaps because cell lethal mutations make homozygosity or hemizygosity for the entire chromosome a rare event. However, our molecular studies confirm that hemizygosity or LOH for the distal short arm does occur frequently, as suggested earlier by our cytogenetic studies.

Our results demonstrating LOH for chromosome 1 are more impressive if we focus on the distal short arm. We detected LOH in only 1 of 15 cases that were informative with the L-myc probe, which maps to 1p32, whereas 5 of 14 informative cases for FUCA (1p34) demonstrated LOH. These results indicate either that L-myc is more proximal than suggested by current mapping data, or that the chromosome 1 deletion is more distal than suggested by the cytogenetic data. In any event, the finding of LOH in less than half of the informative cases at 1p34 indicates that the region consistently deleted most likely is distal to this point. Alternatively, it is possible that chromosome 1p deletions may be restricted to a subset of tumors, such as the advanced stage tumors. In this regard, however, it is interesting that one of our informative cases with LOH was a patient with stage A disease. LOH for chromosome 1p occurs in patients both with and without N-myc amplification (see below), so there is no obvious direct relationship between these two genetic lesions.

## N-MYC AMPLIFICATION

Cytogenetic analysis of human neuroblastomas has revealed evidence of gene amplification, i.e., extrachromosomal double-minute chromatin bodies (DMs) and chromosomally-integrated, homogeneously-staining regions (HSRs), in about a third of primary tumors and ~90% of established cell lines (Table 1) (Biedler, et al, 1980; Brodeur, et al, 1981, Gilbert, et al, 1984). We have determined that virtually every case has amplification of a genomic region including the oncogene N-*myc* (Schwab, et al, 1983; Kohl, et al, 1983; Schwab, et al, 1984; Brodeur, et al, 1984; Seeger, et al, 1985; Brodeur, et al, 1985; Brodeur and Seeger, 1986; Brodeur, et al, 1986). The presence of N-*myc* amplification is associated with advanced stages of disease, rapid progression and a poor prognosis (Brodeur, et al, 1984; Seeger, et al, 1985; Brodeur, et al, 1985; Brodeur, et al, 1986).

We are engaged in a prospective study of N-*myc* amplification in neuroblastomas in the two major groups that treat children with cancer in the United States--the Pediatric Oncology Group (POG) and the Children's Cancer Study Group (CCSG). To date we have studied over 450 primary tumor samples from the two groups. Although the two groups use slightly different staging systems (CCSG: I-IV, IV-S; POG: A-D, IV-S), the patients with low stages and with high stages of disease can be conveniently grouped (Table 2).

Table 2.N-*myc* Amplification in Neuroblastoma Tissue

| Clinical Group | # amplified/total | |
|---|---|---|
| Low Stage Disease (I,II,A,B) | 6/109 | (6%) |
| High Stage Disease (III,IV,C,D) | 95/307 | (31%) |
| Stage IV-S | 2/29 | (7%) |
| Ganglioneuroma | 0/12 | (0%) |

We have confirmed the strong correlation between N-*myc* amplification and advanced stages of disease seen in our earlier studies. In addition, we have identified a small percentage (5-10%) of patients with stages associated with a good prognosis (I, II, IV-S) that have N-*myc* amplification. Our preliminary data indicate that these patients also have rapid tumor progression and a uniformly poor prognosis, similar to those with more advanced stages of disease.

The poor prognostic significance of N-*myc* amplification in neuroblastomas is already being evaluated as one of the variables by which patients with a poor prognosis are selected to undergo autologous bone marrow transplantation. Since conventional therapy alone offers these patients virtually no hope of cure, it is reasonable to subject these individuals to more intensive, experimental approaches. Our preliminary results suggest that patients with low-stage disease who have N-*myc* amplification have a similarly poor prognosis. If this is borne out, it would suggest that these patients also would be appropriate candidates for more innovative approaches to therapy, such as bone marrow transplantation, differentiation therapy, or immunotherapy.

## N-myc Copy Number in Multiple Simultaneous and Consecutive Neuroblastoma Samples

It was not clear if N-*myc* copy number was consistent within an individual tumor, in tumor samples obtained from different sites or at different times. Therefore, we analyzed multiple, simultaneous tumor samples in 31 patients, simultaneous samples of multiple tumor sites in 10 patients, and serial tumor samples over time in vivo in 25 patients (Brodeur, et al, 1987). Our results indicate that N-*myc* copy number is consistent in tumor samples obtained from individual patients. Specifically, all studies of multiple simultaneous or consecutive samples either showed a single copy of N-*myc* in all tissues sampled, or they showed a consistent level of amplification throughout. These results suggest that N-*myc* amplification is an intrinsic biologic property of a subset of tumors that is present at diagnosis, if it is going to occur. N-*myc* amplification is associated with advanced stages of disease, but it does not occur with progressive disease if it is not present at diagnosis. Conversely, the develop-ment of progressive disease is very likely to occur in patients with pre-existing amplification.

## CONCLUSIONS

Mapping of the chromosome 1 deletion in human neuroblastomas should allow identification, cloning and sequencing of the putative neuroblastoma gene. The cloning of this gene or even closely linked genetic sequences would provide probes that could be used for the identification of individuals that are genetically predisposed to develop neuroblas-toma. The identification and characterization of the gene itself could provide insights into mechanisms of causation of the disease as well as innovative therapeutic approaches that could be more specific, more effective, and less toxic than current modalities.

N-*myc* amplification is found in about 30% of primary neuroblastomas from untreated patients. It is associated with advanced stages of disease and rapid tumor progression. Indeed, N-*myc* amplifi-cation is an intrinsic biologic feature of a subset of neuroblastomas that apparently contributes to the poor clinical outcome of these patients. It is not known if amplification is a manifestation of secondary heterogeneity or if it is a feature of a genetically distinct subset of tumors within the group of tumors classified clinically and pathologically as neuroblastoma. This distinction will require other objective biologic or immunologic features which correlate with the presence or absence of N-*myc* amplification.

Our studies were the first to show clinical relevance of oncogene activation in primary human tumors. However, there is recent evidence that amplification of the oncogene c-*erb*-B2 in breast carcinomas is associated with lymph node metastasis and a shorter median disease-free survival (Slamon, et al, 1987). It is likely that other clinical correlations of oncogene activation in specific tumors will be found in the near future. Thus, N-*myc* amplification in neuroblastomas serves as a prototypic model for the clinical application of oncogene research.

## ACKNOWLEDGMENTS

These studies were supported in part by grants from the National Institutes of Health CA-39771, CA-01027 and CA 05587 (GMB); CA22794, CA-27678 and CA-16042 (RCS). Additional support was obtained from the Children's United Research Effort against Cancer and the Fern Waldman Memorial Fund for Cancer Research (GMB). We are grateful to Jonathon Wasson and Sylvia Rayner for their valuable technical contributions.

## REFERENCES

Biedler JL, Ross RA, Shanske S, Spengler BA (1980). Human neuroblastoma cytogenetics: Search for significance of homogeneously staining regions and double minute chromosomes. Progr Cancer Res Ther 12: 81-96.

Brodeur GM: Genetics and cytogenetics of human neuroblastomas (1982). In, Pochedly, Carl (ed): "Neuroblastoma: Clinical and Biological Manifestations," Elsevier North Holland, New York, pp. 183-194.

Brodeur GM (1986). Molecular correlates of cytogenetic abnormalities in human cancer cells: Implications for oncogene activation. Progr Hematol 14: 229-256.

Brodeur GM (1987). Involvement of oncogenes and suppressor genes in human neoplasia. Adv Pediatr 34: (in press).

Brodeur GM, Seeger RC (1986). Gene amplification in human neuroblastomas: Basic mechanisms and clinical implications. Cancer Genet Cytogenet 19: 101-111.

Brodeur GM, Sekhon GS, Goldstein MN (1975). Specific chromosomal aberration in human neuroblastoma. Am J Hum Genet 27: 20A.

Brodeur GM, Sekhon GS, Goldstein MN (1977). Chromosomal aberrations in human neuroblastomas. Cancer 40: 2256-2263.

Brodeur GM, Green AA, Hayes FA, Williams, KJ, Williams DL, Tsiatis AA (1981). Cytogenetic features of human neuroblastomas and cell lines. Cancer Res 41: 4678-4686.

Brodeur GM, Tsiatis AA, Williams DL, Luthardt FL, Green AA (1982). Statistical analysis of cytogenetic abnormalities in human cancer cells. Cancer Genet Cytogenet 7: 137-152.

Brodeur GM, Seeger RC, Schwab M, Varmus HE, Bishop JM (1984). Amplification of N-*myc* in untreated human neuroblastomas correlates with advanced disease stage. Science 224: 1121-1124.

Brodeur GM, Seeger RC, Schwab M, Varmus HE, Bishop JM (1985). Amplification of N-*myc* sequences in primary human neuroblastomas: Correlation with advanced disease stage. Progr Clin Biol Res 175: 105-113.

Brodeur GM, Seeger RC, Sather H, Dalton A, Siegel SE,Wong KY, Hammond D (1986). Clinical implications of oncogene activation in human neuroblastomas. Cancer 58: 541-545.

Brodeur GM, Hayes FA, Green AA, Casper J, Wasson J, Wallach S, Seeger RC (1987). Consistent N-*myc* copy number in simultaneous or consecutive neuroblastoma samples from 60 individual patients. Cancer Res 47: 4248-4253.

Cavenee WK, Dryja TP, Phillips RA, Benedict WF, Godbout R, Gallie BL, Murphree AL, Strong LC, White RL (1983). Expression of recessive alleles by chromosomal mechanisms in retinoblastoma. Nature 305: 779-784.

Cavenee WK, Murphree AL, Shull MM, Benedict WF, Sparkes RS, Kock E, Nordenskjold M (1986). Prediction of familial predisposition to retinoblastoma. New Engl J Med 314: 1201-1207.

Dryja TP, Cavenee W, White R, Rapaport JM, Petersen R, Albert DM, Bruns GA (1984). Homozygosity of chromosome 13 in retinoblastoma. New Engl J Med 310: 550-553.

Fong CT, Morita M, Griffith RC, Brodeur GM (1987). Analysis of human neuroblastomas for loss of heterozygosity for chromosome 1. Proc AACR 28: 52(abstr. 207).

Francke U (1976). Retinoblastoma and chromosome 13. Cytogenet Cell Genet 16: 131-134.

Francke U, George DL, Brown MG, Riccardi VM (1977). Gene dose effect: Intraband mapping of the LDH A locus using cells from four individuals with different interstitial deletions of 11. Cytogenet Cell Genet 19: 197-207.

Franke F, Rudolph B, Lampert F (1986a). Translocation (19;?) in two stage II neuroblastomas. Cancer Genet Cytogenet 2: 129-135.

Franke F, Rudolph B, Christiansen H, Harbott J, Lampert F (1986b). Tumour karyotype may be important in the prognosis of human neuroblastoma. J Cancer Res Clin Oncol 111: 266-272.

Friend SH, Bernards R, Rogelj S, Weinberg RA, Rapaport JM, Albert DM, Dryja TP (1986). A human DNA segment with properties of the gene that predisposes to retinoblastoma and osteosarcoma. Nature 323: 643-646.

Fung YKT, Murphree AL, T'Ang A, Qian J, Hinrichs SH, Benedict WF (1987). Structural evidence for the authenticity of the human retinoblastoma gene. Science 236: 1657-1661.

Gilbert F, Balaban G, Moorhead P, Bianchi D, Schlesinger H (1982). Abnormalities of chromosome 1p in human neuroblastoma tumors and cell lines. Cancer Genet Cytogenet 7: 33-42.

Gilbert F, Feder M, Balaban G, Brangman D, Lurie DK, Podolsky R, Rinaldt V, Vinikoor N, Weisband J (1984). Human neuroblastomas and abnormalities of chromosome 1 and 17. Cancer Res 44: 5444-5449.

Hansen MF, Koufos A, Gallie BL, Phillips RA, Fodstad O, Brogger A, Gedde-Dahl T, Cavenee WK (1985). Osteosarcoma and retinoblastoma: A shared chromosomal mechanism revealing recessive predisposition. Proc Natl Acad Sci USA 82: 6216-6220.

Human gene mapping 8. Helsinki conference (1985). Eigh International Workshop on Human Gene Mapping. Helsinki, Finland, August 4-10, 1985. Cytogenet Cell Genet 40: 1-823.

Kaneko Y, Kanda N, Maseki N, Sakurai M, Tsuchida Y, Takeda T, Okabe I, Sakurai M (1987). Different karyotypic patterns in early and advanced stage neuroblastomas. Cancer Res 47: 311-318, 1987.

Knudson AB Jr, Meadows AT, Nichols WW, Hill R (1976). Chromosome deletion and retinoblastoma. New Engl J Med 195: 1120-1123.

Kohl NE, Kanda N, Schreck RR, Bruns G, Latt SA, Gilbert F, Alt FW (1983). Transposition and amplification of oncogene related sequences in human neuroblastomas. Cell 35: 359-367.

Koufos A, Hansen MF, Copeland NG, Jenkins NA, Lampkin BC, Cavenee WK (1985). Loss of heterozygosity in three embryonal tumours suggests a common pathogenetic mechanism. Nature 316: 330-334.

Lee WH, Bookstein R, Hong F, Young LJ, Shew JY, Lee EYHP (1987). Human retinoblastoma susceptibility gene: Cloning, identification and sequence. Science 235: 1394-1399.

Murphree AL, Benedict WF (1984). Retinoblastoma: Clues to human oncogenesis. Science 223: 1028-1033.

Riccardi VM, Sujansky E, Smith AC, Francke U (1978). Chromosomal imbalance in the aniridia-Wilms' tumor association: 11p interstitial deletion. Pediatr 61: 604-610.

Schwab M, Alitalo K, Klempnauer KH, Varmus HE, Bishop JM, Gilbert F, Brodeur G, Goldstein M, Trent JM (1983). Amplified DNA with limited homology to *myc* cellular oncogene is shared by human neuroblastoma cell lines and a neuroblastoma tumour. Nature 305: 245-248.

Schwab M, Varmus HE, Bishop JM, Grzeschik KH, Naylor SL, Sakaguchi AY, Brodeur G, Trent J (1984). Chromosome localization in normal human cells and neuroblastomas of a gene related to c-*myc*. Nature 308: 288-291.

Seeger RC, Brodeur GM, Sather H, Dalton A, Siegel SE, Wong KY, Hammond D (1985). Association of multiple copies of the N-*myc* oncogene with rapid progression of neuroblastomas. New Engl J Med 313: 1111-1116.

Slamon DJ, Clark GM, Wong SG, Jevin WJ, Ullrich A, McGuire WL (1987). Human breast cancer: Correlation of relapse and survival with amplification of the HER-2/*neu* oncogene. Science 235: 177-182, 1987.

Advances in Neuroblastoma Research 2, pages 17–29
© 1988 Alan R. Liss, Inc.

HUMAN NEUROBLASTOMA METASTASES IN A NUDE MOUSE
MODEL:  TUMOR PROGRESSION AND ONC GENE AMPLIFICATION

Fred Gilbert, Kwei-Lan Tsao,
Faustina LaLatta, Ling Xu,
V.R. Potluri and Gundula LaBadie.

Medical Genetics/Pediatrics, Mount Sinai
School of Medicine, New York, NY  10029

INTRODUCTION

Neuroblastoma, a tumor of childhood, has been sub-divided into five clinical stages, based on the patient's age at diagnosis and the extent of involvement with disease (Evans, 1971).  The analysis of karyotypes prepared from tumors and cell lines has identified a number of recurrent chromosome abnormalities in neuro-blastoma, most frequently deletions and rearrangements involving the short arm of chromosome 1 (1p) and homo-geneously staining regions (HSR) and double minute chromosomes (DMS) (Gilbert, 1984).  The HSR are long, anomalously staining segments, whose chromosomal locations are different in different tumors and can vary as well between cells of the same cell line over time in culture; the DMS are extra-chromosomal, paired chromatin bodies without centromeres, whose number and size can vary between cells of the same cell line and whose staining characteristics are identical to those of the HSR (Biedler, 1976).

The breakdown of HSR can give rise to DMS and both serve as sites for gene amplification, carrying multiple copies of single oncogenes or genes conferring drug resistance on the cell (Biedler, 1976; Balaban-Malen-baum, 1980).  In the case of neuroblastoma, all tumors and cell lines carrying HSR and/or DMS hve been found to contain amplified N-myc (Kohl, 1983; Schwab, 1983).  The latter is a member of the myc oncogene family, similar in sequence to both v-myc, the oncogene defined in the avian myelocytomatosis retrovirus, and its cellular homologue, c-myc (Alt, 1986). Amplification of N-myc in neuroblastoma has been shown to correlate with severity of disease, with very rare examples of amplification in clinical stages with a good prognosis (stages I and IV-S) and a high frequency of amplification (up to two-thirds of cases) in stages with a poor prognosis (stages III and IV) (Brodeur, 1984).

The fact that not every neuroblastoma contains amplified N-myc and the demonstrated association between amplification and metastatic stage IV disease, are both consistent with the hypothesis that oncogene amplification is not a primary event in tumorigenesis (Gilbert, 1983). Rather it is likely to develop following cell transformation and to contribute to the capacity of a tumor cell to grow more rapidly and to spread in the patient.

To confirm the postulated relationship between oncogene amplification and tumor growth and spread, we have developed a mouse model of human tumor metastatsis, using a human neuroblastoma cell line carrying several HSRs and amplified N-myc.

MATERIALS AND METHODS

The human neuroblastoma cell line designated IMR-32 was explanted into culture in 1967 (Tumilowicz, 1970). IMR-5 is a single cell clone established from IMR-32 in 1977 and maintained in culture virtually continuously since (Balaban-Malenbaum, 1977; Balaban-Malenbaum, 1980b). Karyotypes prepared at the time of the original cloning demonstrated that IMR-5 contained two HSRs on 1p in each cell (Balaban-Malenbaum, 1980b).

Cells of IMR-5 ($5x10^6$ cells in a total volume of 0.25 ml of RMPI 1640 without serum) were injected into the tail veins of Balb/c nu/nu mice (ages 6-8 weeks post weaning). The abdomens of the mice post-injection were palpated twice per week and the animals sacrificed when abdominal masses became palpable. A gross autopsy of the abdominal and thoracic cavities was performed to document the extent of involvement with tumor.

Tumor metastases were removed from individual mice, washed in medium RPMI 1640 without serum, minced with scissors and scalpel, and explanted into culture (in

60 mm tissue culture flasks to which 5 ml RPMI 1640, supplemented with 20% fetal calf serum, was added).

The tumor cells that grew out from the explanted metastasis were karyotyped, using previously described techniques (Gilbert, 1984), and expanded for re-injection into another series of nu/nu mice. Tumor cells at each passage were also pelleted and stored frozen, until DNA and RNA extractions could be performed, as per published protocols (Maniatis, 1982). Poly-(A)$^+$ RNA was collected after chromatography of total cellular RNA on oligo-dT cellulose (Maniatis, 1982).

Tumor cell DNAs were digested with Bg1 II, electrophoresed in 0.9% agarose, transferred to nitrocellulose filters, and hybridized with radio-labeled probes for oncogene N-myc (probe NB19, kindly supplied by Fred Alt, Columbia University) and beta-actin (kindly supplied by Ed. Johnson, Mount Sinai), using the protocols outlined in Maniatis (1982).

Poly-(A)$^+$ RNAs were electrophoresed in formaldehyde containing agarose gels (1%), transferred to nitrocellulose, and hybridized with radio-labeled probes for N-myc and histone H3 (pHH3, kindly supplied by Ed. Johnson, Mount Sinai) as per Maniatis (1982).

All hybridized filters were covered with X-Omat AR film (Kodak) and developed after exposure for 24-72 hours at -70°C. Densitometric measurements were made from each autoradiogram (measurements made on an LKB ultroscan XL laser densitometer) and then compared.

RESULTS

Metastases were studied in nine series of nu/nu mice injected intravenously. Of the first three mice injected (series 1), abdominal tumor masses developed in only one (the remaining two mice were tumor-free when sacrificed six months from the time of injection). In the affected mouse, the tumor masses were palpable 60 days following injection. At autopsy, metastatic nodules were identified in both kidneys, in spleen, and multiple abdominal lymph nodes (Table I; Fig. 1).

One kidney nodule and two lymph nodes were minced separately and placed in culture for expansion and chromosome analysis. The cells from the kidney nodule were injected into a second series of mice within one

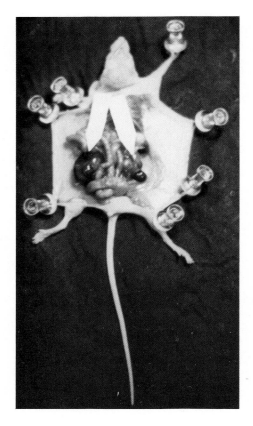

Fig. 1:  Exposed abdominal cavity of athymic mouse of
         series 4, with arrows to metastases in kidney
         (on left) and lymph node (on right).

TABLE I

| Cell Line | Tumors/ Mice | Tumor Sites | Latency | Chromosome Numbers |
|---|---|---|---|---|
| IMR-5 | – | – | – | 47 |
| IMR-5 (VC1) | 1/3 | K,S,LN | 60d | 46–48 |
| IMR-5 (VC2) | 1/5 | K, LN | 35d | 46–48 |
| IMR-5 (VC3) | 1/6 | K,LN | 60d | 46–48 |
| IMR-5 (VC4) | 6/7 | K,LN | 79d | 46–47 |
| IMR-5 (VC5) | 5/5 | K,LN | 78d | nd |
| IMR-5 (VC6) | 7/7 | K,LN | 58d | 45–47 |
| IMR-5 (VC7) | 9/9 | LN | 56d | nd |
| IMR-5 (VC8) | 3/4 | LN | 77d | 45–47 |
| IMR-5 (VC9) | 8/8 | LN | 64d | 45–47 |

Metastases developing after injection of IMR-5 into athymic mice. INJECT $5 \times 10^6$ cells/mouse IV. TUMORS/MICE: number of mice with palpable metastases/number of mice injected. TUMOR SITES: (K) kidney, (S) spleen, (LN) lymph nodes. LATENCY: average number of days following injection before tumors palpable. CHROMOSOME NUMBERS: predominant modes in 100 cells counted.

month following explantation into culture. In only one
of five mice injected (series 2), were abdominal masses
palpable (the remaining four mice were tumor-free at
autopsy six months later). In the involved animal, tumor
masses were palpable 35 days from the time of injection;
after sacrifice, tumor nodules could be identified in one
kidney and multiple abdominal lymph nodes. Two lymph
nodes were explanted into culture.

Cultured cells from one of the lymph nodes of the
series 2 mouse were injected into six new mice (series
3). Tumors in both kidneys and multiple abdominal lymph
nodes developed in a single mouse. Tumor nodules from
two lymph nodes were explanted, grown in culture,
karyotyped, and expanded for re-injection into the next
series of animals.

In series 4 through 9, metastatic nodules in
kidney(s) and/or abdominal lymph nodes were found in
almost all mice injected (Table I). In none of the
autopsies performed were tumor metastases to liver,
intestine, peritoneum, lung, heart, thoracic lymph nodes,
or brain identified by gross examination.

The mean latency period [time in days for intra-
abdominal tumor(s) to become palpable] varied between
56-81 days (with the exception of the single series 2
mouse), and ranged between 45-92 days (Table I). The
latency periods did not change significantly between the
first and ninth series.

The modal chromosome numbers of the parent IMR-5
prior to injection and of selected lines established in
culture from individual metastases, are given in Table I.
The predominant mode (45-47 chromosomes per cell) did
not change from series 1 to 9.

The original IMR-32 cell line, when established in
culture in 1967, had a mode of 48-50 chromosomes with two
large markers (10). The original preparations were
unbanded; in retrospect, it appears that the two markers
were rearranged chromosomes 1 carrying HSRs on their
short arms (W. Nichols, personal communication).

When first cloned in 1977, IMR-5 had a mode of 47
chromosomes with three chromosomes 1, two of which
carried 1pHSRs, and three consistent structural rearrangements: 11q-, 16q+, and 19q+ (Balaban-Malenbaum,
1980b). In 1984, prior to the first injections described

herein, the mode was still 47, and the cells retained the three chromosomes 1 and the rearranged chromosomes 11, 16, and 19 (Fig. 2). However, approximately half of the cells contained an additional HSR, most commonly on 8p, and almost all cells contained a rearranged number 6, with additional 1q material on its short arm (Fig. 2).

Karyotypes prepared from the different metastatic series were less consistent. The modal chromosome numbers did not change appreciably between cells from independent metastases explanted from single animals (data not shown). However, variation in the complement of rearranged markers between cells from individual metastases, as well as between metastases from single animals, was evident in series 1 through 9. Representative karyotypes from cells of series 4, 7, and 9 are given for comparison (Fig. 2). All cells in all metastases retained the three chromosomes 1 (two with HSR) and the 11q-, 16q+ and 19q+ described in the original IMR-5. Almost all cells contained the 6p+ carrying additional 1q material. All cells of the metastic series contained a new rearrangement - a 5p+ with an HSR on the short arm; most cells contained one or more additional HSRs as well (though there was no uniformity as to the chromosomal locations of these HSRs) and many contained additional segments of 1q translocated to different chromosomes within the karyotype. All of the metastatic cells also contained one or more new marker chromosomes, in which the chromosomes of origin of the rearranged segments could not be determined. However, all cells from the metastases were monosomic for chromosome 13; it is possible that all or part of the second number 13 is included in these markers.

By densitometric measurement, the amount of N-myc-specific DNA was approximately 5 fold greater than that of the unamplified beta-actin gene in all lines studied (in IMR-5 pre-injection, as well as in all of the metastatic series) (Table II). The actual number of HSR segments (the sites of amplified N-myc) varied between 3 to 5 per cell within the cells of each line; this within sample variation presumably accounts for the range in the N-myc/beta-actin ratios in the different metastatic series (range, 3.7 to 8.3) (Table II).

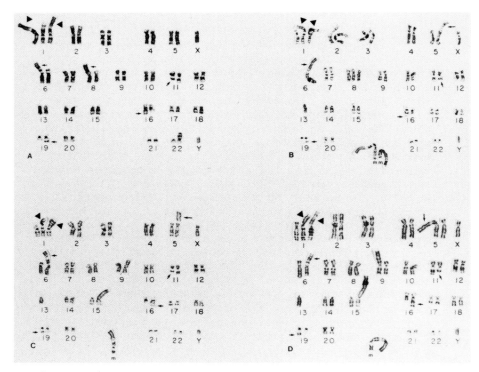

Fig. 2: Karyotypes of a) IMR-5 prior to injection, and
b-d) cells of metastatic series 4, 7, and 9,
respectively. Arrows to HSRs on chromosomes 1
and to the 6p+, 11q-, 16q+, and 19q+ retained in
all lines, and to the 5p+ (HSR) in all cells of
all metastatic series. Individual cells in the
metastases contain one or more additional HSRs
(e.g., 15p+ in VC7, as in C above; 9p+ and 15p+
in VC9, D above), as well as one or more poorly
characterized marker chromosomes (designated m
in B, C, and D above).

TABLE II

| Cell Line | (N-myc)<br>DNA (beta-actin) | (N-myc)<br>mRNA (pHH3) |
|---|---|---|
| IMR-5 | 5.3x | 220x |
| IMR-5 (VC4) | 4.0 | 183 |
| IMR-5 (VC6) | 4.5 | 141 |
| IMR-5 (VC7) | 3.7 | 171 |
| IMR-5 (VC8) | 4.8 | 184 |
| IMR-5 (VC9) | 8.3 | 179 |
| IMR-5 (confluent) | (4.4) | (145) |
| IMR-5 (log) | (4.2) | (265) |
| (log/confluent) | (0.96) | (1.83) |

Densitometric measurements of N-myc DNA and mRNA in metastatic series. N-myc: oncogene amplified in IMR-5. beta-actin, pHH3: non-amplified, single copy genes in IMR-5. DNA, mRNA (poly-A+RNA): prepared and measured densitometrically as described in Methods; each value the average of readings from each of two independent cell pellets prepared from each cell line. (confluent): population of cells that has been confluent, non-dividing for one week in culture. (log): population of cells that has been split 1:2 every three days, actively dividing for two weeks.

The poly-(A)$^+$ RNA specific for N-myc was approximately 180 fold greater than that for the non-amplified histone H3 in IMR-5 and the metastatic series 1 through 9 (Table II). Differences in the mRNA ratios between the metastatic series can, presumably, be accounted for by the variation in the number of HSRs per cell, as noted above, and by differences in the proportion of actively dividing and non-dividing cells in individual populations at the time of sampling. All IMR-5 lines grow predominantly as single cell monolayers, with limited cell division once confluence is attained. When strict attention is paid to growth conditions, it could be shown that the levels of N-myc-specific mRNA in confluent, essentially non-dividing IMR-5 were approximately half those in actively dividing IMR-5 (Table II). [This finding is consistent with previous studies in which a) the induction of active cell division could be associated with the induction of specific oncogene transcription (Kelly, 1983), and b) mRNA coded for by N-myc could be detected in actively dividing fetal brain cells, but not in non-dividing, adult brain (Zimmerman, 1986).]

DISCUSSION

The intravenous injection of cells of a human neuroblastoma line containing HSRs and amplified N-myc into athymic mice, has been shown to result in metastases in the test animals. This is the first demonstration of the metastatic capacity of human neuroblastoma in a mouse model system (see recent reviews of human metastases in athymic mouse systems: Giovanella, 1985; Fidler, 1986).

A comparison of the karyotopes from the neuroblastoma line IMR-5 prior to injection and from the metastatic tumors in nine series of injected animals, showed a) the consistent retention of rearrangements involving chromosomes 1, 6, 11, 16 and 19 (all present in the original IMR-5), and b) additional HSRs (one or more) in all cells of all metastatic series. Interestingly, the absolute number of N-myc gene copies and the levels of N-myc-specific mRNA did not significantly differ between the pre-injection IMR-5 and the cell lines established from the explanted metastatic tumors in all nine series.

If the capacity for metastatic spread is related to the presence of amplified N-myc, then presumably this capacity was present in the cell line prior to the first injection [the original description of the parent line IMR-32, from which IMR-5 was cloned, does not state whether the patient had metastatic stage IV disease (Tumilowicz, 1970)]. However, it is also possible that amplification of sequences other than N-myc also contributes to the cell's ability to metastasize in this test system.

The HSRs in neuroblastoma cell lines are very large and contain more DNA than can be accounted for by the number of N-myc gene copies present (e.g., compare HSR size, measured in Bahr, 1983, with the number of N-myc gene copies in Kohl, 1983; Schwab, 1983); transcriptionally active sequences other than N-myc have already been identified in HSRs and DMS of different neuroblastomas, including IMR-32 (Kohl, 1984). It is, therefore, not unreasonable to predict that the additional HSRs in the metastatic series we have described will contain multiple copies of genes other than N-myc. Studies to prove this are currently in progress.

As to the potential value of a mouse model of metastasis in human neuroblastoma, we have only to look at the current state of treatment of this cancer. Survival statistics for stage IV disease with currently available chemotherapeutic protocols are generally poor. Newer approaches to treatment are needed - perhaps combining immunotherapy with chemotherapy, with or without irradiation and bone marrow transplantation; a mouse model in which metastases develop in a reproducible fraction of animals a given number of days following the injection of tumor cells, would seem to represent a suitable system for testing the efficacy of such therapies.

REFERENCES

Alt FW, DePinho R, Zimmerman K, Legouy E, Hatton K, Ferrier P, Tesfaye A, Yancopoulos G, Nisen P (1986). The human myc gene family. Cold Spring Harbor Symp on Quant Biol 51:931-941.

Bahr G, Gilbert F, Balaban G, Engler W (1983). Homogeneously staining regions and double minutes: chromatin organization and DNA content. J Natl Canc Inst 71:657-661.

Balaban-Malenbaum G, Gilbert F (1977). Double minute chromosomes and the homogeneously staining regions of a human neuroblastoma cell line. Science 198:739-741.

Balaban-Malenbaum G, Gilbert F (1980a). The proposed origin of double minutes from HSR-marker chromosomes in human neuroblastoma cell hybrid cell lines. Canc Genet Cytogenet 2:339-341.

Balaban-Malenbaum G, Gilbert F (1980b). Relationship between homogeneously staining regions and double minute chromosomes in human neuroblastoma cell lines. in Adv in Neuroblastoma Res (Evans AE, ed.) Raven Press, New York. 97-107.

Biedler JL, Spengler BA (1976). Metaphase chromosome anomaly: association with drug resistance and cell-specific products. Science 191:185-187.

Brodeur GM, Seeger RC, Schwab M, Varmus HE, Bishop JM (1984). Amplification of N-myc in untreated human neuroblastoma correlates with advanced disease stages. Science 224:1121-1124.

Evans AE, D'Angio GJ, Randolph J (1971). A proposed staging for children with neuroblastoma. Cancer 27:374-378.

Fidler IJ (1986). Rationale and methods for the use of nude mice to study the biology and therapy of human cancer metastasis. Canc Metastasis Rev 5:29-49.

Gilbert F (1983). Chromosomes, genes and cancer: a classification of chromosome changes in cancer. J Natl Canc Inst 71:1107-1114.

Gilbert F, Feder M, Balaban G, Brangman D, Lurie DK, Podolsky R, Rinaldt V, Vinikoor N, Weisband J (1984).

Human neuroblastomas and abnormalities of chromosomes 1 and 17. Canc Res 44:5444-5449.

Giovanella BC, Fogh J (1985). The nude mouse in cancer research. Adv in Canc Res 44:69-120.

Kelly K, Cochran BH, Stiles CD, Leder P (1983). Cell specific regulation of the c-myc gene by lymphocyte mitogens and platelet-derived growth factor. Cell 35:603-610.

Kohl NE, Kanda N, Schrect RR, Bruns G, Latt SA, Gilbert F, Alt F (1983). Transposition and amplification of oncogene-related sequences in human neuroblastomas. Cell 35:359-367.

Kohl NE, Gee CE, Alt FW (1984). Activated expression of the N-myc gene in human neuroblastomas and related tumors. Science 226:1335-1337.

Maniatis T, Fritsch EF, Sambrook J (1982). Molecular cloning: a laboratory manual. Cold Spring Harbor Laboratory, New York.

Schwab M, Alitalo K, Klempnauer K-H, Varmus HE, Bishop JM, Gilbert F, Brodeur G, Goldstein M, Trent J (1983). Amplified DNA domain with limited homology to the myc cellular oncogene is shared by human neuroblastoma cell lines and a human neuroblastoma tumor. Nature 305:245-248.

Tumilowicz JJ, Nichols WW, Cholon JJ, Greene AE (1970). Definition of a continuous human cell line derived from neuroblastoma. Canc Res 30:2110-2118.

Zimmerman KA, Yancopoulos GD, Collum RG, Smith RK, Kohl NE, Denis KA, Nau MM, Witte ON, Toran-Allerand D, Gee CE, Minne JD, Alt FW (1986). Differentiated expression of myc family genes during murine development. Nature 319:780-783.

ACKNOWLEDGMENTS

The expert editorial assistance of Cathy Peragine is gratefully acknowledged. The studies described were funded under PHS CA 41759 (FG).

Advances in Neuroblastoma Research 2, pages 31–39

BIOLOGICAL CHARACTERISTICS OF N-MYC AMPLIFIED NEUROBLASTOMA
IN PATIENTS OVER ONE YEAR OF AGE

Akira Nakagawara, Keiichi Ikeda, Tohru Tsuda
and Ken Higashi

Department of Pediatric Surgery, Faculty of
Medicine, Kyushu University 60, Fukuoka 812
(A.N, K.I), and Department of Biochemistry,
University of Occupational and Environmental
Health, Kitakyushu 807 (T.T, K.H), Japan

INTRODUCTION

     N-myc oncogene amplification which characteristically
correlates with chromosomal abnormalities such as a homogeneously staining region or double minutes may have an
important role in the regulation of proliferation of neuroblastic tumors in children (Schwab et al., 1984; Emanuel et
al., 1985).  Since the report by Brodeur et al. in 1984,
the clinical significance of N-myc amplification as a
prognostic indicator has been given increasing attention
(Seeger et al., 1985; Nakagawara et al., 1987).  A precise
biological analysis of the poor-prognostic age group has
apparently not been reported.  We extended the analyses of
N-myc amplification to relation with therapy, patterns of
metastasis and invasion, surgery and tumor markers in patients
over one year of age, in conjunction with clinical prognostic
factors.

PATIENTS AND METHODS

     Tumor samples were obtained at the time of surgery,
and stored at - 80 °C until tested.  The preparation of DNA
and the measurement of N-myc copies were performed as
reported (Tsuda et al., 1987).

     Data on patients over one year of age are shown in
Table 1.  Stages of the disease are according to Evans et

Table 1.  N-myc Amplification of Neuroblastoma
in Patients over One Year of Age

|  |  | No. of copies of N-myc | |
| --- | --- | --- | --- |
|  |  | 1 - 10 | 10 < |
| No. of patients |  | 13 | 13 |
| Boy / girl |  | 4 / 9 | 7 / 6 |
| Age :  average |  | 4-y-11-m (1-y-5-m ~ 9-y) | 2-y-11-m (1-y-1-m ~ 11-y) |
| more than 5-y |  | 7 | 1 |
| Primary site | O-S | 8  (5) | 13  (0) |
|  | O-C | 2  (1) | 0 |
|  | O-R | 2  (2) | 0 |
|  | O-P | 1  (1) | 0 |
| Histology | 2-a | 3  (3) | 0 |
|  | 2-b | 2  (1) | 1  (0) |
|  | 2-c | 4  (3) | 2  (0) |
|  | 3-a | 4  (2) | 8  (0) |
|  | 3-b | 0 | 2  (0) |

( ): disease-free survival

O-S: originated from suprarenal region,  O-C: from mediastinum,
O-R: from retroperitoneum,  O-P: from pelvic cavity

2-a: ganglioneuroblastoma, well differentiated type
2-b: ganglioneuroblastoma, composite type
2-c: ganglioneuroblastoma, poorly differentiated type
3-a: neuroblastoma, rosette-fibrillary type
3-b: neuroblastoma, round cell type

al. (1971).

The patients mainly in stages III or IV were prescribed aggressive chemotherapy, according to the Kyushu Protocol for the Advanced Neuroblastoma; cyclophosphamide (CPA) 40 mg/kg/day x 2 days, cisplatinum (CDDP) 20 mg/m$^2$/day x 5 days plus VM-26 100 mg/m$^2$, and adriamycin (ADM) 60 mg/m$^2$ plus DTIC 250 mg/m$^2$/day x 5 days (45 mg/m$^2$ and 200 mg/m$^2$/day x 5 days for poor risk patients, respectively); each high dose therapy was given every three weeks.

For statistical analysis, the life-table technique based on the Kaplan-Meier procedure was used to estimate survival rate. The generalized Wilcoxon test was used to evaluate the significance and the mean was compared using Student's t-test. Differences were considered significant if p values were less than 0.05.

RESULTS

N-myc Amplification of Patients over One Year of Age

As shown in Table 2, N-myc amplification of more than 10 copies was frequently observed in those in stage III or IV neuroblastoma. The amplification was observed in 50 % of patients over one year of age.

Histologically, in the group with 1 - 10 copies of N-myc, 9 of 13 were ganglioneuroblastoma, whereas in case of more than 10 copies, 10 of 13 were neuroblastoma.

All tumors with more than 10 copies of N-myc originated from the suprarenal region, even when children under one year of age were included.

N-myc Amplification and Prognosis

The cummulative survival curves in terms of N-myc amplification in patients over one year of age are shown in

Table 2. Clinical Stages and N-myc Amplification of Neuroblastoma

| Stage | $<$ 1-year-old N-myc (copies) | | 1-year-old $\leq$ N-myc (copies) | | Total rate of amplification |
|---|---|---|---|---|---|
| | 1 - 10 | 10 $<$ | 1 - 10 | 10 $<$ | |
| I | 3 | 0 | 1 | 0 | 0/4 ( 0 %) |
| II | 3 | 0 | 2 | 1 | 1/6 (17 %) |
| III | 2 | 0 | 4 | 4 | 4/10 (40 %) |
| IV | 3 | 0 | 6 | 7 | 7/16 (44 %) |
| IV-S | 4 | 1 | 0 | 1 | 2/6 (33 %) |
| Total | 15 | 1 | 13 | 13 | 14/42 (33 %) |

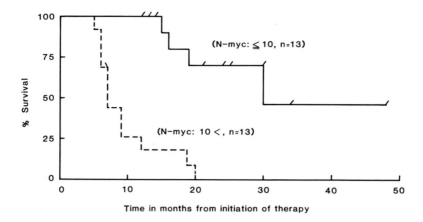

Fig. 1.  Survival Curves and N-myc Amplification of
Neuroblastoma in Patients over One Year of Age.

(/): tumor-free,  (\): recurrent.

Table 3.  Metastatic Pattern and N-myc Amplification of
Neuroblastoma in Patients over One Year of Age.

| Metastatic site | Number of copies of N-myc | | | |
|---|---|---|---|---|
| | 1 - 10 | | 10 < | |
| | At admission | At end-stage or autopsy | At admission | At end-stage or autopsy |
| | ( % ) | ( % ) | ( % ) | ( % ) |
| Bone | 4/13 (31) | 4/4 (100) | 5/13 (38) | 8/10 (80) |
| Orbita | 3/13 (23) | 2/4 ( 50) | 2/13 (15) | 2/11 (18) |
| Bone marrow | 6/13 (46) | 3/3 (100) | 4/13 (31) | 7/9 (78) |
| Liver | 0/13 ( 0) | 1/4 ( 25) | 0/13 ( 0) | 1/10 (10) |
| Skin | 0/13 ( 0) | 0/4 ( 0) | 0/13 ( 0) | 1/11 ( 9) |

Fig. 1. The 48-month survival rate of the group with 1 - 10 copies of N-myc was 47 %, while the rate of the group with more than 10 copies was 0 by 20 months after the initiation of therapy (p < 0.001). The survival intervals for those who died and who had 1 - 10 copies of N-myc was 20.0 ± 3.4 months (mean ± SEM, n=4), while in case of more than 10 copies of N-myc, the survival was 9.4 ± 1.5 months (n=12, p < 0.005).

Metastatic Pattern and Invasiveness

The relationships between metastatic patterns and N-myc amplification in patients over one year of age is shown in Table 3. The patterns of metastasis seemed to be independent of N-myc amplification.

For most children in stage III or IV, preoperative chemotherapy was given, and a total or subtotal removal of the main tumor could be done, independent of the N-myc amplification. However, combined ipsilateral nephrectomy or resection of a part of the liver had to be done in 10 of 13 (77 %) with more than 10 copies of N-myc, while only one combined nephrectomy was required for patients with 1 - 10 copies of N-myc.

Table 4. Quantitative Values of Tumor Markers and N-myc Amplification of Neuroblastoma in Patients over One Year of Age.

| Tumor marker | No. of copies of N-myc | | | | p |
|---|---|---|---|---|---|
| | 1 - 10 | (n) | 10 < | (n) | |
| VMA (mg/day) | 54.3 ± 11.1 | (9) | 4.6 ± 1.0 | (11) | < 0.005 |
| HVA (mg/day) | 71.0 ± 16.5 | (9) | 12.6 ± 4.0 | (11) | < 0.01 |
| LDH (IU/L) | 1039 ± 241 | (11) | 3274 ± 675 | (13) | < 0.01 |
| NSE (ng/ml) | 46 ± 23 | (8) | 148 ± 69 | (4) | NS |
| Ferritin (ng/ml) | 204 ± 87 | (6) | 210 ± 109 | (6) | NS |

Values: Mean ± SEM

Tumor Markers and N-myc Amplification

The relationships between tumor markers and N-myc
amplification of neuroblastoma are shown in Table 4.    The
excretion of urinary VMA was 54.3 ± 11.1 mg/day (mean ± SEM,
n=9) in patients with 1 - 10 copies of N-myc and 4.6 ± 1.0
(n=10) in those with more than 10 copies of N-myc (p < 0.005).
The excretion of urinary HVA was also significantly larger
in the former group.    In contrast, the serum LDH level was
higher in the group with a highly amplified N-myc.    The
cytosomal enzyme neuron-specific enolase (NSE) also had
tended toward an increase in patients with amplified N-myc,
but with no statistical significance, because perhaps of
the small number of cases.    The serum ferritin levels were
not statistically significant.

DISCUSSION

In neuroblastoma, the biological behavior and the prognosis of patients over one year of age differs considerably
from events in much younger patients.    The prognosis of the
former is very poor and metastases occur preferably in bone,
orbita and distant lymph nodes.    The present analysis clearly
showed that the N-myc amplification occurred in a half the
number of patients over one year of age, while it only rarely
occurred in the much younger patients.    The amplification
closely correlated with the prognosis, independent of the
stage of the disease.    Thus, in addition to the patients in
stages III or IV, those in a favorable prognostic stage and
over one year of age should be aggressively treated if their
tumorous N-myc oncogene amplified.

Almost all the patients with amplified N-myc had a
progressive course.    Such tumor progression was also observed in some patients over one year of age and with only 1 -
10 copies of N-myc.    The over-expression of N-myc might be
one cause of the tumor progression.

Bernards et al. suggested that N-myc amplification may
cause down-modulation of the MHC class 1 antigen expression
in the neuroblastoma (1986).    Although MHC antigens are
expected to correlate with the tumor metastasis, our results
showed no relationship between N-myc amplification and pattern
of metastasis of the neuroblastoma in patients over one year
of age.

The invasiveness and rapid tumor progression in those with an amplified N-myc were apparent. Although such tumors responded to aggressive chemotherapy, they recurred after a short interval. Neuroblastoma with an amplified N-myc may readily acquire drug tolerance.

The present study also showed that in those with neuro-blastoma and an amplified N-myc, there was a decreased urinary VMA and HVA and the prognosis was poor. This may be similar to the phenomenon of down-modulation of MHC class 1 antigen expression by N-myc amplification (Bernards et al., 1986).

With regard to the relationship between the poorly developed catecholamine metabolism and the poor-prognosis of those with neuroblastoma, Laug et al. suggested a probable correlation, determined from analyses of the urinary VMA/HVA ratio (1978). Our studies using catecholamine fluorescence and immunohistochemical staining of S-100 protein revealed that the adrenergic differentiation correlated with the histological differentiation of neuroblastoma (Nakagawara et al., 1986). In addition, our preliminary clinical study suggested that the neuroblastomas excreting only dopamine, so-called "dopaminergic neuroblastoma", had a very poor prognosis and an amplified N-myc (in preparation). These data suggest that the immaturity of catecholamine metabolism may correlate with the amplification of the N-myc oncogene in children with neuroblastoma.

To extend the life span of patients over one year of age with neuroblastoma, the N-myc gene or its product modulation may prove to be a new form of therapy.

SUMMARY

1. A genomic amplification of N-myc of neuroblastoma was frequently observed in patients in the advanced stage of the disease, in those with the tumor originating from the suprarenal region, and in those with a histologically un-differentiated neuroblastoma. Thus, N-myc may be one of the most pertinent prognostic factors of neuroblastoma in patients over one year of age.

2. The neuroblastoma patient with 1 - 10 copies of N-myc responded to aggressive multidisciplinary therapy, even

those over one year of age.

3. Rapid invasion and progression of the tumor was evident in children with more than 10 copies of N-myc.

4. N-myc amplification may correlate with immaturity of catecholamine metabolism of neuroblastoma.

## REFERENCES

Bernards R, Dessain S, Weinberg RA (1986). N-myc amplification causes down-modulation of MHC class 1 antigen expression in neuroblastoma. Cell 47:667-674.

Brodeur GM, Seeger RC, Schwab M, Varmus HE, Bishop SM (1984). Amplification of N-myc in untreated human neuroblastomas correlates with advanced disease stage. Science 224: 1121-1124.

Emanuel BS, Balaban G, Boyd JP, Grossman A, Negishi M, Parmiter A, Glick MC (1985). N-myc amplification in multiple homogeneously staining regions in two human neuroblastomas. Proc Natl Acad Sci USA 82:3736-3740.

Evans AE, D'Angio GJ, Randolph J (1971). A proposed staging for children with neuroblastoma. Cancer 27:374-378.

Laug WE, Siegel SE, Shaw KNF, Landing B, Baptista J, Greenstein M (1978). Initial urinary catecholamine concentrations and prognosis in neuroblastoma. Pediatrics 62:77-83.

Nakagawara A, Toyohara T, Nada O, Ikeda K (1986). Catecholaminergic differentiation associated with S100 protein-positive elements in human neuroblastoma. Z Kinderchir 41:275-278.

Nakagawara A, Ikeda K, Tsuda T, Higashi K, Okabe T (1987). Amplification of N-myc oncogene in stage II and IVS neuroblastomas may be a prognostic indicator. J Pediatr Surg 22:415-418.

Nakagawara A, Ikeda K, Tsuda T, Higashi K (1987). N-myc oncogene amplification and prognostic factors of neuroblastoma in children. J Pediatr Surg (in press).

Schwab M, Varmus HE, Bishop JM, Grzeschik K-H, Naylor SL, Sakaguchi AY, Brodeur G, Trent J (1984). Chromosome localization in normal human cells and neuroblastomas of a gene related to c-myc. Nature 308:288-291.

Seeger RC, Brodeur GM, Sather H, Dalton A, Siegel SE, Wong KY, Hammond D (1985). Association of multiple copies of the N-myc oncogene with rapid progression of neuroblastomas. N Engl J Med 313:1111-1116.
Tsuda T, Obara M, Hirano H, Gotoh S, Kubomura S, Higashi K, Kuroiwa A, Nakagawara A, Nagashima N, Shimizu K (1987). Analysis of N-myc amplification in relation to disease stage and histologic types in human neuroblastomas. Cancer (in press).

Advances in Neuroblastoma Research 2, pages 41–49

# EXPRESSION OF N-*myc* BY NEUROBLASTOMAS WITH ONE OR MULTIPLE COPIES OF THE ONCOGENE

Robert C. Seeger, Randal Wada, Garrett M. Brodeur, Thomas J. Moss, Robert L. Bjork, Lawrence Sousa, and Dennis J. Slamon.

Departments of Pediatrics (RCS, RW, TJM, RLB) and Medicine (DJS) and the Jonsson Comprehensive Cancer Center, UCLA School of Medicine, Los Angeles, CA 90024; Departments of Pediatrics and Genetics (GMB), Washington Univ. School of Medicine, St. Louis, MO 63110; Amgen, Inc. (LS), Thousand Oaks, CA; Children's Cancer Study Group, Pasadena, CA 91101.

## INTRODUCTION

Aberrant expresson of proto-oncogenes, which normally are quiescent or regulated, has been implicated in the causation of various malignancies (Bishop, 1983). Schwab et al. (1983) discovered that human neuroblastoma cell lines have multiple copies of a DNA sequence that is related to the v-*myc* and c-*myc* oncogenes and designated it N-*myc*; Kohl et al. (1983) also made similar observations. Brodeur et al. (1984) found that primary untreated neuroblastomas also had amplification of N-*myc* and that this correlated with advanced stage of disease. Seeger et al. (1985) observed that amplification was associated with rapid tumor progression and a poor prognosis.

Thirty percent of all untreated neuroblastomas have amplification of the N-*myc* gene, and these tumors, which can present as local, regional, or metastatic disease, rapidly progress after diagnosis. Another 30%, which do not have amplification of N-*myc* at diagnosis, eventually grow progressively; these tumors present after one year of age and are all metastatic at the time of discovery. The remaining 40% of neuroblastomas, which also do not have amplification of N-*myc*, present as local, regional, or metastatic disease and either spontaneously regress or are nearly always successfully treated. The N-*myc* gene copy number is consistent for a given tumor at different times, which indicates that progression of a non-amplified tumor during therapy is not likely due to development of genomic amplification (Brodeur et al., 1987).

Expression of N-*myc* by these different groups of neuroblastomas has not previously been determined. Genomic amplification has been shown to result in production of high levels of N-*myc* specific mRNA in cell lines and in a few neuroblastomas from patients (Kohl et al., 1984; Schwab et al., 1984; Rosen et al., 1986; Grady-Leopardi et al., 1986). But it is not known, for example, if non-amplified tumors that are metastatic at diagnosis and that subsequently grow progressively overexpress the gene. We developed polyclonal antisera against the N-*myc* protein and demonstrated that it is a doublet protein (62 and 64 kd) that is localized to the nuclear matrix (Slamon et al., 1986). Antisera against N-*myc* specific sequences stain nuclei of neuroblastoma cells overexpressing N-*myc* RNA but not those of HL-60 cells, which overexpress c-*myc* rather than N-*myc*. The current investigation utilized one of these N-*myc* specific antisera to determine expression of the protein in primary untreated neuroblastomas with or without genomic amplification.

**RESULTS**

To date, we have determined the number of copies of N-*myc* in 215 primary untreated neuroblastomas and 7 ganglioneuromas (Table 1). Amplification has not been observed in stage I neuroblastomas or ganglioneuromas.

Expression of N-*myc* by these different groups of neuroblastoma was determined. Initially, a subset of tumors was tested to find the concordance between immunohistologic and biochemical analyses (Table 2). For each tumor, mRNA was assessed by northern analysis using the pNb-1 N-*myc* probe and protein was assessed using a specific antiserum (anti-bGH/N-*myc* II) for immunoblotting and immunohistology. For tumors expressing N-*myc*, northern analysis showed a transcript in the range of 3.2 kb, western analysis showed doublet 62 and 64 kd molecules, and immunostaining localized to nuclei. These experiments indicate that immunohistology is an accurate measure of N-*myc* expression.


Table 1.  Genomic Amplification of N-*myc* Oncogene in Neuroblastoma.

| Stage | Number of tumors | % with genomic amplification |
|---|---|---|
| I | 19 | 0 |
| II | 46 | 10 |
| III | 52 | 39 |
| IV | 80 | 38 |
| IV-S | 18 | 6 |
| Ganglioneuroma | 7 | 0 |

Table 2.  Concordance Between Immunohistological and Biochemical Analyses for Expression of N-*myc*.

| Number of gene copies of N-*myc* | Number tumors tested | % concordance |
|---|---|---|
| 1 | 14 | 93 |
| >10 | 5 | 100 |

One hundred twenty-six tumors have been evaluated immunohistologically (Table 3).  All 25 with >10 gene copies of N-*myc* stained strongly, and 3 of 4 with 3-10 copies did so.  The staining pattern of amplified tumors was quite similar with marked heterogeneity of expression between individual cells always being present; this gives the appearance of "stars in the sky."  None of these tumors had focal areas of highly expressing neuroblasts among other non-expressing neuroblasts.  As with amplification, expression is independent of the stage of the tumor at diagnosis (Table 4).

Eighteen of 97 non-amplified tumors of all stages

also expressed N-*myc*; with few exceptions, however, the
amount was less than that seen in amplified tumors. Three
tumors that were stroma-rich had nodules of strongly
staining neuroblasts. The remaining 15 tumors, which
appeared to be stroma-poor and undifferentiated, had
uniform staining of the tumor cells throughout. Single
copy primary tumors that did not stain included 29 that
had metastasized widely (Table 4).

Table 3. Immunohistologic Staining of Primary
Neuroblastomas with Anti-N-*myc* Serum in Relationship to
Gene Copy Number.

| Staining | Gene Copy Number | | | Total |
|---|---|---|---|---|
| | 1 | 3-10 | >10 | |
| 0 | 79* | 1 | 0 | 80 |
| 1 | 14 | 2 | 3 | 19 |
| 2 | 4 | 0 | 10 | 14 |
| 3 | 0 | 1 | 12 | 13 |
| Total | 97 | 4 | 25 | 126 |

*Number of tumors

Table 4. Expression of N-*myc* in Relationship to Stage and
Genomic Amplification.

| Stage | Non-amplified | | Amplified | |
|---|---|---|---|---|
| | Number of tumors | % with expression | Number of tumors | % with expression |
| I | 12 | 8 | 0 | 0 |
| II | 26 | 27 | 4 | 100 |
| III | 19 | 26 | 12 | 92 |
| IV | 31 | 6 | 13 | 100 |
| IV-S | 11 | 27 | 1 | 100 |
| Ganglioneuroma | 5 | 0 | 0 | 0 |

**DISCUSSION**

Oncogenes can be activated from their normal quiescent or regulated state by 1) gene amplification; 2) increased expression of a single gene; or 3) gene alteration resulting in a product with increased oncogenic potential (Bishop, 1983). Our investigations of N-*myc* demonstrated that genomic amplification occurs in untreated primary tumors, particularly those that are widespread at diagnosis (Brodeur et al., 1984) and that a high gene copy number is associated with rapid tumor progression (Seeger et al., 1985). These clinical observations, the homology of N-*myc* to c-*myc* and v-*myc* (Schwab et al., 1983), and the ability of N-*myc* alone or in cooperation with c-Ha-*ras* to transform cells (Schwab et al., 1985; Small et al., 1987), strongly suggest that N-*myc* has an important role in determining the tumorigenicity of human neuroblastomas. Oncogene amplification has been identified in a variety of other human tumors and cell lines, but no large clinical studies were reported until recently. Slamon et al. (1987) studied 189 primary breast cancers and found that HER-2/*neu* was amplified in 30% of tumors and that amplification predicted significantly shorter time to relapse and survival. Thus, genomic amplification is a mechanism of oncogene activation that correlates with highly malignant tumor behavior.

We have studied expression of N-*myc* in 126 neuroblastomas by immunohistology and in a subset by immunohistology, immunoblotting, and northern analysis. Tumors with more than ten copies of the N-*myc* gene all expressed it at a high level. Tumors with low level amplification (3-10 copies) are infrequent and so only four have been studied; of interest, one did not detectably express N-*myc*, which suggests that low copy number sometimes is insufficient to activate the gene.

Although amplification of N-*myc* is an important mechanism of overexpression, one-half of neuroblastomas that are aggressive do not have amplification at diagnosis (Seeger et al., 1985) or when progression occurs (Brodeur et al., 1987). We hypothesize other mechanisms for this group of tumors: 1) non-amplified N-*myc* can be overexpressed and/or abnormally expressed; and 2) other oncogenes can be activated and/or suppressor genes can be lost.

We observed expression of N-*myc* by non-amplified tumors: 1) most often, these tumors were stroma-poor and undifferentiated, and all tumor cells expressed low or moderate levels; 2) occasionally, however, these tumors consisted of infrequent nests of highly expressing neuroblasts among non-expressing stroma; it is not known if these subpopulations are amplified or not. Retinoblastoma (Lee et al., 1984), small cell lung carcinoma (Nau et al., 1986), and neuroblastoma cell lines (Alt et al., 1986; Sadee et al., 1987; Wada et al., 1987) with non-amplified N-*myc* can express the gene but in lower levels than cell lines with amplification. N-*myc* also is expressed by non-amplified primary Wilms' tumors (Alt et al., 1986). It is possible that N-*myc* overexpression, without amplification, may play a role in determining malignancy (perhaps in concert with other oncogenes). Expression of an abnormal N-*myc* product also may result in malignant behavior; and further studies of the molecular nature of the N-*myc* protein in non-amplified, agressive neuroblastomas are required.

Our studies also indicate that there are many aggressive neuroblastomas that do not express N-*myc*. Clearly, other oncogenes must be active in such tumors. Other members of the *myc* family may be activated in neuroblastomas that do not have activated N-*myc*; indeed, a neuroblastoma cell line (SK-N-SH) that has neither N-*myc* nor c-*myc* amplified overexpresses c-*myc* (Alt et al., 1986; Sadee et al., 1987). In model systems, transformation by *ras* oncogenes as well as oncogenes encoding various protein kinases can induce the metastatic phenotype (Egan et al., 1987a; Egan et al., 1987b). These classes of genes are important to examine since all of the poor prognosis patients whose neuroblastomas do not have amplification of N-*myc* have metastatic disease. In addition, N-*ras* was first isolated from the SK-N-SH cell line. Identification of missing supressor genes in neuroblastoma may also provide insight into tumor behavior (Brodeur et al., 1988).

Assessment of N-*myc* expression by immunohistology is likely to be useful for prognostication since it identifies all tumors with more than ten copies; it may also be helpful for some non-amplified tumors, although clinical correlations are needed to ascertain this. Immunohistologic analysis is rapid, uses small samples, and can be performed on cell populations where tumor cells are relatively infrequent such as in bone marrow (Moss et al., 1988).

In summary, we have demonstrated that neuroblastomas with genomic amplification of N-*myc* express high levels of the protein and that some non-amplified tumors also express significant amounts. Increased expression of the gene product by amplified and aggressive tumors further supports an important role for N-*myc* in determining tumor behavior.

### ACKNOWLEDGEMENTS

These studies were supported in part by USPHS grants awarded by the National Cancer Institute, DHHS: CA22794, CA27678, CA16042, CA36011 (RCS); CA39771, CA01027, CA05587 (GMB); and CA36827 (DJS). Additional support was obtained from the Children's United Research Effort against Cancer and the Fern Waldman Memorial Fund for Cancer Research (GMB).

### REFERENCES

Alt FW, DePinho R, Zimmerman K, Legouy E, Hatton K, Ferrier P, Tesfaye A, Yancopoulos G, Nisen P (1986). The human *myc* gene family. Cold Spring Harbor Symp Quant 51 Pt 2:931–941.

Bishop JM (1983). Cellular oncogenes and retroviruses. Ann Rev Biochem 52:301–354.

Brodeur GM, Seeger RC, Schwab M, Varmus HE, Bishop JM (1984). Amplification of N-*myc* sequences in primary human neuroblastomas. Science 224:1121–1124.

Brodeur GM, Hayes FA, Green AA, Casper JT, Wasson J, Wallach S, Seeger RC (1987). Consistent N-*myc* copy number in simultaneous or consecutive neuroblastoma samples from sixty individual patients. Cancer Res 47:4248–4253.

Brodeur GM, Fong C, Morita M, Griffith R, Hayes FA, Seeger RC (1988). Molecular analysis and clinical significance of N-*myc* amplification and chromosome 1 abnormalities in human neuroblastomas. Prog Clin Biol Res in press.

Egan SE, McClarty GA, Jarolim L, Wright JA, Spiro I, Hager

G, Greenberg AH (1987a). Expression of H-*ras* correlates with metastatic potential: Evidence for direct regulation of the metastatic phenotype in 10T1/2 and NIH 3T3 cells. Mol Cell Biol 7:830–837.

Egan SE, Wright JA, Jarolim L, Yanagihara K, Bassin RH, Greenberg AH (1987b). Transformation by oncogene encoding protein kinases induces the metastatic phenotype. Science 238:202–204.

Grady-Leopardi E, Schwab M, Ablin AR, Rosenau W (1986). Detection of N-*myc* oncogene expression in human neuroblastoma by *in situ* hybridization and blot analysis: relationship to clinical outcome. Cancer Res 46:3196–3199.

Kohl NE, Kanda N, Schreck RR, Bruns G, Latt SA, Gilbert F, Alt FW (1983). Transposition and amplification of oncogene-related sequences in human neuroblastomas. Cell 35:359–367.

Kohl NE, Gee CE, Alt FW (1984). Activated Expression of the N-*myc* gene in human neuroblastomas and related tumors. Science 226:1335–1337.

Lee W-H, Murphree AL, Benedict WF (1984). Expression and amplification of the N-*myc* gene in primary retinoblastoma Nature 309:458–462.

Moss TJ, Law YM, Slamon DJ, Brodeur GM, Seeger RC (1988). N-*myc* protein expression by neuroblastoma cells that have metastasized to bone marrow. Prog Clin Biol Res in press.

Nau MM, Brooks BJ Jr, Carney DN, Gazdar AF, Battey JF, Sausville EA, Minna JD (1986). Human small-cell lung cancers show amplification and expression of the N-*myc* gene. Proc Natl Acad Sci USA 83:1092–1096.

Rosen N, Reynolds CP, Thiele CJ, Biedler JL, Israel MA (1986). Increased N-*myc* expression following progressive growth of human neuroblastoma. Cancer Res 46:4139–4142.

Sadee VC, Yu ML, Richards PN, Preis MR, Schwab FM, Brodsky FM, Biedler, JL (1987). Expression of neurotransmitter receptors and *myc* protooncogenes in subclones of a human neuroblastoma cell line. Cancer Res 47:5207–5210.

Schwab M, Alitalo K, Klempnauer K-H, Varmus HE, Bishop JM, Gilbert F, Brodeur G, Goldstein M, Trent J (1983). Amplified DNA with limited homology to *myc* cellular oncogene is shared by human neuroblastoma cell lines and a neuroblastoma tumor. Nature 305:245–248.

Schwab M, Ellison J, Busch M, Rosenau W, Varmus HE, and Bishop JM (1984). Enhanced expression of the human gene N-*myc* consequent to amplification of DNA may contribute to malignant progression of neuroblastoma. Proc Natl Acad Sci USA 81:4940–4944.

Schwab M, Varmus HE, Bishop JM (1985). Human gene N-*myc* contributes to neoplastic transformation of mammalian cells in culture. Nature 316:160–162.

Seeger RC, Brodeur GM, Sather H, Dalton A, Siegel SE, Wong KY, Hammond D (1985). Association of multiple copies of the N-*myc* oncogene with rapid progression of neuroblastomas. N Engl J Med 313:1111–1116.

Slamon DJ, Boone TC, Seeger RC, Keith DE, Chazin V, Lee HC, Souza IM (1986). Identification and characterization of the protein encoded by the human N-*myc* oncogene. Science 232:768–772.

Slamon DJ, Clark GM, Wong SG, Levin WJ, Ullrich A, McGuire WL (1987). Human breast cancer: correlation of replase and survival with amplification of the HER-2/*neu* oncogene Science 235:177–182.

Small MB, Hay N, Schwab M, Bishop JM (1987). Neoplastic transformation by the human gene N-*myc*. Mol Cell Biol 7:1638–1645.

Wada R, Seeger R, Brodeur G, Slamon D, Rayner S, Tomayko M, Reynolds CP (1988). Neuroblastoma cell lines that express one copy of the N-*myc* oncogene. Prog Clin Biol Res in press.

Advances in Neuroblastoma Research 2, pages 51–56
© 1988 Alan R. Liss, Inc.

DISCUSSION

Chairman:        Garrett Brodeur

Discussants:     G. Brodeur, F.Gilbert,
                 A. Nakagawara, Robert Seeger

Dr. Matthay, UCSF, asked Dr. Nakagawara about the 2/16 IVS patients with amplified N-myc; were they studied at diagnosis, how were they selected and what was their outcome. Dr. Nakagawara said the first patient's tumor had 13 copies of N-myc, was 1 month of age with very aggressive bilateral adrenal disease with metastases to liver and bone marrow. He was treated with small doses of vincristine and cyclophosphamide but died 7 days later of tumor lysis syndrome with very high uric acid. The second patient was 14½ years old with a small right adrenal tumor, completely excised which had 20 copies of N-myc. He had a local recurrence 6 months later with progressive disease involving bone, scalp and orbit. He felt this second patient's disease was bad because of the age.

Dr. Knudson, Philadelphia, asked how the process of amplification starts and why N-myc. Could it occur at any gene or was it N-myc because it was being expressed in the target tissue? Bearing on this he also asked how often HSR's or DM's occurred which did not contain N-myc? Dr. Brodeur replied that this was impossible to answer at this time. However, the observation that the amplification occurred in only a subset of tumor and was stable when it occurred suggests this is a propensity or capability of a subset of tumors (for unknown reasons). Secondly, N-myc is only about 10 kb long, while the amplified region is 500–1000 kb but the amplified region between different tumors is surprisingly conserved. Bert Vogelstein studied about 12 primary tumors and found each amplified about 80% of the same domain. Thus there seems to be something specific about amplification of this region. There are 2 cell lines from St. Jude with cytogenetic evidence of gene amplification that could not be shown to include N-myc, C-myc, L-=myc, H-ras, N-ras, C-sis, C-erb B1, or C-erb 2.

R. Seeger:  Are those cell lines neuroblastoma?

Brodeur:  One is unequivocally a neuroblastoma by clinical and histological criteria. I'm not positive of the other.

   Fred Gilbert (Mt. Sinai, New York) commented that neuroblastoma was a relative anomaly among tumors in that other tumors in which amplification had been identified there is no uniformity about which oncogenes were amplified whereas in neuroblastoma, in all cases of which he was aware, it was always N-myc. The second point was that the amplification units always contained sequences from around N-myc on chromosome 2p while HSR's are usually on chromosomes other than 2. Finally, there is evidence from Sam Latt's and Fred Alt's lab that some of the amplified sequences are found in some NBL's but not others so the common thread between all the amplifications is N-myc. Dr. Brodeur replied that if N-myc is in the middle of the amplification unit the ends may vary and what is at the ends may be important. It will also be interesting to study the ends in terms of recombination breakpoints to gain insight into the mechanism of amplification. Dr. Gilbert went on to say that if N-myc amplification was a passive marker of the stage of differentiation and a myc family member was enhancing expression of all tumor cells then he would expect to see amplification of myc in all tumor cells and that isn't the case. So the amplification of N-myc is very interesting and maybe there is something specific about the region surrounding N-myc, perhaps a not yet identified oncogene and perhaps N-myc is only a marker for this. The size of the amplification unit is very large and an HSR may be as large as chromosome 1, or 10% of the genome, so there is the potential for a very large number of copies of N-myc. Since 30 copies of N-myc would only account for .1% of this then 99.9% of the HSR is something else.

   Dr. Uriel Littauer (Weizman) asked if the mechanism of overexpression of N-myc RNA in single copy gene tumors was due to stabilization of the mRNA. Dr. Seeger replied he had no data on this. Secondly, Dr. Littauer asked if there was any data on down regulation of specific differentiation pathways such as the NGF receptor. Dr. Seeger again had no data.

   Dr. John Kemshead (London) asked if there was difficulty in identifying N-myc RNA or protein in tumor biopsy specimens as they had found them extremely labile. He also asked if they had identified the degradation products of the N-myc protein. Dr. Seeger replied that not every tumor specimen had good RNA but if frozen quickly was adequate. Multiple copy specimens were easier to see than single copy ones. With respect to degradation products they have not been studied consistently but there are often low molecular weight bands seen, especially in multiple copy tumors.

Dr. Kemshead then asked the panel to comment on the specificity of N-myc amplification in that it had now been reported in one astrocytoma, one rhabdomyosarcoma and was over-expressed in some Wilms' tumors. Dr. Brodeur replied that it was also amplified in retinoblastoma and small cell carcinoma of the lung. However, N-myc is the only amplified oncogene that has been identified in neuroblastomas; it is amplified, commonly in these tumors and has not been shown to be as consistently, or specifically amplified in any other tumors. Dr. Seeger pointed out that the overexpression of N-myc seemed to be limited to neuroblastoma and had not been seen in other lines. Dr. Kemshead said this was contrary to their experience even though both groups felt they had specific antisera.

Dr. Bernard Mirkin (Minneapolis) asked Dr. Nakagawara about the catecholamine pattern with low or high amplification. Dr. Nakagawara said that he had only reported VMA and HVA in this study (end metabolites) as they wanted to correlate N-myc amplification with down regulation of the catecholamine pathway. In another study however, where they had measured all the catecholamines and metabolites, there were six cases which showed high dopamine but everything distal to this was low and all the patients died. Of those tested (3/16) all had highly amplified N-myc. Dr. Mirkin wondered if the conclusion was that the gene products, enzymes were down regulated in NBL. He had seen some evidence for this in mouse NBL's grown in NGF. Audrey Evans (Philadelphia) commented that clinically there are patients without excess catecholamine secretion who are at both ends of the spectrum--either mature benign ganglioneuromas or immature neuroblastomas. The catecholamine secretion may have nothing to do with N-myc per se but with the degree of differentiation of the tumor. Dr. Tom Moss (Los Angeles) then asked Dr. Nakagawara what correlation there was between the VMA/HVA ratio of N-myc amplification. Dr. Nakagawara replied that was only a nonsignificant tendency to a positive correlation (as reported in March 7, 1987 Lancet). Dr.

Evans commented that was some prognostic importance of the VMA/HVA ratio but more to the lack of secretion.

Dr. Marie Favrot (Lyon, France) asked Dr. Brodeur now many primary tumors with amplified N-myc had been studied after induction therapy at second look surgery. Dr. Brodeur replied that in every case with two exceptions, N-myc amplification was seen at second look if seen initially, although sometimes to a lesser degree. The two exceptions, when examined retrospectively, were explained histologically in that there was little if any tumor tissue in abundant stroma. Otherwise there has been extreme consistency in N-myc copy number, although there could be exceptions to the rule. N-myc expression could change with treatment or with differentiation and that has been shown by Carol Thiele (NCI) and Mark Israel (NCI). Conceivably since DM's are not integrated into chromosomes and are unstable they could be lost, but this has not been seen.

Thierry Philip (Lyon, France) asked if this stability could be explained by a selection of bad cases for second surgery. Dr. Brodeur said that in POG, any patient with a residual mass after induction therapy had second look surgery and that the only patients who didn't were those with progressive disease. Dr. Philip then said that after four courses of chemotherapy there are histologic changes in the tumor and asked how did one know if one was analyzing the right portion of the tumor. Dr. Brodeur replied that amplification did not change in the genome with differentiation, even though expression did.

Robert Castleberry (Alabama) asked if there were any patients with amplified N-myc at diagnosis who had gone on to have ganglioneuroma at second look surgery. Dr. Seeger replied that in CCSG they hadn't done yet a molecular biology-pathology correlation but from immunohistochemical stains samples from delayed surgery were often very stromatous with few blast cells. They had not yet evaluated serial samples immunohistochemically.

T. Philip then asked if we could rely on second-look surgery (where primary surgery not otherwise indicated) for assessment of amplification. Dr. Seeger didn't feel the question could be answered yet. Dr. Brodeur was concerned that N-myc copy number would not be assessable reliably, based on his studies of serial tumor samples from the same patients over time. Some patients with N-myc amplification at diagnosis had false-negative results from second-look tissue, due to the parity or absence of malignant cells.

A. Green (St. Jude's) pointed out that if the primary tumor completely resolved with chemotherapy, the patient would not get second-look surgery, and also not in the face of progressive disease. Therefore the second-look surgery results are selected, potentially biased and we must be careful in interpreting those results.

Dr. Israel felt that the same arguments about degree of stroma at second-look could suggest that we are actually seeing a greatly increased N-myc amplification in these selected cells but only it is masked by the lack of cellularity. Dr. Brodeur replied that what they saw at diagnosis held up at second-look except in the two cases that were recognized as representing the "false-negative." The sample at diagnosis seems more important then subsequent samples. Nevertheless, subsequent samples can usually be compared to the original, nonselected result, even if the tumor histology is altered by treatment.

Dr. Gilbert commented that in his mouse model they see considerable changes in the karyotype without changes in N-myc amplification or expression so N-myc may not be the only (or best) marker. Also, when the primary tumor is analyzed, it has been growing for months to years so it is already selected.

Dr. Brodeur "amplified" this by saying that there are many patients with progressive disease without amplification of N-myc so there must be other genes or factors that are very important. It is not the only prognostic variable. Dr. Evans pointed out that in fact 50% of children with progressive disease don't have amplified or overexpressed N-myc.

Dr. Seeger commented that only three of thirteen single copy N-myc overexpressors went on to die so maybe there are two sets of single copy overexpressors. One subset may be imparting a very malignant phenotype but the larger subset seems to have benign disease.

When asked about amplification of other oncogenes, Dr. Brodeur said that they had looked at over 12 oncogenes for amplification or overexpression in neuroblastoma but hadn't found any that occurred with any frequency. Also, one doesn't see chromosome 1p deletion in all tumors with N-myc amplification. They do not know yet how chromosome 1p changes correlate with N-myc amplification or with prognosis. They need more cases.

Dr. Lipinski (Villejuif, France) asked what is known about N-myc expression in fetal tissues. Dr. Brodeur said Fred Alt had reported expression in murine brain, kidney and lung. Dr. Kemshead had seen the same.

Chris Frantz (Rochester) commented that since we haven't really identified the crucial gene in neuroblastoma that we can't say that all NBL's haven't lost the "neuroblastoma" gene. Dr. Brodeur agreed but said that we can say that obvious large deletion of 1p aren't seen in all Stage IV patients and are rarely seen in low stage patients. Dr. Frantz replied that we don't see large deletions in most Wilms' tumor or retinoblastoma patients either. Dr. Brodeur expanded to say that in over 50% of Wilms' tumors appeared to have normal karyotypes but turned out to have two copies of the same chromosome homology by whatever mechanism. This suggests cytogenetics is important to focus on the right portion of a chromosome, and even to suggest a mechanism for rearrangement, but that molecular studies are needed to really understand what is going on.

Nao Ikegaki (Philadelphia) asked for comments on the heterogeneity of N-myc expression between cells of the same tumor or line. Dr. Seeger said that they do see so much heterogeneity in cell lines that sections can look like a starry sky. Possible explanations include changes of expression with the cell cycle or unequal segregation of DM's at division. He sees the same in tumors. This doesn't support a clonal explanation because one would then expect to see nests of expressing cells but this situation is still compatable with either cell cycle variation or DM's. Dr. Brodeur said they certainly have seen DM's vary from one to over a hundred per cell. Dr. Gilbert said they had seen an inverse correlation between DM's and HSR's and certainly a heterogeneity of chromosomes themselves.

Advances in Neuroblastoma Research 2, pages 57–69
© 1988 Alan R. Liss, Inc.

# CHARACTERIZATION OF HUMAN NEUROBLASTOMA CELL LINES THAT LACK N-*myc* GENE AMPLIFICATION

Randal K. Wada, Robert C. Seeger, Garrett M. Brodeur, Dennis J. Slamon, Sylvia A. Rayner, Mary M. Tomayko, and C. Patrick Reynolds.

Departments of Pediatrics (R.K.W., R.C.S., S.A.R., M.M.T., and C.P.R.) and Medicine (D.J.S.) and the Jonsson Comprehensive Cancer Center, UCLA School of Medicine, Los Angeles, CA 90024; Department of Pediatrics (G.M.B.), Washington University School of Medicine, St. Louis, MO 63110

## INTRODUCTION

Amplification of the N-*myc* oncogene in human neuroblastomas is associated with advanced tumor stage (Brodeur *et al.*, 1984) and rapid disease progression (Seeger *et al.*, 1985). As 60% of Stage IV tumors lack detectable amplification, yet 90% eventually develop progressive disease (Voute, 1984; Seeger *et al.*, 1985), other mechanisms in addition to gene amplification may be involved in N-*myc* activation. Most neuroblastoma cell lines available for study have amplification of the N-*myc* gene, and many of the lines that lack N-*myc* amplification previously thought to be neuroblastomas have been identified as primitive neuroectodermal tumor (PNET) lines (Donner *et al.*, 1985, Reynolds *et al.*, 1988). Thus, there is a need for neuroblastoma cell lines that lack N-*myc* amplification to study other mechanisms of disease progression. We have established cell lines from two neuroblastoma patients who had poor clinical outcomes, yet whose tumors lacked N-*myc* amplification as defined by Southern analysis. Here we describe the characteristics of these lines, and demonstrate that they have higher amounts of N-*myc* protein and mRNA than non-neuroblastoma lines.

**MATERIALS AND METHODS**

Establishment and Culture of Cell Lines

Patient 1 (SMS-IHN): Tumor tissue was obtained at surgery, minced in Puck's saline A with 10 mM HEPES and 1 mM EDTA (Puck's-EDTA), washed once with Puck's-EDTA, and resuspended in growth medium consisting of RPMI-1640 with 15% Fetal Calf Serum (FCS), 100 IU penicillin/ml, and 100 ug streptomycin/ml. Cell suspensions were placed into tissue culture flasks at 1-2 million cells/ml, and were passed into new flasks with fresh medium using Puck's-EDTA (Reynolds et al., 1986). Once established the cell line could also be maintained in Leibovitz's L15 with 15% FCS and 50 ug/ml of gentamycin.

Patient 2 (LA-N-6): Whole bone marrow was harvested in 30 U/ml of preservative-free heparin and treated by sedimentation, filtration, incubation with monoclonal antibodies, and then goat anti-mouse immunoglobulin coated magnetic beads (Seeger et al., 1987). Heta starch (HES) sedimentation, the initial step in this process, serves to pellet clumps of tumor cells. The tumor-enriched HES pellet was washed in Dulbecco's Phosphate Buffered Saline without $Ca^{++}$ or $Mg^{++}$ (PBS) and resuspended in Leibovitz's L15 growth medium with 15% FCS and 50 ug/ml gentamycin. Cells were plated and passaged as described above for Patient 1. Established cells could also be grown in RPMI-1640 with 10% FCS.

Analysis of G6PD isoenzymes by Robert Sparkes, M.D., University of California, Los Angeles, showed both cell lines had the B G6PD isotype, ensuring that they were not contaminated by HeLa cells. Metaphase spreads of SMS-IHN and LA-N-6 showed predominant karyotypes of 44X and 47X, respectively. Both cell lines lack double minute chromosomes, homogeneously staining regions, chromosome 1 p deletions, and 11;22 translocations.

Growth Rate: Human neuroblastoma cell lines NGP and NLF (Brodeur et al., 1981); SMS-KCNR (Reynolds et al., 1986); LA-N-5 (Seeger et al., 1982); SK-N-SH (Biedler et al., 1973) and human PNET cell lines SK-N-MC (Biedler et al., 1973); CHP-100 (Schlesinger et al., 1976); CB-AGPN (Reynolds et al., 1988) were maintained in vitro at 37° C in a humidified 5% $CO_2$ atmosphere in RPMI 1640 with 10% FCS. All cell lines were tested and found to be free of mycoplasma. To determine growth rate $5 \times 10^4$ cells were seeded into 35 mm tissue culture dishes and removed every 2 days by successive rinses with Pucks-EDTA (Reynolds, et al, 1986), suspended in 0.06% trypan blue and counted with a hemocytometer. Doubling times were determined to be the inverse of the slope of the best fit line calculated by linear regression of the log (base 2) of the cell counts (Merchant et al., 1964).

For injection into nude mice, cultured neuroblastoma cells were removed from tissue culture flasks using Pucks-EDTA, resuspended in PBS, and freed of clumps by gentle pipetting with a pasteur pipet. Cell number and viability were determined by trypan blue exclusion and $10^8$ cells were injected through 22 gauge needles subcutaneously between the scapula of 6 to 12 week old nu/nu mice. Mice were housed in a laminar flow caging system, and food, bedding, and water were autoclaved. Mice were examined once a week and the tumor lag time recorded as the number of days between injection of cells and appearance of a palpable mass.

Differentiation Markers and N-myc

*Quantitation of Cell Surface Antigens*: Cells were stained using concentrated tissue culture supernatent (10x) from the hybridoma HSAN 1.2 (Smith and Reynolds, 1987), W6/32 (Parham et al., 1979), or a non-binding control monoclonal antibody, followed by FITC-labeled goat anti-mouse Ig, and fluorescence was quantitated using flow cytometry as described elsewhere in this volume (Reynolds, et al., 1988). Electronic gates for positive antibody binding were determined based on controls for each cell line such that controls showed 2% or less positive cells. The binding index was calculated as the % cells positive X mean fluorescence channel/100.

*Catecholamine Fluorescence*: Glyoxylic acid-induced catecholamine fluorescence of touch preps from nude mouse tumors was determined as previously described (Reynolds et al., 1981).

*Southern Analysis*: DNA was isolated, digested with restriction endonuclease Eco R1, fractionated on agarose gels and transferred to nitrocellulose paper, where it was hybridized to the isotopically labeled plasmid N-myc probe pNb1 and washed under stringent conditions (Brodeur et al., 1984).

*Northern Analysis*: Total RNA was isolated by the

guanidine isothiocyanate method (Chirgwin et al., 1979), run on formaldehyde-agarose gels and northern blotted (Lehrach et al., 1980) prior to hybridization with labeled pNb1. Slot blots of total RNA were performed as described by Davis et al., (1986).

*Western Analysis*: Total cellular protein was isolated and fractionated on 7% SDS-polyacrilamide gels (Slamon et al., 1986), transferred to nitrocellulose, and immunostained (Davis et al., 1986) with the N-*myc* specific, polyclonal antiserum anti-bGH/N-*myc*II (Slamon et al., 1986). Primary antiserum was used at a 1:400 dilution. A biotinylated goat anti-rabbit serum at a 1:200 dilution served as the secondary antibody. This was followed by incubation with avidin-biotin-alkaline phosphatase complexes, and development with an alkaline phosphatase substrate kit (Vector Laboratories; Burlingame, CA). All incubations and washes were carried out using a modified Omniblot processing system, with a wash flow rate of 35 ml/minute (Oste et al., 1986; Wada and Seeger, in preparation).

*Immunocytology*: Cultured cells were placed onto coverslips by cytocentrifugation and fixed serially with 2% paraformaldehyde in Dulbecco's PBS at pH 6.5 and pH 11, followed by methanol, at $4^0$ C for 10 minutes each. Non-specific antigenic sites were blocked with 10% normal goat serum in PBS prior to overnight incubation with primary antiserum (anti-bGH/N-*myc*II) at 1:4000 dilution. This was followed by incubation with biotinylated goat anti-rabbit serum, phenylhydrazine treatment, reaction with avidin-biotin-peroxidase complexes, and visualization of bound peroxidase with diaminobenzidine/$H_2O_2$ (Slamon et al., 1986).

**RESULTS**

Clinical Summaries

Patient 1: A 2 y.o. boy presented to his physician with a two day history of a limp and complaints of left leg pain. Physical exam was significant for tenderness of the left anterior thigh, decreased extension of his hip, and a 3cm x 4cm firm, non-tender facial mass overlying the left zygomatic arch. A skeletal survey showed a mass in the left zygoma and lytic lesions in the right humerus and left femur. A bone scan demonstrated increased uptake in the left femur, right humerus, left kidney, lumbar vertebrae 2-3, and the posterior region of the right 8-9th ribs. Biopsy of the left femoral region revealed a small round cell malignant tumor. VMA was slightly elevated in a 24 hour urine collection (10 mg/24 hours). A bone marrow biopsy showed clumps and sheets of non-hematopoietic tumor cells which demonstrated positive catecholamine fluorescence and neurite outgrowth in tissue culture. Subsequently an intravenous pyelogram revealed a right suprarenal mass, and the diagnosis of Stage IV neuroblastoma was made. The patient received several courses of cytoxan/adriamycin, during which his marrow cleared and the primary tumor decreased in size. The patient underwent laparotomy 6 months after diagnosis to remove the primary tumor ( a ganglioneuroblastoma at surgery), at which time the cell line SMS-LHN was established. Two months after surgery the patient developed metastatic disease in his bone marrow and died of progressive disease fifteen months after diagnosis.

Patient 2: A 5 y.o. boy initially presented with cervical lymphadenopathy, anemia, and weight loss, but his diagnosis remained unclear until eight months later when a right adrenal mass was detected by ultrasound. HVA and VMA were elevated (458 ug/mg of creatinine and 262 ug/mg of creatinine, respectively), and a bone marrow biopsy showed nests of small round cells compatible with neuroblastoma. A bone scan revealed metastases to bone, retro-orbital space, and the right thorax. The patient received 5 courses of cytoxan/adriamycin but still had persistent tumor and metastases. He then began cis-platinum and VM-26, and received 3 courses of cis-platinum, but because of an anaphylactic reaction to his first dose of VM-26, this was discontinued and substituted with 1 course of VP-16. At this point a CT scan showed some decrease in the primary tumor and resolution of his bone metastases, although his marrow remained positive for tumor cells. Five months after diagnosis the patient was referred for possible autologous bone marrow transplant with ex vivo tumor purging. Prior to his marrow harvest the patient was maintained on alternate regimens of cytoxan, vincristine, and DTIC. Bone marrow was harvested for transplant, however there was near total replacement of marrow with tumor, and it could not be adequately purged. The tumor-enriched fraction of the marrow harvest was placed into culture and gave rise to the cell line LA-N-6. The patient developed progressively increasing metastatic disease, and died thirteen months after diagnosis.

Growth Characteristics in vitro and in vivo: In culture the predominant cell in LA-N-6 was a small tear-drop-shaped cell with processes. SMS-LHN was composed mostly of more

compact, stellate cells, which have a greater tendency to grow
in clusters than does IA-N-6. Figure 1 compares the doubling
times in tissue culture for IA-N-6 and SMS-IHN with SK-N-SH (N-
*myc* non-amplified) and SMS-KCNR (N-*myc* multi-copy). IA-N-6 and
SMS-IHN had doubling times of 4.3 days and 9.3 days,
respectively; which are significantly longer (p<0.01) than
those seen in the N-*myc* amplified cell line SMS-KCNR (1.8
days), or in the SK-N-SH cell line (1.8 days).

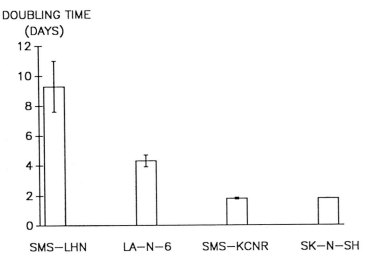

Figure 1.  Doubling times in tissue culture.

In nude mice the average lag times between cell injection
and formation of palpable tumor are 187 days for IA-N-6 and 141
days for SMS-IHN, compared to lag times of 31 days for SMS-KCNR
and 29 days for SK-N-SH.

*Differentiation Markers*:  Flow cytometry demonstrated that
these cell lines possess cell surface antigen profiles that
distinguish them from primitive neuroectodermal tumors (PNET).
In the PNET cell lines CB-AGPN and SK-N-MC, the intensity of
staining with the anti-HIA A,B,C antibody W6/32 is greater than
that with the anti-neuroblastoma antibody HSAN 1.2.    In
contrast IA-N-5 and SMS-KAN, neuroblastoma lines with N-*myc*
amplification, show very strong staining with HSAN 1.2, and
very weak anti-HIA staining. The non-amplified cell lines IA-N-
6 and SMS-IHN have cell surface antigen patterns similar to

multi-copy neuroblastoma (Figure 2). The adrenergic nature of the two cell lines was confirmed as both cell lines form tumors with marked catecholamine fluorescence when grown in nude mice.

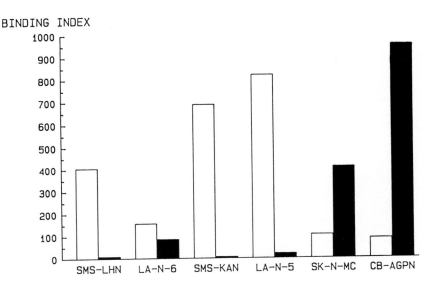

Figure 2. Measurement of cell surface antigen density by flow cytometry.

Oncogene Studies

Figure 3 (Southern analysis) shows a comparison of the N-*myc* amplified (140 copies) NGP neuroblastoma line with IA-N-6, SMS-IHN, and the non-amplified neuroblastoma line SK-N-SH. Relative intensity was quantitated by laser densitometry, which confirmed the lack of N-*myc* amplification in IA-N-6 and SMS-IHN.

On northern analysis both IA-N-6 and SMS-IHN express the same 3.2kb N-*myc* mRNA transcript as the multi-copy cell lines NLF and NGP. The relative amounts of expression are displayed in Figure 4. The intensity of expression in the non-amplified neuroblastoma lines is intermediate between that in the lymphoblastoid cell line LCL, and the amplified neuroblastoma lines.

Western analysis revealed that IA-N-6, SMS-IHN, and SK-N-

SH express a doublet molecule of approximately 62–64kd identical to that observed in the N-*myc* amplified line IA-N-5. Again, their level of expression is intermediate between the amplified neuroblastoma lines and HL-60 (promyelocytic leukemia) or Colo 320 (colon carcinoma), which express c-*myc* but not N-*myc*. Expression of the N-*myc* protein is greater in the non-amplified neuroblastoma cell lines than in the PNET cell lines CHP-100 and CB-AGPN, Figure 5.

Visualization of N-*myc* expression by immunocytology showed that as in multi-copy cell lines, N-*myc* was localized to the nucleus. Both non-amplified cell lines showed N-*myc* staining, although to a lesser extent than in amplified lines.

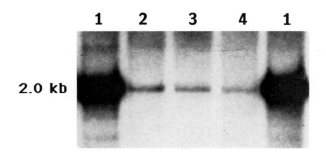

Figure 3. Southern analysis of N-*myc* copy number: lanes 1) NGP (140 copies), 2) IA-N-6, 3) SMS-IHN, 4) SK-N-SH.

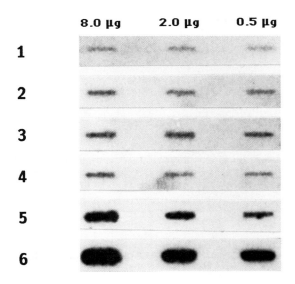

Figure 4.  Slot blot analysis of N–myc mRNA expression:    lanes
1) LCL, 2) SK–N–SH, 3) SMS–LHN, 4) LA–N–6, 5) NLF, 6) NGP.

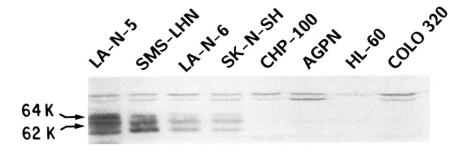

Figure 5.  Western analysis of N–myc protein expression.

DISCUSSION

IA-N-6 and SMS-IHN were established from neuroblastoma patients with typical presentations and poor clinical outcome; however, unlike most neuroblastoma cell lines, they lack amplification of N-*myc*. In this respect IA-N-6 and SMS-IHN are representative of many of advanced stage neuroblastoma patients. Cell surface antigen patterns (Reynolds *et al.*, 1988) of these lines distinguish them from PNET lines, which also do not show N-*myc* amplification. In addition, the 11;22 chromosomal translocation found in most PNET cell lines (Whang-Peng *et al.*, 1984) was absent in IA-N-6 and SMS-IHN. Relative to non-neuroblastoma lines (including PNET cell lines), these lines overexpress N-*myc* at both the mRNA and protein levels, although not to the extent seen in amplified neuroblastoma lines. Thus, their clinical histories, cell surface antigen phenotypes, karyotypes, and N-*myc* expression demonstrate that, like SK-N-SH, IA-N-6 and SMS-IHN are neuroblastoma cell lines that express N-*myc* without N-*myc* gene amplification. However, unlike SK-N-SH, the growth rates of these two cell lines *in vitro* and in nude mice are markedly slower than N-*myc* amplified cell lines.

The mechanisms of N-*myc* overexpression in neuroblastoma lines which lack genomic N-*myc* amplification have not yet been explored, but we have shown that the sizes of their mRNA and protein products are similar to those of multi-copy lines. It is possible that point mutations, alterations of control elements leading to increased message production, or decreased degradation may play a role in increasing N-*myc* protein in these cell lines.

An increase in tumor N-*myc* production may be related to aggressive behavior in neuroblastomas. Measurements of N-*myc* expression by *in situ* hybridization of tumor mRNA showed that neuroblastomas and ganglioneuroblastomas with a favorable course did not have elevation of N-*myc* expression, while those with a fatal outcome usually did, even in the absence of gene amplification (Grady-Leopardi *et al.*, 1986). This is supported by northern analyses of paired neuroblastoma cell lines, derived from the same patients at diagnosis and later at disease progression, which showed increased expression of N-*myc* in the post-chemotherapy/relapse cell lines (Rosen *et al.*, 1986). Although N-*myc* expression alone may not be sufficient to produce highly aggressive tumor behavior, it is likely to play an important role.

Induction of differentiation in neuroblastoma cells results in a down-regulation of N-*myc* that occurs within 24 hours of adding the differentiation inducer, and precedes both cell cycle arrest and neurite outgrowth (Thiele *et al.*, 1985). This suggests that if N-*myc* expression can be decreased, there may be a corresponding improvement in tumor behavior. Ultimately, understanding the mechanisms of N-*myc* expression could lead to its manipulation for therapeutic benefit. The LA-N-6 and SMS-LHN cell lines will serve as useful tools to explore this issue further.

## ACKNOWLEDGEMENTS

This study was supported in part by grants CA44904 (CPR); CA39771, CA01027, CA05587 (GMB); CA22794, CA16042 (RCS), CA09120 (RKW), from the National Cancer Institute, DHHS. LCDR Reynolds is assigned to the UCLA School of Medicine from the Navy. The views expressed in this article are those of the authors and do not reflect the official policy or position of the Department of the Navy, Department of Defense, nor the U. S. Government. We thank Dr. June Biedler for providing the SK-N-SH and SK-N-MC cell lines, and Dr. Harvey Schlesinger for providing the CHP-100 cell line.

## REFERENCES

Biedler JL, Helson L, Spengler BA (1973). Morphology and growth, tumorigenicity, and cytogenetics of human neuroblastoma cells in continuous culture. Cancer Res 33:3751-3757.

Brodeur GM, Green AA, Hayes FA, Williams KJ, Williams DL, Tsiatis AA (1981). Cytogenetic features of human neuroblastomas and cell lines. Cancer Res 41:4678-4686.

Brodeur GM, Seeger RC, Schwab M, Varmus HE, Bishop JM (1984). Amplification of N-*myc* sequences in primary human neuroblastomas. Science 224:1121-1124.

Chirgwin JM, Przybyla AE, MacDonald RJ, Rutter WJ (1979). Isolation of biologically active ribonucleic acid from sources enriched in ribonuclease. Biochemistry 18:5294.

Davis LG, Dibner MD, Batty JF (1986). "Basic Methods in Molecular Biology." New York, New York: Elsevier, pp 311-314.

Donner L, Triche TJ, Israel MA, Seeger RC, Reynolds CP (1985).

A panel of monoclonal antibodies which discriminate neuroblastoma from Ewing's sarcoma, rhabdomyosarcoma, neuroepithelioma and hematopoietic malignancies. Prog Clin Biol Res 175:347–366.

Grady-Leopardi EF, Schwab M, Albin AR, Rosenau W (1986). Detection of N-myc oncogene expression in human neuroblastoma by in situ hybridization and blot analysis: Relationship to clinical outcome. Cancer Res 46:3196–3199.

Lerach H, Diamond D, Wozney J, Boedtker H (1977). RNA molecular weight determinations by gel electrophoresis under denaturing conditions, a critical reexamination. Biochemistry 16:4743.

Merchant DJ, Kahn RH, Murphy WH (1964). "Handbook of cell and organ culture." 2nd ed. Minneapolis: Burgess.

Oste CC, Mullenbach G, Tabrizi A, Compton S (1986). The Omniblot Processing System: Optimizing Procedures for Plaque and Bacterial Colony Lifts. BioTechniques 4(4):368–375.

Parham P, Barnstable CJ, Bodmer WF (1979). Use of a monoclonal antibody (W6/32) in structural studies of HLA-A,B,C antigens. J Immunol 123:342–349.

Reynolds CP, German DC, Weinberg AG, et al. (1981). Catecholamine fluorescence and tissue culture morphology. Techniques in the diagnosis of neuroblastoma. Am J Clin Pathol 75:275–282.

Reynolds CP, Biedler JL, Spengler BA, Reynolds DA, Ross RA, Frenkel EP, Smith RG (1986). Characterization of human neuroblastoma cell lines established before and after therapy. JNCI 76:375–387.

Reynolds CP, Brodeur GM, Tomayko MM, Donner L, Helson L, Seeger RC, Triche TJ (1988). Biological classification of cell lines derived from human extra-cranial neural tumors. Prog Clin Biol Res (in press, this volume).

Rosen N, Reynolds CP, Thiele CJ, Biedler JL, Israel MA (1986). Increased N-myc expression following progressive growth of human neuroblastoma. Cancer Res 46:4139–4142.

Schlesinger HR, Gerson JM, Moorhead PS, Maguire H, Hummeler K (1976). Establishment and characterization of human neuroblastoma cell lines. Cancer Res 36:3094–3100.

Seeger RC, Danon YL, Rayner SA, Hoover F (1982). Definition of a Thy-1 determinant on human neuroblastoma, glioma, sarcoma, and teratoma cells with a monoclonal antibody. J Immunol 128:983–989.

Seeger RC, Brodeur GM, Sather H, Dalton A, Siegel SE, Wong KY, Hammond D (1985). Association of multiple copies of the N-myc oncogene with rapid progression of neuroblastomas. N Engl J Med 313:1111–1116.

Seeger RC, Reynolds CP, Moss TJ, Lenarsky C, Feig SA, Selch M, Ugelstad J, Wells J (1987). Autologous bone marrow transplantation for poor prognosis neuroblastoma. In: Dicke K, (ed): "Autologous Marrow Transplantation: Proceedings of the Third International Symposium," Gulf Printing, in press.

Slamon DJ, Boone TC, Seeger RC, Keith DE, Chazin V, Lee HC, Souza IM (1986). Identification and characterization of the protein encoded by the human N-myc oncogene. Science 232:768-772.

Smith RG and Reynolds CP (1987). Monoclonal antibody recognizing a human neuroblastoma-associated antigen. Diag Clin Immunol (in press).

Thiele CJ, Reynolds CP, Israel MA (1985). Decreased expression of N-myc precedes retinoic acid-induced morphological differentiation of human neuroblastoma. Nature 313:404-406.

Thiele CJ, McKeon C, Triche TJ, Ross RA, Reynolds CP, Israel MA (1987). Differential proto-oncogene expression characterizes histopathologically indistinguishable tumors of the peripheral nervous system. J Clin Invest, 80:804-811.

Voute PA (1984). In Sutow WW, Fernbach DJ, Vietti TJ (eds): "Clinical Pediatric Oncology," St. Louis: Mosby, p 559.

Whang-Peng J, Triche TJ, Knutsen T, Miser J, Kao-Shan S, Tsai S, Israel MA (1986). Cytogenetic characterization of selected small round cell tumors of childhood. Cancer Genet Cytogenet 21:185-208.

Advances in Neuroblastoma Research 2, pages 71–88
© 1988 Alan R. Liss, Inc.

# ANALYSIS OF A NOVEL LOCUS FREQUENTLY CO-AMPLIFIED WITH N-MYC IN HUMAN NEUROBLASTOMA

Kate T. Montgomery[*] and Peter W. Melera

Graduate Program in Molecular Biology, Memorial
Sloan-Kettering Cancer Center, N.Y, NY 10021
*Present address:  Dept. of Molecular
Pharmacology, Albert Einstein College of
Medicine, BX, NY 10461

During the past 5 years, molecular evidence has proven
unequivocally that amplification of the N-myc gene is common in human neuroblastoma cell lines, and in human neuroblastoma tumors of Stage III and Stage IV (Schwab et al.,
1983;  Kohl et al., 1983;  Brodeur et al., 1984;  Michitsch
et al., 1984;  Schwab et al., 1984a;  Seeger et al., 1985;
Brodeur and Seeger, 1986;  Brodeur et al., 1986).  Amplification occurs during tumor progression - it is not the
primary oncogenic event.  The N-myc gene is abundantly
expressed in these tumors and cell lines (Schwab et al.,
1984b;  Kohl et al., 1984), and seems to be the "target"or
core gene in the amplification unit.  However, the genomic
domain amplified in neuroblastoma is much larger than the
N-myc gene, and includes hundreds of kilobase pairs of
DNA.  This enormous size is, in fact, a characteristic of
all amplification units, both in drug resistant cultured
cells, and in other tumor systems.  There must be some
controlling factor other than the presence of the gene
required for a selective advantage, that dictates the size
of amplification units.  It seems very likely that this
factor is a mechanistic one, but we know so little about
how amplification occurs that we cannot easily understand
what this mechanistic requirement might be.  A logical
possibility suggested by Heintz et al., 1983 and based on
their observation that DNA synthesis for each amplicon
initiates in the same region, is that the initial amplified
unit is the equivalent of a normal replicon.  However, this
is not very helpful, since the characteristics of a normal
replicon are still undefined.

Recently, Looney and Hamlin (1987) report the cloning of 2 amplicons from Methotrexate resistant CHO cells. In these amplicons, the DHFR gene is located near one end of the amplified domain, not in the center. So the active gene does not necessarily occupy a central location in the amplicon. In this paper, we describe a locus frequently co-amplified with N-myc in human neuroblasoma tumors and cell lines which we believe may play a mechanistic role in gene amplification. We present our observations of the amplification of this locus, and propose models for how amplification might occur based on these observations.

We began our characterization of the amplified domain in human neuroblastoma by kinetic purification of a fraction of genomic DNA highly enriched for sequences present from 10 to 300 times within the genome of the neuroblastoma cell line BE(2)-C, which exhibited cytological evidence (HSRs) for amplified DNA sequences (Biedler and Spengler, 1976). We believed that this heterogeneous set of genomic DNA sequences should contain the sequences that encoded genes critical to the maintainance of the neuroblastoma phenotype, as well as sequences co-amplified with these hypothetical genes. We found that when the heterogeneous probe was radioactively labeled, it hybridized specifically with a complex series of fragments in BE(2)-C DNA (Figure 1, lane 1). The complex set of hybridizing fragments was not seen in normal human DNA (lane 4), nor in DNA from non-neuroblastoma tumor cell lines (Montgomery et al., 1983). However, the BE(2)-C derived probe cross-hybridized with a similar set of fragments in DNA isolated from the vast majority of neuroblastoma cell lines (Montgomery et al., 1983), each independently derived from different patients, and with fragments amplified in the one tumor DNA analysed (lane 5 and Montgomery, 1986). We concluded that the visible bands represent ECO RI fragments amplified only in neuroblastoma cells, though present in all DNAs. Later experiments using individually isolated amplified fragments to probe similar filters support this conclusion. The fragments are present at single copy levels in unamplified DNA. The fact that these studies showed for the first time that similar fragments are amplified in different cell lines and patients, led us to propose that the sequences co-amplified with whatever expressed genes are present are not randomly selected, but probably consist largely of sequences flanking the critical gene(s) prior to amplification (Montgomery et al., 1983).

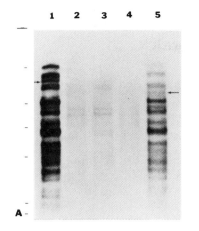 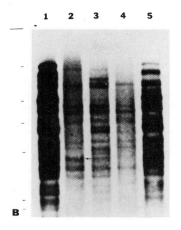

Figure 1. Preparation of genomic DNA from cell lines and
tissues, restriction enzyme digestion protocols, gel electrophoresis, transfer to nitrocellulose, and hybridization
techniques have been described (Montgomery et al., 1983).
The probe for this experiment was the heterogeneous set of
DNA sequences repeated from 10 to 300 times in DNA from the
cell line BE(2)-C, purified essentially as described by
Brison et al. (1982), and labeled by nick translation. For
the gel, 20ug of each DNA was digested with ECO RI and electrophoresed. Lane 1: BE(2)-C; lane 2: IMR-32; lane 3:
Y-79 (retinoblastoma); lane 4: human placenta; lane 5:
NOS-JJI (neuroblastoma tumor DNA provided by R. Seeger).
Panel B is a darker exposure of Panel A.


This has since been proven by chromosomal in situ hybridization studies using amplified fragments for probes, by
Southern analysis of human/rodent somatic cell hybrid DNAs
in several labs (Kanda et al., 1983; Schwab et al.,
1984b; Shiloh et al., 1985), and by gel renaturation
studies (Kinzler et al., 1986).

Clearly, the kinetically purified genomic fraction
represented a probe which could be used to screen a
neuroblastoma cDNA library made from poly (A+) RNA from the
BE(2)-C cell line, and to identify amplified sequences
expressed in neuroblastoma cells. We did this and identified a number of related cDNA clones which hybridized with

an abundant message in amplification positive cells
(Michitsch et al., 1984). This gene is now known as N-myc
(Schwab et al., 1983; Kohl et al., 1983; Melera et al.,
1985).

The locus which we describe in this paper was
identified through a clone, pBE(2)-C-77, obtained from the
cDNA library as described above. This clone, p77, provides
an interesting and novel view of the amplified domain
because it exhibits different characteristics of hybridization with neuroblastoma DNAs from the probes described
by others (Kanda et al., 1983; Kohl et al., 1984; Shiloh
et al., 1986). When p77 was used to probe a Southern
transfer of ECO RI digested genomic DNAs isolated from
neuroblastoma BE(2)-C and from placenta, it hybridized with
a 19.5kb ECO RI fragment clearly amplified in BE(2)-C, and
also present at single copy level in placenta (Figure 2).

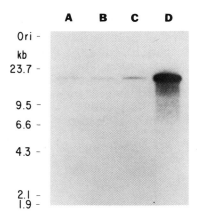

Figure 2. DNAs were digested with ECO RI. Lane A: 10ug
human placental DNA; lane B: 0.05ug BE(2)-C DNA; lane
C: 0.1ug BE(2)-C DNA; lane D: 1ug BE(2)-C DNA. The size
markers were lambda DNA digested with HIND III.

In screening 8,000 cDNA clones, only one of the p77
type was isolated, while 6 of the N-myc (pBE(2)-C-59 or
p59) type clones were found. Furthermore, despite the fact

that p77 was isolated from a cDNA library and is clearly
derived from an amplified DNA fragment, Northern analysis
has not revealed an RNA molecule corresponding to it. We
determined the sequence of the 1200bp insert in p77, and
found no open reading frame and no homology with any
sequence reported in the Genbank database (Montgomery,
1986). Based on these observations, it is reasonable to
suggest that p77 does not represent the transcript of a
true Pol II gene amplified in these cells. It is certainly
clear that the p77 sequence is not over-expressed in
neuroblastoma cells, as would most likely be the case if it
were an amplified gene, and so elevated expression of this
gene plays no role in the neuroblastoma phenotype.

It is possible that p77 is simply a piece of amplified
DNA we cloned inadvertantly. If so, this probe is analogous to "probe 8" (Kanda et al., 1983), and other cloned
genomic fragments described elsewhere, and it may be of use
in continuing to define the amplified domain in neuroblastoma cells. A more interesting thought is that p77 may
represent some other kind of RNA molecule transcribed from
the amplified region, with an as yet unidentified role.
Of particular significance here is the fact that the hetero-
eneous genomic probe used to find this clone is uniquely
capable of identifying any transcript from the amplified
domain, even if it were extremely rare. No other cDNA
screening method would be likely to have picked up such a
clone, so it is entirely possible we have identified a
unique type of molecule. We report here the results of a
number of studies using this probe for the amplified domain
in human neuroblastoma cells.


RESULTS

Chromosomal Localization and Derivation of p77.

In situ hybridizations using our cDNA clone for the 3'
end of N-myc (p59) or using p77 showed that both hybridize
specifically to the HSR in a clonal derivative of the cell
line, SK-N-BE(2), BE(2)m17 (Figure 3). Furthermore, a
panel of DNAs from human/rodent somatic cell hybrids were
screened with p77, and it was found that like N-myc, this
sequence is located on choromosome 2p in normal cells
(Barker, Montgomery, Melera and Ruddle, unpublished
observations).

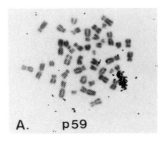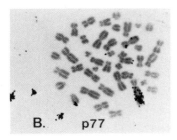

Figure 3. Chromosome preparations from a clonal derivative of the neuroblastoma cell line BE(2) known as BE(2)m17 were hybridized in situ with $^3$H-labeled clones p59 (left panel) and p77 (right panel). Grains were clustered over the long HSR seen in this cell line in both cases. (Hybridization done by B. Spengler in J.L. Biedler's laboratory, protocol previously described in Montgomery et al., 1983).

Frequency of Amplification:

To determine the frequency of p77 amplification in neuroblastoma tumors and cell lines, we probed Southern blots of a number of DNAs with the three different probes used in our studies. Table 1 summarizes the results. The first column lists the neuroblastoma cell lines or tumors we have analysed, column 2 shows whether or not we saw the complex banding pattern with kinetically purified genomic probes from amplified cell lines, column 3 shows whether or not N-myc (p59) was amplified, and column 4 shows whether p77 was amplified. When the heterogeneous amplified probe gave positive results, p59 also did, in every case. Thus, whenever N-myc is amplified, a similar (but not identical) set of cross-hybridizing fragments are also amplified. p77 however, was NOT co-amplified with p59 in every case, and it was never amplified independently of p59. Thus, like a number of other probes for the amplified domain which have been described, p77 is amplified in a subset of neuro-blastoma tumors and cell lines. It should be pointed out that p77 is not amplified in IMR-32, from which most of the other probes have been isolated, so this probe clearly is derived from a different area of the potentially amplifi-able region in neuroblastoma cells and tumors.

TABLE 1. Summary of Results of Southern Hybridizations with Neuroblastoma Amplified Sequence Probes and p59 and p77

| Cell Line[e]/Tissue | Amp. Probe | p59 | p77 |
|---|---|---|---|
| SK-N-BE(1) | + | + | ?[a] |
| BE(2)-C | + | + | + |
| NAP(D) | + | + | + |
| CHP-234 | + | + | + |
| KAN | + | + | + |
| KAN | + | + | + |
| KCN | + | + | - |
| KCNR | ND | + | - |
| SK-N-MC | - | - | - |
| MCIX-C | - | - | - |
| SH-SY5Y | - | ?[a] | ?[a] |
| SMS-MSN | + | + | + |
| IMR-32 | + | + | - |
| Y-79 | + | + | - |
| LA-N-1 | ND | + | + |
| NGP | ND | + | - |
| NMB | ND | + | - |
| NOS-JJI[b] | + | + | + |
| NOS-ZZ2[b] | - | - | - |
| NOS-S2[b] | - | - | - |
| NOS-M8[b] | - | - | - |
| 371-H21[c] | - | - | - |
| 82-79-04[c] | - | - | - |
| #4, 8, 35, 43, 50, 52[d] | ND | + | + |
| #33[d] | ND | + | ?[a] |
| #2, 5, 6, 7, 9, 10, 11, 15, 16, 17, 21, 28, 38, 39, 41[d] | ND | - | - |

ND : Not done
a : Results not definitive
b : Tumor sample provided by R. Seeger, Children's Cancer Study Group
c : Tumor sample provided by Tumor Procurement Service, Memorial Sloan Kettering Cancer Center
d : Tumor DNAs provided by G. Brodeur, and described in Brodeur et al., 1984
e : Neuroblastoma cell lines used in these studies were provided by J.L. Biedler, and have been described elsewhere (Biedler et al., 1983).

One thing in particular is interesting about these results: p77 is amplified in only 7 of 14 cell lines studied (50%), whereas it is amplified in 7 of 8 (87.5%), or perhaps in all 8 (100%), of the tumors which amplify N-myc. Our sample size is small, but p77's more consistant amplification in tumors than in cell lines is unique. In contrast, probe 8 was reported by Shiloh et al. (1986) to be amplified in 8 of 11 cell lines (73%) and in 14 of 25 tumors (56%) which amplify N-myc, while G21 is amplified in 9 of 11 cell lines (82%) and 16 of 25 tumors (64%). While the cell lines we analysed differed from those reported by Shiloh and co-workers, our tumor DNAs were largely the same, provided to us by G. Brodeur. Thus it seems that p77 may exhibit a truly distinct amplification frequency from probes 8 and G21.

## Gene Copy Number of the p77 Locus Relative to N-myc

A series of "dot blots" were done to compare the gene copy number of the N-myc locus and the p77 locus in several cell lines and in the tumor DNA designated NOS-JJI. The results of these experiments are shown in Table 2.

TABLE 2. Gene Copy Number of p59 and p77 in a Variety of Neuroblastoma DNAs, By Dot Blot Analysis[a]

| Cell Line/Tissue | p59 | p77 |
|---|---|---|
| Placenta | 1 | 1 |
| SH-SY5Y | 1-1.5 | 1-1.5 |
| BE(2)-C | 133 | 200 |
| SK-N-BE(1) | 23.5 | 1-2 |
| CHP-234 | 98 | 195 |
| NAP(D) | 60 | 91 |
| NAP(H) | 64 | 110 |
| NOS-JJI | 66 | 59 |
| KAN | 117 | 348 |
| KANR | 26 | 39 |
| KCN | 66 | 1 |
| IMR-32 | 18 | 1 |
| SMS-MSN | 21 | 34 |
| Y-79 (retinoblastoma) | 18 | 1 |

[a]. DNA was denatured in NaOH (.3M NaOH, 6X SSC), heated to 80°C for 10 minutes, and applied to nitrocellulose in a 96 well dot blot apparatus (Schleicher and Schuell). Filters were baked at 80°C under vacuum, and hybridized with radioactive probes by standard techniques (Montgomery et al., 1983). Following exposure to X-ray film, dots were cut out and bound radioactivity was counted in scintillation fluor. A placental standard was included in each experiment to normalize for single copy, and background counts subtracted from each sample.

The data confirm our observation that p77 is not amplified with N-myc (p59) in every case - for example, in IMR-32 and in the retinoblastoma line, Y-79. Interestingly, the gene copy number of p77 is from 1.5 to 3 times higher than that of p59 in every cell line tested where they are clearly both amplified. The consistant over-amplification of this locus is surprising, since it does not seem to encode a gene product which might be selected for, and it is clearly not necessary for the neuroblastoma phenotype or for progression of the tumor. Probes 8 and G21 have varied in their level of amplification relative to N-myc. There are two logical explanations for the consistant over ampli-fication of the p77 locus. Either the presence of the N-myc gene within the amplification unit of these cell lines becomes detrimental to cell growth and cells where N-myc has been excised from some amplicons are selected for, or there is a mechanistic reason for the p77 locus to be replicated more frequently than N-myc. Current data does not allow us to choose between these possibilities, or to be certain there is not some other explanation. In con-trast to the cell line data, the level of amplification of N-myc in the tumor sample, NOS-JJI, does not differ from that of p77. Possibly this is due to the many fewer cell divisions which have occurred in vivo in this tumor, than in the cell lines grown in culture for years. Then, what-ever conditions favor the exclusion of N-myc from some amplicons or, alternatively, enhance the re-replication of the p77 locus, are largely inoperative. We have not been able to measure the relative levels of amplification of p59 and p77 in other tumor samples, so cannot draw further conclusions.

## Rearrangement of the p77 Locus Occurs in 2 Cases

As shown in Figure 4, the p77 probe hybridizes with unique novel ECO RI fragments in two cases. In each case, the unique fragment is amplified as well as the normal 19.5kb fragment. When other restriction enzymes were used, novel fragments were still observed, so the extra bands don't simply reflect point mutations resulting in new ECO RI sites in some amplicons. Since one of the rearrange-ments occurs in a tumor DNA, we must assume it is not the result of excessive genomic plasticity related to long term culture in vitro.

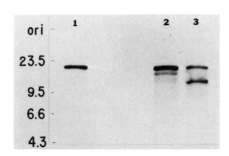

Figure 4. Each lane contains 2ug of DNA digested with ECO RI. Lane 1: BE(2)-C DNA; lane 2: CHP-234 DNA; lane 3: NOS-JJI DNA.

To further characterize these rearrangements, we went back to the genome of the cell line from which p77 was derived, BE(2)-C, and cloned approximately 35kb of genomic flanking region. Using portions of these larger clones, we derived a restriction map for the "normal" locus and localized the breakpoints in the rearranged DNAs. The respective maps are shown in Figure 5.

The mapping studies reveal that the breakpoints lie on either side of the p77 fragment, and the divergent sequences extend in either direction away from p77. This suggests that this locus may have a tendency to recombine in a rather complex way. In these two cases, this recombination event must have taken place early in the course of amplification, since the novel amplicon as well as the normal one continued to amplify following recombination. At this point, we can only hypothesize about the exact mechanism of recombination. However, we have identified novel PST I fragments in both CHP-234 and in NOS-JJI which span the breakpoints. The first step in continuing to characterize these rearrangements will be to clone these fragments, and using them, determine the origin of the divergent sequences. Are they derived from the amplified domain as well? Are they related, or do the sequences linked with the p77 locus in CHP-234 differ from those linked in NOS-JJI? These questions should be relatively easy to answer.

THE 77 LOCUS

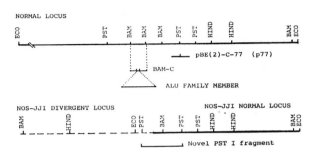

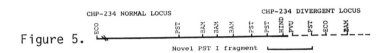

Figure 5.

In the course of our study of the p77 locus in BE(2)-C, we found that it includes an ALU family member. The complete "BAM C" fragment shown in Figure 5 was sequenced. The sequence of the ALU family member which lies within it is shown in Figure 6.

```
BAM C ALU:       aGCcaGtCaa GGTGGCTCAt g CTGTAATC tgAGCACTTT
ALU CONSENSUS:   GGCTGGGCGT GGTGGCTCAC ACCTGTAATC CCAGCACTTT

                 tGGAGGCCGA GGcaaGTGGA TCACCTGAGa TCAGGAGTTC
                 GGGAGGCCGA GGTGGGTGGA TCACCTGAGG TCAGGAGTTC

                 AAGACCAGCC TGGCCAAaAg aaTGAAACCt tGTCcCTACT
                 AAGACCAGCC TGGCCAACAT GGTGAAACCC CGTCTCTACT

                 AAAAgTACAA AAAATTAaCCG GatGcaGTGG CaCGtGCCTG
                 AAAAATACAA AAAATTAGCCG GGCGTGGTGG CGCGCGCCTG

                 TAgTCCCAGC TACTCaGGAG GCTGAGGCAG GAGgATtGCT
                 TAATCCCAGC TACTCGGGAG GCTGAGGCAG GAGAATCGCT

                 TGAACCCtGG AGGctGAGGT TGCAGTGAGC tgAGATCaat
                 TGAACCCAGG AGGTGGAGGT TGCAGTGAGC CGAGATCGCG

                 gtgACTGCAC TCCAGCCTGG GtgACgGAGC aAGACTCtgT
                 CC ACTGCAC TCCAGCCTGG GCAACAGAGC GAGACTCCAT

                 gTCcAAAAAA AAAAAgAAA gAAAA
                 CTCAAAAAAA AAAAAAAAAA AAAAA
```

Small letters in the BAM C ALU sequence denote divergence from the consensus sequence.

Figure 6.

BAM-C ALU is 84% homologous to the consensus ALU sequence (Jelinek and Schmid, 1982) and 75% homologous to the BLUR 8 sequence. Since ALU sequences have been implicated in a variety of recombination events (Jagadeeswaren et al., 1982; Ottolenghi and Giglioni, 1982; Lehrman et al., 1985; Lehrman et al., 1986; and Nicholls et al., 1987), it seemed possible that the presence of this sequence was related to the recombination we observe. However, as can be seen in Figure 5, the breakpoints lie beyond the ALU sequence in both cases, and the ALU sequence is not directly involved in the rearrangement in either case.

## DISCUSSION

We have proposed two models to explain the selection of sequences to be amplified with N-myc in human neuroblastoma (Montgomery, 1986). These models (Figue 7) are based on concepts of gene amplification described by Schimke (1982) and reviewed by Stark and Wahl, 1984 and Hamlin et al., 1984. They presume that the initial event of amplification occurs when one origin of replication fires asynchronously, resulting in the unscheduled replication of a portion of the genome. If this over-replication results in a proliferative advantage for a sub-population of cells, further unscheduled replication of the region will be selected for, and a population of cells containing many copies of this region of the genome may arise. The models also presume that an amplicon is equivalent to a replicon, as suggested by Heintz et al., 1983. It is likely that the amplified sequences pass through an extrachromosomal phase, since they ultimately may be found in extrachromosomal double minute chromosomes, or integrated into an apparently random assortment of expanded chromosomal loci (Biedler et al. 1983).

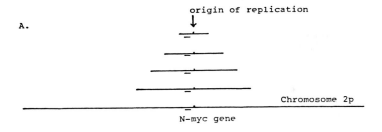

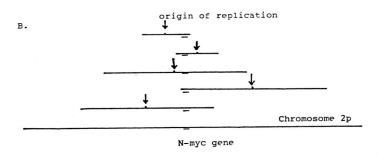

Figure 7. In each model, the bottom line represents a portion of chromosome 2p. Each of the other lines represents the amplified domain in one neuroblastoma cell line or tumor. The core of each domain is proposed to be the activated origin of replication, and the N-myc gene is included in each case.


In Model A, the amplified sequences in every tumor are nested around a central core sequence, which represents the origin of replication involved in the replication of the single gene critical to the progressive neuroblastoma phenotype, N-myc. This suggests a fixed origin of repli- cation for the N-myc-containing replicon/amplicon. In this model, the variation observed in amplified sequences inclu- ded in various cell lines and tumors reported by us and others might simply reflect the distance traversed by the replication forks when this region first undergoes un- scheduled replication, unless some unusual recombination event occurs as has been suggested for IMR-32 (Shiloh et al., 1985; Latt et al., 1986).

Model B postulates a variety of origins of replication, implying the potential activation of different origins of replication in different tumors. This model permits a much greater diversity of sequences in the amplification unit, since the bulk of the sequences included could extend in either direction from the N-myc gene.

Support for Model B is derived from our use of kinetically purified heterogeneous probes enriched in amplified sequences from different cell lines. As demonstrated in Figure 1, the BE(2)-C probe contains many sequences homologous to the amplified sequences in both BE(2)-C and in NOS-JJI, but only a few which are also amplified in IMR-32 (lane 2) or in the retinoblastoma cell line Y-79 (lane 3), though N-myc is amplified in each case. The darker exposure in panel B shows that the differences are not merely a reflection of lower copy number. Other cell lines and probes show different degrees of cross-hybridization (Montgomery, 1986).

We believe our data on the 77 locus can be interpreted in the context of Model B, and can be used to extend this model. These interpretations are hypothetical, but they suggest some interesting future experiments, and are therefore useful. The observations are summarized below.

1. The 77 locus is amplified in 7 of 8 tumor DNAs which amplify N-myc, and it may also be amplified in DNA #33. (Table 1)
2. The 77 locus is amplified in only 50% (7 of 14) of the cell line DNAs studied. (Table 1)
3. The 77 locus is present in higher copy number than N-myc in every cell line where they are co-amplified. (Table 2)
4. Rearrangements occur near to the p77 sequence in at least 2 cases, but the novel sequences extend in opposite directions from p77. (Figure 5)
5. p77 was isolated from a cDNA library screened with a unique type of probe consisting of amplified sequences. It would not have been identified by +/- cDNA screening since the transcript is exceedingly rare, and not elevated in neuroblastoma so far as we can determine.

We make the following hypothetical proposals to extend Model B, based on this data: 1) There are several potential origins of replication which may fire to initiate unscheduled DNA replication of the N-myc region; 2) The 77 locus is closely linked to an origin of replication active in 50% of the neuroblastomas amplifying N-myc; 3) The 77 locus lies fairly close to N-myc, so that is always/almost always included in the initial amplification unit, and it is amplified with N-myc in most/all tumors; 4) Any time an origin of replication is activated on the other side of N-myc from p77, the 77 locus may be excluded from the unit, either initially or during long term culture because there is no selective pressure to maintain this non-functional element in the amplicon; 5) If the origin near to the 77 locus is active in the amplification, this locus may become more highly amplified than N-myc, due to repeated firings of the origin followed by recombinations which do not include the entire unit. Thus, the representation of any given sequence within the amplified domain of a tumor or cell line depends, in this model, upon its location both relative to N-myc and relative to the origin of replication which initiates the amplification. In at least two cases as described here, one might hypothesize that the replication forks did not extend very far out from the p77 "origin", and the newly replicated DNA strands recombined to create the novel amplicons we have observed. The model is hypothetical, but fits our data so far, seems to fit that of other labs as far as we can tell, and suggests a number of experiments to test it.

A further interesting possibility relates to the origin of the p77 clone. Since we find no evidence that it represents the transcript of a normal Pol II gene, perhaps it is an RNA molecule of the sort which has been postulated to be involved in priming of DNA replication (Kornberg, 1980). Our cDNA library probe was uniquely appropriate for identifying a clone derived from such a molecule. Clearly, this genomic region may be useful for further efforts at characterizing the mechanisms for amplification in human neuroblastoma. We believe the data reported here support the possibility that the 77 locus may play an important mechanistic role in the amplification of N-myc in human neuroblastoma. In addition, this region may be useful for studies of normal eukaryotic DNA replication.

ACKNOWLEDGEMENTS

This work was supported in part by grants from NIH to Sloan-Kettering Institute for Cancer Research and from the Special Projects Committee of the Society of the Memorial Sloan-Kettering Cancer Center, the Milton Schamach Foundation, and the Jeanette Warren Davison Fund for Cancer Research to P.W.M.

REFERENCES

Biedler JL, Meyers MB, Spengler BA (1983). Homogeneously staining regions and double minute chromosomes, prevalent cytogenetic abnormalities of human neuroblastoma cells. Adv Cell Neurobiol 4:267-307.
Biedler JL, Spengler BA (1976). Metaphase chromosome anomaly: association with drug resistance and cell-specific products. Science 191:185-187.
Brison O, Ardeshir F, Stark GR (1982). General method for cloning amplified DNA by differential screening with genomic probes. Mol Cell Biol 2:578-587.
Brodeur GM and Seeger RC (1986). Gene amplification in human neuroblastomas: basic mechanisms and clinical implications. Cancer Genet Cytogenet 19:101-111.
Brodeur GM, Seeger RC, Sather H, Dalton A, Siegel SE, Wong KY, Hammond D (1986). Clinical implications of oncogene activation in human neuroblastomas. Cancer 58:541-545.
Brodeur GM, Seeger RC, Schwab M, Varmus HE, Bishop JM (1984). Amplification of N-myc in untreated human neuroblastomas correlates with advanced stage disease. Science 223:1121-1124.
Hamlin JL, Milbrandt JD, Heintz NH, Azizkhan JC (1984). DNA sequence amplification in mammalian cells. Int Rev Cytol 90:31-82.
Heintz NH, Milbrandt JD, Greisen KS, Hamlin JL (1983). Cloning of the initiation region of a mammalian chromosomal replicon. Nature 302:439-441.
Jagadeeswaran P, Tuan D, Forget BG, Weissman SM (1982). A gene deletion ending at the midpoint of a repetitive DNA sequence in one form of hereditary persistance of fetal haemoglobin. Nature 296:469-470.
Jelinek WR, Schmid CW (1982). Repetitive sequences in eukaryotic DNA and their expression. Ann Rev Biochem 51:813-844.

Kanda N, Schreck R, Alt F, Bruns G, Baltimore D, Latt S (1983). Isolation of amplified DNA sequences from IMR-32 human neuroblastoma cells: facilitation by fluorescence-activated flow sorting of metaphase chromosomes. Proc Natl Acad Sci USA 80:4069-4073.

Kinzler KW, Zehnbauer BA, Brodeur GM, Seeger RC, Trent JM, Meltzer PS, Vogelstein B (1986). Amplification units containing N-myc and C-myc genes. Proc Natl Acad Sci USA 83:1031-1035.

Kohl NE, Gee CE, Alt FW (1984). Activated expression of the N-myc gene in human neuroblastomas and related tumors. Science 226:1335-1337.

Kohl NE, Kanda N, Schreck RR, Bruns G, Latt SA, Gilbert F, Alt FW (1983). Transposition and amplification of oncogene-related sequences in human neuroblastomas. Cell 35:359-367.

Kornberg A (1980). "DNA Replication." San Francisco: W.H. Freeman and Company, pp367-368.

Lehrman MA, Schneider WJ, Sudhof TC, Brown MS, Goldstein JL, Russell DW (1985). Mutation in LSL receptor: Alu-Alu recombination deletes exons encoding transmembrane and cytoplasmic domains. Science 227:140-146.

Lehrman MA, Russell DW, Goldstein JL, Brown MS (1986). Exon-Alu recombination deletes 5 kilobases from the low density lipoprotein receptor gene, producing a null phenotype in familial hypercholesteronemia. Proc Natl Acad Sci USA 83:3679-3683.

Looney JE, Hamlin JL (1987). Isolation of the amplified dihydrofolate reductase domain from methotrexate-resistant chinese hamster ovary cells. Mol Cell Biol 7:569-577.

Melera PW, Michitsch RW, Montgomery KT, Biedler JL, Scotto KW, Davide JP (1985). Studies on the expression of the amplified domain in human neuroblastoma cells. Adv Neuroblastoma Res 3:115-129.

Michitsch RW, Montgomery KT, Melera PW (1984). Expression of the amplified domain in human neuroblastoma cells. Mol Cell Biol 4:2370-2380.

Montgomery KT (1986). Studies in gene amplification in human neuroblastoma. Ph.D. thesis presented to Cornell University Graduate School. University Microfilms International, Ann Arbor, MI.

Montgomery KT, Biedler JL, Spengler BA, Melera PW (1983). Specific DNA sequence amplification in human neuroblastoma cells. Proc Natl Acad Sci USA 80:5724-5728.

Nicholls RD, Fischel-Ghodsian N, Higgs DR (1987). Recombination at the human alpha-globin gene cluster: sequence features and topological constraints. Cell 49:369-378.

Ottolenghi S, Giglioni B (1982). The deletion in a type of delta$^O$-beta$^O$ thalassemia begins in an inverted Alu I repeat. Nature 300:770-771.

Schimke RT (1982). "Gene Amplification" Cold Spring Harbor, Cold Spring Harbor Laboratory, pp317-333.

Schwab M, Alitalo K, Klempnauer KH, Varmus HE, Bishop JM, Gilbert F, Brodeur G, Goldstein M, Trent JM (1983). Amplified DNA with limited homology to myc cellular oncogene is shared by human neuroblastoma cell lines and a neuroblastoma tumour. Nature 305:245-248.

Schwab M, Ellison J, Busch M, Rosenau W, Varmus HE, Bishop JM (1984a). Enhanced expression of the human gene N-myc consequent to amplification of DNA may contribute to malignant progression of neuroblastoma. Proc Natl AcadSci USA 81:4940-4944.

Schwab M, Varmus HE, Bishop JM, Grzeschik K-H, Naylor SL, Sakaguchi AY, Brodeur G, Trent J (1984b). Chromosome localization in normal human cells and neuroblastomas of a gene related to c-myc. Nature 308:288-291.

Seeger RC, Brodeur GM, Sather H, Dalton A, Siegel SE, Wong KY, Hammond D (1985). Association of multiple copies of the N-myc oncogene with rapid progression of neuroblastomas. N Engl J Med 313:1111-1116.

Shiloh Y, Korf B, Kohl NE, Sakai K, Brodeur GM, Harris P, Kanda N, Seeger RC, Alt F, Latt SA (1986). Amplification and rearrangement of DNA sequences from the chromosomal region 2p24 in human neuroblastomas. Cancer Res 46:5297-5301.

Shiloh Y, Shipley J, Brodeur GM, Bruns G, Korf B, Donlon T, Schreck RR, Seeger R, Sakai K, Latt SA (1985). Differential amplification, assembly, and relocation of multiple DNA sequences in human neuroblastomas and neuroblastoma cell lines. Proc Natl Acad Sci USA 82:3761-3765.

Stark GR, Wahl GM (1984). Gene Amplification. Ann Rev Biochem 53:447-491.

Advances in Neuroblastoma Research 2, pages 89–90
© 1988 Alan R. Liss, Inc.

DISCUSSION

Chairman:       H. C. MaGuire

Discussants:    R. K. Wada, K. T. Montgomery

Dr. Frantz (Rochester) asked Dr. Wada how the cell lines he described were started and grown. The cell line LANG was started by Dr. Lee. It was obtained from bone marrow infiltrated by tumor and purified by a technique developed by Dr. Seeger and Dr. Wells. The marrow is purified by differential centrifugation and filtration and then purged with magnetic immunobeads. One of the centrifugation steps results in a pellet which has greater than 95% tumor cells. It was grown in L-15 medium. The cell line LHN was isolated from a primary tumor after multiple courses of chemotherapy and initially was grown in RPM1 1640 and 10% serum, then carried in L-15 medium.

Dr. Mary C. Glick (Philadelphia) commented to Dr. Lipinski that she and Dr. Fred Troy showed that neuroblastoma cells contain NCAM and polysialics and that NBL cells in the marrow also contained many polysials in Ewing's. Dr. Lipinski replied that they did not find polysial acids on Ewing's tumors and didn't know about neuroblastomas. She also asked if their antibodies were to NCAM itself or to the polysialic acids. Dr. Lipinski replied that they used several antibodies including a rabbit polyclonal and mouse monoclonal against NCAM and got similar results.

Dr. Frantz then asked what the known function of NCAM was and why it might be suspected of playing a role in oncogenesis. He also asked what the difference was between the 120kd and 180kd species in terms of function. Dr. Lipinski replied, quoting the work of Dr. Joseph Edelman of New York, that the NCAM molecule is involved in recognition between neural cells and between neural and other cells. The degree of glycosylation might play a role in metastatic behavior in that during development the level of sialation changes tremendously and these changes are correlated with the migration properties of the cells. An hypothesis would be that the type of NCAM expressed could determine the type of metastatic behavior, although there is no strong evidence for this. Dr. Frantz asked whether both forms of NCAM were from same NCAM gene. Dr. Lipinski said all forms, the 120,

140 and 180kd were all from the NCAM gene. The 120kd is peculiar in that it has no transmembrane portion and is believed to be very easily cleaved.

Dr. Littauer (Weizman) asked if there was any difference in the phosphoinositol linkage between Ewings cells and normal cells. Dr. Lipinski said they hadn't looked.

Dr. Cohen (NCI) asked Dr. Wada what the status of c-MYC expression in his two cell lines was. He said it had not been looked at. Dr. Thiele (NCI) said that LHN did express c-MYC similar to PNETs. Dr. Brodeur asked how this compared to SKNSH for instance. Dr. Thiele said it was similar to SKNSH but elevated over neuroblastomas where it is not expressed.

Dr. Kemshead (London) to Dr. Lipinski: He agreed with the immunostaining but not with the interpretation because with the same antibodies and immunostaining one can get similar results with rhabdomyosarcomas and Wilms' tumors so one can't use it as a criteria for PNETs. Dr. Lipinski replied that one also finds positive staining of rhabdomyosarcomas or Wilms' tumors with other cell surface antibodies that are absent in Ewing's (and PNETs). Also the karyotypic change, the t11, 22, is very specific to both Ewings and PNET. Kemshead agreed with the cytogenetic argument but felt it was a difficult matter to say that similar antigen profiles equated with similar cell origins.

Dr. M.B. Meyers (Memorial Sloan Kettering) to Dr. Montgomery: Is your speculation about the position of 77 based on data such as homology to known origins or replications? Dr. Montgomery replied, "no", that there are no known origins identified in eukaryotic cells and that this is purely speculative based on the relative amplification of 77 compared with N-myc.

Dr. Frantz (Rochester) asked if there were any changes of N-myc with cell cycle or differentiation. Dr. Wada (California) said he hadn't done such experiments. Dr. Reynolds commented that γHN is the only neuroblastoma so far which responded to retinoic acid by complete growth inhibition with differentiation to viable mature cells, even 14 weeks after removal of retinoic acid. Molecular studies had not yet been done.

Advances in Neuroblastoma Research 2, pages 91–101
© 1988 Alan R. Liss, Inc.

# N-*myc* PROTEIN EXPRESSION BY NEUROBLASTOMA CELLS THAT HAVE METASTASIZED TO BONE MARROW

Thomas J. Moss, Yuk M. Law, Dennis J. Slamon, Garrett M. Brodeur, Robert C. Seeger.

Departments of Pediatrics (TJM, YML, RCS) and Medicine (DJS) and the Jonsson Comprehensive Cancer Center, UCLA School of Medicine, Los Angeles, CA 90024; Departments of Pediatrics and Genetics (GMB), Washington Univ. School of Medicine, St. Louis, MO 63110; Children's Cancer Study Group, Pasadena, CA 91101.

## INTRODUCTION

The N-*myc* gene, when amplified in neuroblastomas, is associated with advanced stage of disease at diagnosis (Brodeur et al., 1984) and with a poor prognosis (Seeger et al., 1985). Immunohistologic and immunochemical analyses of primary neuroblastomas with an antiserum specific for the N-*myc* protein have shown that those tumors with genomic amplification overexpress it and that some non-amplified ones also do so (Seeger et al., 1988).

For patients with stage IV disease, bone marrow is a ready source of tumor cells at diagnosis, during therapy, and at relapse. Analysis of N-*myc* gene copy number and expression could provide prognostic information and therapeutic response data. We previously demonstrated that bone marrow metastases from approximately 30% of patients have genomic amplification of N-*myc* at diagnosis (Lee et al., 1986). The purpose of this study was to develop immunocytology for assessing expression of N-*myc* by bone marrow metastases. We found that staining with anti-N-*myc* serum alone is sufficient to assess expression when tumor cell clusters or more than 10% tumor cells are present; however, if fewer tumor cells are present, it is advantageous to identify them by immunostaining with monoclonal antibodies against neuroblastoma cell surface antigens.

## MATERIALS AND METHODS

*Cell lines and bone marrow specimens.* Four cell lines (LA-N-1, LA-N-2, LA-N-5, and SMS-KAN), which have amplification of the N-*myc* gene (Reynolds et al., 1988), were used to develop immunocytologic analysis of N-*myc* protein expression. These cell lines were maintained in Leibovitz's L15 medium supplemented with 15% fetal calf serum, gentamicin and glutamine (L15-FCS) at 37° C. Cells were detached with 0.1 mM EDTA in phosphate buffered saline (PBS), washed twice with L15, and then resuspended in L15-FCS.

Bone marrow from patients with neuroblastoma was aspirated, anticoagulated (heparin, 100 units/ml), and sent to us immediately from cooperating institutions. Upon receipt (approximately 24 hrs after aspiration), samples were diluted with Hank's Balanced salt solution (HBSS) containing 2% FCS, and mononuclear cells were isolated by equilibrium density centrifugation. Twice washed mononuclear cells were resuspended in L15-FCS.

*Antibodies.* Rabbit antisera against the N-*myc* protein were made using proteins produced by bacteria expressing fragments of cloned N-*myc* cDNA, and the N-*myc* specific serum, anti-bGH/N-*myc* II, was used in these experiments (Slamon et al., 1986). Four monoclonal antibodies (459, HSAN 1.2, 390, and 126-4) were used to immunostain cell surface antigens. Their production and specificity have been described previously (Rosenblatt et al., 1982; Seeger, et al., 1982; Schulz et al., 1984; Smith and Reynolds, 1987).

*Immunoperoxidase staining.* For immunostaining only N-*myc* protein, cells in L15-FCS were cytocentrifuged onto coverslips; for combined immunostaining of N-*myc* protein and cell surface antigens, they were incubated with a mixture of monoclonal antibodies 390, 459, HSAN1.2, 126-4, (20 mcg/ml of each antibody for $10^6$ cells; room temperature; 30 min), washed once with L15-2% FCS, and then cytocentrifuged onto coverslips. Cells on coverslips were fixed with 2% paraformaldehyde in PBS (4 °C, pH 6.5 for 10 min followed by pH 11.0 for 10 min) and then absolute methanol (4 °C, 15 min). This was followed by incubation for 1 hr at 37 °C in PBS supplemented with 10% horse serum, 10% goat serum, and 2% bovine serum albumin to block non-specific protein and immunoglobulin binding. Anti-N-*myc* serum (1:4000 dilution in PBS-2% goat serum) was applied to coverslips overnight at room temperature in a moist chamber. The next day, biotinylated secondary antibodies (Vector Laboratories) were applied to coverslips: 1) goat anti-rabbit serum (1:300 dilution, one hr) when staining only N-*myc*; 2) goat anti-rabbit serum followed by 45 min with a mixture of goat anti-rabbit and horse anti-mouse sera (1:300 dilution) when staining both N-*myc* and cell surface antigens. Endogenous peroxidase was blocked with phenylhydrazine (45 min, 37 °C, $10^{-2}$ M), and then avidin-biotin-peroxidase complexes were added (one hr, room temperature; Vector Laboratories). Bound peroxidase was visualized with diaminobenzidene/$H_2O_2$ (1 mg/ml in 50 mM citrate buffer pH 5.0, 0.3% $H_2O_2$, 10 min, room temperature). Dehydration with ethyl alcohol (95% and then 100%) was followed by xylene and then mounting of coverslips with Cytoseal.

## RESULTS

Immunostaining of four different neuroblastoma cell lines that have amplification of the N-*myc* gene with anti-N-*myc* serum bGH/N-*myc* II yielded similar results. Reactivity was localized to nuclei, and the intensity varied markedly from cell to cell (Figure 1A). Immunostaining both cell surface antigens and N-*myc* resulted in membrane and nuclear reactivity for cells expressing N-*myc* and in membrane reactivity for those expressing little or no N-*myc* (Figure 1B). Greater than 95% of cells were labeled with the mixture of monoclonal antibodies 390, 459, HSAN 1.2, and 126-4, and so tumor cells could be identified even though they did not express N-*myc*.

Eleven bone marrow specimens from patients have been stained with anti-N-*myc* serum alone or in combination with monoclonal antibodies against cell surface antigens. Immunostaining with only anti-N-*myc* serum was done when marrow contained greater than 10% tumor cells, and double staining was done if tumor cells or clumps were rare. An example of a double-stained marrow specimen is shown in Figure 2. The relationship between N-*myc* protein expression and gene copy number in bone marrow metastases is summarized in Table 1. All metastases with genomic amplification stained significantly, and two of five without amplification also did so.

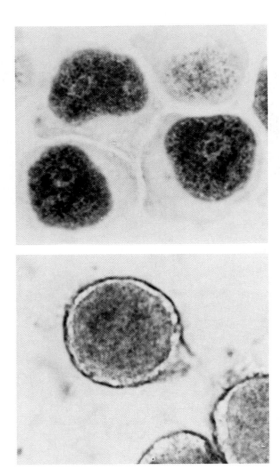

Figure 1. Immunoperoxidase staining of LA-N-5 human neuroblastoma cells with anti-N-*myc* serum bGH/N-*myc* II. Immunostaining with anti-N-*myc* serum alone demonstrates that the protein is localized to the nucleus and that there is marked heterogeneity in expression between cells (1A). Immunostaining with both anti-N-*myc* serum and monoclonal antibodies against cell surface antigens demonstrates uniform staining of cell surfaces and

heterogeneous staining of nuclei. One cell with double staining and overexpression is shown (1B). All staining visualized in both 1A and 1B is due to antibody binding as no counterstain was employed.

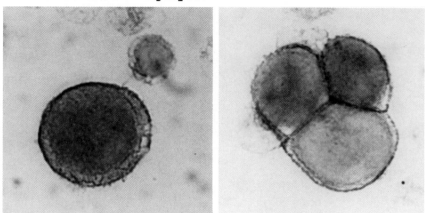

Figure 2. Immunostaining N-*myc* protein and cell surface antigens of neuroblastoma bone marrow metastases. Neuroblastoma cells are distinguished from normal cells by their cell surface reactivity with monoclonal antibodies 390, 459, HSAN 1.2, and 126-4; this permits assessment of N-*myc* expression by single tumor cells (2A) and infrequent tumor cell clumps (2B). All staining visualized in 2A and 2B is due to antibody binding as no counterstain was employed.

Table 1. N-*myc* gene copy number and expression by bone marrow metastases[*].

| Expression | Gene Copy Number | |
|---|---|---|
| | 1 | >10 |
| 0 | 3[**] | 0 |
| 1 | 1 | 2 |
| 2 | 1 | 2 |
| 3 | 0 | 2 |

[*]Each specimen was tested for gene copy number by Southern analysis and for expression by immunostaining with anti-N-

*myc* serum.   Expression of 0 indicates that staining with antiserum was not present or no greater than that with pre-immune normal serum.

**Number of patients.

## DISCUSSION

Expression of N-*myc* by neuroblastoma cells in bone marrow   can   be   determined   by   immunocytology. Immunoperoxidase staining with anti-N-*myc* serum alone is sufficient for marrow specimens with obvious tumor cell clusters or more than 10% tumor cells. Marrow obtained at diagnosis from most patients with stage IV disease meets these criteria, but, if not, immunostaining for cell surface antigens can identify infrequent neuroblastoma cells.   Since our previous study indicated that a primary tumor and its bone marrow metastases are concordant with respect to N-*myc* genomic amplification (Brodeur et al., 1987), it should be possible to evaluate N-*myc* expression of amplified tumors without removal or biopsy of the primary.   Additional studies of non-amplified primary and metastatic tumor cells from the same patient are necessary to determine concordance of N-*myc* expression for this group.

Our initial studies indicate that all metastases with amplification of N-*myc* express the protein and that some without amplification also do so.   This is similar to what we have found for primary tumors (Seeger et al., 1988). The clinical significance of expression by non-amplified tumor   cells   remains   to   be   determined;   however, overexpression secondary to genomic amplification of N-*myc* appears to be an important cause of aggressive tumor behavior. The considerable evidence supporting this latter conclusion includes the following:   1) Most continuously growing   neuroblastoma   cell   lines   have   genomic amplification of N-*myc* and synthesize large quantities its mRNA (Kohl et al., 1984; Schwab et al., 1984), and even those that are not amplified express the gene (Alt et al., 1986; Sadee et al., 1987; Wada et al., 1988).   2) Cell lines established from the same patients after tumor progression express more N-*myc* mRNA than lines developed at diagnosis (Rosen et al., 1986).   3) Cell lines with amplification of N-*myc* grow faster *in vitro* and in nude mice than non-amplified ones (Reynolds et al, 1988). 4) Treatment of neuroblastoma cell lines *in vitro* with retinoic acid rapidly causes decreased expression of N-*myc*, which is followed by fewer cells in S+G$_2$+M (Thiele et al, 1985). 5) Transfection of N-*myc* alone or together with c-Ha-*ras* into non-transformed cells results in tumorigenic cells (Schwab et al., 1985; Small et al., 1987). 6) Amplification and overexpression of N-*myc* is highly correlated with widespread disease at diagnosis and rapid progressive growth during therapy (Seeger et al, 1988). 7) Last, c-*myc*, which is related to N-*myc*, is integrally involved in the regulation of cell proliferation in that its expression is necessary for cells to enter S phase (Armelin et al., 1984; Kelley et al., 1983; Persson et al., 1984; Persson and Leder, 1984; Studzinski et al., 1986; Heikkila et al., 1987).

Prognostic factors obtained at diagnosis include age of the patient and clinical stage, serum neuron specific enolase (Zeltzer et al., 1983), serum ferritin (Hann et al., 1985), histopathology (Shimada et al., 1984), and N-*myc* gene copy number (Seeger et al., 1985). In this study, we have demonstrated that expression of N-*myc* by bone marrow metastases can be assessed with immunostaining, and so this technique can now be tested for its ability to predict outcome. If immunostaining does provide prognostic information, it will be an important test to perform at diagnosis. In addition, serial evaluations of bone marrow metastases may identify tumor cell population changes with respect to N-*myc* expression that correlate with response to therapy.

Recently, pilot investigations suggest that high-dose chemotherapy, total body irradiation (TBI), and bone marrow transplantation (BMT) may improve the survival of patients with poor prognosis neuroblastoma (August et al., 1984; Philip et al., 1986; Hartmann et al., 1986; Seeger et al., 1988). However, some patients still develop progressive disease. Studies which utilize Southern and immunostaining analyses will determine if patients whose tumors have genomic amplification and/or increased expression of N-*myc* can be treated successfully by this approach. If they are not adequately treated, new therapies aimed at regulation of the gene or eradication of the cells will need to be developed.

**ACKNOWLEDGEMENTS**

These studies were supported in part by USPHS grants awarded by the National Cancer Institute, DHHS: CA22794, CA27678, CA16042, CA36011 (RCS); CA39771, CA01027, CA05587 (GMB); and CA36827 (DJS). Additional support was obtained from the Children's United Research Effort against Cancer and the Fern Waldman Memorial Fund for Cancer Research (GMB).

**REFERENCES**

Alt FW, DePinho R, Zimmerman K, Legouy E, Hatton K, Ferrier P, Tesfaye A, Yancopoulos G, Nisen P (1986). The human *myc* gene family. Cold Spring Harbor Symp Quant 51 Pt 2:931–41.

Armelin HA, Armelin MCS, Kelly K, Stewart T, Leder P, Cochran BH, Stiles CD (1984). Functional role for c-*myc* in mitogenic response to platelet-derived growth factor Nature 310:655–660.

August CS, Serota FT, Kock PA, Burkey E, Schlesinger H, Elkins WL, Evans AE, D'Angio GJ (1984). Treatment of advanced neuroblastoma with supralethal chemotherapy, radiation, and allogeneic or autologous marrow reconstitution. J Clin Oncol 2:609–616.

Brodeur GM, Seeger RC, Schwab M, Varmus HE, Bishop JM (1984). Amplification of N-*myc* sequences in primary human neuroblastomas Science 224:1121–1124.

Brodeur GM, Hayes FA, Green AA, Casper JT, Wasson J, Wallach S, Seeger RC (1987). Consistent N-myc copy number in simultaneous or consecutive neuroblastoma samples from sixty individual patients. Cancer Res 47:4248–53.

Hann HW, Evans AE, Siegel SE, Wong KY, Sather H, Dalton A, Hammond D, Seeger RC (1985). Prognostic importance of serum ferritin in patients with Stages III and IV neuroblastoma: the Childrens Cancer Study Group experience. Cancer Res 45:2843–8.

Hartmann O, Benhamou E, Beaujean F, Pico JL, Kalifa C, Patte C, Flamant F, Lemerle J (1986). High-dose busulfan and cyclophosphamide with autologous bone marrow transplantation support in advanced malignancies in children: a phase II study. J Clin Oncol 4:1804–1810.

Heikkila R, Schwab G, Wickstrom E, Loke SL, Pluznik DH, Watt R, Neckers IM (1987). A c-*myc* antisense oligodeoxynucleo- tide inhibits entry into S phase but not progress from G0 to G1. Nature 328:445-9.

Kelly K, Cochran BH, Stiles CD, Leder P (1983). Cell-specific regulation of the c-*myc* gene by lymphocyte mitogens and platelet-derived growth factor. Cell 35:603-610.

Kohl NE, Gee CE, Alt FW (1984). Activated Expression of the N-*myc* gene in human neuroblastomas and related tumors. Science 226:1335-1337.

Lee HC, Brodeur GM, Reynolds CP, Sather H, Seeger RC (1986). Genomic amplification of N-*myc* in neuroblastoma cells that have metastasized to bone marrow. Proc Amer Soc Clin Oncol 5:25.

Persson H, Hennighausen L, Taub R, DeGrado W, Leder P (1984). Antibodies to human c-*myc* oncogene product: evidence of an evolutionary conserved protein induced during cell proliferation Science 225:687-693.

Persson H, Leder P (1984). Nuclear localization and DNA binding properties of the protein expressed by c-*myc* oncogene. Science 225:718-721.

Philip T, Bernard JL, Zucher JM, et al. (1987). High dose chemoradiotherapy with bone marrow transplantation as consolidation treatment in neuroblastoma: an unselected group of stage IV patients over one year of age. J Clin Oncol 5:266-271.

Reynolds CP, Brodeur GM, Tomayko MM, Donner L, Helson L, Seeger RC, Triche TJ (1988). Biological classification of cell lines derived from human extra-cranial neural tumors. Prog Clin Biol Res in press.

Rosen N, Reynolds CP, Thiele CJ, Biedler JL, Israel MA (1986). Increased N-*myc* expression following progressive growth of human neuroblastoma. Cancer Res 46:4139-4142.

Rosenblatt H, Seeger RC, Wells J (1982). A monoclonal antibody reactive with neuroblastoma but not normal bone marrow. Clin Res 31:68A.

Sadee VC, Yu ML, Richards PN, Preis MR, Schwab FM, Brodsky FM, Biedler, JL (1987). Expression of neurotransmitter receptors and *myc* protooncogenes in subclones of a human neuroblastoma cell line. Cancer Res 47:5207-5210.

Schulz G, Cheresh DA, Varki NM, Yu A, Staffileno LK, Reisfeld RA (1984). Detection of Ganglioside GD2 in tumor tissues and sera of neuroblastoma patients. Cancer Res 44:5914-20.

Schwab M, Ellison J, Busch M, Rosenau W, Varmus HE, and Bishop JM (1984). Enhanced expression of the human gene N-*myc* consequent to amplification of DNA may contribute to malignant progression of neuroblastoma. Proc Natl Acad Sci USA 81:4940–4944.

Schwab M, Varmus HE, Bishop JM (1985). Human gene N-*myc* contributes to neoplastic transformation of mammalian cells in culture. Nature 316:160–162.

Seeger RC, Danon YL, Hoover F, Raynor SA (1982). Definition of a Thy-1 determinant on human neuroblastoma, glioma, sarcoma, and teratoma cells with a monoclonal antibody. J Immunol 128:983–989.

Seeger RC, Brodeur GM, Sather H, Dalton A, Siegel SE, Wong KY, Hammond D (1985). Association of multiple copies of the N-*myc* oncogene with rapid progression of neuroblastomas. N Engl J Med 313:1111–1116.

Seeger RC, Reynolds CP, Moss TJ, Lenarsky C, Feig SA, Selch M, Ugelstad J, Wells J (1988). Autologous bone marrow transplantation for poor prognosis neuroblastoma. In: Dicke K, Spitzer G, Zander A. eds. Autologous Bone Marrow Transplantation: Proceedings of the Third International Symposium. Houston: Gulf Press in press.

Seeger RC, Wada R, Brodeur GM, Moss TJ, Bjork RL, Sousa L, and Slamon DJ (1988). Expression of N-*myc* by neuroblastomas with one or multiple copies of the oncogene. In Evans AE, D'Angio G, Seeger RC, (eds): Advances in Neuroblastoma Research, New York: Alan Liss; in press.

Shimada H, Chatten J, Newton WA Jr, Sachs N, Hamoudi AB, Chiba T, Marsden HB, Misugi K (1984). Histopathologic prognostic factors in neuroblastic tumors: definition of subtypes of ganglioneuroblastoma and an age-linked classification of neuroblastomas. JNCI 73:405–16.

Slamon DJ, Boone TC, Seeger RC, Keith DE, Chazin V, Lee HC, Souza IM (1986). Identification and characterization of the protein encoded by the human N-*myc* oncogene. Science 232:768–772.

Small MB, Hay N, Schwab M, Bishop JM (1987). Neoplastic transformation by the human gene N-*myc*. Mol Cell Biol 7:1638–45.

Smith RG, Reynolds CP (1987). Monoclonal antibody recognizing a human neuroblastoma-associated antigen Diag Clin Immunol (in press).

Studzinski GP, Brelvi ZS, Feldman SC, Watt RA (1986).

Participation of c-*myc* protein in DNA synthesis of human cells. Science 234:467-470.

Thiele CJ, Reynolds CP, Israel MA (1985). Decreased expression of N-myc precedes retinoic acid-induced morphological differentiation of human neuroblastoma. Nature 313:404-6.

Wada R, Seeger R, Brodeur G, Slamon D, Rayner S, Tomayko M, Reynolds CP (1988). Neuroblastoma cell lines that express one copy of the N-*myc* oncogene. Prog Clin Biol Res (in press).

Zeltzer PM, Marangos PJ, Sather H, Evans A, Siegel S, Wong KY, Dalton A, Seeger R, Hammond D (1985). Prognostic importance of serum neuron specific enolase in local and widespread neuroblastoma. Prog Clin Biol Res 175:319-29.

Advances in Neuroblastoma Research 2, pages 103–120
© 1988 Alan R. Liss, Inc.

MODULATION OF N-myc EXPRESSION, BUT NOT TUMORIGENICITY,
ACCOMPANIES PHENOTYPIC CONVERSION OF NEUROBLASTOMA CELLS
IN PROLONGED CULTURE

Richard W. Michitsch[*†], June L. Biedler[+] and
Peter W. Melera[*]

Molecular[*] and Cell Biology[+] Programs, Memorial
Sloan-Kettering Cancer Center, New York,
NY 10021

INTRODUCTION

Alterations in cellular oncogenes resulting in either
deregulated expression of the proto-oncogene or changes in
the structure of the encoded protein have been implicated
in the genesis of malignant disease (Bishop, 1985). These
alterations are thought to activate the proto-oncogene and
confer a growth advantage to the cell. The precise role of
these genes in the normal growth of the cell and their
activation resulting in increased proliferative capacity,
however, is not yet understood.

Amplification and overexpression of the N-myc gene has
been reported in a number of neuroblastoma cell lines and
tumors (Schwab et al., 1983; Kohl et al., 1983; Michitsch
et al., 1984). The increase in N-myc gene copy number in
neuroblastoma tumors correlates with the disease stage
(Brodeur et al., 1984; Seeger et al., 1985). That is, N-
myc gene amplification is more frequent in the advanced
stages of the disease, suggesting an involvement of this
proto-oncogene in the metastatic potential or proliferative
capacity of the cell. However, the normal function(s) of
N-myc has not been determined, although evidence suggests a
role in the early stages of multiple differentiation pathways of the cell (Zimmerman et al., 1986). Our studies of
N-myc expression in neuroblastoma cells also suggest an involvement in differentiation, rather than transformation,
and show that high levels of N-myc expression may not always
be indicative of the tumorigenic phenotype.

MATERIALS AND METHODS

Cell Lines and Culture:

Neuroblastoma cell lines used in this study have been described previously (Biedler et al., 1983), and include the HSR-containing cell lines BE(2)-C, LA-N-1, LA 1-5S, and LA 1-15N. Normal control tissue used was human placenta. Cells were maintained in a 50:50 mixture of Eagle's Minimal Essential Medium and Ham's F-12 (GIBCO) supplemented with 15% fetal bovine serum and fed twice weekly. Cells were removed from the flask with 0.025% trypsin (GIBCO) and passed into new culture flasks when confluent. Subclones LA 1-5S and LA 1-15N were initially established in microtiter plates from single cells derived from limiting dilutions of LA-N-1 cells, based on their distinct morphologies. The clonal origin of cells was verified microscopically soon after plating.

Preparation and Analysis of DNA and RNA:

Preparation of high molecular weight DNA, total cytoplasmic RNA, and poly(A)$^+$ RNA was carried out as described previously (Lewis et al., 1982; Melera et al., 1982; Montgomery et al., 1983). DNA and RNA transfer experiments were performed as described by Southern (1975) and Thomas (1980), with modifications (Lewis et al., 1982). Dot-blot analysis of DNA and RNA were done using the Schleicher and Schuell 96-well microsample filtration manifold. High molecular weight DNA was dissolved in buffer containing 56.6 mM Tris-Cl, pH 7.4, 0.2 M NaOH, and 6.6 x SSC, heated at 80°C for 10 min, and the solution neutralized by addition of 2 M Tris-Cl to a final concentration of 0.24 M. The samples were added to the manifold wells and bound to nitrocellulose membranes under vacuum. Total cytoplasmic RNA was dissolved in buffer containing 1 M NaCl, 6% formaldehyde and 30 mM NaPO$_4$, heated to 55°C for 15 min, then added to the manifold wells. Nitrocellulose filters were baked under vacuum at 80°C for 2 h, and hybridized with DNA probes [$^{32}$P]-labeled to a specific activity of 0.5-2.0 x 10$^8$ cpm/µg DNA (Rigby et al., 1977). N-myc DNA and RNA levels were quantitated by liquid scintillation counting of the nitrocellulose dots, with comparison to single-copy gene and expression levels, as indicated in the figure legends.

Methylation and 5-azacytidine Studies:

To determine the methylation status of N-myc locus, restriction digests with the enzymes Msp I and Hpa II were performed according to manufacturer's suggestions. The DNA was electrophoresed through 0.8% agarose gels, transferred to nitrocellulose membranes, and hybridized with $[^{32}P]$-labeled probes. The effects of 5-aza-cytidine (5-aza-C) on N-myc expression and methylation of the N-myc gene was determined by incubating cells (150 cm$^2$ flasks; 60-70% confluent) with $10^{-5}$ M 5-aza-C (Sigma) dissolved in 0.15 M NaCl at 37°C for 48 h. The flasks were washed 3 times with medium with no drug, then incubated for 24 h at 37°C in medium without 5-aza-C. RNA and DNA were prepared as described previously.

Soft Agar Assay:

Varying dilutions of LA 1-5S and LA 1-15N cells in culture medium were mixed with two parts of 0.5% agar (final concentration 0.33% agar), and 1 ml of the cell:agar suspension was overlayed on a 5 ml 0.5% solid agar base. The plates were incubated 14 days at 37°C, at which time the number of colonies was determined by counting with an inverted microscope. Colony formation was expressed as a percentage of the total number of cells plated.

RESULTS

Subclones derived from the neuroblastoma cell line LA-N-1 were initially established from single cells and exhibited distinct morphologies (Fig. 1). One subclone, designated LA 1-5S, contains relatively large, elongated cells which adhere strongly to the substrate. The other line, LA 1-15N, contains cells which are smaller, more rounded, and weakly substrate-adherent. Biochemical characteristics of the two cell types also differ, with 5S cells exhibiting biochemical properties more similar to a melanocytic/Schwannian phenotype, while 15N cells show neuroblastic characteristics (Table 1).

Studies were undertaken to correlate N-myc gene copy number and expression in the subclones and to determine if N-myc expression might be altered in association with the observed changes in cellular phenotype. Cells from both

LA-N-1 AND CLONAL SUBLINES

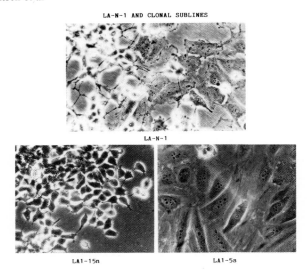

LA-N-1

LA1-15n                    LA1-5s

Figure 1.  Cell cultures of LA-N-1, LA 1-15N, and LA 1-5S.
Subclones of the parental neuroblastoma cell line LA-N-1
(Panel A) were initially established as single-cell iso-
lates of LA-N-1 cells.  One subclone, designated LA 1-15N
(Panel B), contains cells which are small, rounded, and
weakly substrate-adherent, while the other subclone, LA 1-
5S (Panel C), contains larger, elongated cells, which
attach strongly to the substrate.  Both subclones exhibit
distinct enzymatic activities (see Table 1 and Ross et al.,
this volume).

subclones were seeded from liquid nitrogen storage, and
after one month in culture aliquots were harvested and DNA
and RNA prepared.  Northern blot analysis of poly(A)$^+$ RNA
from the subclones showed that LA 1-15N cells had about a
fivefold higher steady-state amount of the 3.0 kb N-myc
transcript (Michitsch et al., 1984) than did LA 1-5S cells
(Fig. 2).  Relative N-myc expression in the cells was determined by visual comparison of hybridization intensities resulting from probing equal quantities of poly(A)$^+$ RNA with
the N-myc specific cDNA clone, pBE(2) C-59 (Michitsch et
al., 1984).  Southern blot analysis of DNA taken from these
cells revealed that LA 1-15N cells contained less than one-
half the N-myc gene copy number of LA 1-5S cells (Fig. 3).
Therefore, although LA 1-5S cells contained more N-myc

TABLE 1. Biochemical Phenotype of LA 1-5S and LA 1-15N
Subclones[a]

| Cell Line | Enzyme Activity | | |
|---|---|---|---|
| | Tyrosinase | Tyrosine Hydroxylase | Dopamine-β-Hydroxylase |
| | (pmol/h/mg) | (pmol/h/mg) | (nmol/h/mg) |
| LA 1-15N | N.D. | 320 ± 76.1 | 0.61 |
| LA 1-5S | 0.14 ± 0.07 | N.D. | N.D. |

N.D. = Not detected
[a] Data taken from Ross et al., this volume.

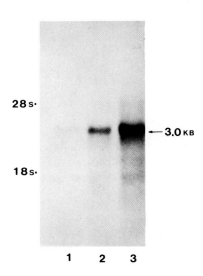

Figure 2. N-myc expression in neuroblastoma cells maintained in culture 1.5 months. poly(A)$^+$ RNA prepared from
cell lines (BE(2)-C, LA 1-5S, and LA 1-15N was electrophoresed through a 1.5% agarose-formaldehyde gel, transferred to nitrocellulose membrane, and hybridized with the
559 base pair DNA insert from clone pBE(2)-C-59 containing

the 3'-end of N-myc mRNA (Michitsch et al., 1984), [$^{32}$P]-labeled to a specific activity of 1.0 x 10$^8$ cpm/μg DNA.   5 μg poly(A)$^+$ RNA were loaded in each lane.   Lane 1, LA 1-5S; 2, LA 1-15N; 3, BE(2)-C.   Ribosomal RNA markers were used as indicated at the left of the figure.

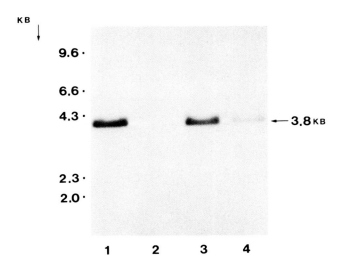

Figure 3.   N-myc amplification in neuroblastoma cells. Eco RI-digested genomic DNA from cell lines BE(2)-C, LA 1-5S, and LA 1-15N, and human placental tissue were electro-phoresed through a 0.8% agarose gel, transferred to nitro-cellulose membrane, and hybridized with the 559 base pair DNA insert from clone pBE(2)-C-59, [$^{32}$P]-labeled to a specific activity of 1.0 x 10$^8$ cpm/μg DNA.   20 μg Eco RI-digested DNA was loaded in each lane.   Lane 1, BE(2)-C; 2, human placenta; 3, LA 1-5S; 4, LA 1-15N.   Hind III-digested lambda phage DNA was used as markers and is indicated at the left of the figure.

genes than LA 1-15N cells, the steady-state level of N-myc mRNA in LA 1-5S cells was approximately one-fifth that found in LA 1-15N cells.   The subclones were then expanded, and the Northern and Southern analysis repeated 1.5 months later (total time in culture 2.5 months).   The results were the same as those shown in Figures 2 and 3 (data not shown).

Both subclones were maintained in culture and seven months after the initial seeding N-myc DNA and RNA amounts were again determined. N-myc mRNA levels were found to have increased in LA 1-5S cells and were approximately equal to N-myc expression levels in LA 1-15N cells (Fig. 4). Southern blot analysis of DNA from these cells showed that the relative N-myc gene copy number had not detectably changed from five months earlier (data not shown), thus ruling out the possibility that the increase in N-myc steady-state mRNA levels was due to an increase in the LA 1-5S cell N-myc gene copy number.

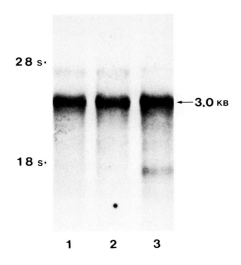

Figure 4. N-myc expression in neuroblastoma cells maintained in culture 7 months. poly(A)$^+$ RNA prepared from cell lines BE(2)-C, LA 1-5S, and LA 1-15N was electrophoresed through a 1.5% agarose-formaldehyde gel, transferred to nitrocellulose membrane, and hybridized with the 559 base pair DNA insert from clone pBE(2)-C-59, [$^{32}$P]-labeled to a specific activity of 1.0 x 10$^8$ cpm/μg DNA. Lane 1, 10 μg LA 1-5S; 2, 10 μg LA 1-15N; 3, 5 μg BE(2)-C. Ribosomal RNA markers are indicated at the left of the figure.

Finally, after remaining in culture for 11 months, the subclones were once again harvested, RNA and DNA prepared, and dot-blot analysis performed to quantitate N-myc gene copy number and RNA levels. The results (Table 2) show that the LA 1-5S cells have 120 copies of the N-myc gene,

TABLE 2. N-myc Gene Copy Number and Relative Expression

| Cell Line | N-myc Genes | N-myc Expression |
|-----------|-------------|------------------|
| LA 1-5S   | 120         | 70               |
| LA 1-15N  | 34          | 40               |
| BE(2)-C   | 140         | 150              |
| SH-SY5Y   | 1           | 1                |
| SH-EP     | 1           | N.D.             |

N.D. = Not detected

while LA 1-15N cells contain 34 copies. N-myc mRNA levels in LA 1-5S cells were found to be almost double that of the LA 1-15N cells (Fig. 5, left panel). Hence, during 11 months in culture, LA 1-5S cells had increased their N-myc expression level approximately 10-fold without a concomitant change in their N-myc gene copy number. In contrast, the level of N-myc expression in the LA 1-15N cells did not change to any appreciable level during this time period nor did the N-myc expression level in the control line BE(2)-C become elevated. The results show that the steady-state level of N-myc RNA in some neuroblastoma cell lines can vary widely with time in culture and that such variation can occur without an alteration in N-myc gene copy number.

c-myc expression in the N- and S-type cells was also determined. As seen in Figure 5 (right panel) and Table 3, c-myc mRNA was barely detectable in total cytoplasmic RNA from either LA 1-5S, LA 1-15N, or BE(2)-C (all of which contain a single copy c-myc gene), while the neuroblastoma cell line SH-SY5Y, with single copy N- and c-myc genes, exhibits readily detectable c-myc transcripts. Hence, in these neuroblastoma cell lines the steady-state expression level of the c-myc proto-oncogene did not vary proportionally in any obvious way with that of N-myc.

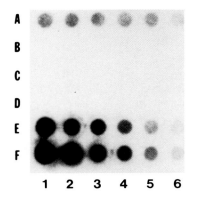
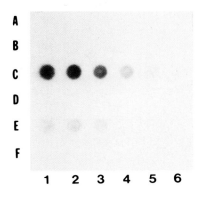

Figure 5. Quantitation of N- and c-myc expression in neuroblastoma cells. Total cytoplasmic RNA prepared from neuroblastoma cell lines was spotted on nitrocellulose membranes and hybridized with the 559 base pair DNA insert from clone pBE(2)-C-59, [$^{32}$P]-labeled to a specific activity of 0.5 x $10^8$ cpm/µg DNA (left panel), or the third exon of the human c-myc gene (see Michitsch et al., 1984, for a detailed description of this probe), [$^{32}$P]-labeled to a specific activity of 0.5 x $10^8$ cpm/µg DNA (right panel). Decreasing concentrations of RNA were spotted in both panels, as indicated by the numbers in the vertical lanes: 1, 20 µg; 2, 10 µg; 3, 5 µg; 4, 2.5 µg; 5, 1.25 µg; 6, 0.625 µg. The cell lines from which the samples were prepared are indicated by letters in the horizontal rows: (left panel) A, LA 1-15N; B, SK-N-SH; C, SH-SY5Y; D, SH-EP; E, LA 1-5S; F, BE(2)-C. (Right panel) A, LA 1-15N; B, LA 1-5S; C, SH-SY5Y; D, SH-EP; E, SK-N-SH; F, BE(2)-C.

In an attempt to determine if the 10-fold increase in expression of N-myc, observed in LA 1-5S cells in prolonged culture, is accompanied by acquisiton of the tumorigenic phenotype, soft agar cell colonization studies were performed. Previous experiments had demonstrated a positive correlation between the growth of LA 1-15N cells in soft agar and their ability to induce tumors in nude mice (see

TABLE 3.  c-myc Gene Copy Number and Relative Expression

| Cell Line | c-myc Genes | c-myc Expression |
|-----------|-------------|------------------|
| LA 1-5S   | 1           | 1                |
| LA 1-15N  | 1           | N.D.             |
| BE(2)-C   | 1           | N.D.             |
| SH-SY5Y   | 1           | 32               |
| SH-EP     | Not done    | N.D.             |

N.D. = Not detected


Table 4).  No such correlation had been observed for LA 1-5S cells, however, since they did not colonize in soft agar


TABLE 4.  Growth of Cells in Soft Agar Versus Their Ability to Form Tumors in Mice

| Cell Line | Plating Efficiency (% colonies formed/ plated cells) | Tumor Frequency[a] |
|-----------|------------------------------------------------------|--------------------|
| LA 1-15N  | 28.8%  | 100%     |
| LA 1-5S   | 1.4%   | 0%       |
| LA 1-5S (in culture 11 months) | 0.06% | Not done |

[a] See Biedler et al., this volume, for details.


nor form tumors in the nude mouse assay.  LA 1-5S cells, taken from prolonged culture, and which exhibited N-myc expression levels 2-fold higher than LA 1-15N cells, also failed to grow in soft agar, suggesting that increased N-myc expression alone is not sufficient to confer a tumorigenic phenotype on these cells.

The methylation status of the N-myc gene and its

flanking DNA was determined as a potential means to explain the discrepancies between the N-myc gene copy number and mRNA steady-state levels in the LA 1-5S cells. DNA from BE(2)-C, LA 1-5S, and LA 1-15N was digested with Msp I and Hpa II, the DNA transferred to nitrocellulose membranes and probed with [$^{32}$P]-labeled DNA representing the 5'-end of the N-myc gene, including the first exon. The results (Fig. 6) show that hybridization patterns produced by

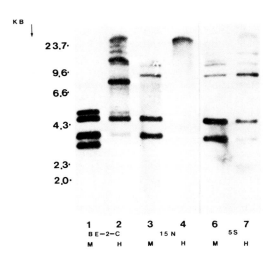

Figure 6. Methylation patterns of the 5'-end of the N-myc gene in neuroblastoma cell lines BE(2)-C, LA 1-15N, and LA 1-5S. 5 μg genomic DNA prepared from BE(2)-C and LA 1-5S cells and 10 μg from LA 1-15N cells were digested with the restriction enzyme Msp I or Hpa II, electrophoresed through a 0.8% agarose gel, and transferred to nitrocellulose membrane. The filter was probed with a DNA fragment isolated from a lambda bacteriophage library (Michitsch, 1986), which included the first exon of the N-myc gene and sequences 5'-ward. The probe was [$^{32}$P]-labeled to a specific activity of 0.5 x 10$^8$ cpm/μg DNA. Lane 1, BE(2)-C; Msp I. 2, BE(2)-C; Hpa II. 3, LA 1-15N; Msp I. 4, LA 1-15N; Hpa II. 6, LA 1-5S; Msp I. 7, LA 1-5S; Hpa II. Hind III-digested lambda phage DNA markers are shown on the left.

Hpa II-digested DNA from BE(2)-C and LA 1-5S cells are more
similar than those exhibited by LA 1-15N DNA. Similarities
are also seen between LA 1-5S and BE(2)-C Hpa II-digested
DNA probed with the second and third exons of the N-myc
gene (Michitsch, 1986), while the pattern in LA 1-15N DNA
is different (data not shown). The relative decrease of
bands hybridizing to the probe in the LA 1-15N DNA as compared to BE(2)-C and LA 1-5S Hpa II-digested DNA indicates
a greater degree of methylation of the internal cytosine
residue of the CCGG recognition sequence in the N-myc gene
of the LA 1-15N cells. Also of interest are the Msp I
cleavage patterns, which suggest that the distribution of
CCGG sites at the 5' end of the amplified N-myc genes in
LA 1-5S and LA 1-15N cells are the same, and yet differ
from that in BE(2)-C DNA (Fig. 6, lanes 1, 3, 6). These
results suggest that the N-myc amplified locus in LA 1-15N
cells is hypermethylated as compared to that in BE(2)-C or
LA 1-5S cells even though the steady-state level of N-myc
RNA is greatest in the LA 1-15N cell line (Table 2). Moreover, they argue against the generalized concept that
hypermethylation is associated with a reduction in gene expression (Razin et al., 1984). Variations in the degree of
methylation also exist among the amplified N-myc genes in
the different cell lines, as seen when comparing intensities of the hybridizing bands in Hpa II-digested DNA (Fig.
6).

To determine if changes in N-myc expression and/or
methylation pattern could be induced by treatment with a
known differentiation agent, neuroblastoma cells were incubated with 5-azacytidine, and the RNA and DNA prepared from
them analyzed. Total cytoplasmic RNA was spotted onto
nitrocellulose filters and probed with the second exon-con-
taining region of the N-myc gene. The results (Fig. 7)
show that for LA 1-15N and BE(2)-C no difference in N-myc
expression was detected between the 5-azacytidine-treated
cells and untreated controls (the greater intensity seen in
rows A and B is due to a longer exposure for the LA 1-15N
autoradiogram). When comparing treated and untreated LA 1-
5S cells, however, there was a 2.5-fold decrease in N-myc
expression associated with drug treatment. Therefore,
treatment with 5-azacytidine results in decreased N-myc expression in LA 1-5S cells, but has no effect on N-myc expression in LA 1-15N or BE(2)-C cells.

Hpa II/Msp I digestions of 5-azacytidine treated and

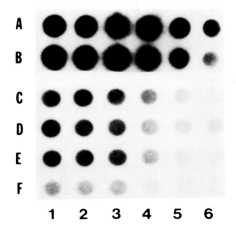

Figure 7. N-myc expression in 5-azacytidine treated and
untreated neuroblastoma cells. Total, cytoplasmic RNA
prepared from cell lines LA 1-15N, BE(2)-C, and LA 1-5S,
pretreated with the differentiation agent, 5-azacytidine
($10^{-5}$ M), or untreated, was spotted on nitrocellulose membranes and hybridized with the second exon of the N-myc
gene (Michitsch, 1986), [$^{32}$P]-labeled to a specific activity of 0.5 x $10^8$ cpm/μg DNA. Decreasing concentrations of
RNA were spotted on the membranes and are indicated by
numbers in the vertical lanes:  1, 20 μg; 2, 10 μg; 3, 5
μg; 4, 2.5 μg; 5, 1.25 μg; 6, 0.625 μg.  RNA from the cell
lines incubated in the presence or absence of 5-azacytidine,
indicated by letters, are in the following horizontal rows:
A, LA 1-15N; (-) 5-aza-C.  B, LA 1-15N; (+) 5-aza-C.  C,
BE(2)-C; (-) 5-aza-C.  D, BE(2)-C; (+) 5-aza-C.  E, LA 1-5S;
(-) 5-aza-C.  F, LA 1-5S; (+) 5-aza-C.

untreated BE(2)-C DNA were hybridized with [$^{32}$P]-labeled
probes representing the first, second, and third exons of
N-myc (Fig. 8).  When comparing hybridization patterns of
DNA from treated and untreated cells and probing with the
first exon and 5'-flanking sequences of the N-myc gene, the
Hpa II pattern is identical with the exception of one hy-
bridizing band at 2.2 kb (note the arrow) observed in the
Hpa II digest of 5-azacytidine-treated cells (Lane 3,

Fig. 8). This band is not seen in the untreated cells
(Lane 1, Fig. 8), suggesting that methylation at a
specific site in the 5'-end of the gene had been inhibited. Probing with the second exon failed to show hybridization pattern differences. However, at the third
exon a faint band at 0.8 kb (Lane 11, Fig. 8), not apparent in the Hpa II-digested DNA from untreated cells (Lane
9, Fig. 8), is observed, suggesting another potential

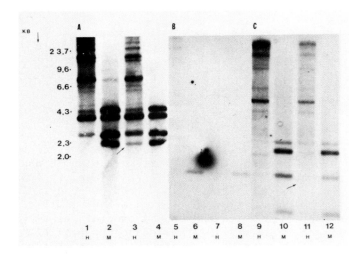

Figure 8. Methylation patterns of BE(2)-C restriction-
digested DNA prepared from 5-azacytidine treated and untreated cells. Genomic DNA from BE(2)-C cells was digested
with Msp I or Hpa II, electrophoresed through a 0.8%
agarose gel, and transferred to nitrocellulose membranes.
The filters were probed with the first exon of the N-myc
gene and sequences 5'-ward (panel A), the second exon of
the N-myc gene (panel B), and the third exon of the N-myc
gene (panel C). The probes were [$^{32}$P]-labeled to the
following specific activities: first exon, $1.0 \times 10^8$ cpm/
µg DNA; second exon, $0.5 \times 10^8$ cpm/µg DNA; third exon,
$0.7 \times 10^8$ cpm/µg DNA. Restriction digests and presence or
absence of 5-aza-C are indicated in the following lanes:
1, Hpa II: no drug. 2, Msp I: no drug. 3, Hpa II: 5-
aza-C. 4, Msp I: 5-aza-C. 5, Hpa II: no drug. 6,

Msp I: no drug. 7, Hpa II: 5-aza-C. 8, Msp I: 5-aza-C. 9, Hpa II: no drug. 10, Msp I: no drug. 11, Hpa II: 5-aza-C. 12, Msp I: 5-aza-C. Hind III-digested lambda phage DNA markers were used as indicated at the left of the figure.

inhibition of methylation. When comparing hybridization patterns of 5-azacytidine treated and untreated LA 1-5S DNA, no major differences were observed with any of the three probes used (data not shown). Therefore, although N-myc expression decreased in 5-azacytidine-treated LA 1-5S cells, it was apparently not due to a change in the methylation status of the internal cytosine residues within the Hpa II/Msp I recognition sequences (CCGG) of the amplified N-myc genes. These results, in combination with those indicating no change in N-myc gene methylation with time in culture (Fig. 6), argue against hypomethylation of the N-myc locus as the basis for the increased expression of N-myc in the cell lines tested.

DISCUSSION

Initial studies of N-myc gene copy number and expression showed that LA 1-5S cells contained at least twice as many N-myc genes but only one-fifth the N-myc RNA as LA 1-15N cells. When these parameters were measured after the subclones had been in culture for extended periods of time, it was found that the N-myc expression level in LA 1-5S cells increased, and by the end of almost one year, was about twice that of the LA 1-15N cells. No change in relative gene copy number was detected over that time. Additionally, LA 1-5S cells, regardless of their steady-state level of N-myc RNA or time in culture, failed to colonize in soft agar, while LA 1-15N cells, whose N-myc expression is consistently elevated, did so routinely throughout the culturing period. When both subclones were treated with the differentiation agent 5-azacytidine, the level of N-myc RNA decreased approximately 2.5-fold in LA 1-5S cells, but remained unchanged in the LA 1-15N sub-clone. The results suggest that the LA 1-5S subclone represents a neural crest-derived cell that, in culture, may revert to a more primitive phenotype in which N-myc expression is elevated without acquisition of the tumorigenic phenotype. The uncoupling of N-myc expression from

tumorigenicity, together with its sensitivity to the
differentiation agent 5-aza-cytidine in LA 1-5S cells, suggests a role for N-myc in normal cellular differentiation.
These results, while considered preliminary in nature, are
consistent overall with those reported by 1) Ross et al.
(1983), who described a similar cellular heterogeneity
within the neuroblastoma cell line SK-H-SH; 2) Bernards
et al. (1986), who concluded from a study of N-myc amplification and the expression of MHC Class 1 antigen in
neuroblastoma, that elevated N-myc expression may be
associated with maintenance of the undifferentiated state,
and 3) Zimmerman et al. (1986), who showed high level N-myc
expression to be restricted to specific tissue types and
developmental stages in the mouse.

Ross et al. (1983) have established two subclones from
the neuroblastoma cell line SK-N-SH. The neuroblast-like
subclone SH-SY5Y expresses tyrosine hydroxylase and
dopamine-β-hydroxylase activities and is not tumorigenic
(see Biedler et al., this volume), while the epithelial-
like subclone, SH-EP, expresses tyrosinase activity and is
tumorigenic. Neither subclone carries amplified N-myc
genes or overexpresses N-myc RNA (Table 2). The SH-SY5Y
subline, however, does overexpress c-myc (Table 3). Upon
maintenance in culture, a percentage of the neuroblast-like
cells displayed an epithelial morphology, while some epithelial cells showed a neuroblastic morphology, suggestive
of a bidirectional morphological interconversion. Concomitant with the morphological changes were coordinate
changes in the biochemistry of the subcloned cells. Preliminary observations suggest that LA 1-5S and LA 1-15N
cells may also be capable of such interconversion as well,
although at very low frequency (Biedler and Spengler,
unpublished observations). However, the increasing steady-
state level of N-myc mRNA in LA 1-5S cells may reflect a
similar, but not as extensive a conversion in culture from
a cell type beginning, but not committed to, a differentiation pathway and one more primitive and nondifferentiated,
and characterized by elevated N-myc expression and sensitivity to differentiation agents like 5-azacytidine. The
functional role played by the N-myc proto-oncogene in this
primitive setting and the impact of its overexpression on
the neuroblastoma phenotype remain to be determined.

Note added in proof: The appropriate designations for the

LA-N-1 derived subclones described in this study are LA1-5S and LA1-15N.

## ACKNOWLEDGMENTS

This work was supported in part by grants from the National Institutes of Health to the Sloan-Kettering Institute for Cancer Research and from the Special Projects Committee of the Society of the Memorial Sloan-Kettering Cancer Center, the Milton Schamach Foundation, and the Jeanette Warren Davison Fund for Cancer Research to P.W.M.

## REFERENCES

Bernards R, Dessain SK and Weinberg RA (1986). N-myc amplification causes down-modulation of MNC class 1 antigen expression in neuroblastoma. Cell 47:667-674.
Biedler JL, Meyers MB and Spengler BA (1983). Homogeneously staining regions and double minute chromosomes, prevalent cytogenetic abnormalities of human neuroblastoma cells. In Advances in Cellular Neurobiology (4) pp 267-307. Academic Press.
Bishop JM (1985). Viral oncogenes. Cell 42:23-38.
Brodeur GM, Seeger RC, Schwab M, Varmus HE and Bishop JM (1984). Amplification of N-myc in untreated human neuroblastoma correlates with advanced disease stage. Science 224:1121-1124.
Kohl NE, Kanda N, Schreck RR, Bruns G, Latt SA, Gilbert F and Alt FW (1983). Transposition and amplification of oncogene related sequences in human neuroblastomas. Cell 35:359-367.
Lewis JA, Biedler JL and Melera PW (1982). Gene amplification accompanies low level increases in the activity of dihydrofolate reductase in antifolate resistant Chinese hamster lung cells containing abnormally banding chromosomes. J Cell Biol 94:418-424.
Melera PW, Hession CA, Davide JP, Scotto KW, Biedler JL, Meyers MB and Shanske J (1982). mRNA directed overproduction of multiple dihydrofolate reductases from a series of independently derived sublines containing amplified dihydrofolate reductase genes. J Biol Chem 251:12939-12949.
Michitsch RW (1986). Isolation and characterization of the N-myc gene. Ph.D. Thesis. Graduate School of Medical

Sciences, Cornell University, New York, NY.

Michitsch RW, Montgomery KT and Melera PW (1984). Expression of the amplified domain in human neuroblastoma cells. Mol Cell Biol 4:2370-2380.

Montgomery KT, Biedler JL, Spengler BA and Melera PW (1983). Specific DNA sequence amplification in human neuroblastoma cells. Proc Natl Acad Sci USA 80:5724-5728.

Razin A, Cedar H and Riggs AD (1984). Introduction and general overview. In DNA Methylation. Biochemistry and Biological Significance, pp 1-10. Springer-Verlag.

Rigby PW, Dieckman M, Rhodes C and Berg P (1977). Labeling deoxyribonucleic acid to high specific activity in vitro by nick-translation with DNA polymerase I. J Mol Biol 114:237-251.

Ross RA and Biedler JL (1985). Presence and regulation of tyrosinase activity in human neuroblastoma cell variants in vitro. Cancer Res 45:1628-1632.

Ross RA, Spengler BA and Biedler JL (1983). Coordinate morphological and biochemical interconversion of human neuroblastoma cells. J Natl Cancer Inst 71:741-747.

Schwab M, Alitalo K. Klampnauer K-H, Varmus HE, Bishop JM, Gilbert F, Brodeur G, Goldstein M and Trent J (1983). Amplified DNA with limited homology to myc cellular oncogene is shared by human neuroblastoma cell lines and a neuroblastoma tumor. Nature 305:245-248.

Seeger RC, Brodeur GM, Sather H, Dalton A, Siegel SE, Wong KY and Hammond D (1985). Association of multiple copies of the N-myc oncogene with rapid progression of neuroblastoma. N Engl J Med 313:111-1116.

Southern EM (1975). Detection of specific sequence among DNA fragments separated by gel electrophoresis. J Mol Biol 98:503-517.

Thomas PS (1980). Hybridization of denatured RNA and small DNA fragments transferred to nitrocellulose. Proc Natl Acad Sci USA 77:5201-5205.

Zimmerman KA, Yancopoulos GD, Collum RG, Smith RK, Kohl NE, Denis KA, Nau MM, Witte ON, Toran-Allerand D, Gee CE, Minna JD and Alt FW (1986). Differential expression of myc family genes during murine development. Nature 319:780-783.

**Advances in Neuroblastoma Research 2, pages 121–131**
© **1988 Alan R. Liss, Inc.**

REARRANGEMENT DYNAMICS INVOLVED IN GENE AMPLIFICATION IN HUMAN NEUROBLASTOMA CELLS

Hiroyuki Shimatake, Takanobu Kikuchi, Chizuru Abe-Nakagawa, Naotoshi Kanda and Yoshiaki Tsuchida Department of Molecular Biology, Toho University School of Medicine, Tokyo 143, (H.S.,T.K.,C.A-N.) Department of Anatomy, Tokyo Women's Medical College, Tokyo 162, (N.K.) Department of Surgery, National Children's Hospital, Tokyo 154, (Y.T.)

INTRODUCTION

It is not well understood how gene amplification takes place in malignant cells. The onion-skin model has been proposed to explain gene amplification in drug resistant cells (Schimke, 1984 and Stark and Wahl, 1984). This model does not necessarily explain gene amplification in neuroblastoma cells because several genes are amplified in almost equal amount in the same homogeneously staining region (HSR) and because none of the gene amplification has been observed to take place at the original site of the gene (Kanda et al., 1983, 1987 and Schwab et al., 1984).

In a preliminary observation we found that the clone 8 had been rearranged in neuroblastoma cell line TNB-1. It is known that the clone 8 is rearranged in cell line NB-9 (Kohl et al., 1983) and two more additional cell lines of neuroblastoma (Shiloh et al., 1986). Thus, the clone 8 is likely to be a hot spot for gene rearrangement, even though the clone represents only a minor fraction in gene amplification unit of thousand kilo bases (Kanda et al., 1983). There could well be a possibility that specific signals for DNA rearrangement is located in the clone 8 and that the rearrangement event triggers gene amplification which leads to clinically agrressive form of neuroblastoma. We, therefore, set out to analyse rearranged region of the clone 8 in TNB-1 cell line.

MATERIALS AND METHODS

Cell Lines and Tumors

Human neuroblastoma cell line TNB-1 was cultured in MEM medium supplemented with 10 % fetal calf serum. Six human neuroblastoma xenografts TNB-4, TNB-6, TNB-9, TNB-10, TNB-11 and MNB were maintained by xenotransplantation in nude mice. These cells and xenografts were derived from the neuroblastoma tumors in stage III and IV patients, as described previosly (Tsuchida et al., 1984).

Hybridization Analysis

DNA fragments digested with restriction endonucleases were separated by electrophoresis on 0.8% agarose gel and transferred to a nitrocellulose membrane (Southern, 1985). Hybridization with $^{32}$P-labeled probe was done at 65°C for 16 hr in aqueous hybridization buffer containing 6xSSC. The membrane was then washed with 0.1xSSC at 60°C. Radiolabelling of the probe DNA was done by nick-translation (Rigby et al., 1977).

Chromosomal localization of clone 8, T and N-myc gene was analysed by in situ hybridization technique (Harper and Saunders, 1981) with a slight modification (Kanda et al., 1983).

Genomic Cloning and Sequence Analysis

Standard cloning techniques were used (Maniatis, 1982). Genomic DNA was completely digested with endonuclease EcoR I and electrophoresed throgh 0.8% agarose gel. DNA fragments eluted by electrophoresis were cloned into the EcoR I site of the lambda gt11 vector. Positive plaques were purified three times and phage DNA was prepared (Benton and Davis, 1977). DNA fragments containing the rearrangement junction were inserted to M13 phage vectors mp18 and mp19 (Yanisch-Perron et al., 1985). DNA sequencing was done by the dideoxy chain termination method (Sanger et al., 1980).

## RESULTS AND DISCUSSION

Southern blot analysis of TNB-1 DNA showed that there were two bands of clone 8: 3.8 kb and 2.1 kb by Eco RI digestion and 1.75 kb and 1.70 kb by Hind III digestion, respectively (Fig. 1). Although Hind III digestion on Figure 1 did not show two bands clearly, higher percentage agarose gel electrophoresis revealed two separate bands in equi-molar ratio (data not shown). EcoR I did not show equal intesity of the two bands. This was probably due to an unequal efficiency of transfer for Southern blotting.

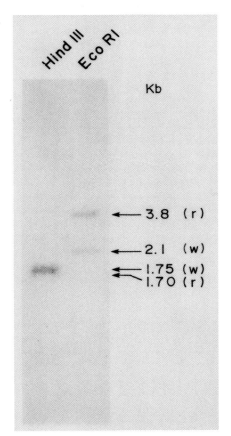

Figure 1. Southern blot analysis of the clone 8 in human neuroblastoma TNB-1 cells. Samples of 2 μg DNA digested with endonuclease Hind III or EcoR I were separated by electrophoresis in 0.8 % agarose gel and transferred to a nitrocellulose membrane, and hybridized to the nick-translated IMR-clone 8 probe (1.75Kb Hind III fragment)

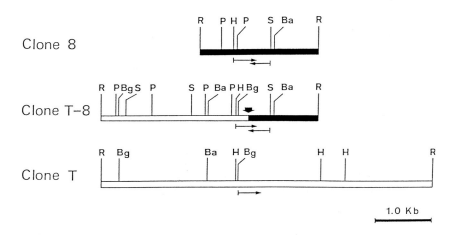

Figure 2. Restriction map of the wild type clone 8, the rearranged clone T-8 and the wild type clone T. The wild type clone T obtained as a 5.6 Kb EcoRI fragment was derived from TNB-9 genome. Restriction map of the clone T in TNB-9 cells was the same as in normal pracenta by Southern blot analysis and the fragment was amplified in the cells. The sequences of clone 8 and clone T were indicated by closed boxes and open boxes, respectively. Sequencing strategy for the three clones is shown by horizontal arrows. Restriction endonuclease sites are as follows: Ba, BamHI; Bg, BglII; H, HindIII; P, PstI; R, EcoRI; S, SacI.

We found that 2.1 kb on EcoR I and 1.75 kb on Hind III digestion represented wild type pattern and that 3.8 kb on EcoR I and 1.70 kb on Hind III represented rearranged pattern. We, therefore, cloned both wild type and rearranged species of clone 8 from TNB-1 cells in order to analyse a structure of rearrangement site at a DNA sequence level (Fig. 2). Rearrangement took place in a segment between BamH I and Hind III restriction sites. Unknown DNA which replaced a portion of clone 8 was designated as clone T (Fig. 2). Wild type T was cloned to find out an exact point of rearrangement in the clone 8 (see below).

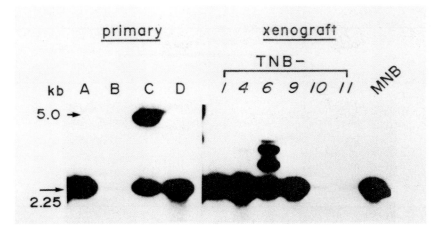

Figure 3. The amplified clone T in human neuroblastoma xenografts and primary tumors. Each sample of 10 μg DNA was digested with HindIII and EcoRI, electrophoresed on a 0.8 % agarose gel, and transferred to nitrocellulose membrane. The membrane was hybridized to [32]P-labeled 2.2Kb EcoRI/HindIII fragment of clone T.

Southern blot analysis of a variety of neuroblastoma cells with clone T as a hybridization proberevealed that the clone T also coamplified with N-myc gene (Fig. 3). Three out of four primary tumors and five out of seven xenografts showed an amplified pattern of clone T. This data indicated that a distance between the N-myc gene and clone T was as close as the distance between the N-myc gene and the clone 8. Some of the lanes (C and 6) of the Figure 3 showed an altered pattern of digestion, which was due to a partial digestion for Southern blot analysis but not due to a rearranged pattern. Thus clone T did not show any rearrangement pattern as opposed to clone 8 which represented a hot spot for gene rearrangement involved in gene amplification (Shiloh et al., 1986). Amplification pattern in a series of the neuroblastoma cell lines was sammarized (Table 1). Coamplification frequency suggested the following possibilities. A distance of clone 8 and clone T on chromosome 2 could be either very close if these clones are located on the same side with respect to

Table 1.  Gene Amplification in Human Neuroblastoma Cells

| Neuroblastoma cells | Gene amplification | | | | |
|---|---|---|---|---|---|
| | N-myc | clone 8 | clone T | DMs | HSR |
| TNB-1 | + | + | + | - | + |
| TNB-4 | + | - | + | + | - |
| TNB-5 | + | - | ND | + | - |
| TNB-6 | + | + | + | + | - |
| TNB-9 | + | + | + | - | + |
| TNB-10 | - | - | - | - | + |
| TNB-11 | + | ND | - | - | - |
| MNB | + | + | + | - | + |

DMs; double minutes, HSR; homogeneously staining region
ND; not done

the N-myc gene or could be very far if these are on the opposite side. If the latter is the case, then the clone 8 and T rearrangement site may well represent a junction between two amplificaion units (Kikuchi et al., 1987).

TNB-1 cell was known to contain two HSRs on chromosome 12 (Kaneko et al.,1985). Because of the presence of two forms of the clone 8 in this cell, it was not clear whether wild type of the clone 8 was contained in one HSR and rearranged form was in another HSR or whether both forms were located on the same HSR. In situ hybridization (Fig. 4) revealed the latter was the case. All of the clones N-myc, 8 and T were present on each of the HSRs. These two chromosomes containing HSR were likely to represent equivalent chromosomes created by unequal distribution at mitosis. In wild type chromosome, both the clone 8 and T were located on chromosome 2p very close to a normal location of the N-myc gene (data not shown). These genes located close to each other, therefore, must have been moved as one unit to other chromosome to amplify.

Southern blot analysis indicated that the wild type clone T was not amplified in TNB-1 cell, but only the rearranged form of the clone T was amplified (Fig. 5). The reciprocal form of the rearrangement between the clone 8 and T was not amplified in the cell line (data not shown).

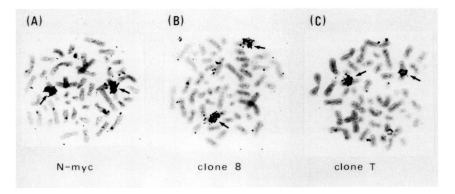

Figure 4. Chromosome localization the N-myc gene (A), clone 8 (B) and clone T (C) in metaphase TNB-1 cells. Probes used for <u>in situ</u> hybridization were 2.0Kb EcoRI fragment of NB-19-21 (Kikuchi et al., 1987) of the N-myc gene, 0.6Kb EcoRI/HindIII fragment of the clone 8 and 2.2Kb EcoRI/HindIII fragment of the clone T, respectively.

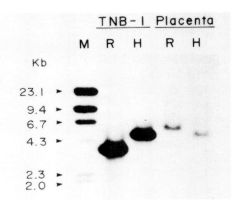

Figure 5. Southern blot analysis of TNB-1 and normal human placenta DNA. 5 µg of TNB-1 DNA and 10 µg of placenta DNA were digested with EcoRI and HindIII.  3' portion of the clone T (HindIII to EcoRI fragment, see Fig. 2) was used for a hybridization probe. R: EcoRI digest, H: HindIII digest, M: Lambda DNA  HindIII-digest.

## A

```
                                                                        70
AACATATTGG GGTAATTTGT TACGCAGCCA TAGTAACTGG ACCACCACCA TTCAGAGCTA CAGTGGAAGC
                        replaced by clone T   ------ ---******
                                                                       140
AGCCTTTATA AATTCCTATT TTTATTATTG TATCATAGAA AACAGGCAGT ATAAATTCTT ATATTCAGAA
                                                                       210
TTGTTTTCTC CAGGCATTTT GAACATTCTT GACCATCTTT TTTATTACCT ACCCCTCTTT TTCATATAGC
                                                                       280
AAGTGGTTTT GTTTCAGTCT ACTAAAAAAA AAAAAATCAC AGACCTTGTT AACAAGAAAA CCTGAGATCA
                        replaced by 9-J   --------- ******
                                                                       350
ATTTCACAGA CAGGAAGGAG GTGCAGCGAA GCAAGGAACC TGGGCGGGAG GCTGAGAAAG CGAGCCTGAG
```

## B

```
clone T       CATTCAGTTTGAAAAAAAAAAAAAAAGAACTGAAATGTGTACACGTCCTTGA
              ―――――――――――――――――――――――――――――――――――――――――――――――――――――
clone 8-A   ATAGTAACTGGACCACCACCATTCAGAGCTACAGTGGAAGCAGCCTTTATA
                                        ――――――――――――――――――――――――――――――――
                                  ✻✻✻✻✻

clone 8-B   GTCTACTAAAAAAAAAAAAAAATCACAGACCTTGTTAACAAGAAAACCTGAGA
            ―――――――――――――――――――――――――――――――
NB-9-J5     · · · · · · · · · · · · · · · · · · ·GTAGAA??????
```

Figure 6.(A) Nucleotide sequence of the wild type clone 8.
------ denotes the replacement of the clone 8 by the clone
T in TNB-1 cell and by the 9-J in NB-9 cell, respectively.
Note that sequences downstream to the hexamer is conserved
in either rearrangement. (B) Comparison of the nucleotide
sequences spanning the junction regions in TNB-1 and NB-9
cells. Rearranged sequence was indicated by black bar.
* denotes the hexamer sequence AGANCT.

These analyses excluded a possible insertion mechanism
that the clone 8 was inserted into the clone T or vice
versa. Whether these two clones were located nearby in the
wild type chromosome and a possible deletion joined these
two clones was not clarified by the present experiment.
Alternatively, these clones might represent end segments
of the whole amplification unit. It will be interesting to
investigate these possibilities by further experiments.

In order to find an exact point of rearrangement between clone 8 and T, we have determined DNA sequences in the relevant regions (Fig. 6A). The clone 8 and the clone T showed exactly the same nucleotide sequence with respect to the 3' region of the hexamer sequence AGANCT at nucleotide 54-59. Upstream to the hexamer was replaced by clone T in the rearranged form of the clone 8. Although several features including stem and loop structure and AT rich region were apparent near the rearrangement site, significance of these features was not clear. Comparison of the nucleotide sequence of the wild type clone 8 and clone T revealed that the rearrangement occurred at the short homology of the hexamer(Fig. 6B). Latt et al.(1986) reported the clone 8 rearrnagement at nucleotide 251-256.

It is interesting to point out that the clone 8 rearrangement in Tokyo and in Boston shares several features in common. Both rearrangement event took place within a short stretch of the clone 8. In both cases, upstream region was replaced by other DNA segments (clone T or 9-J) and downstream region of the clone 8 was conserved. Hexamer sequence (AGANCT) was involved in both cases, although it was not clear in Boston case whether the short homology recombination was the case as in our case in Tokyo (Kikuchi et al., 1987).

ACKNOWLEDGMENTS

We are grateful to Dr. Samuel A. Latt for kind offer of the clone 8. We would also like to thank Mr. Tetsuo Tsukahara for critically reading this manuscript.

REFERENCES

Benton WD, Davis RW (1977). Screening lambda gt recombinant clones by hybridization to single plaques in situ. Science 196:180-182
Harper ME, Saunders GF (1981). Localization of single copy DNA sequences on G-banded chromosome by in situ hybridization. Chromosoma (Berl.) 83:431-439.
Kanda N, Schreck RR, Alt FW, Bruns G, Baltimore D, Latt SA (1983). Isolation of amplified DNA sequences from IMR-32 human neuroblastoma cells: Facilitation by fluorescence-activated flow sorting of metaphase chromosomes. Proc

Natl Acad Sci 80:4069-4073.

Kanda N, Tsuchida Y, Hata J, Kohl NE, Alt FW, Latt SA, Utakoji T (1987). Amplification of IMR-32 clones 8, G-21 and N-myc in human neuroblastoma xenografts. Cancer Res 47:3291-3295.

Kaneko Y, Tsuchida Y, Maseki N, Takasaki N, Sakurai M, Saito S (1985). Chromosome findings in human neuroblastomas xenografted in nude mice. Jpn J Cancer Res (Gann) 76:359-364.

Kikuchi T, Abe-Nakagawa C, Kanda N, Shimatake H (1987). Gene amplification and chromosome abnormality in human neuroblastoma-Cloning and sequence analysis of rearrangement junction in the amplified clone 8. Jpn J Cancer Res 78:119.

Kohl NE, Kanda N, Schreck RR, Bruns G, Latt SA, Gilbert F, Alt FW (1983). Transposition and amplification of oncogene-related sequences in human neuroblastomas. Cell 35:359-367.

Latt SA, Shiloh Y, Sakai K, Brodeur G, Donlon T, Korf B, Shipley J, Bruns G, Heartlein M, Kanda N, Alt F, Seeger R (1986). Novel DNA rearrangement phenomena associated with DNA amplification in human neuroblastomas and neuroblastoma cell lines. In Ramel C, Lambert B, Magnussen (eds): "Genetic toxicology of environmental chemicals, Part A, Basic principles and mechanisms of action." New York: Alan R. Liss, pp 601- 612.

Maniatis T, Fritsch EF, Sambrook J (1982). "Molecular Cloning." New York: Cold Spring Harbor Laboratory.

Rigby PWJ, Dieckmann M, Rhodes C, Berg P (1977). Labeling deoxyribonucleic acid to high specific activity in vitro by nick translation with DNA polymerase I. J Molec Biol 113:237-251.

Sanger F, Coulson AR, Barrell BG, Smith AJH, Roe BA (1980). Cloning in single stranded bacteriophage as an aid to rapid DNA sequencing. J Molec Biol 143:161-178.

Schimke RT (1984). Gene amplification in cultured animal cells. Cell 37:705-713.

Schwab M, Alitalo K, Klempnauer KH, Varmus HE, Bishop JM, Gilbert F, Brodeur G, Goldstein M, Trent J (1983). Amplified DNA with limited homology to myc cellular oncogene is shared by human neuroblastoma cell lines and a neuroblastoma tumour. Nature 305:245-248.

Schwab M, Varmus HE, Bishop JM, Grzeschik K-H, Naylor SL, Sakaguchi AY, Brodeur G, Trent J (1984). Chromosome localization in normal human cells and neuroblastomas of a gene related to c-myc. Nature 308:288-291.

Shiloh Y, Shipley J, Brodeur GM, Bruns G, Korf B, Donlon T, Schreck RA, Seeger R, Sakai K, Latt SA (1985). Differential amplification, assembly, and relocation of multiple DNA sequences in human neuroblastomas and neuroblastoma cell lines. Proc Natl Acad Sci 82:3761-3765.

Shiloh Y, Korf B, Kohl NE, Sakai K, Brodeur GM, Harris P, Kanda N, Seeger RC, Alt F, Latt SA (1986). Amplification and rearrangement of DNA sequences from the chromosomal region 2p24 in human neuroblastomas. Cancer Res 46:5297-5301.

Southern EM (1975). Detection of specific sequences among DNA fragments separated by gel electrophoresis. J Molec Biol 98:503-517.

Stark GR, Wahl GM (1984). Gene amplification. Ann Rev Biochem 53:447-491.

Tsuchida Y, Yokomori K, Iwanaka T, Saito S (1984). Nude mouce xenograft study for treatment of neuroblastomas: effects of chemotherapeutic agents and surgery on tumor growth and cell kinetics. J Pediatr Surg 19:72-76.

Yanisch-Perron C, Vieira J, Messing J (1985). Improved M13 phage cloning vectors and host strains: Nucleotide sequences of M13mp18 and pUC19 vectors. Gene 33:103-119.

Advances in Neuroblastoma Research 2, pages 133–144
© 1988 Alan R. Liss, Inc.

EXPRESSION AND LOCALIZATION OF THE NMYC PROTEIN IN HUMAN
NEUROBLASTOMA CELLS: ANALYSIS OF THE EFFECT OF GAMMA INTER-
FERON TREATMENT AND DISTRIBUTION OF THE NMYC PROTEIN IN THE
NUCLEUS

Naohiko Ikegaki[1], Katarina Polakova[1,3], Laura
Prince[2], Roger H. Kennett[1]
Department of Human Genetics, University of Penn-
sylvania, School of Medicine, Philadelphia, PA
19104[1], Department of Biomedical Science, Drexel
University, Philadelphia, PA 19104[2], Cancer
Research Institute, Slovak Academy of Science,
Bratislava, Czechoslovakia[3]

INTRODUCTION

The NMYC gene is often found to be amplified in neuroblastoma tumors and cell lines (Schwab et al., 1983; Kohl et
al., 1983; Michitsch et al., 1984). The degree of amplification of the gene correlates well with the disease stage of
this neoplasm (Brodeur et al., 1984; Seeger et al., 1985).
In those tumors of cell lines that show NMYC gene amplification, the gene is expressed at high levels (Schwab et al.,
1984; Kohl et al., 1984). Moreover, the NMYC gene has been
shown to cooperate with an activated RAS gene in tumorigenic
conversion of primary rat fibroblasts (Schwab et al., 1985;
Yancopoulos et al., 1985). These observations suggest that
the overexpression of NMYC protein may play an important
role in development of tumors.

To investigate the expression and properties of the NMYC
gene product, we have prepared a panel of monoclonal antibodies reacting with different epitopes of the NMYC gene product,
and reported the identification and initial characterization
of the NMYC protein in human neuroblastoma cells (Ikegaki et
al., 1986). The NMYC protein is a relatively labile nuclear
protein, and has DNA-binding activity in vitro (Slamon et al.,
1986; Ikegaki et al., 1986; Ramsay et al., 1986). In a continuing effort to characterize the NMYC protein, we have been
focussing on the following aspects of its expression in human
neuroblastoma cells: 1) Response of NMYC expression to treatment with gamma interferon (IFN); 2) Specific localization of
the NMYC protein in the nucleus.

The administration of gamma IFN causes downmodulation of CMYC expression and enhancement of MHC class I and/or II expressions in several cell types (Pfizenmaier et al., 1985; Yarden & Kimchi, 1986; Sariban et al., 1987). The NMYC gene amplification coincides with the decreased expression of MHC class I gene in a rodent system (Bernards et al., 1986). The expression of HLA class I genes in human neuroblastoma cells can be enhanced by the administration of gamma IFN (Lampson & Fisher, 1984). These observations led us to examine the effect of gamma IFN on the expression of both NMYC protein and MHC Class I antigen in comparison to the case of CMYC protein and MHC Class I antigen.

We have previously shown nuclear localization of the NMYC protein in neuroblastoma cells by biochemical fractionation and immunofluorescence methods. Since the precise function of NMYC protein has not been defined, the determination of fine localization of NMYC protein in the nucleus should contribute toward a better understanding of NMYC function.


RESULTS


## Effect of gamma IFN on MYC and HLA Class I expression

First, we examined the effect of gamma IFN on CMYC protein and HLA antigen expression to confirm the observation made at mRNA levels (Yarden & Kimchi, 1986; Sriban et al., 1987). For this purpose, we choose two human cell lines, Colo320HSR and VUP-1, that express relatively high levels of CMYC protein, and have either neural characteristics or neural crest origin, respectively. The latter feature was taken into consideration in attempt to make a valid comparison of the results of CMYC in these lines and NMYC in neuroblastoma lines. Colo320HSR is a neuroendocrine tumor line and has about 20 copies of CMYC genes per haploid (Alitalo et al., 1983). VUP-1 is an uveal melanoma cell line and may have a few extra CMYC genes per haploid genom (Siracky et al., 1982; K.P., N.I. & R.K unpublished data). Figure 1 shows the dose response of the CMYC protein and HLA Class I antigen expression to gamma IFN treatment. The HLA Class I expression was significantly enhanced even at 10 units gamma IFN per ml, while the CMYC expression was reduced by 50% at 1000 units gamma IFN per ml in both cell lines.

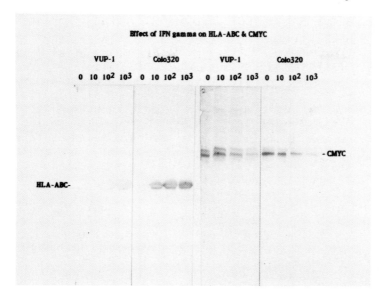

Figure 1. Dose response of the CMYC protein and HLA Class I
antigen expression to gamma IFN treatment.  Cells were grown
or four days in the presence of different concentrations of
gamma IFN as indicated (units per ml).  Extracts were made
from cytoplasmic/membrane and nuclear fractions at $5 \times 10^7$
cells equivalent per ml (Ikegaki et al., 1986).  Aliquots
equivalent to $5 \times 10^6$ cells from cytoplasmic/membrane and nuclear fractions were subjected to immunoblotting analysis
using "anti-HLA-ABC" monoclonal antibody (purchased from
Cooper Biomedical) for HLA-ABC antigen and anti-panMYC monoclonal antibody, NCM II 143 (Ikegaki et al., 1986) for CMYC
protein, respectively.


We next examined the response of the NMYC protein and
HLA Class I antigen expression to gamma IFN treatment in
neuroblastoma lines. We choose four well characterized neuroblastoma lines, SK-N-SH, IMR5 (a clone of IMR32), CHP134 &
CHP404.  Except for SK-N-SH which has a single copy of the
NMYC gene and expresses the gene at low levels, the other
lines have amplified NMYC genes and express the corresponding
protein at high levels (Ikegaki et al., 1986).  As shown in

Figure 2, gamma IFN at 1000 unit per ml markedly enhanced HLA Class I expression in all four cell lines. In contrast, NMYC expression was unchanged even at the dose of gamma IFN (1000 units per ml) that reduced CMYC expression by about 50%.

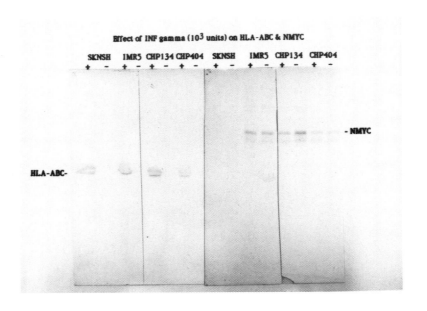

Figure 2. Effect of gamma IFN on HLA-ABC antigen and NMYC protein expression in human neuroblastoma cells. Cells were grown for three days in the presence ($10^3$ units per ml) or absence of gamma IFN. Immunoblotting assay was performed essentially as Fig. 1 except that anti-NMYC monoclonal antibody, NCM II 100 was used to detect NMYC protein.


To confirm these observations, we also studied the time course of the response of CMYC, NMYC and HLA Class I expression to gamma IFN. Figure 3 showed the response of NMYC and HLA Class I expression to gamma IFN in CHP404 cells. The HLA Class I expression was enhanced significantly in a time dependent manner, while the NMYC expression remained unchanged throughout the three day period. Figure 4 shows the time dependent response of CMYC and HLA Class I expression to gamma

IFN in Colo320 cells. The HLA Class I expression was again enhanced markedly, in contrast the CMYC expression was reduced by about 50% by day three.

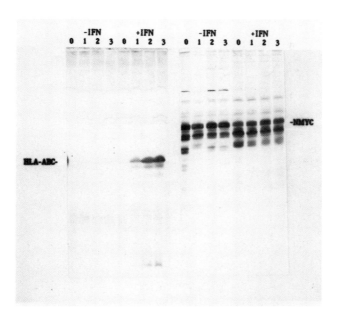

Figure 3. Time course of the response of NMYC protein and HLA-ABC antigen expression to gamma IFN. CHP404 cells were grown for three days in the presence of gamma IFN ($10^3$ units per ml). At the end of each day a portion of cells were harvested. Extracts were made and immunoblotting was performed as Fig. 1 except that NCM II 100 antibody was used to detect NMYC protein.

It seemed that the enhancement of Class I expression and the reduction of CMYC expression were inversely correlated. However we noticed in a separate experiment that the enhancement of Class I expression by IFN is a somewhat earlier event than the reduction of CMYC expression (data not shown). Thus, these events would appear to be independent responses to the gamma IFN treatment.

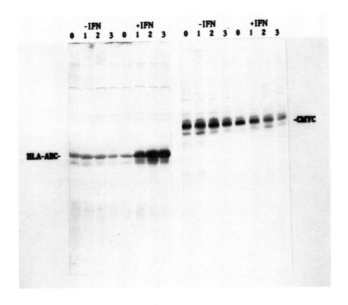

Figure 4. Time course of the response of HLA-ABC antigen and
CMYC protein expression to gamma IFN. Colo320 cells were
grown for three days in the presence of gamma IFN (103 units
per ml). At the end of each day, a portion of cells were
harvested. Extracts were made and immunoblotting was performed as in Fig. 1.


    Gamma IFN is known to exhibit cytostatic effects on some
tumor cell lines (Clements & McNurian, 1985). Both CMYC and
NMYC have been implicated in cell growth (Kelly et al., 1983;
Bernards et al., 1986). In addition, our data showed that
gamma IFN reduced CMYC expression but did not do so for NMYC.
Thus it was of interest to examine the effect of gamma IFN on
cell growth in the context of NMYC and CMYC protein expression. Figure 5 shows the cell growth profiles of each representative of CMYC (Colo320 HSR) and NMYC (CHP404) expressing
cell lines in the presence of 1000 units gamma IFN per ml.
The growth of Colo320 was inhibited by 60% compared to the
control culture that has been grown in the absence of gamma
IFN; in contrast, gamma IFN reduced the growth of CHP404
cells by only 15%. This result suggested the close associat-

ion between the reduction of MYC expression and cytostatic
effects of gamma IFN.

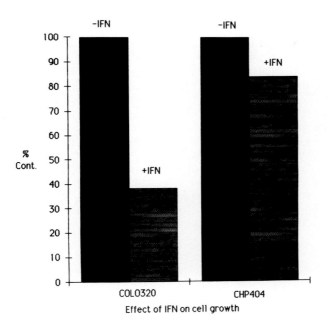

Figure 5. Effect of gamma IFN on the growth of cells expressing either CMYC (Colo320) or NMYC (CHP404). Cells were grown
for three days in the presence of $10^3$ units per ml gamma IFN.
The number of cells was counted and compared to the control
in which cells were grown in the absence of IFN.

## Fine localization of NMYC protein in neuroblastoma cells

We have previously shown the nuclear localization of
NMYC protein in neuroblastoma cells by biochemical fractionation and immunofluorescence. These methods provided a
general impression of the localization of NMYC protein in the
cell. To extend this observation and attempt to search for a
more precise localization of the protein in the nucleus, we
decided to employ an immunohistochemical staining method,

since these methods tend to give sharper resolution of staining than immunofluorescence. Figure six A shows the result of initial experiments, in which the formaldehyde-fixed cells were permeabilized by methanol/acetone(1:1), followed by immunoperoxidase assay. Some particulate structures are clearly stained in the nucleus of the cells. This result is of particular interest because the CMYC protein has been shown to colocalize with small nuclear ribonucleoprotein particles (Spector et al., 1987). To confirm this observation, we used another permeabilization method (use of a detergent, TritonX-100), because it is known that different fixation and/or permeabilization methods can occasionally give different staining patterns. As shown in Figure six B, this method gives a diffuse nuclear staining pattern, though some areas of the nucleus showed darker staining than other areas. Thus the precise subnuclear localization of NMYC protein still remains an open question. Despite these results, the following observations were made: 1) there is a heterogeneity in the expression of NMYC protein in individual cells; 2) the NMYC protein is disassociated from mitotic chromatins.

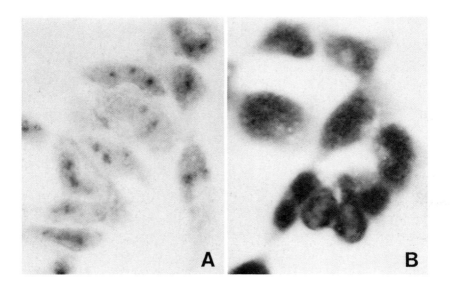

Figure 6. Immunohistochemical detection of NMYC protein in human neuroblastoma cells. CHP404 cells were grown on glass slides for two days. Cells were fixed by formaldehyde (3.7%)

and permeabilized by either methanol/acetone(1:1), chilled on
dry ice (A) or TritonX-100, 2.5% (B). Immunoperoxidase assay
(Jonak, 1980) was performed using a mixture of three monoclonal antibodies: NCM II 100 (anti-NMYC), NCM II 143 and
NCM II 274 (anti-panMYC). 200X

DISCUSSION

Differential susceptibilities of CMYC and NMYC expressions
to gamma IFN

The results clearly demonstrate that treatment of cells
with gamma IFN has different effects on the expression of
CMYC and NMYC: CMYC expression can be suppressed substantially, but NMYC expression is not reduced in response to
physiological doses of gamma IFN. In addition, the cytostatic effect of gamma IFN appears to be correlated with the
expression levels of CMYC and NMYC, suggesting that the level
of MYC expression may serve as a marker for monitoring the
growth status of tumor cells. This result also suggests that
those tumors that express CMYC, rather than NMYC might respond well to the gamma IFN treatment in vivo. Since a
majority of neuroblastomas express NMYC, this result stimulates questions regarding the relationship between NMYC expression and the efficiency of IFN treatment of neuroblastoma. The results do imply, however, that if other biological
response modifiers are found to downmodulate NMYC expression,
then they may be more effective for therapy of neuroblastomas.
In this regard, investigations are currently examining the
effects of other biological response modifiers on the expression of NMYC and growth status of neuroblastoma cells.

What accounts for the difference in the susceptibilities
of CMYC and NMYC expressions to gamma IFN? A clue may be
seen from the recent study in developmental expression of the
MYC gene family (Zimmerman et al., 1986). Three members of
the family, C, N and LMYC show distinctive patterns of tissue
specific expression during development of mouse, suggesting
that each gene has different transcription controlling regions. This could account for the difference in the susceptibilities of CMYC and NMYC to gamma IFN. An IFN-produced intracellular signal may act differentially on these controlling
regions. Another explanation is that the stabilities and/or

translation of CMYC and NMYC mRNAs would be differentially regulated in the presence of gamma IFN, since IFN is known to affect stability and translation of mRNA (Clemens & McNurian, 1985).

## Expression of the NMYC protein in individual cells

Immunohistochemical staining of the NMYC protein in cultured neuroblastoma cells revealed that the NMYC expression was not homogeneous among individual cells. A simple explanation for these observations is that the NMYC protein expression is cell cycle dependent. Thus the heterogeneity in NMYC expression may be due to the differences in cell cycle stages of individual cells. This idea is supported by the observation that mitotic cells show relatively homogeneous staining.

## ACKNOWLEDGMENTS

We would like to thank Dr. J. Vilcek for providing us recombinant human gamma interferon produced by Biogen. This work is supported by the Seligson Foundation and grants CA14489 and CA24263 from the USPHS.

## REFERENCES

Alitalo K, Schwab M, Lin CC, Varmus HE, Bishop JM (1983). Homogeneously staining chromosomal regions contain amplified copies of an abundantly expressed cellular oncogene (CMYC) in malignant neuroendocrine cells from a human colon carcinoma. Proc Natl Acad Sci USA 80:1707-1711.
Bernards R, Dessain SK, Weinberg RA (1986). NMYC amplification causes down-modulation of MHC Class I antigen expression in neuroblastoma. Cell 47:667-674.
Brodeur GM, Seeger RC, Schwab M, Vermus HE, Bishop JM (1984). Amplification of NMYC in untreated human neuroblastomas correlates with advanced disease stage. Science 224:1121-1124.
Clemens MJ, McNurian MA (1984). Regulation of cell proliferation and differentiation by interferons. Biochem J 226:345-360.
Ikegaki N, Bukovsky J, Kennett RH (1986). Identification and characterization of the NMYC gene product in human

neuroblastoma cells by monoclonal antibodies with defined specificities. Proc Natl Acad Sci USA 83:5929-5933.

Jonak ZL (1980). Peroxidase-conjugated antiglobulin method for visual detection of cell-surface antigens, in: Monoclonal Antibodies Hybridomas: A New Dimension in Biological Analyses (Kennett RH, McKearn TJ, Bechtol KB, eds.) Plenum Press, New York, pp 378-380.

Kelly K, Cochran BH, Stile CD, Leder P (1983). Cell-specific regulation of the CMYC gene by lymphocyte mitogens and platelet-derived growth factor. Cell 35:603-610.

Kohl NE, Knada N, Scheck RR, Bruns G, Latt SA, Bilbert F, Alt FW (1983). Transposition and amplification of oncogene-related sequence in human neuroblastomas. Cell 35:603-610.

Kohl N, Gee CE, Alt FW (1984). Activated expression of the NMYC gene in human neuroblastomas and related tumors. Science 226:1335-1337.

Lampson LA, Fisher CA (1984). Weak HLA and beta2-microglobulin expression of neuronal cell lines can be modulated by interferon. Proc Natl Acad Sci USA 81:6476-6480.

Michitsch RW, Montogomery KT, Melera P (1984). Expression of the amplified domain in human neuroblastoma cells. Mol Cell Biol 11:2370-2380.

Pfizenmaier K, Bartsch H, Scheurich P, Seliger B, Ucer U, Vehmeyer K, Nagel GA (1985). Differential gamma-interferon response of human colon carcinoma cells: Inhibition of proliferation and modulation of immunogenicity as independent effects of gamma-interferon on tumor growth. Cancer Res 45:3503-3509.

Ramsay G, Stanton L, Schwab M, Bishop JM (1986). Human proto-oncogene NMYC encodes nuclear proteins that bind DNA. Mol Cell Biol 6:4450-4457.

Sariban E, Mitchel T, Griffin J, Kufe DW (1987). Effect of interferon-gamma on proto-oncogene expression during induction of human monocytic differentiation. J Immunol 138:1954-1958.

Schwab M, Alitalo K, Klempnauer K, Vermus HE, Bishop JM, Gilbert F, Brodeur G, Goldstein M, Trent J (1983). Amplified DNA with limited homology to MYC cellular oncogene is shared by human neuroblastoma cell lines and a neuroblastoma tumor. Nature 305:245-248.

Schwab M, Ellison J, Bush M, Rosenau W, Vermus HE, Bishop JM (1984). Enhanced expression of the human gene NMYC consequent to amplification of DNA may contribute to malignant progression of neuroblastoma. Proc Natl Acad Sci USA 81:4940-4944.

Schwab M, Vermus HE, Bishop JM (1985). Human NMYC gene contributes to neoplastic transformation of mammalian cells in culture. Nature 316:160-162.

Seeger RC, Brodeur GM, Sather H, Dalton A, Siegel SE, Wong KY, Hammond D (1985). Association of multiple copies of the NMYC oncogene with rapid progression of neuroblastomas. New Engl J Med 313:1111-1116.

Siracky K, Blasko M, Borovansky J, Kovarik J, Svec J, Vrba M (1982). Human melanoma cell lines: morphology, growth, and alphamannosidase characteristics. Neoplasma 29:661-669.

Slamon DJ, Boone TC, Seeger RC, Keith DE, Chazin V, Lee HC, Souza LM (1986). Identification and characterization of the protein encoded by the human NMYC oncogen. Science 232:768-772.

Spector DL, Watt RA, Sullivan NF (1987). The VMYC and CMYC oncogene proteins colocalize in situ with small nuclear ribonucleoprotein particles. Oncogene 1:5-12.

Yancopolos GD, Nisen PD, Tesfaye A, Kohl N, Goldfarb MP, Alt FW (1985). NMYC can cooperate with RAS to transform normal cells in culture. Proc Natl Acad Sci USA 82:5455-5459.

Yarden A, Kimchi A (1986). Tumor necrosis factor reduces CMYC expression and cooperates with interferon-gamma in HeLa cells. Science 234:1419-1421.

Zimmerman KA, Yancopoulos GD, Collum RG, Smith RK, Kohl NA, Denis KA, Nau MM, Witte ON, Toran-Allerand D, Gee CE, Minna JD, Alt FW (1986). Differential expression of MYC family genes during murine development. Nature 319:780-783.

Advances in Neuroblastoma Research 2, pages 145–149
© 1988 Alan R. Liss, Inc.

DISCUSSION

Chairman:       A. Knudson

Discussants:    T.J. Moss, R.W. Michitsch,
                H. Shimatake, N. Ikegaki

Dr. Knudson asked Dr. Ikegaki if the fact that the levels of N-MYC could be modulated without respect to the state of differentiation implied that N-myc is not important in neuroblastoma and that we are looking at the wrong gene in the amplification unit? He replied that he couldn't answer the question directly but that when N-myc was introduced into murine fibroblasts, they tended to grow more aggressively, so it seems to have some role in cell growth. If they could control N-myc expression by some other means they could possibly answer the question.

Dr. Bruce Bostrum (Minnesota) asked Dr. Ikegaki about the site of synthesis of N-myc protein, whether in the nucleus or cytoplasm. Dr. Ikegaki presumed it was made in the cytoplasm and then transported to the nucleus, but the transportation signal remains to be found. Dr. Bostrum replied that if so, N-myc protein should be found in the cytoplasm. Dr. Moss commented that, since the monoclonal Ab is directed against only a portion of the protein, that portion may not always be available for binding. For instance, of 6 antibodies developed by Seeger only three stained immunohistologically. Perhaps the protein's structure in the cytoplasm is different than that in the nucleus. Nao also said that when C-myc is microinjected into the cytoplasm it is rapidly transported into the nucleus so cytoplasmic levels may be very low.

Dr. Lipinski asked if anyone had transfected single copy NBL cells with amplified N-myc, as found in HSR's or DM's, and assessed subsequent function. Dr. Moss replied that experiments had been done that showed that N-myc could serve as an oncogene in conjunction with H-ras and convey a malignant phenotype. He wondered if anyone had done experiments using antigens to N-myc in a cell with amplified N-myc to see if the malignant phenotype could be reversed. Dr. Thiele (NCI) replied that in Mark Israel's lab they were doing experiments transfecting N-myc along with the DHFR gene into single or multiple copy N-myc NBLs and PNETs. These clones were just being analyzed so results were not available.

Dr. Moss commented that they had seen several instances where a reported single copy NMYC tumor had given intense although heterogeneous immunohistological staining. He felt it is important to make sure that the sample for immunohistochemical staining is taken from the same area of the tumor that was analyzed for N-myc copy number, because one is comparing a single cell assay with a population assay. Single copy status could be mistakenly made because of dilution of the sample by stromal cells. He noted one case which had single copy of the primary, 10 copies in the marrow metastases, and intense but heterogeneous immunohistochemical staining in the primary.

Someone asked if Dr. Moss was suggesting that immunoperoxidase is more reliable than DNA analysis for determining this prognostic marker? Dr. Moss replied that care must be taken either way. With bone marrows, Southern analysis can only be done with greater than 10% involvement because it is a population based assay. Before submitting samples for DNA analysis they always examine a frozen section morphologically to make sure there are adequate numbers of tumor cells. In terms of immunohistochemistry, care must be taken to get very fresh tissue. Every technique has its shortcomings. However, with very light involvement of marrow, say 1%, it appears that one can rely on the immunohistochemistry, at least in cases of high copy number or high expression.

Dr. Israel (NCI) asked Dr. Shimatake if their hypothesized consensus sequences were seen in any other examples of rearrangements. Dr. Shimatake replied that by computer assisted searching they could not find any homologous recombination sequences.

A participant (Sloan Kettering) asked what was known about variation of N-myc expression through the cell cycle. Dr. Moss replied that it was not yet known. Possibly cell cycle variation explained some of the heterogeneity in immunochemical staining although Dr. Reynolds' idea of nonuniform segregation of DMs was also a possibility. Dr. Kemshead (London) said that very preliminary data from the MRC at Cambridge showed no variation in N-myc expression with the cell cycle. He also commented that they had seen a case with very heterogeneous immunohistochemical staining that didn't have DM's so this couldn't be the only explanation.

Dr. Gilbert (New York) asked Dr. Knudson whether, since both Wilms' tumor and retinoblastoma can have single copies of N-myc yet relatively overexpress it, the function of the NBL gene and other "antioncogenes" is to regulate N-myc and related genes. Dr. Knudson replied that he didn't think so. Firstly, N-myc is elevated in the target cell itself. Secondly, other growth factors such as IGFII are elevated in Wilms' tumor so one would have to postulate that the regulating gene is controlling several different genes. It seems easier to say that those genes are turned up as an expression of the target cell. However, the fact that the overexpressed gene can be amplified suggests it is important. Dr. Gilbert replied that since N-myc is a DNA-binding protein, and presumably acts by modulating the expression of a series of other genes, the elevation of other factors may point to N-myc expression as a primary event.

Dr. Shimatake, commenting about the cell cycle, said that N-myc drops during S phase but is high during $G_1$ and $G_2$.

Peter Melera (Rye, New York) commented on another possibility regarding N-myc amplification. c-MYC can be greatly upregulated without the necessity for amplication. One reason why amplification does occur (e.g., DHFR) is to accommodate for a relative deficiency of the product. Perhaps N-myc is amplified because of a fault in the pathway producing the normal levels necessary for the stage of differentiation, and the amplification is a secondary adaptive phenomena. Dr. Moss replied that, using IV-S as a model, the fact that cases with N-myc amplification do less well suggests its importance.

Dr. Melera replied that he did not mean that N-myc is not the target, but that it was amplified because the cells couldn't attain adequate levels.

Dr. Brodeur (St. Louis) noted that N-myc can be overexpressed in retinoblastoma, NBL and Wilms' tumor but that each disease is associated with a deletion of a different chromosome. The retinoblastoma gene is the only one cloned and found on chromosome 13g. It is expressed in some NBL cells although when it is there is no change in N-MYC expression.

Dr. Frantz (Rochester) asked Dr. Moss about the rapid half-life of N-myc protein and RNA, and how that affected immunohistochemical staining. Dr. Moss replied that stained cells still show staining after 24-48 hours at 4°C. but much less after one week. He said stained marrow cells were good for at least 24 hours, and stained LAN 5 cells in the marrow for 24-48 hrs. He hadn't worked with the RNA.

Dr. Reynolds (Los Angeles) asked Dr. Michitsch about his cell lines: did the cell morphology (flat vs round) remain the same over 11 mos, did the growth rate change and what were the cytogenetic correlates. Dr. Michitsch replied that there was not a change in morphology, and although growth rates were not formerly assessed, there appeared not to be a change. Dr. Biedler (New York) commented on the cytogenetics; that the 5S cells actually had longer HSR's than the 15N cells.

Dr. Knudson, referring to the dynamics of amplification, asked: If single cell clones with very few HSR's or DMs are grown, do they reproduce the full spectrum of amplification units or is the characteristic stable. Dr. Biedler replied that this hadn't really been looked at.

Someone clarified that there was no change in gene amplification in 5S cells or 15-N cells over 11 months in culture, although N-myc RNA did increase. Someone asked if there were cases with increased N-myc mRNA without increased N-myc protein. Dr. Moss didn't know of any. Dr. Ikegaki said the RNA and protein levels were usually well correlated.

Dr. Knudson asked if, in single copy NBL with overexpression, was the gene always normal in all its parts or was there evidence for a truncated gene, for example. Dr. Moss replied that Dr. Wada had done some Western analyses but that with immunohistocytology they were only looking at a small portion of the protein so they wouldn't see small changes.

A questioner asked Dr. Michitsch if the failure of LAN 5 cells with increased N-myc to grow in soft agar was expected and whether any other changes were noted. Dr. Michitsch replied that LAN5 cells had initially had a poor plating efficiency and tumor formation, so they didn't know what to expect. They did not see any other changes in morphology or growth rate.

Dr. Bernard L. Mirkin (Minnesota) asked Dr. Michitsch about the one cell line--5S--which showed a 2.5 fold decrease in N-myc after 5-azacytidine, compared with 15N which showed no change. Was this a function of duration of exposure to 5-azacytidine. Dr. Michitsh replied that all cultures were exposed for 48 hours. Dr. Mirkin then asked if it was possible that the 15N cells could have a transportation defect, or developmentally regulated different kinetics such as the 5-azacytidine was not reaching the nucleus but that in fact the 15N cell nucleus could be just so susceptable? Dr. Michitsch replied he hadn't looked at azacytidine kinetics at all. Dr. Knudson asked if Dr. Michitsch had looked at any other methylated genes as a control but he had not.

Dr. Evans asked Dr. Ikegaki to speculate on why γ interferon should increase HLA expression in both c-MYC and N-myc expressing cells but only affect the levels of c-MYC. He replied that transcriptional control of the 2 myc genes must be different because they have different developmental patterns; N-myc in brain, kidney and lung and c-MYC everywhere. Dr. Evans asked if expression of N-myc and c-MYC were completely unrelated to HLA gene expression. Dr. Ikegaki quoted Weinberg's recent publication that showed N-myc amplification downregulated HLA Class I antigen expression but there is no evidence for gamma interferon effecting N-myc expression.

Dr. Duerst (Rochester): regarding the fact that the cell line LAN1 is tetraploid is there any evidence for increased N-myc expression? Dr. Moss replied that LAN5 consistently stained the best but LAN1 also stained very strongly. SKNSH in comparison stained much less well.

Advances in Neuroblastoma Research 2, pages 151–163
© 1988 Alan R. Liss, Inc.

# N-MYC: STUDIES ON GENE AMPLIFICATION / EXPRESSION AND THE DEVELOPMENT OF A NON-ISOTOPIC TECHNIQUE FOR GENE MAPPING.

J.A.Garson[1], J.van den Berghe[2],
P.Sheppard[3], J.T.Kemshead[1].

1. ICRF Oncology Laboratory, ICH, London.
2. Mothercare Unit, ICH, London.
3. Cam.Res.Bioch.Harston Cambridge.

## INTRODUCTION.

An exponential growth in research into the molecular biology of cancer has occurred over the last few years. This has provided us with significant new insights into the fundamental nature and complexities of the neoplastic process. The previously distinct fields of viral oncogenesis, chemical carcinogenesis, cytogenetics and molecular genetics have converged around the central unifying concept of the oncogene. Despite this impressive step forward in understanding of basic mechanisms, clinical oncology in general has yet to benefit significantly from these advances. However, clinical correlations are now being made and in the case of neuroblastoma (NBL) at least, these may bear directly upon the management of the cancer patient (Brodeur et al.1984).
Northern and Southern blot analysis of RNA and DNA from malignant cells cannot answer questions about the heterogeneity of amplification or expression of a gene that may occur between individual cells. To this end we have attempted to define conditions that allow in situ hybridisation of DNA/RNA probes to frozen sections so that the morphology of the material is maintained for histological analysis. Whilst we have been successful at this using a 2.1 Kb probe to a highly repeated sequence (- 2000 copies)

present on the Y chromosome we have not yet been
able to increase the sensitivity to the point that
either a single copy or multiple copies of the N-
myc gene can be identified in frozen biopsy
samples (Cooke et al. 1982). However in
undertaking this study we have defined conditions
that allow the identification of a unique sequence
as small as 1Kb on chromosomes using a non-
isotopic procedure. Unlike other methods this
technique is entirely compatible with prior Giemsa
banding so permitting in situ experiments on
routinely G-banded clinical material (Garson et
al.1987). The details of this technique will be
reviewed along with data on the expression of the
N-myc gene obtained using a heteroantiserum raised
against a synthetic peptide sequence.

## METHODS.

### In Situ Hybridisation.

DNA probes were labelled with biotin-11-dUTP
by standard nick translation and unincorporated
nucleotides removed by ethanol precipitation in
the presence of 20ug of glycogen. Biotin labelled
probes were stored at 100ng/ul in 10mM Tris-Cl pH
7.6, 1mM EDTA at $-20^{\circ}$C. These have been shown to
remain stable for at least 1 year.
Chromosome preparations of cultured cells
were made by conventional methods and slides
incubated for 2-10 minutes at $37^{\circ}$C in phosphate
buffered saline pH 7.4 (PBS) containing $1 \times 10^{-7}$%
trypsin. Following a further 1 hour incubation in
PBS at $60^{\circ}$C, G-banding was completed by staining
the slides for 8 minutes with 2% Giemsa in pH 6.8
phosphate buffer. G-banded metaphases were
located and photographed under pH 6.8 buffer.
Giemsa stain was removed with ethanol and the
slides treated for 1 hour at $37^{\circ}$C with DNAase-free
RNAase at 100ug/ml in 2 x SSC (1 x SSC = 0.15M
NaCl, 0.015M Na Citrate). Before hybridisation
chromosomes were dehydrated through an ethanol
series. 50 - 100ng of biotinylated probe in 10ul
of hybridisation buffer was applied to each slide
under sealed glass coverslips. Hybridisation
buffer contained 50% deionised formamide, 10%
dextran sulphate, 2 x SSC, 0.1 mM EDTA, 0.05mM

Tris-Cl pH7.5 and 100ug/ml of denatured sonicated salmon sperm DNA. The chromosomal DNA and probe were denatured together at 80°C for 10 mins. Hybridisation was performed at 42°C for approximately 16 hours and the slides subsequently washed in 2 x SSC for 30 mins, 0.1 x SSC at 42°C for 30 mins, 2 x SSC for 15 mins and finally in TNM-A (0.1M Tris-Cl pH7.5, 0.1M NaCl, 2mM MgCl$_2$, 0.05% Triton X-100, 3% bovine serum albumin) for 15 mins. Hybridized probe was detected by incubating slides for 20 min with 0.01mg/ml streptavidin conjugated alkaline phosphatase in TNM-A. Excess conjugate was removed by washing, 3 x 5 mins, in TNM (TNM-A without albumin) then once in pH 9.5 buffer (0.1M Tris-Cl pH 9.5, 0.1M NaCl, 50mM Mg Cl$_2$). Incubation with 150ul of chromogenic substrate was performed in subdued light for 4 - 5 hours. The substrate solution was made by adding 4.4ul of nitroblue tetrazolium (NBT) (at 75mg/ml in 70% dimethylformamide) and 3.3ul of 5-bromo-4-chloro-3-indolyl phosphate (BCIP) (at 50mg/ml in dimethylformamide) to 1ml of pH 9.5 buffer. 1mM levamisole was included to inhibit any endogenous alkaline phosphatase activity. Colour development was terminated by washing for 5 mins in 20mM Tris-HCl pH 7.5, 5mM EDTA and the slides mounted in aqueous mountant (Dako). Metaphases were viewed under phase contrast illumination and results scored by two independent observers. The preparations are permanent and can be viewed repeatedly without fading. Biotinylated pBr322 was used as a negative control in parallel experiments.

## Antiserum to the N-myc Gene Product.

An antiserum to the N-myc gene product was produced in sheep by Cambridge Research Biochemicals. This was raised against a synthetic peptide, representing a sequence in the hydrophylic region of the protein. The peptide was linked to the carrier, keyhole limpet haemocyanin to increase its immunogenicity. The serum was affinity purified using the immunizing peptide prior to use. Antibody binding to tissue was visualized using an indirect technique involving biotin anti-sheep Ig, and streptavidin /

biotin peroxidase complex. Controls for non-specific binding employed the use of the antiserum pre-incubated with an excess of synthetic peptide.

## RESULTS.

### In Situ Hybridisation to the HSR in the NBL Kelly Cell Line using a Biotinylated N-myc Probe pNb-1.

G-banding of the Kelly cell line revealed a pseudodiploid karyotype, 60% of cells having 46 chromosomes. All cells were apparently nullisomic for chromosome 17 and part of the long arm of chromosome 7 (being 7q-, -7) and trisomic for chromosome 22 and part of the long arm of chromosome 1 (being 1q+, +1p-q+). Additionally, all cells carried three marker chromosomes, a small telocentric, a medium metacentric, both of unidentified origin and a large sub-telocentric with an extensive central HSR occupying approximately 85% of the chromosome. Giemsa banding of this marker showed one dark and one light band distal to the HSR, and a pale region with a centromere and a small pale short arm proximal to the HSR. This pattern is consistent with the HSR having inserted at 17q21. Ninety percent of cells carried two copies of this HSR bearing marker chromosome. Sixty percent of cells had an 11q+ chromosome and 40% had 2 copies of the metacentric marker chromosome. Some variation in chromosome number occurred in chromosomes 2 to 15 and X but not in chromosomes 4, 8, 12, 16, and 18 to 22 where 2 copies were present in every cell examined.

Under bright field illumination, after hybridisation with the biotinylated N-myc probe, HSRs stained purple while non-HSR bearing chromosomes remained completely unstained. The purple colouration of HSRs was also seen in those preparations which had not been previously stained with Giemsa. The intensity of staining of HSRs was greatly enhanced by phase contrast illumination which also permitted visualization of the unstained chromosomes (Fig.1). The in situ procedure did not appear to significantly affect chromosome morphology. Although the Giemsa staining of HSRs in this cell line was quite

homogeneous, well marked striations were evident
in many HSRs after in situ hybridisation with N-
myc. Striations were visible most frequently in
those metaphases with well elongated chromosomes,
dividing the HSR into several (usually 5)
alternating stained and unstained blocks.
Hybridisation with biotinylated lambda DNA, used
as a negative control under identical conditions,
produced no staining of the HSRs or of any other
chromosome.

Figure 1. In situ hybridisation of a N-myc probe
to HSRs in chromosome 17 shows a periodicity in
the hybridisation pattern.

**CHROMOSOME 17**

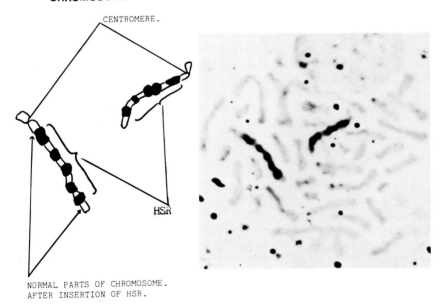

NORMAL PARTS OF CHROMOSOME.
AFTER INSERTION OF HSR.

## Identification of a Single Gene Copy by a Non-Isotopic In Situ Hybridisation Technique.

For single copy detection of the B-nerve
growth factor (NGF) gene a genomic, 7Kb insert
probe in pBr322 was used. This was labelled with
biotin-11-dUTP by standard nick translation and
purified by ethanol precipitation. The single
strand length of the biotinylated fragments was

300-600 base pairs as determined by
glyoxal/agarose gel electrophoresis (data not
presented). Metaphase spreads from human
peripheral blood lymphocytes were prepared,
conventionally G-banded and photographed (Fig. 2).
Slides were destained with ethanol, treated with

Figure 2. 7Kb sequence hybridizes to a single copy
of the B-NGF gene on Chromosome 1p13.

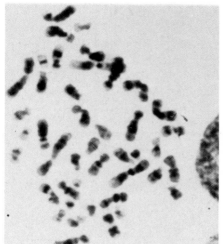
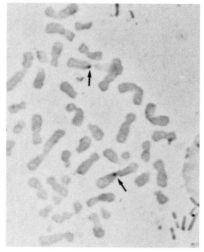

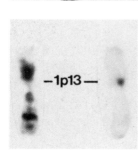

RNAase and In situ hybridisation
performed. The previously
photographed metaphases were
relocated by bright field
microscopy. Discrete deposits of
purple precipitate at the sites
of hybridisation were observed.
These deposits, referred to as
"grains", were most clearly
visualized by standard phase
contrast illumination (Fig.2).
Of 52 metaphases examined, 27 (51%) had at least
one grain deposited on band p13 of chromosome 1.
The background staining was minimal with an
average of only 2.5 grains per metaphase.Signal to
noise ratios were calculated by dividing the total
number of grains at 1p13 by the expected number of
grains per band, assuming a random grain
distribution and using a standard 311 G-band

ideogram. The optimal signal to noise ratio of
100:1 was achieved with a probe concentration of
50ng/10ul; higher concentrations only increased
the background observed.
     The localization of the B-NGF gene to
chromosome band 1p13 by this non-isotopic method
is consistent with a previous autoradiographic
study on normal human chromosomes, which reported
specific labelling over bands 1p13-1p22.

Figure 3. Localization of a single copy of the N-
myc gene to 2p24 using a 1 Kb insert (pNb1).

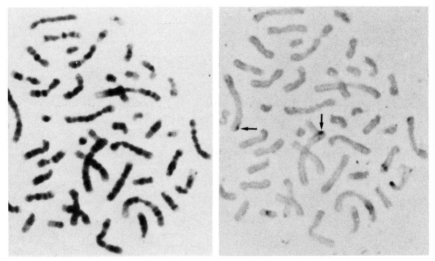

The high signal to noise ratio
obtained with the 7Kb B-NGF
target sequence suggested that
even smaller unique sequences
might be detectable using this
technique. We therefore
proceeded to biotinylate the
plasmid pNB-1, which contains a
1Kb EcoR1-BamH1 fragment of the
N-myc oncogene in pBr322.
The biotinylated probe was hybridized in situ to
human metaphase chromosomes as described above
(Fig.3). Of 100 metaphases examined, 20 had at
least 1 grain deposited on band p24 of chromosome
2. The overall signal to noise ratio, although
lower than that obtained with the larger B-NGF

probe, remained acceptable at approximately 20:1
(Fig.4). Optimal probe concentration with
biotinylated pNb-1 was somewhat higher
(100ng/10ul) than with the B-NGF probe. Schwab et
al. using a tritiated probe in situ, have
previously mapped the N-myc gene to the region
2p23-2p24. The present study shows a signal peak
at band 2p24 only, thus demonstrating the superior
spatial resolution that can be obtained by
avoiding the silver grain scatter inevitably
associated with even the thinnest autoradiographic
emulsion.

Figure 4. Signal to noise ratio obtained using
pNb1 to identify a single copy of the N-myc gene.

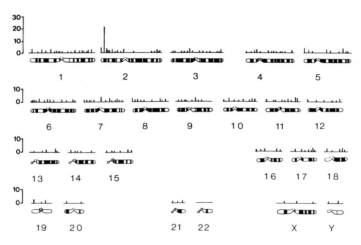

        Single copy localization was also achieved
with a third probe containing a 2.5Kb insert. The
overall signal to noise ratio obtained in this
case was 34:1. Plotting signal to noise ratio
against size of the hybridising sequence of these
3 probes gives an approximately linear
relationship over the range 1Kb-7Kb (Fig.5).
Although extrapolation beyond this range must
remain speculative, the slope of the line suggests
that unique sequences even smaller than 1Kb may be
detectable. The lower detection limit of this in
situ technique thus appears, unlike earlier non-
isotopic systems, to be comparable to that of high
specific activity tritiated probes which can

detect as little as 0.5 Kb of target sequence. In
addition to this extraordinary sensitivity (1Kb =
approximately 10-18g of DNA), streptavidin-
alkaline phosphatase detection has the added
advantage of being a simple one step procedure, in
contrast to alternative antibody based indirect
immunoperoxidase methods.

Figure 5, Linear
relationship between probe
size and signal to noise
ratio.

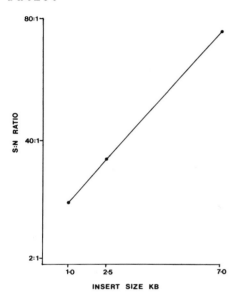

Whether this
technique can be
adapted to analyze
gene amplification in
either the interphase
nucleus or ultimately
in frozen sections
remains to be
elucidated. In
addition our attempts
at in situ
hybridisation to RNA
in tissue sections
have not proved
successful.
Northern blot analysis
on tissues would
suggest this failure
is due to the quality
of the material under
review. Biopsy or
autopsy material has
not been obtained in a
sufficiently fresh
state to prevent
degradation of mRNA.

As an alternative approach to studying N-myc
gene expression we have examined tissues with an
antiserum to a synthetic peptide sequence present
in the gene product. Studies with this reagent
have revealed heterogeneity in N-myc gene
expression in individual cells in both cell lines
(Kelly) and fresh biopsy samples. Using this
reagent we have also confirmed an earlier
observation that N-myc amplification/over
expression can occur in rhabdomyosarcoma (Garson
et al.1986). Whilst 15 primary medulloblastomas
examined have not shown amplification,

approximately 50% appear to over express the N-myc gene product.

While the use of the antiserum to study gene expression is less complex than mRNA analysis these studies are not without difficulty. The short half life of the N-myc gene product (approx, 30min) means that if tissue is badly preserved false negatives may be obtained. The fact that we have been able to identify the N-Myc gene product in this instance possibly reflects our success in obtaining freshly frozen biopsy material.

Table 1. N-myc protein analysis by immunohistology with an antiserum to a synthetic peptide in the hydrophylic region of the protein.

| Tumour | Positive/Total |
|--------|----------------|
| Neuroblastoma | 5/14 (3 Equiv) |
| Rhabdomyosarcoma | 1/12 |
| Retinoblastoma | 1/3 |
| Medulloblastoma | 6/12 (1 Equiv) |
| Lymphoma | 0/3 |

## DISCUSSION.

In situ hybridisation using radioactive probes, while offering high sensitivity, suffers several disadvantages including prolonged autoradiographic exposure times and limited spatial resolution. To overcome these difficulties several non-radioactive systems have been introduced using a variety of immunogenic, fluorescent and enzymatic labels but none have achieved the sensitivity of the technique described above. This exploits the specific and essentially irreversible interaction between biotin and streptavidin ($K_D = 10^{-15}$M) (Leary et al 1983), together with a highly sensitive, one step enzyme amplification system. It produces a permanent preparation which can be viewed without resort to special reflection contrast (Landegent et al 1985) or fluorescent microscopy (Bauman et al. 1981). The technique is compatible with prior G-banding, providing better definition than either pre-Lipsol or post-Wrights banding, so permitting

the use of routinely G-banded clinical material
for in situ experiments.

The excellent spatial resolution provided by
this technique has revealed a previously
undescribed periodic microstructure within HSRs.
The striations observed here have not been
reported in earlier autoradiographic studies of
HSRs in either drug resistant or tumour cell lines
(Schwab et al. 1984). Although the nature of the
non hybridising DNA between the blocks of N-myc
bearing sequences remains unknown, recent
molecular studies on the HSR of the human
neuroblastoma cell line IMR-32 may be relevant
(Shiloh et al 1985). They demonstrated that the
IMR-32 HSR located on chromosome 1 was constructed
not only of amplified DNA from the immediate
region of the N-myc gene at 2p23-24, but also from
distant sequences located more proximally at 2p13.
They postulated a novel relocation-rejoining
process to account for their findings. The
alternating hybridising and non-hybridising HSR
segments seen here may represent direct
morphological evidence of a similar complex
amplification, relocation and splicing mechanism
operating in the Kelly cell line. Alternatively,
the repeating blocks of non N-myc sequences might
represent amplified satellite DNA, as described
previously in methotrexate resistant mouse cell
lines (Bostock & Clark 1980). That the observed
striations may reflect local variations in probe
accessibility or chromatin compaction, also
remains a possibility that can not at present be
excluded. From photomicrographic measurements we
estimate the size of the N-myc amplicon in the
Kelly cell line to be approximately $1.5 \times 10^3$ Kb.
This figure is in broad agreement with previous
estimates of amplicon size in other neuroblastoma
cell lines (Brodeur & Seeger 1986). These
observations have been made whilst attempting to
develop in situ hybridisation techniques that are
sensitive enough to detect N-myc amplification in
frozen sections. We have not been successful in
this aim to date. In addition, due to the
inadequate preservation of our biopsy material we
have been unsuccessful at in situ studies looking
for overexpression of N-myc mRNA. As an
alternative we have explored the use of an

antiserum to a synthetic peptide sequence present in the gene product. This has shown over-expression of the N-myc gene product in neuroblastoma, rhabdomyosarcoma and medulloblastoma. However our preliminary data on the use of this reagent suggests that this approach is also complicated by the labile nature of the protein in vivo (- 30mins). The analysis of N-myc amplification and overexpression in tissue sections is therefore complex and to understand the variation that may occur on a cell to cell basis more detailed studies are necessary.

## ACKNOWLEDGEMENTS.

This work was supported by the Imperial Cancer Research Fund. We thank S. Watts for preparing this manuscript.

## REFERENCES.

Bauman JGJ, Wiegant J, Duijn P, Lubsen NH, Sondermeijer PJA, Henning W, Kubli E (1981). Rapid and high resolution detection of in situ hybridization to polytene chromosomes using fluorochrome labelled RNA. Chromosoma 84:1-18.

Brodeur G, Seeger R, Schwab M, Varmus V, Bishop J (1984). Amplification of N-myc in untreated human neuroblastomas correlates with advanced disease stage. Science 224:1121-1125.

Brodeur GM, Seeger RC (1986). Gene amplification in human neuroblastomas: Basic mechanisms and clinical implications. Cancer Genet Cytogenet 19:101-111.

Bostock CJ, Clark EM (1980). Satellite DNA in large marker chromosomes of methotrexate resistant mouse cells. Cell 19:709-715.

Garson JA, McIntyre P, Clayton J, Kemshead, JT (1986). N-myc oncogene amplification in rhabdomyosarcoma at relapse. Lancet i. 1496.

Garson JA, van den Berghe JA, Kemshead JT (1987).
High resolution in situ hybridization technique
using biotinylated N-myc oncogene probe reveals
periodic structure of HSRs in human
neuroblastoma. Cancer Genet Cytogenet. In Press.

Landegent JR, Jansen in de wal N, Ommen GJB, Baas
F, De vijlder JM, van duijn P, van der ploeg M
(1985). Chromosomal localization of a unique
gene by non autoradiographic in situ
hybridization. Nature 317:175-177.

Leary JJ, Brigati DJ, Ward DC (1983). Rapid and
sensitive colorimetric method for visualizing
biotin labelled DNA probes hybridized to DNA or
RNA immobilized on nitrocellulose Bio blots.
Proc Natl Acad Sci USA 80:4045-4049.

Schwab M, Alitalo K, Klempnauer KH, Varmus HE,
Bishop JM, Gilbert F, Brodeur G, Goldstein M,
Trent J (1984). Amplified DNA with limited
homology to myc cellular oncogene is shared by
human neuroblastoma cell lines and a
neuroblastoma tumour. Nature 305:245-248.

Shiloh Y, Shipley J, Brodeur GM, Bruns G, Korf B,
Danlon T, Schrek RR, Seeger R, Sakai K, Latt SA
(1985). Differential amplification assembly and
relocation of multiple DNA sequences in human
neuroblastomas and neuroblastoma cell lines.
Proc Natl Acad Sci USA 82:3761-3765.

Advances in Neuroblastoma Research 2, pages 165–173
© 1988 Alan R. Liss, Inc.

THE neu GENE IN 4 HUMAN NEUROBLASTOMA CELL LINES

Henry C. Maguire Jr., Erica Sibinga, David Weiner
and Mark Greene

Department of Pathology and Laboratory Medicine
University of Pennsylvania School of Medicine
Philadelphia, PA 19104

INTRODUCTION

Ethylnitrosourea (ENU) is a point mutagen and carcinogen (Rajewski,1983; Singer and Kusmierek,1982). When it was given to BDIX rats on the 15th day of their gestation, these rats developed neuroblastomas in high incidence as adults (Schubert et al.,1982).

Shih et al.(1981) tested the ability of samples of DNA, taken from 4 different ENU-induced rat neuroblastomas, to induce the malignant phenotype when transfected into NIH-3T3 cells. Three of these tumors gave positive results, thereby implying that an oncogene, now designated neu, was responsible for the rat neuroblastomas. When the donor DNA was digested with Hind III, Bam I or XhoI (but not with Eco RI) the ability to induce malignant transformation was lost.

Polyclonal and monoclonal antibodies, induced by immunization with neu transfected cells, have identified the neu encoded product as a transmembrane protein, p185. Cloning and sequence data demonstrate that neu has strong homology with the epidermal growth factor (EGF) receptor (Padhy et al.,1982; Drebin et al.,1984; Schechter et al.,1984). P185 has tyrosine kinase activity, and its organization suggests that it is a receptor for an as yet unidentified growth factor (Stern et al.,1986). Our laboratory has studied the tissue distribution of p185 during fetal development and in the newborn period (Kokai et al.,1987). P185 appears in the CNS on gestational day 14, lasts for 2 days, and then rapidly disappears. It is noteworthy that peak expression of p185 and highest susceptibility

of the rat CNS to neuroblastoma induction by ENU both occur
on day 15 of gestation; probably, expression of the neu gene
renders it physically accessible to ENU.

The neu induced malignant phenotype requires surface
expression of the oncogene product, p185. Thus, monoclonal
antibodies, with specificity for extracellular domains of p185,
that down-regulated p185 expression also profoundly inhibited
the ability of neu transformed cells to grow on semi-solid
media, or to form tumors in nude mice or in syngeneic rats
(Drebin et al.,1985; Drebin et al.,1986).

The rat neu oncogene is derived from the neu proto-oncogene by a single point mutation that specifies an A→T
transversion at nucleotide position 2012 (12). This results
in a valine→glutamic acid change at amino acid residue 664, a
site located in the presumptive transmembrane region of the
molecule. Exactly how this substitution of a hydrophilic for a
hydrophobic amino acid perturbs the molecule in situ, leading
to acquisition of the malignant phenotype, is not understood.

The human neu gene (also called HER-2 and erbB-2) has
been identified and sequenced. It is located on chromosome
17q21, near to erbA, and shows about 90% homology with the rat
neu. Recent studies by several groups have shown amplification
of neu gene sequences and mRNA in human tumor cell lines
(stomach carcinoma, breast carcinoma, salivary gland carcinoma)
and in human tissue samples (King et al.,1985; Coussens et
al.,1985; Semba et al.,1985; Fukushige et al.,1986; Yokota et
al.,1986; Van der Vijver et al.,1987; Kraus et al.,1987); this
amplification is restricted to cancers arising from secretory
epithelia. In one investigation of breast carcinomas, substantial amplification of the neu gene in breast tumor tissue
correlated with a poorer patient prognosis (Slamon et al.,1987).

We have examined neu in the genomic DNA derived from 4
human neuroblastoma cell lines. As compared to human placental
DNA, neu was increased about twofold. A large amplification
of neu, comparable to that which has been noted with N-myc in
many of these lines and in other neuroblastomas, was not seen.


METHODS

1. Four neuroblastoma cell lines that had been stored in liquid nitrogen were obtained from Dr. Audrey Evans (CHOP);
   these were CHP 100 (a peripheral neuroectodermal tumor),

IMR-5, CHP 134B and CHP 382. The cells were thawed and transferred to culture flasks in the routine way. They were maintained in HY media supplemented with 10% FBS, 1% gluta-mine, 1% OPI (oxaloacetic acid, pyruvic acid, insulin) and penicillin/streptomycin. Aliquots of 50-100 x $10^6$ neuro-blastoma cells were harvested by trypsinization, washed 3 times in physiological saline and stored at -70°C.

2. DNA and RNA extractions of tumor cells were performed following the methods outlined in Maniatis et al. (1982) Briefly, cells were lysed in guanidinium thiocyanate, layered on a cesium chloride gradiant and fractionated at 32,000 RPM for 18 hours. The DNA rich band and RNA rich pellet were removed and worked up separately. The RNA pellet was dried, subject to two rounds of precipitation in absolute ethanol and then dissolved in Tris-EDTA (TE) buffer. The DNA was purified by successive extractions with phenol, chloroform and diethyl ether, and then dialyzed against several changes of TE buffer. Ten µg DNA was digested with 20 units of Hind III or 20 units Eco RI. The RNA or DNA fragments were electrophoresed in 1% agarose gel, transferred to a Gene Screen Plus® nylon matrix, and hybridized and rehybridized with probes that were labelled with $^{32}$P. Autoradiographs of DNA preparations were analyzed with a soft laser densitometer (LKB).

Probes - the neu probe represented nucleotide sites 959-1376 of the rat neu-oncogene; the beta actin probe and the N-myc probe have been described (Spiegelman et al., 1983; Schwab et al., 1983). The neu probe was oligo labeled, and the beta actin and N-myc probes were labeled by nick translation.


RESULTS

Four neuroblastoma cell lines were examined for possible amplification of the neu gene. We used a rat neu gene probe that had approximately 90% homology with the human neu gene; preliminary experiments had shown that this rat neu probe would hybridize with human neu DNA and RNA, and would identify highly amplified neu and increased neu expression in a cell line where that was known to occur. The results of one experiment in which a matrix having Hind III digests of CHP-100, IMR-5 and placenta was probed with neu is shown in Figure 1.

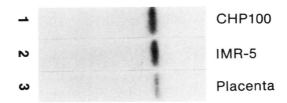

Figure 1.

There was an approximately two-fold increase in neu detected in
the neuroblastoma cell lines as against control human placental
DNA. Digests of CHP 134B, CHP 382 and placental DNA gave a
similar increase in neu; again, removing the neu probe and
rehybridizing with an actin probe demonstrated comparable DNA
in the 3 lanes. The densitometric measurements made from
radio-autographs of the neu hybridized neuroblastoma and
placental DNA digests are summarized in Table I.

|          | EcoRI | Hind III |
|----------|-------|----------|
| Placenta | 1.0   | 1.0      |
| 382      | 2.4   | 2.5      |
| CH 134B  | 2.2   | 1.8      |
| IMR 5    | 2.3   | 2.4      |
| CHP 100  | 2.8   | 4.3      |

TABLE I. Hybridization of the neu probe to digests of DNA from
neuroblastoma cell lines and from human placenta, the values are
normalized to placenta DNA=1.0.

With both Eco RI and Hind III digests about a two-fold increase in neu is seen in the neuroblastomas as against a human
placental DNA standard.

    In a separate experiment, Eco RI and Hind III digests of
DNA from each of the four neuroblastoma cell lines and from a
placenta standard were probed with N-myc.  Three of the four
neuroblastoma cell lines viz. CHP 382, IMR-5 and CHP 134B,
showed many-fold amplification of N-myc (Figure 2.).

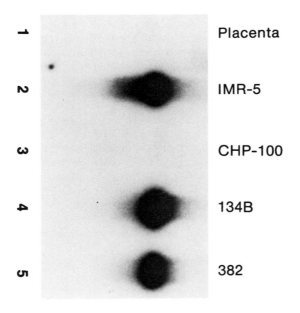

Figure 2.

Amplification of N-myc and its increased mRNA expression in CHP
134, as well as increased mRNA expression of c-myc (with no
amplification or increased mRNA expression of N-myc) in CHP 100
has been reported (Kohl et al., 1983; Nisen et al., 1986).

Studies of RNA from the four neuroblastoma cell lines were done utilizing Northern blots and hybridization with the neu probe. No substantial increase in neu m-RNA expression was found.

DISCUSSION

Analysis of DNA extracted from 4 human neuroblastoma cell lines indicated an approximately twofold increase in neu, when compared to human placental DNA. A substantial amplification of neu, that has been seen in a subset of malignant tumors of secretory cell origin was not found (Table I). Three of the 4 cell lines had a many fold amplification of N-myc. Substantial amplification of N-myc was initially described in neuroblastoma cell lines and has since been observed in neuroblastoma tumor tissue, where it connotes a poor prognosis. Transfection experiments have demonstrated that increased N-myc expression can contribute to the malignant phenotype (Bernards, R. et al.,1986). Thus, transfection of multiple copies of N-myc into the rat ENU-induced neuroblastoma, B-104, substantially increased the growth rate, invasiveness and lethality of B-104 tumors in nude mice. It is likely that a similar event occurs in the human disease. We hypothesize that a subset of human neuroblastomas arise, as do the rat ENU-induced neuroblastomas, from a carcinogen-induced pertinent mutation in the neu gene, the result being an unregulated increase in the activity of the tyrosine kinase domain of the human p185 neu-encoded gene product and malignant transformation.

The role of increased neu expression in the initiation and accentuation of the malignant phenotype is unclear. In the case of the rat neu oncogene, transfectants with 50-100 copies of the proto-oncogene and with the expected high expression of the gene product did not result in the malignant phenotype, whereas a single copy of the neu oncogene, without increased expression, is associated with characteristic in vitro and in vivo changes of malignancy (Bargmann et al., 1986). However, it has recently been reported that transfection of a construct, that markedly increases expression of the human neu (erbB-2), leads to malignant transformation of NIH 3T3 transfected cells (DiFiore et al., 1987).
The human and rat neu gene products have a similar organization and have a close homology. Limited experience suggests that monoclonal antibodies having high reactivity for extracellular domains of the rat p185 react, with rather low affinity, with epitopes on the human p185. Thus, although

there is some cross-reactivity, it would clearly be desirable to have monoclonals specifically raised against epitopes on the human p185, and especially against epitopes on the extra-cellular domain of this protein. These antibodies could be unique diagnostic and therapeutic tools if, as in the rat neuroblastoma, some human tumors require the neu gene-encoded product on the cell surface for maintenance of the malignant phenotype. The generation of antibodies against the human p185 is under way in our laboratory.

In summary, we have found that there is no substantial increase in gene copies or of mRNA expression of neu in four human neuroblastoma cell lines. This suggests that insofar as an abnormal neu contributes to the malignant phenotype of human neuroblastomas, it is by a product of the mutated proto-onco-gene. ENU induced rat neuroblastomas provide a well-studied precedent for this.

REFERENCES

Bargman CI, Hung MC, Weinberg RA (1986). Multiple independent activations of the neu oncogene by a point mutation altering the transmembrane domain of p185. Cell 45:649-657.
Bernards R, Dessain SK, Weinberg RA (1986). N-myc amplifi-cation causes down-modulation of MHC Class I antigen expression in neuroblastoma. Cell 47:667-674.
Coussens L, Yang-feng TL, Liao Y-C, Chen E, Gray A, McGrath J, Seeburg PH, Libermann TA, Schlessinger J, Francke U, Levinson A, Ullrich A (1985). Tyrosine kinase receptor with extensive homology to EGF receptor shares chromosomal loca-tion with neu oncogene. Science 230:1132-1139.
Di Fiore PP, Pierce JH, Kraus MH, Segatto O, King CR, Aaronson SA (1987). ErbB-2 is a potent oncogene when overexpressed in NIH-3T3 cells. Science 237:178-182.
Drebin J, Stern DF,Link VC, Weinberg RA, Greene MI (1984). Monoclonal antibodies identify a cell surface antigen associ-ated with an activated cellular oncogene. Nature 312:545-548.
Drebin JA, Link VC, Stern DF, Weinberg RA, Greene MI (1985). Down-modulation of an oncogene protein product and reversion of the transformed phenotype by monoclonal antibodies. Cell 41:695-706.
Drebin JA, Link VC, Weinberg RA, Greene, MI (1986). Inhibition of tumor growth by a monoclonal antibody reactive with an on-cogene-encoded tumor antigen. Prod Natl Acad Sci 82:9129-9133.

Fukushige S-I, Matsubara K-I, Yoshiba M, Sasaki M, Suzuki T, Semba K, Toyoshima K, Yamamoto T (1986). Localization of a novel v-erbB-related gene, c-erbB-2, on human chromosome 17 and its amplification in a gastric cancer cell line. Mol. and Cell. Biol 6:955-958.

King CR, Kraus MH, Aaronson SA (1985). Amplification of a novel v-erbB-related gene in a human mammary carcinoma. Science 229:974-976.

Kohl NE, Kanda N, Schreck RR, Bruns G, Latt SA, Gilbert F, Alt FW (1983). Transposition and amplification of oncogene related sequences in human neuroblastomas. Cell 35:359-367.

Kokai Y, Cohen J, Drebin JA, Greene MI. Stage and tissue specific expression of the neu oncogene in rat development. Submitted for publication.

Kraus MH, Popescu NC, Amsbaugh SC, King CR (1987). Overexpression of the EGF receptor-related proto-oncogene erbB-2 in human mammary tumor cell lines by different molecular mechanisms. EMBO Journal 6:605-610.

Maniatis T, Futseb EF, Sambrook J (1982). Molecular Cloning: A Laboratory Manual. Cold Spring Harbor Laboratory Publications.

Nisen PD, Zimmerman KA, Cotter SV, Gilbert F, Alt FW (1986). Enhanced expression of the N-myc gene in Wilm's Tumors. Cancer Research 46:6217-6222.

Padhy LC, Shih C, Cowing D, Finkelstein R, Weinberg RA (1982). Identification of a phosphoprotein specifically induced by the transforming DNA of rat neuroblastomas. Cell 28:865-871.

Rajewski MF (1983). Structural modifications and repair of DNA in neuro-oncogenesis by N-Ethyl-N-nitrosourea. Recent Results in Cancer Research 84:63-76.

Schechter AL, Stern DF, Vaidyanathan L, Decker SJ, Drebin JA, Greene MI, Weinberg RA (1984). The neu oncogene: an erb-B-related gene encoding a 185,000 - Mr tumour antigen. Nature 312: 513-516.

Schubert D, Heinermann S et al. (1974). Clonal cell lines from the rat central nervous system. Nature 249:224-227.

Schwab M, Alitalo K, Klempnauer KH, Varmus HE, Bishop JM, Gilbert F, Brodeur G, Goldstein M, Trent J (1983). Amplified DNA with limited homology to myc cellular oncogene is shared by human neuroblastoma cell lines and a neuroblastoma tumor. Nature 305:245-248.

Semba K, Kamata N, Toyoshima K, Yamamoto T (1985). A v-erbB-related protooncogene, c-erbB-2, is distinct from the c-erbB-1/epidermal growth factor-receptor gene and is amplified in a human salivary gland adenocarcinoma. Proc Natl Acad Sci 82:6497-6501.

Shih C, Padhy LC, Murray M, Weinberg R (1981). Transforming genes of carcinomas and neuroblastomas introduced into mouse fibroblasts. Nature 290:261-264.

Singer B, Kusmierek JT (1982) Chemical Mutagenesis. Am. Rev. Biochem. 52:655-693.

Slamon DJ, Clark GM, Wong SG, Levin WJ, Ulbrich A, McGuire WL (1987). Human breast cancer: correlation of relapse and survival with amplication of the HER-2/neu oncogene. Science 235:177-182.

Spiegelman BM, Frank M, Green H (1983). Molecular cloning of mRNA from 3T3 adipocytes. J Biol Chem 258:10083-10089.

Stern DF, Hefferman PA, Weinberg RA (1986). p185, a product of the neu proto-oncogene, is a receptor-like protein associated with tyrosine kinase activity. Mol Cell Biol 6:1729-40.

Van de Vijver M, Vande Bersslaer R, Devilee P, Correlisse C, Petersen J, Nusse R (1987). Amplication of the neu (c-erb-B-2) oncogene in human mammary tumors is relatively frequent and is often accompanied by amplification of the linked c-erb-A oncogene. Mol & Cell Biol 7:2019-2023.

Yokota J, Toyoshima K, Sugimura T, Yamamoto T, Terada M, Battifora H, Cline MJ (April 5, 1986). Amplification of c-erbB-2 oncogene in human adenocarcinomas in vivo. Lancet 765-767.

Advances in Neuroblastoma Research 2, pages 175–184
© 1988 Alan R. Liss, Inc.

# CHROMOGRANIN A EXPRESSION IN CHILDHOOD PERIPHERAL NEUROECTODERMAL TUMORS

Mark J. Cooper,[1] Lee J. Helman,[1] Audrey E. Evans,[2] Sudha Swamy,[1] Daniel T. O'Connor,[3] Lawrence Helson,[4] and Mark A. Israel[1]

[1]Pediatric Branch, National Cancer Inst., Bethesda, MD 20892, [2]Children's Hospital of Philadelphia, PA 19104, [3]University of California & VA Medical Center, San Diego, CA 92161 and [4]ICI Americas, Wilmington, DE 19897

## INTRODUCTION

Primitive neuroectodermal tumors of childhood (PNET) constitute a spectrum of genetically distinct disorders which may be particularly amenable to analysis by molecular genetic techniques. Histologically identical neuroblastoma and peripheral neuroepithelioma are two PNETs that can be distinguished not only on the basis of clinical presentation, but also by differences in proto-oncogene expression, karyotypic abnormalities, HLA expression, and neurotransmitter biosynthetic enzyme profiles (Thiele, et al., 1987). To analyze molecular events involved in neural crest development that may be important in the understanding of these tumors, we have initiated experiments to characterize the spectrum of expression among neural crest tumors of specific genes of interest. For these experiments we have utilized cDNA molecular probes which were known to be expressed in normal adult adrenal medulla but not in primitive neuroblastoma (Helman, et al., 1987a). Our aim was to determine whether patterns of gene expression that may reflect discrete stages in differentiation along a neuro-

endocrine pathway could be found among neuroblastoma cell lines and tumors.  The distribution
of expression of such molecular probes has
recently been reported in normal and malignant
human tissues (Helman, et al., 1987a), and other
such genes have recently been characterized.  One
such gene encodes chromogranin A (Helman, et al.,
1987b), the major acidic protein of neurosecretory chromaffin granules.

In experiments described below, we found
that chromogranin A is expressed at very high
levels in some neuroblastoma cell lines and
tumors.  These levels are similar to those found
in pheochromocytoma and normal adrenal medulla.
In contrast, chromogranin A mRNA was not detected
in other neuroblastoma cell lines and not in any
of seven neuroepithelioma tumor cell lines that
we examined.  These findings contrast with the
pattern of expression of neuron-specific enolase,
a protein that tends to be ubiquitously expressed
in most neuroblastoma and neuroepithelioma cell
lines as well as other malignancies of the
peripheral nervous system, including pheochromocytoma.  Furthermore, we were able to detect
chromogranin A in neuroblastoma cells using
standard immunohistochemical techniques, and some
patients with neuroblastoma have elevated serum
chromogranin A levels.

MATERIALS AND METHODS

Cell Lines

All cell lines were grown in RPMI 1640
supplemented with penicillin, streptomycin,
glutamine, and 15% fetal calf serum.

Northern Analysis

Total cellular RNA was made by the method of
Chirgwin (Chirgwin, et al., 1979) and 30 ug of
total cellular RNA were electrophoresed in 1%

agarose formaldehyde gels, transferred to Nytran membranes, and hybridized to nick translated cDNA probes (specific activity $\cong 10^8$ cpm/ug) for human neuron-specific enolase (kindly provided by E. Ginns, NIH) or human chromogranin A (Helman, et al., 1987b). Filters were hybridized as previously described (Helman, et al., 1987a). Autoradiograms were exposed for 1-14 days at -70°C using Kodak XOMAT film.

Immunohistochemistry

    Cell lines were grown on Lab Tech slides (Miles Scientific) for several days prior to fixation with 2% paraformaldehyde for 5 minutes. Slides were incubated overnight with either a mouse anti-human chromogranin A IgG monoclonal antibody (LK2H10, Boerhinger Mannheim) or a mouse anti-mouse H2 IgG monoclonal antibody (kind gift of Dr. David Sachs, Immunology Branch, NCI). Standard avidin-biotin complex immunoperoxidase techniques were used to detect immunologic reactivity of these antibodies (Vector laboratories).

Serum chromogranin A

    Detection of serum chromogranin A was performed by radioimmunoassay as previously reported (O'Connor and Bernstein, 1984; O'Connor and Deftos, 1986).

RESULTS

    Expression of neuron-specific enolase, a sensitive but nonspecific marker of the neuronal phenotype, can be detected in pheochromocytoma, a neuroendocrine malignancy of the adrenal medulla (Fig. 1, lane 1), and also in three neuroblastoma cell lines (Fig. 1, lanes 3-5) and two neuroepithelioma cell lines (Fig. 1, lane 6-7). No expression is detected by this assay in lung (Fig. 1, lane 2) or most other non-neuronal tissues (data not shown). As with neuron-

specific enolase, chromogranin A mRNA is also
easily detected in pheochromocytoma, but not in
normal lung. In contrast, however, chromogranin
A is detected only in some neuroblastoma cell
lines (Fig. 1, lanes 4,5) but not in all (Fig. 1,
lane 3), and it is not detected in two neuroepithelioma cell lines (Fig. 1, lanes 6,7). Chromogranin A expression is also not detected in five
other neuroepithelioma cell lines in which identical amounts of RNA were examined (data not
shown).

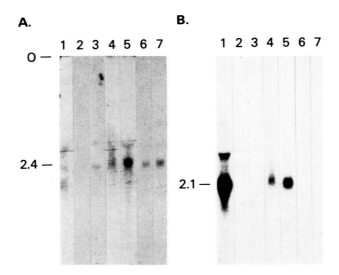

Figure 1. Northern analysis of human tissues
and cell lines. A. Neuron-specific enolase, B.
Chromogranin A. Lane 1, pheochromocytoma; lane
2, lung; lanes 3-5 neuroblastoma cell lines;
lanes 6,7, neuroepithelioma cell lines.


The chromogranin A gene protein product can
be detected in normal and malignant chromaffin
tissues by standard avidin-biotin peroxidase
linked immunohistochemical techniques (Lloyd and
Wilson, 1983). To determine whether chromogranin

A could be immunologically detected in cell lines
of neuroblastoma, a neuroblastoma cell line in
which chromogranin A mRNA had previously been
detected was grown on glass slides, fixed, and
evaluated for chromogranin A expression using a
mouse monoclonal antibody (Fig. 2, panel B). In
this experiment, dark cytoplasmic staining of
cells indicated the expression of chromogranin A
protein. The specificity of this reaction was
demonstrated in a parallel experiment in which a
control mouse monoclonal antibody for mouse H2
determinants was used (Fig. 2, panel A). As
expected, cell lines which do not express chromogranin A mRNA do not stain for chromogranin A
(data not shown).

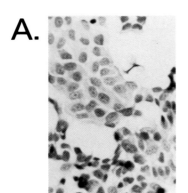 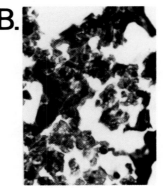

Figure 2. Immunoperoxidase staining for chromogranin A in a neuroblastoma cell line. A. 34-4-
20, mouse anti-mouse H2 monoclonal antibody. B.
LK2H10, mouse anti-human chromogranin A monoclonal antibody.

To extend our analysis of chromogranin A
expression in neuroblastoma, we evaluated pathologic tumor specimens for chromogranin A mRNA.
As expected, chromogranin A mRNA is seen in pheochromocytoma (Fig. 3, lane 1). However, sharply
contrasting levels of chromogranin A mRNA are
detected in the representative neuroblastoma
tumor specimens shown here (Fig. 3, lanes 2,3).

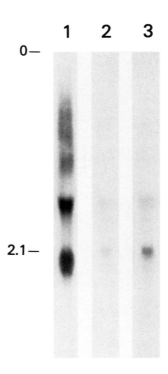

Figure 3.   Northern analysis of pheochromocytoma
and neuroblastoma tumors for chromogranin A.
Lane 1, pheochromocytoma; lane 2-3, neuroblastoma
tumors.

These findings indicate that differences in the level of chromogranin A expression are observed in neuroblastoma tumor specimens, similar to the differences in chromogranin A expression previously noted in neuroblastoma cell lines. Experiments to detect chromogranin A in pathologic specimens by immunohistochemical techniques are currently underway.

Chromogranin A can be detected in the serum of patients with small cell cancer of the lung, pheochromocytoma, and other neuroendocrine tumors (Sobol, et al., 1986; O'Connor and Deftos, 1986), although elevated serum chromogranin A levels have not previously been reported in patients with neuroblastoma. As we were able to detect chromogranin A mRNA in some examples of neuroblastoma cell lines and tumors but not in any neuroepithelioma cell lines, we were interested in evaluating serum from neuroblastoma patients for chromogranin A. In preliminary experiments, we have found that serum from patient 1 (Figure 3, lane 2) has a serum chromogranin A level of 33 ng/ml (normal range, 18-52 ng/ml), whereas patient 2, with increased chromogranin A mRNA in tumor tissue (Figure 3, lane 3) has a remarkably elevated serum chromogranin A level of 284 ng/ml.

DISCUSSION

Multiple prognostic factors that predict clinical outcome have been identified in patients with neuroblastoma. In addition to age > 2 years and advanced stage (Evans, et al., 1971, Breslow and McCann, 1971), poor prognostic factors include amplification of the N-myc oncogene (Brodeur, et al., 1984), elevated serum ferritin levels (Hann, et al., 1980), and elevated serum neuron-specific enolase levels (Zeltzer, et al., 1983). Good prognostic factors include a high urinary vanilmandelic acid: homovanillic acid ratio (Laug, et al., 1978), and histologic evidence of Schwannian differentiation (Shimada, et al., 1985). The appropriate biologic context in which to place these prognostic factors

remains unclear. Some of these factors may
reflect tumor burden, whereas other factors may
relate more directly to the biology of the tumor
as manifested by tissue invasiveness and metastatic potential. One appealing concept is that
some of these prognostic factors and the corresponding clinical behavior which they predict may
also be related to the degree of differentiation
of the tumor.

In this report we present data indicating
that a gene normally expressed in adult adrenal
medulla is expressed in some neuroblastoma cell
lines and tumors, but not in any neuroepithelioma
cell lines. These data contrast to neuron-
specific enolase, which is expressed in most
examples of primitive neuroectodermal tumors.
It is possible that neuroblastoma tumors that
express chromogranin A mRNA have achieved a
greater degree of neuroendocrine differentiation
than chromogranin A negative tumors. These data
may be of clinical significance since evidence of
neuroblastoma tumor maturation can predict
improved survival (Shimada, et al., 1985; Evans,
et al., 1987). To pursue this possibility, we
have begun to analyze serum samples from neuroblastoma patients for chromogranin A. Although
the data are preliminary, abnormal chromogranin A
levels have been detected in the serum of
patients whose tumor specimens express chromogranin A mRNA, whereas normal serum chromogranin
A levels have been noted in patients whose tumors
are chromogranin A negative. The diagnostic and
prognostic value of elevated serum chromogranin A
levels in patients with neuroblastoma is under
study.

REFERENCES

Breslow, N, and McCann, B (1971). Statistical
  estimation of prognosis for children with
  neuroblastoma. Cancer Res 31:2098-2103.
Brodeur, GM, Seeger, RC, Schwab, M, Varmus, HE,
  and Bishop, MJ (1984). Amplification of N-myc
  in untreated human neuroblastomas correlates

with advanced disease stage. Science 224:1121-1124.

Chirgwin, JM, Przybyla, AE, MacDonald, RJ, and Rutter, WJ (1979). Isolation of biologically active ribonucleic acid from sources enriched in ribonuclease. Biochemistry 18(24):5294-5299.

Evans, AE, D'Angio, GJ, Propert, K, Anderson, J, and Hann, HW (1987). Prognostic factors in neuroblastoma. Cancer 59:1853-59.

Evans, AE, D'Angio, GJ, and Randolph, JA (1971). A proposed staging for children with neuroblastoma, Children's Cancer Study Group A. Cancer 27:374-378.

Hann, HWL, Levy, HM, and Evans, AE (1980). Serum Ferritin as a guide to therapy in neuroblastoma. Cancer Res 40:1411-13.

Helman, LJ, Thiele, CJ, Linehan, WM, Nelkin, BD, Baylin, SB, and Israel, MA (1987a). Molecular markers of neuroendocrine development and evidence of environmental regulation. Proc Natl Acad Sci USA. 84:2336-2339.

Helman, LJ, Ahn, TG, Allison, A, Levine, MA, and Israel, MA (1987b). Cloning and sequence of human chromogranin A. Submitted.

Laug, WE, Siegel, SE, Shaw, KNF, Landing, B, Baptista, J, and Gutenstein, M (1978). Initial urinary catecholamine metabolite concentrations and prognosis in neuroblastoma. Pediatrics 62:77-83.

Lloyd, RV and Wilson, BS (1983). Specific endocrine tissue markers defined by a monoclonal antibody. Science 222:628-630.

O'Connor, DT, and Bernstein, KN (1984). Radioimmunoassay of chromogranin A in plasma as a measure of exocytotic sympathoadrenal activity in normal subjects and patients with pheochromocytoma. N Engl J Med 311(12):764-770.

O'Connor, DT, and Deftos, LJ (1986). Secretion of chromogranin A by peptide-producing endocrine neoplasms. N Engl J Med 314(18):1145-1151.

Shimada, H, Aoyama, C, Chiba, T, and Newton, WA (1985). Prognostic subgroups for undifferentiated neuroblastoma: Immunohistochemical study with anti-S-100 protein antibody. Human Pathology 16(5):471-476.

Sobol, RE, O'Connor, DT, Addison, J, Suchocki, K,

Royston, I, and Deftos, LJ (1986). Elevated serum chromogranin A concentrations in small-cell lung carcinoma. Arnals of Internal Medicine 105:698-700.

Thiele, CJ, McKeon, C, Triche, T J, Ross, RA, Reynolds, CP, and Israel, MA (1987). Differential proto-oncogene expression characterizes histopathologically indistinguishable tumors of the peripheral nervous system. J Clin Invest, In press.

Zeltzer, PM, Marangos, PJ, Parma, AM, Sather, H, Palton, A, Siegel, S, Seeger, RC (1983). Raised neuron-specific enolase in serum of children with metastatic neuroblastoma. Lancet 13:361-363.

Advances in Neuroblastoma Research 2, pages 185–194
© 1988 Alan R. Liss, Inc.

DEVELOPMENTALLY REGULATED GENES IN NEUROBLASTOMA

Carol J. Thiele, Lorraine Cazenave,
Joseph B. Bolen,* and Mark A. Israel

Molecular Genetics Section, Pediatric Branch
and *Laboratory of Tumor Virus Biology,
National Cancer Institute, National
Institutes of Health, Bethesda, MD  20892

INTRODUCTION

A number of clinical observations suggest that human
neuroblastoma (NB) tumors may arise in association with
alterations in the  regulation of normal differentiation.
Neuroblastoma in situ, a term used to describe the observation of nests of neuroblasts in the adrenal glands of
infants and young adults autopsied for reasons other than
malignancy, occurs at a frequency which predicts an incidence of NB 40–50 times higher than that clinically
observed (Beckwith and Perrin, 1963; Guin, et al., 1969).
There are documented cases of spontaneous as well as
chemotherapy associated maturation of NB to benign gang-
lioneuronoma (Fox, et al., 1959; Griffin and Bolande,
1969; Evans, et al., 1976).  Stage IVS NB, which presents
as widely disseminated disease in infants usually under
one year of age, frequently resolves without aggressive
anti-cancer therapy (D'Angio, et al., 1971, Evans, et al.,
1980).  Furthermore, NB cell lines can be induced by a
variety of biologic response modifiers to differentiate
morphologically and biochemically in vitro (Prasad, 1980;
Sidell, 1982; Sidell, 1983).  These findings suggest that
NB tumors have not lost or significantly altered the
structural genes important for normal cell growth and
differentiation but rather the regulation of these genes
may be altered in these cells.

To facilitate the evaluation of regulatory mechanisms
involved in the differentiation of NB tumor cells, we
initiated studies to identify and isolate genes regulated

during retinoic acid (RA) induced differentiation of NB
cell lines. In this report we describe the identification
and characterization of several genes that are differentially regulated during RA-induced maturation of human NB.


MATERIALS AND METHODS


Cells and RNA Isolation

Human NB cell line SMS-KCNR (Reynolds, et al., 1986)
was cultured in vitro and treated with 5 uM trans-retinoic
acid (RA) (Sigma Chemical Co., St. Louis) to induce morphological differentiation. Total RNA was isolated from
control (KCNR) and cells treated with RA for 14 days (RA-
KCNR) and fractionated on oligo-d(T)-cellulose columns to
enrich for poly(A) containing RNA species as previously
described (Thiele, et al., 1986).


cDNA Synthesis and Sequence Complexity Analysis

High specific activity ($3x10^8$ cpm/ug) complementary
DNA (cDNA) was synthesized using AMV reverse transcriptase
and $^{32}$P-dCTP (3000Ci/mmol) from a poly(A) RNA template
isolated from RA-KCNR according to Hedrick, S. et al.
(Hedrick, et al., 1984).


Analysis of Hybridization Kinetics

Analytical RNA/cDNA hybridization reactions were
prepared in 0.5 M phosphate buffer pH 7.4, 2mM EDTA (PE)
and 0.2% sodium dodecyl sulfate (SDS) with 10pg $^{32}$P-
labeled RA-KCNR cDNA and 1 ug of poly(A) RNA from KCNR or
RA-KCNR cells. These reactions were aliquoted into micro-
capillary tubes, heat sealed, boiled 10 min. and incubated
at 68°C for varying periods of time. In all cases, $R_0T$
values were corrected to standard salt conditions
(Britten, et al., 1974). At the end of the incubation,
reaction mixtures were diluted into 0.12M PE buffer and
loaded onto a hydroxyapatite columns at 60°C. Single-
stranded DNA which eluted in 0.12M PE and double-stranded
DNA which eluted off the column in 0.12mM PE at 95°C were
precipitated with an equal volume of 10% trichloroacetic

acid containing 1% sodium pyrophosphate and carrier tRNA at 4°C for 15 min. and the precipitates were collected on Millipore filter and counted in 10ml Aquasol (NEN, MA.).

## In Vitro Translation and 2D Gel Analysis

1 ug of poly(A) RNA isolated from KCNR and RA-KCNR was incubated in a rabbit reticulocyte lysate (Promega Biotec, Wisconsin) with $^{35}$S-Methionine (Amersham, IL.) according to manufacturer's instructions for 60 min. at 30°C. Equal amounts (cpm) of the resulting reaction products were analyzed by 2D-polyacrylamide gel electrophoresis (PAGE) essentially as described by O'Farrell (O'Farrell, 1975).

## cDNA Cloning and Isolation

1 ug of poly(A) RNA from RA-KCNR was used to prepare double-stranded cDNA by the method of Gubler and Hoffman (Gubler and Hoffman, 1983). dsDNA was cloned into PUC9 by G-C tailing and transformed into E. coli strain DH1. Approximately 25,000 ampicillin resistant colonies were screened by hybridizing replicated filters with $^{32}$P-labeled RA-KCNR cDNA and $^{32}$P-labeled KCNR cDNA probes according to Mariatis (Mariatis, et al., 1982).

Clones which hybridized to a greater extent with the $^{32}$P-RA-KCNR cDNA, thus reflecting genes whose expression was increased during RA induced differentiation, and those clones which hybridized to a greater extent $^{32}$P-labeled KCNR cDNA, representing genes whose expression was decreased during differentiation were subjected to a second round of differential cDNA screening as described above. Plasmid DNA was isolated from clones which retained this hybridization pattern. These plasmid DNAs were nick-translated to high specific activity (Rigby, et al., 1977) and used to analyze Northern blots.

RESULTS AND DISCUSSION

Analysis of Hybridization Kinetics

Analysis of hybridization kinetics provides information concerning the sequence complexity and distribution
frequency of poly(A) RNAs that characterize a given cell
type. This type of analysis is particularly useful for
comparing the relatedness of poly(A) RNAs from two different cell types. A graph of the heterologous hybridization
reaction between RA-KCNR cDNA and KCNR poly(A) RNAs(o-o)
as well as the homologous hybridization reaction between
RA-KCNR cDNA and RA-KCNR poly(A) RNAs (o-o) is shown in
Fig. 1.

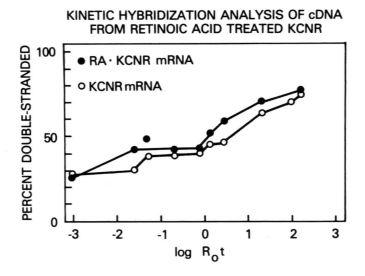

Figure 1. Kinetic hybridization analysis between [32]p-
labeled RA-KCNR cDNA and KCNR mRNA(o-o) or RA-KCNR mRNA
(o-o).

The shape of the curves are similar suggesting a remarkable similarity in the mRNA populations of these two cell types. However, the kinetics of the reaction are different suggesting that different RNA species are not in the same relative abundance in the two populations. This analysis indicates that RA affects the steady-state levels of RNAs and possibly induces new gene transcription.

2-D PAGE Analysis of Proteins in RA-Treated NB Cells

Another method to analyze changes in RNA expression induced by RA is to identify and characterize their protein products. We incubated poly(A) RNAs from KCNR and RA-KCNR cells in a reticulocyte lysate and analyzed the resulting products by 2-D PAGE (Fig. 2). The same amount (cpm) of $^{35}$S-Methionine labeled proteins translated from KCNR and RA-KCNR poly(A)RNAs are pictured in the Panels A and B, respectively. The bracketed areas of each autoradiogram are enlarged to the right. While the general pattern of protein spots is similar in both KCNR and RA-KCNR translation reactions, the circled and numbered areas indicate examples of differences between the gels. Proteins corresponding to spots 1-4 are examples of proteins whose expression is decreased after RA treatment while spots 5-8 indicate proteins whose expression has increased in the differentiated state. Spot 9 has an appearance which may indicate a protein whose isoelectric point has shifted after RA treatment. The shift in the isoelectric point of this protein may be due to the loss or addition of a few peptides, since glycosylation and most other post-translational modifications which alter a protein's charge do not occur in vitro in reticulocyte lysate mediated protein synthesis. These data support the results of the hybridization kinetic analysis and demonstrate that the changes induced by RA reflect changes in the amounts and perhaps types of proteins being produced by NB cells.

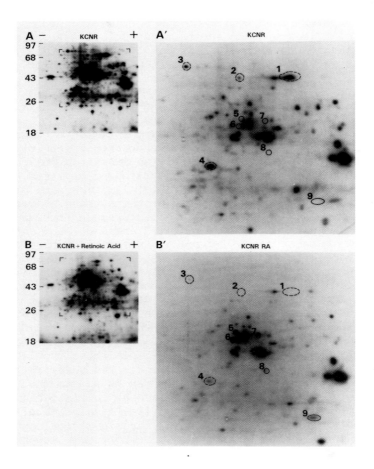

Figure 2. 2D-gel electrophoresis of $^{35}$S-Methionine labeled proteins from KCNR(A) and RA-KCNR(B) mRNA translated in vitro in rabbit reticulocyte lysate. Panels A' and B' are enlargements of the bracketed areas in Panels A and B. The circled and numbered spots indicate proteins that are differentially regulated after RA treatment of KCNR cells.

Isolation of cDNAs Differentially Expressed in RA-Treated
NB Cells

We prepared a cDNA library from RA-KCNR poly(A) RNAs
and used differential cDNA hybridization to identify
bacterial colonies which carried plasmids encoding genes
differentially expressed in morphologically differentiated
NB cells.  Fig. 3 illustrates four such genes.  The data
in panels A and B demonstrate genes in which the steady-
state levels of their mRNA are increased during RA
treatment.  Panel A describes a gene, C1, which encodes a
mRNA of approximately 3.4kb.  The expression of C1 is
first detected in 30 ug of total RNA at day-4 (lane 3) of
RA treatment.  Panel B identifies a gene, G1, which
encodes a 5.4kb mRNA that is first detected at day-2 (lane
2) of RA treatment and is maximally expressed by day-4
(lane 3).  Previously we have shown that after 2 days of
RA treatment NB cells are growth arrested and there are no
obvious signs of morphological differentiation in the NB
cells.  After 4 days in RA, 75% of the NB cells have
extended processes and by day-6 an extensive network of
processes has been established (Thiele, et al., 1985).  In
this preliminary analysis, G1 appears to be expressed
prior to the dramatic phenotypic changes in the RA differentiated NB cells, while C1 appears to be expressed
coincident with these changes.

Panels C and D (Fig.3) are examples of genes whose
expression is decreased during RA-induced differentiation
of NB cells.  F10 encodes a 2.2kb mRNA which seems to be
markedly decreased at day-10 (Panel C, lane 3), while G3
encodes an approximately 1.2kb mRNA which is markedly
reduced at day-2 of RA treatment (Panel D, lane 2).  Thus,
G3 may be a gene associated with the altered growth rate
of the NB cells.

CONCLUSIONS

We have characterized the populations of RNAs in RA
differentiated NB cell lines and shown after 14 days of
RA treatment marked changes in gene expression can be
detected.  These changes may be recognized by both
increases and decreases of particular genes and their
protein products.

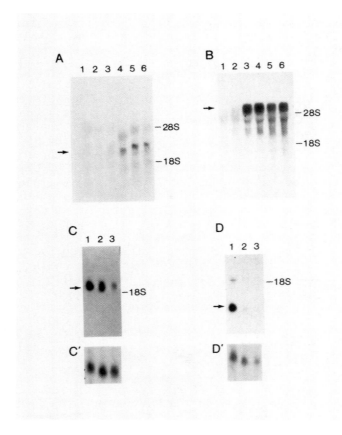

Figure 3. Northern blots of KCNR and RA-KCNR RNA hybridized with plasmid DNAs encoding genes differentially
regulated after RA treatment. Panels A and B are Northern
blots containing 30ug of KCNR RNA (lane 1), 2 days RA-KCNR
(lane 2), 4 days RA-KCNR (lane 3), 6 days RA-KCNR (lane
4), 9 days RA-KCNR (lane 5) and 12 days RA-KCNR (lane 6)
and hybridized with $^{32}$P-labeled C1 and G1 plasmid DNA,
respectively. Panels C and D are Northern blots containing 30ug of KCNR RNA (lane 1), 2 days RA-KCNR RNA (lane 2)
and 10 days RA-KCNR RNA (lane 3), hybridized with $^{32}$P-
labeled F10 and G3 plasmid DNAs, respectively and panels
C' and D' are the above Northern blots re-hybridized with
$^{32}$P-labeled actin plasmid DNA.

Since RA treatment of NB cell lines causes both growth arrest and differentiation of tumor cells (Thiele, et al., 1985), the types of genes which we have isolated may encode proteins which are important for these two crucial cell processes. Such genes might encode proteins associated with cell growth or genes whose products are associated with specific neural features such as neuro-transmitter biosynthetic enzymes, receptors or ion channels. Currently we are characterizing the primary structural features of these genes and determining their pattern of expression in normal cells as well as tumor cell lines.

REFERENCES

Beckwith, JB, Perrin, EV (1963). In situ neuroblastomas: A contribution to the natural history of neural crest tumors. Am J Pathol 43:1089-1104.

Britten, RJ, Graham,DE and Neufeld, BP (1974). Analysis of repeating DNA sequences by reassociation. Meths Enzymol 29:363-418.

D'Angio, GJ, Evans, AE, Koop, CE (1971). Special pattern of widespread neuroblastoma with a favourable prognosis. Lancet 1:1046-1049.

Evans, AE, Gerson, J, Schnaufer, L (1976). Spontaneous regression of neuroblastoma. Natl Cancer Inst Monogr 44:49-54.

Evans, AE, Chatten, J, D'Angio, GJ, et al. (1980). A review of 17 IV-S neuroblastoma patients at the Children's Hospital of Philadelphia. Cancer 45:833-839.

Fox, F, Davidson, J, Thomas, LB (1959). Maturation of sympathicoblastoma into ganglioneuroma. Cancer 12:108-116.

Griffin, ME, Bolande, RP (1969). Familial neuroblastoma with regression and maturation to ganglioneurofibroma Pediatrics 43:377-382.

Gubler, V, and Hoffman, BJ, (1983). Gene 25:263-269.

Guin, GH, Gilbert, EF, Jones, B (1969). Incidental neuroblastoma in infants. Am J Clin Pathol 51:126-136.

Hedrick, SM, Cohen,DI, Nielson, EA, and Davis, MM (1984). Isolation of cDNA clones encoding T-cell specific membrane-associated proteins. Nature 308:149-153.

Maniatis, T, Fritsch, EF and Sambrook, J (1982). Molecular cloning: A laboratory manual (Cold Spring

Harbor Laboratory, Cold Spring Harbor, New York).

O'Farrell, PH (1975). High resolution two-dimensional electrophoresis of proteins. J Biol Chem 250:4007.

Prasad, KN (1980). Control mechanisms of malignancy and differentiation in cultures of nerve cells. In Evans, AE, (ed): "Advances in neuroblastoma research," New York: Raven Press, pp 135-144.

Reynolds, CP, Beidler, JL, Spengler, VA, Reynolds, DA, Ross, RA, Frenkel, RA, and Smith, RG, (1986). Characterization of human neuroblastoma cell lines established before and after therapy. J Natl Cancer Inst 76: 375-387.

Rigby, PW, Dieckmann, M, Rhodes, C, Berg, P, (1977). Labeling deoxyribonucleic acid to high specific activity in vitro by nick translation with DNA polymerase I. J Mol Biol 113(1):237-251.

Sidell, N (1982). Retinoic acid-induced growth inhibition and morphologic differentiation of human neuroblastoma cells in vitro. J Natl Cancer Inst 68:589-596.

Sidell, N, Altman, A, Haussler, MR, et al. (1983). Effects of retinoic acid (RA) on the growth and phenotypic expression of several human neuroblastoma cell lines. Exp Cell Res 148:21-30.

Thiele, CJ, Reynolds, CP, and Israel, MA, (1985). Decreased expression of N-myc precedes retinoic acid induced morphological differentiation of human neuroblastoma. Nature (London) 313:404-406.

Thiele, CJ, Whang-Peng, J, Kao-Shan, CS, et al. (1986). Translocation of the c-sis oncogene in peripheral neuroepithelioma. Cancer Genet Cytogenet 21:185-208.

Advances in Neuroblastoma Research 2, pages 195–199
© 1988 Alan R. Liss, Inc.

DISCUSSION

Chairman:     Bernard Mechler

Discussants:  J.T. Kemshead,  H.C. McGuire,
              M.J. Cooper,  C.J. Thiele

Dr. Seeger (Los Angeles) asked Dr. Cooper if retinoic acid, like dexamethasone, also induced chromogranin transcription in LAN5 cells. Dr. Cooper didn't know for LAN5 cells but said it was not the case for CNR cells. However he said there was considerable plasticity between cell lines in terms of pattern of differentiation. For example, the clone PE9, which is related to chromogranin, was the only one of four dexamethasone inducible genes to be stimulated by retinoic acid. Chromogranin itself was not induced by retinoic acid.

Dr. Brodeur (St. Louis) commented on Dr. McGuire's data on the two fold amplification of the Neu oncogene in neuroblastoma. He quoted Dr. Gilbert's cytogenetic data showing an increased frequency of duplication of chromosomes 17q in neuroblastoma cell lines and suggested that this might account for the modest two-fold amplification. Dr. McGuire stated that cytogenetic analysis had not been done on his cases. Dr. Brodeur said that he had not seen Neu amplified in several hundred cases although they could have missed a 2-fold amplification.

Dr. Reynolds (Los Angeles) noted that there are relatively few single copy N-myc neuroblastoma cell lines available, and asked Dr. Cooper which ones he used. Dr. Cooper said both SKN F1 and SKN AS were provided by Dr. Helson at Memorial Sloan Kettering. Both were derived from adrenal tumors and produced catecholamines. Dr. Reynolds claimed that he had evidence that these two cell lines were more like peripheral neuroepitheliomas (PNETS) than neuroblastoma Dr. Cooper replied that he found no evidence to suggest they were PNETs. Dr. Seeger (UCLA) noted that these lines were negative for N-myc expression but positive for c-MYC, as found in PNETS. Dr. Cooper agreed that they did have that oncogene expression pattern but that PNETS had several other distinguishing markers, including 11:22 translocation, production of cholinergic neurotransmitters, HLA expression, and,

perhaps, absence of expression of thes . chromaffin genes,
features that were not seen in th 2 neuroblastoma cell
lines.

Dr. Barbara A. Spengler (Rye, New York) asked Dr.
Thiele which cell lines she had used. Dr. Thiele
answered SKNAS and LAN 5, both of which had amplified
N-myc.

Dr. Mirkin (Minnesota) commented to Dr. Cooper that
in some animals, such as reptiles, where the adrenal
medulla develops without being enveloped by the adrenal
cortex, there is still development of a chromaffin-like
cell. So the issue is whether it is the presence of
cortical tissue or secretion of corticosteroids that is
responsible for the phenomena observed. Dr. Mirkin asked
if Dr. Cooper had observed the production of methyl
transferase enzymes in conjunction with chromogranin as
would be expected. Dr. Cooper replied that the cell
lines had been sent to Dr. Ross for analysis of
neutrotransmitters, including methyl transferase, and
that none were found. One explanation for this could be
that these enzymes were induced at a later stage than
these cell lines represent.

Dr. Reynolds (Los Angeles) commented that he had
found dopamine and norepinephrine, but not epinephrine,
in several neuroblastoma lines.

Dr. Knudson (Philadelphia) said that the idea of
differing levels of differentiation in neuroblastoma was
very interesting. He had postulated several years ago
that there might be three genes responsible for tumors of
the adrenal medulla: a neuroblastoma gene, a
pheochromocytoma gene and a gene for pheochromocytoma as
it occurs in the MEN2 syndrome. Now Dr. Cooper seems to
be saying there may be more than one NBL tumor. So,
perhaps there are different neuroblastoma genes, not just
different alleles. Is the gene underlying Stage I and II
neuroblastoma different from the one associated with
Stage III and IV tumors? Dr. Cooper replied that all the
data were from Stage IV tumors, but that they planned to
look at Stage I and II tumors. He believes that early
stage disease may represent a different pattern of gene
expression and a different level of differentiation.

Dr. Michitsch (New York) asked Dr. Cooper if
malignant pheochromocytoma might show a transition in the
differentiation markers being studied and so extend the

model of differentiation. Dr. Cooper replied that Dr.
Kelman in their lab had studied 9 to 12 pheochromocytoma
tumor specimens and that one was clearly malignant. The
clone PE9, of the chromaffin related genes, was not
expressed only in the one malignant cell line, so PE9,
might be different between benign and malignant
pheochromocytomas.

Dr. Evans commented about the definition of Stage
IVs Neuroblastoma. Everyone has seen babies with
extensive tumor, with metastases to skin and liver only
and recognized that they are different, and that they
might have a good outlook. In fact, spontaneous
regressions often occur in these babies. She noted cases
reported today of IV-S in a 10 year old and several case
of IV-S with amplified N-myc. Since this staging system
has the same shortcomings of any staging system there
will be cases which fit the clinical definition of IV-S
but which biologically are anything but IV-S. In the
patient with clinical IV-S disease, but with amplified
N-myc in the tumor, diligent search should be made for
evidence of Stage IV disease. Spontaneous resolution may
not occur with IVS disease if accompanied by unfavorable
laboratory features such as elevated ferritin or
amplified N-myc. These children may be incorrectly
staged, not by mistake but by virtue of the imperfect
staging system.

Dr. Dini (Genoa, Italy): The Italian Cooperative
Group recorded two cases of Stage IV-S neuroblastoma in
infants, 6 and 8 months old, with N-myc amplification and
both are free of disease after 23 and 14 months from
diagnosis. One tumor had low amplification (five
copies), the other, high (40 copies). So N-myc
amplification in Stage IV-S is not synonymous with Stage
IV. Dr. Evans asked if the patient with highly amplified
N-myc was treated. Dr. Dini replied that both were
treated with a specific protocol for IVS using low doses
of drugs. Dr. Evans commented that it would be
interesting to see if the IV-S patient with highly
amplified N-myc who was not retreated still had a
spontaneous regression. Dr. Seeger asked Dr. Dini if
they had looked at expression of N-myc in these two
cases. He suggested that if the amplification unit did
not include the whole gene it might not be expressed, and
that before it was concluded that N-myc amplification was
not a bad prognostic factor, N-myc expression should be
measured. Dr. Dini replied that expression was not

measured due to technical difficulties with the tumor samples.

Someone asked if there was any follow-up on IV-S patients with amplified N-MYC. Dr. Seeger replied that the one patient they had had who had amplified N-myc (40 copies) at diagnosis had developed progressive disease and died.

Dr. Bostrom (Minnesota) asked Dr. Cooper if any other cell lines, such as PNET,s had been studied to see if the chromogranin-like genes were induced by dexamethasone. Dr. Cooper replied that TC32 had been examined and the genes were not induced. Dr. Thiele commented that SKNSH cell line does have a detectable level of chromogranin, which is dramatically decreased by treatment with retinoic acid.

Dr. Bernhard Mechler (Mainz, Germany) asked Dr. Cooper if they had more DNA probes which showed differential expression. With further probes and more tumors more stages of differentiation might emerge. Dr. Cooper replied that of several hundred thousand clones screened, twenty fit the criterion of being on pheochromocytoma and not on KCNR. Most of these were duplicates and four were finally isolated.

Dr. Mark Israel (Bethesda) commented that further screening is being done in his lab and that they do have further candidates. He wanted a large battery of tumors to examine; if differentiation is a spectrum, they should be able to define many stages of differentiation. They were trying to work out techniques to analyze tissue samples because there were not enough cell lines to see the full spectrum.

Dr. Israel also commented that in other tumors that are known to have glucocorticoid receptors, like breast cancers, dexamethasone does not turn on chromogranin; the regulation is obviously complex.

Dr. K.T. Montgomery (New York) commented that there is evidence that dexamethasone may act to stabilize some RNA's and that it should be ascertained whether the transcription rate or RNA half-life is increased before assigning the site of regulation.

Dr. Reynolds (Los Angeles): There are a number of agents that induce morphological differentiation. Any of these changes can be duplicated by c-AMP. Dr. Thiele replied that cyclic AMP does cause some similar changes in patterns of protooncogene expression but that detailed analyses of effects on developmental genes or neuronally specific genes are not yet complete.

# BONE MARROW TRANSPLANTATION

Advances in Neuroblastoma Research 2, pages 203–213
© 1988 Alan R. Liss, Inc.

# BONE MARROW TRANSPLANTATION FOR POOR PROGNOSIS NEUROBLASTOMA

Robert C. Seeger, Thomas J. Moss, Stephen A. Feig, Carl Lenarsky, Michael Selch, Norma Ramsay, Richard Harris, John Wells, Harland Sather, and C. Patrick Reynolds.

Departments of Pediatrics (RCS, TJM, SAF, CL, CPR), Medicine (JW), and Radiation Oncology (MS) and the Jonsson Comprehensive Cancer Center, UCLA School of Medicine, Los Angeles, CA 90024; the Department of Pediatrics (NR), University of Minnesota School of Medicine, Minneapolis, MN 55455; the Department of Pediatrics (RH), University of Cincinnati College of Medicine, Cincinnati, OH 45229; and the Children's Cancer Study Group (HS), Pasadena, CA 91101.

## INTRODUCTION

Neuroblastoma, a neoplasm of the sympathetic nervous system, is the most common extracranial tumor of childhood (Young and Miller, 1975). With conventional therapy that includes chemotherapy, local irradiation, and surgery, the disease-free survival for 60% of patients ranges from 0% to 20% (Breslow and McCann, 1971; Evans, 1980; Hayes and Green, 1983; Shimada et al., 1984; Hann et al., 1985; Seeger et al., 1985; Evans et al., 1987). Recent pilot studies of intensive chemotherapy and total body irradiation followed by allogeneic or autologous bone marrow transplantation (BMT) have given encouraging results (August et al., 1984; Philip et al., 1986; Hartmann et al., 1986; Seeger et al., 1987). We report data from two studies in which 58 patients with advanced neuroblastoma underwent intensive four-drug chemotherapy, total body irradiation, and autologous or allogeneic BMT.

**RESULTS AND DISCUSSION**

**CCG-322P.   Intensive multimodal therapy and bone marrow transplantation for newly diagnosed or unresponsive metastatic neuroblastoma.** In our initial study (patient entry January, 1983 to October, 1985), we investigated toxicity and efficacy of VM-26, doxorubicin, L-phenylalanine mustard, cisplatin, and total body irradiation (VAMP-TBI) followed by allogeneic or autologous BMT (Table 1). Thirty-one patients, who all were diagnosed after one year of age and who had stage IV (n=29) or stage III (n=2) disease, were given VAMP-TBI and transplanted.

Table 1.   Pre-transplant Intensive Chemoradiotherapy Regimen (VAMP-TBI)[*].

day -9: cisplatin, 90 mg/m$^2$ IV
day -8: no therapy
day -7: teniposide, 150 mg/m$^2$ IV; doxorubicin, 45 mg/m$^2$ IV
day -6: L-phenylalanine mustard, 140 mg/m$^2$, IV
day -5: L-phenylalanine mustard, 70 mg/m$^2$, IV
day -4: teniposide, 150 mg/m$^2$, IV
day -3: TBI, 3.33 Gy, 5-8 cGy/min
day -2: TBI, 3.33 Gy, 5-8 cGy/min
day -1: TBI, 3.33 Gy, 5-8 cGy/min

[*]For patients <2 yrs old or weighing <12 kg, the doses of cisplatin, teniposide, L-phenylalanine mustard, and doxorubicin are calculated according to weight assuming 1 m$^2$ = 26 kg (eg., cisplatin, 3.5 mg/kg; doxorubicin, 1.7 mg/kg; L-phenylalanine mustard, 5.4 mg/kg and 2.7 mg/kg; teniposide, 5.8 mg/kg).

Twelve patients received bone marrow from HLA-MLC matched, non-identical siblings (median of 3 x 10$^8$ and range of 2-4 x 10$^8$ nucleated marrow cells/kg).  These patients were given methotrexate after BMT for prophylaxis of graft versus host disease (10 mg/m$^2$ on days 1, 3, 6, 11, and then weekly to 100 days).

Nineteen patients received cryopreserved autologous marrow.  Autologous marrow was used for restoration of hematopoiesis only if tumor cells were not detected in an aliquot of the cryopreserved specimen by immunoperoxidase staining with anti-cell surface monoclonal antibodies (mixture of antibodies 390, 459, HSAN 1.2, and 126-4) and anti-neuron specific enolase serum; analysis of $3 \times 10^5$ bone marrow mononuclear cells gives a 95% probability of detecting one neuroblastoma cell among $10^5$ normal cells (Moss et al., 1985; Moss et al., 1987). Marrow was prepared for cryopreservation by equilibrium density centrifugation over Ficoll-Hypaque (patients 1-15) (Wells et al., 1979); by sedimentation and filtration (patient 16); or by sedimentation, filtration, incubation with monoclonal antibodies (390, 459, HSAN 1.2, BA-1, and RB21-7), and then goat anti-mouse immunoglobulin coated magnetic beads (patients 17-19) (Reynolds et al., 1986; Seeger et al., 1987). Recipients of autologous marrow were given a median of $7 \times 10^7$ nucleated marrow cells/kg (range 2 - $54 \times 10^7$ cells/kg).

Severe oral mucositis and enteritis was observed in all patients after treatment with VAMP-TBI. Total parenteral nutrition via central venous catheter was necessary after BMT for all patients because of mucositis, enteritis, and anorexia; for those surviving the first month after transplantation, the median time until parenteral nutrition was discontinued was two months. Skin desquamation was significant in the allogeneic but not in the autologous BMT group.

Early mortality was greatest in the allogeneic group (p = 0.003). Six deaths occurred during the first month after transplantation among the twelve patients undergoing allogeneic BMT. The causes of these early deaths, which all occurred prior to documented engraftment, were renal failure (1), hepatic veno-occlussive disease (2), disseminated aspergillosis (1), disseminated candidiasis (1), and bacterial sepsis (1). Graft versus host disease was not observed in any of the allogeneic marrow recipients. Among the 19 patients receiving autologous marrow, there were no deaths in the first month post transplantation. One patient, who failed to recover platelets even though megakaryocytes were present in the marrow, died from a cerebral hemorrhage three months after BMT (patient 17); and one, who engrafted, died of bacterial sepsis due to suspected child abuse seven months after transplantation (patient 8). Methotrexate given for prophylaxis of graft versus host disease was the most likely cause of the added toxicity with allogeneic BMT, as toxicity would be increased if renal clearance was impaired secondary to chemotherapy (eg., cisplatin), radiation, and/or nephrotoxic antimicrobials.

Survival was significantly better for the 16 patients transplanted before (6 allogeneic and 10 autologous) than for the 15 transplanted after (6 allogeneic and 9 autologous) development of progressive disease (p = 0.004). Estimated survival was 53% at 54+ months for the former group (6 are tumor-free from 25+ to 54+ months after BMT), whereas it was only 7% at 31+ months for the latter. These data indicate that this intensive chemoradiotherapy regimen (VAMP-TBI) must be given relatively soon after diagnosis and before development of progressive disease in order to increase the liklihood of long-term survival.

**CCG-321P3. Treatment of poor prognosis neuroblastoma before disease progression with intensive multimodal therapy and bone marrow transplantation.** In our current study (patient entry October, 1985 to present), we are determining the toxicity and efficacy of aggressive induction chemotherapy followed by VAMP-TBI and BMT. For those requiring autologous BMT, we are investigating the removal of neuroblastoma cells *ex vivo*.

*Induction phase.* The induction therapy for this study is that developed by Green et al. (1986), which utilizes cyclophosphamide, cisplatin, doxorubicin, and teniposide. The estimated progression-free survival for 28 patients after five months is 85%; however, at one year it is 36% for those not undergoing BMT. Although the initial response to this chemotherapy is good, most patients eventually develop progressive disease; based upon this exprience, we recommend beginning the BMT phase of therapy no later than 5 months after diagnosis.

*BMT phase: allogeneic BMT.* Six patients have undergone allogeneic BMT. Two deaths occurred before it was apparent from this study and CCG-322P that delayed clearance of methotrexate is a major contributor to toxicity. Although closely monitored and rescued with leucovorin, a third patient had toxic complications after the day +18 dose of methotrexate that lead to death. It is likely that even partial impairment of renal function secondary to VAMP-TBI and/or other agents results in prolonged elevated levels of methotrexate ($>4 \times 10^{-8}$ M). The three patients who had no complications cleared methotrexate normally; the last of these three was not given doxorubicin and was given only two doses of methotrexate. Based upon our experience, the following changes have been made for recipients of allogeneic marrow: 1) doxorubicin is not given in the pre-transplant regimen; 2) methotrexate is given in a lower dose (5 $mg/m^2$) on only days +3 and +6, and levels are monitored at 24 hrs and, if necessary, at 36 and 48 hrs with adjustments in dosage and/or leucovorin rescue.

*BMT phase: autologous BMT with ex vivo removal of tumor cells from autologous marrow.* Ex vivo purging of autologous marrow utilizes sedimentation, filtration, and monoclonal antibody coated magnetic beads. To plan the purging procedure, numbers of normal and tumor cells in posterior iliac crest marrow are determined three to ten days before the large-scale harvest (Moss et al., 1987). Sufficient marrow then is obtained from the large-scale harvest to provide approximately $10^8$ marrow cells per kg after *ex vivo* purging.

Whole marrow is mixed 1:1 with 3% hetastarch and allowed to sediment, after which supernatant cells are filtered through nylon wool, washed, and mixed with magnetic beads that have been coated with a mixture of monoclonal antibodies via goat anti-mouse immunoglobulin (1:1 bead to total cell ratio). Attachment of monoclonal antibodies to the beads, which is a modification of our previous method of first binding them to cells and then to beads (Seeger et al., 1985; Reynolds et al., 1986), increases the speed of purging and decreases non-specific cell loss because cell washing steps are not required. Following one-half hour of rotation with immunobeads, tumor cells attached to beads are removed with samarium cobalt magnets; the immunobead depletion step is repeated if the pre-harvest marrow contained more than one tumor cell per $10^4$ normal cells. Total cell recovery is approximately 66% after sedimentation and filtration and 50% after each magnetic immunobead step; thus, approximately 35% of the initial cells are recovered after sedimentation, filtration, and one cycle of magnetic immunobeads. An aliquot of marrow ($10^8$ cells/kg) that is treated only by sedimentation and filtration is cryopreserved as a backup in case antibody treated marrow does not engraft.

Marrow from 31 patients has been treated *ex vivo* using sedimentation, filtration, and magnetic immunobeads. Twenty-two (71%) of these marrows had detectable tumor by immunocytology before purging (range, 0.7 to 1800 tumor cells per $10^5$ marrow cells; median, 3.6 per $10^5$), and none had detectable tumor afterwards. Thus, we have demonstrated in a clinical setting that this method can remove three or more logs of tumor cells. Monitoring with immunocytology is essential for assessing the efficacy of purging and for interpretting the results of clinical trials.

Twenty-one autologous marrow transplants have been performed. Two therapy-related deaths due to hepatic veno-occlusive disease occurred. The first three patients, whose marrows were treated with monoclonal antibodies 459, BA-1, and 126-4, had slow engraftment, and two died of infection (*P. carinii* pneumonia and candida sepsis). Although this combination of antibodies was highly efficient for tumor cell removal while preserving CFU-G,M and total cells, the suprisingly poor engraftment suggested that these antibodies were removing hematopoietic stem cells. Therefore, subsequent marrows were treated with a different combination of antibodies, 459, BA-1, 390, and HSAN 1.2, which were equally as effective in removing tumor cells. Sixteen of 17 marrows treated this latter mixture of antibodies have reconstituted hematopoiesis completely; the one exception restored myeloid and erythroid cells but not platelets even though megakaryocytes were present. Thus, the mixture of monoclonal antibodies 459, BA-1, 390, and HSAN 1.2 effectively removes tumor cells without removing pluripotent hematopoietic stem cells.

The outcome for 17 patients receiving autologous marrow treated by sedimentation, filtration, and magnetic beads coated with antibodies 459, BA-1, 390, and HSAN 1.2 is encouraging. The follow-up is 1+ to 14+ months with a median of 7+ months. One death occurred as a result of therapy (veno-occlusive disease), and one patient developed progressive disease at 11 months. This study is too new to reach conclusions about efficacy; however, the estimated disease-free survival at 12+ months of 70% is encouraging.

**Combined results (CCG-322P and CCG-321P3) for bone marrow transplantation before disease progression.** Forty-three patients, who received VAMP-TBI and were transplanted before tumor progression, have an estimated survival of 56% at 54+ months after BMT (Figure 1A).

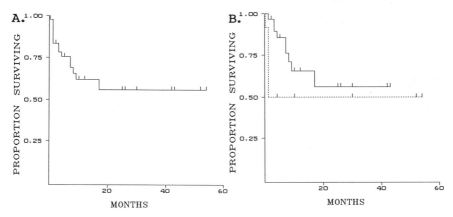

Figure 1. Survival after BMT of patients transplanted before tumor progression: (A) all patients, n = 43, median time of followup = 7 months; (B) autologous BMT (——), n = 31, median time of followup = 7 months; allogeneic BMT (------), n = 12, median time of followup = 3 months. After initially receiving conventional chemotherapy (various regimens), 43 patients whose tumors were not growing progressively were given VAMP-TBI followed by autologous or allogeneic marrow. Analysis includes patients who died from therapy-related complications, infections, and progressive disease.

Of the 12 receiving allogeneic marrow, 6 had fatal therapy-related complications in the first three months after BMT; however, only one of the survivors has relapsed. Thus, whereas toxic complications were unacceptable, relapse-free survival was encouraging. It appears that recent modifications to the protocol have decreased toxicity to an acceptable level; now, it will be important to monitor relapse-free survival. Thirty-one patients received autologous marrow, and therapy-related deaths in this group included two from hepatic veno-occlusive disease and one from poor engraftment. Estimated survival for the allogeneic group is 50% and for the autologous group is 56% (Figure 1B).

The estimated disease-free survival for all patients who survived therapy related toxicities is 45% at 54+ months after BMT (Figure 2). Although 6 patients are long-term disease-free survivors (25+ to 54+ months), the rate of relapse indicates the need for further improvement.

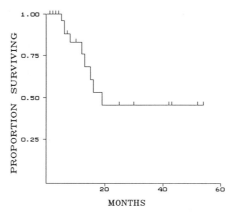

Figure 2. Disease-free survival after BMT for 33 patients who were transplanted before tumor progression and who survived the BMT phase (6 allogeneic and 27 autologous BMT). This analysis excludes patients who died from therapy related complications and infections (n = 10).

## SUMMARY

These studies suggest that intensive chemoradiotherapy (eg., VAMP-TBI), if given relatively soon after diagnosis and before development of progressive disease, improves long-term survival for patients with advanced neuroblastoma. Although this particular therapy is not useful for those who already have developed progressive disease, other intensive regimens may warrant testing in this latter group of patients.

Our current study is testing aggressive induction chemotherapy, ex vivo purging of autologous marrow, and VAMP-TBI followed by BMT. Because of the increasing risk of progressive disease with time after diagnosis, we recommend beginning the BMT phase by 20 weeks after diagnosis. This should result in 85% of newly diagnosed patients entering the BMT phase without progressive disease; and, with fewer toxic deaths, 90% should survive the BMT phase. Thus, approximately 70% of patients could be disease-free survivors 8-9 months after diagnosis.

Because a significant number of patients still develop progressive disease during induction or after BMT, efforts are being made to improve induction and pre-transplant therapies and to identify prognostic factors. If modifications of the current regimens do not decrease the rate of progressive disease, it may be necessary to develop additional or different therapy for patients identified to be at high risk. Hopefully, new strategies will further increase the percentage of patients with tumor-free survival.

### ACKNOWLEDGEMENTS

This study was supported in part by grants CA12800, CA27678, CA16042, and CA21737 from the National Cancer Institute, DHHS and by a grant from Concern II. LCDR Reynolds is assigned to the UCLA School of Medicine from the Department of the Navy; the views expressed in this article are those of the authors and do not reflect the official policy or position of the Department of the Navy, Department of Defense, nor the U. S. Government. We thank Dr. P. Marangos for providing anti-neuron specific enolase serum, Dr. R. Reisfeld and Hybritech Inc. for providing monoclonal antibodies 126-4 and BA-1 respectively, and Dr. J. Ugelstad and Sintef for providing magnetic beads.

### REFERENCES

August CS, Serota FT, Kock PA, Burkey E, Schlesinger H, Elkins WL, Evans AE, D'Angio GJ (1984). Treatment of advanced neuroblastoma with supralethal chemotherapy, radiation, and allogeneic or autologous marrow reconstitution. J Clin Oncol 2:609-616.
Breslow N, McCann B (1971). Statistical estimation of prognosis of children with neuroblastoma. Cancer Res 31:2098-2103.
Evans AE, D'Angio GJ, Propert K, Anderson J, Hann HW

(1987). Prognostic factors in neuroblastoma. Cancer 59:1853–1859.

Evans AE (1980). Staging and treatment of neuroblastoma. Cancer 45:1799–1802.

Green AA, Hayes FA, Rao B (1986). Disease control and toxicity of aggressive 4 drug therapy for children with disseminated neuroblastoma. Proc Am Soc Clin Soc Oncol 5:210.

Hann HW, Evans AE, Siegel SE, Wong KY, Sather H, Dalton A, Hammond D, Seeger RC (1985). Prognostic importance of serum ferritin in patients with Stages III and IV neuroblastoma: the Childrens Cancer Study Group experience. Cancer Res 45:2843–2848.

Hartmann O, Benhamou E, Beaujean F, Pico JL, Kalifa C, Patte C, Flamant F, Lemerle J (1986). High-dose busulfan and cyclophosphamide with autologous bone marrow transplantation support in advanced malignancies in children: a phase II study. J Clin Oncol 4:1804–1810.

Hayes FA, Green AA (1983). Neuroblastoma. Ped Annals 12:366–374.

Moss TJ, Seeger RC, Kindler-Rohrborn A, Marangos PJ, Rajewsky MF, Reynolds CP (1985). Immunohistologic detection and phenotyping of neuroblastoma cells in bone marrow using cytoplasmic neuron specific enolase and cell surface antigens. Prog Clin Biol Res 175:367–78.

Moss TJ, Xu G, Rayner SA, Reynolds CP, Heitjan D, Seeger RC (1987). Immunohistologic detection of infrequent neuroblastoma cells and autologous bone marrow transplantation (BMT). Proc Amer Assoc Cancer Res 28:219.

Philip T, Bernard JL, Zucher JM, et al. (1987). High dose chemoradiotherapy with bone marrow transplantation as consolidation treatment in neuroblastoma: an unselected group of stage IV patients over one year of age. J Clin Oncol 5:266–271.

Reynolds CP, Seeger RC, Vo DD, Black AT, Wells J, Ugelstad J (1986). Model system for removing neuroblastoma cells from bone marrow using monoclonal antibodies and magnetic immunobeads. Cancer Res 46:5882–5886.

Seeger RC, Reynolds CP, Vo DD, Ugelstad J, Wells J (1985). Depletion of Neuroblastoma Cells from bone marrow with monoclonal antibodies and magnetic immunobeads. Prog Clin Biol Res 175:443–458.

Seeger RC, Brodeur GM, Sather H, Dalton A, Siegel SE, Wong

KY, Hammond D (1985). Association of multiple copies of the N-myc oncogene with rapid progression of neuroblastomas. N Engl J Med 313:1111-1116.

Seeger RC, Reynolds CP, Moss TJ, Lenarsky C, Feig SA, Selch M, Ugelstad J, Wells J (1988). Autologous bone marrow transplantation for poor prognosis neuroblastoma. In: Dicke K, Spitzer G, Zander A. eds. Autologous Bone Marrow Transplantation: Proceedings of the Third International Symposium. Houston: Gulf Press in press.

Shimada H, Chatten J, Newton WA Jr, Sachs N, Hamoudi AB, Chiba T, Marsden HB, Misugi K (1984). Histopathologic prognostic factors in neuroblastic tumors: definition of subtypes of ganglioneuroblastoma and an age-linked classification of neuroblastomas. J Natl Cancer Inst 73:405-416.

Wells JR, Sullivan A, Cline MJ (1979). A technique for the separation and cryopreservation of myeloid stem cells from human bone marrow. Cryobiology 16:201-210.

Young Jr. LL, Miller RW (1975). Incidence of malignant tumors in United States children. J Peds 86:254-258.

Advances in Neuroblastoma Research 2, pages 215–223
© 1988 Alan R. Liss, Inc.

BONE MARROW TRANSPLANTATION (BMT) FOR ADVANCED NEUROBLASTOMA
(NBL):   A MULTICENTER POG PILOT STUDY.

J. Graham-Pole, A.P. Gee, S. Gross, J. Casper, M. Graham,
W. Harvey, N. Kapoor, P. Koch, N. Mendenhall, D. Norris,
T. Pick, and P. Thomas

University of Florida, Gainesville; Brooke Army Medical
Center, San Antonio; Cleveland Clinic, Cleveland; Cook
Children's Hospital, Fort Worth; Johns Hopkins
University, Baltimore; Montreal Children's Hospital,
Montreal; University of Oklahoma, Oklahoma; University
of Wisconsin, Milwaukee, and The Pediatric Oncology
Group.

INTRODUCTION

Although combination chemotherapy has improved the
survival duration of children with disseminated neuroblastoma
(NBL), most still die of their disease. The concept that
"more is better" has led to the use of marrow-ablative
chemotherapy and radiation supported by allogeneic or
autologous bone marrow infusions (August et al, 1984, Philip
et al, 1986, Seeger et al, 1987). A high response rate and
in some cases longterm disease-free survival have been
reported.

Although using autologous marrow avoids the limitations
of allogeneic marrow (donor non-availability and
graft-versus-host disease: GVHD), it is limited in NBL by
the high incidence of neoplastic infiltration. If this were
overcome, all such patients might potentially benefit by
autologous marrow infusions. The technology of in vitro
immunomagnetic purging (IMP) seems to be an effective method
for eliminating cancer cells from marrow, and has been
extensively tested in NBL (Treleaven et al, 1984). We report
our early experience with the use of a high-dose chemotherapy
plus fractionated total body irradiation (FTBI) regimen with
and without IMP to treat 50 patients with metastatic NBL at

eight institutions on a Peditric Oncology Group (POG) pilot protocol.

PATIENTS AND METHODS

A. Patient Preparation

50 consecutive patients aged 1 to 14 (median 4) years with metastatic NBL were treated on a POG pilot protocol (8340) with a regimen of high dose melphalan 60mg/m$^2$ IV daily for 3 days, FTBI (200 cGy twice daily for 3 days), with or without irradiation of local lesions (150 cGy twice daily for 5 days), followed by autologous or allogeneic marrow infusions. Thirty-eight had their marrows treated in vitro by IMP at the University of Florida (UF) and cryopreserved until needed. Bone marrows collected from non-UF patients were transported on ice and returned in liquid nitrogen containers. Seven other patients received autologous non-purged marrows and 5 received allogeneic BMT. 24 patients were initially diagnosed and treated at the BMT centers, and 26 were referred from other centers for BMT. 29 patients were treated during first complete (CR) or partial (PR) remission, and 21 in second CR or PR. Most patients were initially treated with combinations of cyclophosphamide, adriamycin, cis-platinum and VM-26 or VP-16 (CECA). Cyclophosphamide or cis-platinum in high doses, vincristine and/or VP-16, were mostly used for reinduction following relapse. Marrow was collected when patients were in clinical remission, with grossly normal marrow aspirates and biopsies (more than 75% cellularity and less than 5% blasts). Approximately 15ml/kg marrow was aspirated under general anesthesia from the posterior iliac crests with sterile technique, using syringes loaded with TC199 tissue culture medium plus heparinized saline (50 units/ml). It was filtered through steel mesh screens and transferred to 600ml blood bags. We aimed to collect a minimum of 10$^8$ /kg nucleated cells for processing. Patients receiving allogeneic BMT also received prophylaxis against graft-versus-host-disease (GVHD) in the form of prednisone 40mg/m$^2$ day +7 to +21, tapering over 1 week, plus methotrexate 15mg/m$^2$ day +1, 10mg/m$^2$ day +3 and +11, then 10mg/m$^2$ weekly until day +100.

Figure 1: Magnetic Bone Marrow Purging Apparatus used at the University of Florida

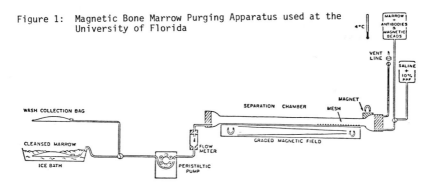

## B.  Immunomagnetic purging procedure

Figure 1 shows a schema of this procedure, which aims to selectively remove cancer cells from the marrow while leaving hematopoietic cells intact. We used a panel of 6 monoclonal antibodies directed against NBL cell-surface antigens,* and a monodisperse suspension of magnetic polystyrene microspheres**. Murine antibodies were used, prepared against human fetal brain. $IgG_1$ antibodies were purified on immobilized protein A, and IgM antibodies by FPLC. Extensive reactivity was demonstrated against fresh NBL cells in vitro, but not against normal hematopoietic cells, using both immunofluorescence and colony forming assays. The beads have a diameter of 4.5um, contain approximately 20% by weight of magnetite, and each gram has a surface area of about $5m^2$. They were sterilized with ethanol, diluted to a concentration of 1 mg/ml in 0.1M phosphate-buffered saline (PBS), pH 7.7 at 4°C, and incubated with antibody at a concentration of 3.4mg immunoglobulin per 100 mg of beads for 16 hours at 4°C. They were washed with PBS to remove unbound antibody.

We developed a new system in our laboratory for separating the bead-coated NBL cells from the marrow. The nucleated cells were sedimented using Hespan (Hetastarch), either in 50 ml syringes (marrow volumes <400 ml) or using an Erytrenn blood cell separator (volumes >400 ml). They were then incubated with the optimal concentration of antibody, known to saturate all binding sites at low levels of marrow infiltration, for 30 minutes at 4°C with frequent mixing,

*    Supplied by John Kemshead, Ph.D., Imp Cancer Research Fund, London
**  Supplied by Professor Ungelstad, Ph.D., Trondheim, Norway

centrifuged at 220 g for 10 minutes, and washed twice in PBS. A low-ceilinged disposable chamber (23 x 1.5 x 0.3cm) placed over a carrier containing samarium cobalt permanent magnets, produced a graded magnetic field such that the field strength increased as the marrow flowed through the chamber. From the chamber, the purged marrow was drawn through a flow meter using a peristaltic pump to the collection packs, which were kept on ice.

We monitored the efficiency of the purging procedure by indirect immunofluorescence and by clonogenic outgrowth in the Courtenay assay for neoplastic cells, and by CFU-C, CFU-E, and CFU-GEMM assays using a modification of the methods described by Fausner and Messner. Before freezing, samples were taken for nucleated cell counts and sterility checks. 30ml aliquots were transferred into Stericon freezing bags on ice, adding an equal volume of freezing mixture containing 20% dimethyl sulphoxide and 20% purified protein fraction. The bags were heat-sealed, transferred to aluminum storage cannisters, and frozen in a programmable cryofreezer using predetermined freezing ramps. The marrow viability was routinely in excess of 80%. For reinfusion into the patient, it was thawed rapidly at the bedside within its sealed bag in a 37°C water bath.

C.  Treatment and Supportive Care

All patients were nursed in isolation with strict precautions to reduce contamination (careful hand washing, restricted visiting, gowns, gloves and masks for dressing changes, and antifungal regimens for mucosal surfaces). Central venous catheters were placed to facilitate blood drawing, blood component and antibiotic therapy, and total parenteral nutrition. All blood products were irradiated to at least 1500 cGy to prevent GVHD from transfused lymphocytes. Systemic antibiotics were given for fever developing during the neutropenic phase, after collecting appropriate cultures. Amphotericin was added if fever persisted for 7 days. The nurse: patient ratio was approximately 1:2, and several support personnel were available, including social workers, occupational and physical therapists, child psychologists and teachers. Patients were discharged when they were clinically stable, afebrile, off systemic antibiotics, and taking adequate nutrition by mouth. This was most often between 4 and 6 weeks after the marrow infusion. They were then seen frequently but received no further specific therapy.

Table 1    **Major Complications**

| | |
|---|---|
| Engraftment* time > 10 weeks | 4 |
| Fatal sepsis | 3 |
| Grade 3-4 GVHD | 2 |
| Severe nephrotoxicity | 2 |
| CNS hemorrhage | 1 |
| | |
| Total Fatalities | 6  (12%) |
| allogeneic | 2 |
| autologous | 4 |

*Sustained WBC > $1000/mm^3$

RESULTS

Table 1 documents the major toxicity of this pilot study. There were a total of six (12%) fatalities relating to the BMT procedure, 2 among the 5 allogeneic, and 4 among the 45 autologous, BMT recipients. Three were in first CR/PR patients and three in second CR/PR patients. Among patients treated in initial remission, one died 19 days after an autologous BMT with systemic aspergillosis, and another suffered a fatal intracerebral hemorrhage 4 months after an autologous BMT. He had a normal blood count and no evidence of his cancer, and was suspected of having a congenital vascular malformation. A third patient developed fungal encephalitis complicating severe GVHD two months after allogeneic BMT. Among those transplanted after relapse, four failed to engraft for more than 10 weeks following BMT. Two died respectively of pneumopericarditis plus renal failure, and encephalopathy due probably to disseminated herpes zoster infection. The other two are alive and clinically free of disease 4 and 8 months post-BMT. One has a weak graft, no longer requires blood components, and is free of infections. The third death in this group was in a patient with severe GVHD following allogeneic BMT who died from pulmonary aspergillosis.

Other major complications included progression of pre-existing renal insufficiency in two patients who had received considerable prior cis-platinum therapy as well as local abdominal irradiation before BMT. One patient developed the clinical picture of hepatic veno-occlusive

disease, from which he recovered completely, and one
developed successively pseudomonas sepsis and pneumocystis
carinii pneumonia, from both of which he also recovered. All
patients suffered from mucositis for approximately 10-14
days, and were anorexic for 3-8 weeks.

Patients undergoing autologous BMT received a mean of
$1.63 \pm 1.02 \times 10^8$/kg nucleated cells, and re-engrafted a
mean of $41.0 \pm 22.6$ days later (as defined by a sustained
white blood cell count $\geq 1000$/cu.mm.).

Figure 2

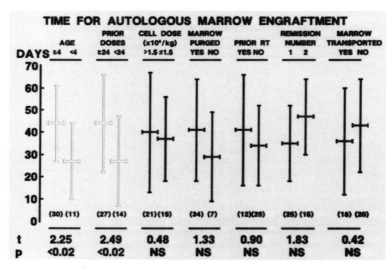

Figure 2 shows the time to engraftment as a function of
factors that might influence marrow recovery, excluding
patients who received allogeneic BMT or who died within 3
weeks of autologous BMT. Significantly faster engraftment
times were seen in children under 4 compared with those over
4 years old, and in those who had received less than 24 doses
of myelosuppressive chemotherapy (CECA) when compared to
those who had received more than 24 doses. On the other
hand, there were no significant differences in engraftment
times between patients receiving either purged or unpurged
marrow, patients receiving or not receiving local irradiation
before marrow harvest, patients whose marrow was transported
to and from UF as opposed to UF BMT patients, or between
patients receiving more or less than $1.5 \times 10^8$/kg nucleated
marrow cells at the time of autologous BMT.

Table 2                    **Disease-Free Survival**

|  | **Stratum 1 and 2** | **Stratum 3 and 4** |
|---|---|---|
| Patients | 29 | 21 |
| DFS | 16 (55.2%) | 6 (28.6%) |
| F/U* from BMT | 7 (2 – 32) mos. | 8 ( 4 – 21) mos. |
| F/U from Dx | 17 (8 – 42) mos. | 34 (16 – 61) mos. |

*median (range) follow-up of disease-free survivors

Table 2 shows the current disease-free survival of all 50 patients. Excluding the six treatment-related deaths, 16 of 26 (61.5%) first CR or PR (stratum 1 and 2) patients, and 6 of 18 (33.3%) second CR or PR (stratum 3 and 4) patients, are currently disease-free a median of 9 months post-BMT ($X_2$ = 3.38, P=0.07). Sites of relapse have included the abdomen, skeleton and marrow in all but one case, and in only one patient has the marrow been the sole site of relapse.

Figure 3 shows the actuarial disease-free survival of these patients, compared with that of standard maintenance chemotherapy as used in the two most recent POG protocols for metastatic NBL (8104 and 8441).

**FIGURE 3**

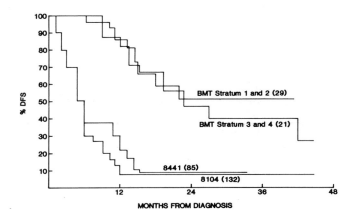

DISEASE-FREE SURVIVAL PROBABILITY
(POG Stage D > 1 yr.)

DISCUSSION

This pilot project shows the feasibility of hematologic support using allogeneic or autologous marrow infusions for children with disseminated NBL undergoing marrow-ablative therapy with curative intent. Since only six patients have so far remained disease-free for more than one year after BMT, and since two patients have relapsed more than one year after BMT, it is premature to draw any conclusions about the ultimate outcome of this study. Because chemotherapy regimens for inducing and maintaining remissions without the use of BMT are steadily improving, we consider that a phase 3 multicenter trial must now be conducted to compare directly BMT with the best available alternative therapy. The POG is about to embark on such a study.

In view of the greater toxicity encountered by those patients who were transplanted after an initial relapse (particularly non-engraftment), and the higher number of post-BMT relapses in this group, BMT is probably best used in NBL patients in first remission who have biological features putting them at the highest risk of relapse. However, the frequency of post-BMT relapses we and others have seen even in patients transplanted in first remission underscores the need for improvements in treatment regimens for NBL both for induction and for conditioning for BMT.

Although we cannot prove that IMP eliminates the risk of reseeding with malignant cells, extensive testing indicates that it consistently removes all NBL cells detectable by currently available assays. However, marrow collected from patients who have suffered prior relapse and who have been heavily pretreated seems to have lower hematopoietic potential, even when the nucleated cell count is adequate. We encountered no difficulties with transporting marrow for in vitro treatment. The viability of hematopoietic cells is such that marrow can be shipped throughout the United States for this purpose. However, such feasibility studies as ours are essential, since autologous marrow infusions are being used increasingly to protect against myeloablative treatment regimens.

Our purging technology compares favorably in both safety and efficacy with other in vitro physical and non-physical methods. No complement source is needed, no toxin is introduced, and normal hematopoietic cells are completely unaffected. It is also adaptable to removing other cells from the marrow, including both neoplastic cells and T-lymphocyte subsets. Since the latter are important in mediating reactions between donor and recipient in allogeneic BMT, IMP may also prove an ideal in vitro method for preventing GVHD following allogeneic BMT.

REFERENCES:

August CS, Serota FT, Koch PA, Burkey E, Schlesinger H, Elkins WL, Evans AE, and D'Angio GJ. Treatment of advanced neuroblastoma with supralethal chemotherapy, radiation and allogeneic or autologous marrow reconstitution. J Clin Oncol 2, 609, 1984.

Philip T: Autologous bone marrow transplantation for very bad prognosis neuroblastoma. In Evans et al (eds): Advances in Neuroblastoma Research, Liss (NY) 1985, pp 568-586.

Seeger R, Lenarsky C, Moss T, Feig S, Selch M, Ramsay N, Harris R, Reynolds CP, Siegel S, Sather H, Hammond D and Wells J. Bone marrow transplantation (BMT) for poor prognosis neuroblastoma.

Treleaven JG, Gibson FM, Ugelstad J, Rembaum A, Philip T, Caine CD, and Kemshead JT. Removal of neuroblastoma cells from bone marrow with monoclonal antibodies conjugated to magnetic microspheres. Lancet i, 70, 1984.

ACKNOWLEDGEMENTS:

This work was funded in part by grants from the Pediatric Oncology Group (CA 29281), the American Cancer Society (CH-33), Dynal A.S. of Oslo and Stop Children's Cancer Inc.

Advances in Neuroblastoma Research 2, pages 225–236
© 1988 Alan R. Liss, Inc.

# VERY LONG DELAY TO ENGRAFTMENT AFTER ABMT IN NEUROBLASTOMA PATIENTS AND EFFECT OF CD8 MONOCLONAL ANTIBODY IN VIVO THERAPY

M.C. FAVROT (1), T. PHILIP (1), V. COMBARET (1),
P. BIRON (1), J. MORISSET (2), A. BERNARD (2)
(1) Centre Léon Bérard, Lyon, France
(2) Institut G. Roussy, Villejuif, France
Supported by grant INSERM 486022

INTRODUCTION

Whereas non engraftment is a major complication of allogenic bone marrow transplantation (BMT), it is very rarely observed after an autologous BMT. However, delays to normal hematological recovery have been reported; in acute leukemia, such delay seems more frequently observed in the group of patients grafted for an acute myeloid leukemia than in those grafted for an acute lymphoid leukemia (Gorin et al., 1986). In the 174 patients with solid tumor treated in our Institute since 1983 by high dose chemotherapy with or without TBI followed by an autologous BMT, we observed 14 delays to engraftment and 2 non engraftments, 15 of these cases being those of children suffering from stage IV neuroblastoma (Philip et al., 1987 a,b). We shall review hereafter these 15 neuroblastoma cases. The clinical factors possibly responsible for these delays to hematological recovery will be analyzed, as well as the hematological and immunological features of circulating and BM regenerating cells. Six patients, including 5 of the neuroblastoma cases, were treated by continuous infusion of $CD_8$ monoclonal antibody; the effect of such immunotherapy on the hematological and immunological reconstitution in the 5 neuroblastoma cases will be analyzed.

MATERIALS AND METHODS

## Patients and Chemotherapy

All patients were children under 12 with stage IV neuroblastoma. Induction therapy varied between patients: a first group received 6 courses of CADO, a second group received VP16-CDDP, and the last group received in alternance CDDP-containing regimen and ifosfamide-containing regimen. They were then included either in our current LMCE protocol of in the pilot double autograft program (Philip et al., 1987 a,b). In the single autograft program, patients received VCR, high dose Melphalan (180 mg/m²) and TBI (12 Grays in 6 fractions). In the double autograft program, the first conditioning regimen included BCNU, VM26 and Cis-platinum. The second one was similar to that of the single augograft program.

## Autologous Bone Marrow Graft

Bone marrow was harvested at the end of induction therapy. When patients entered a double autograft program, BM for the second autograft was harvested after the first autograft hematological reconstitution. BM grafts were treated by immunomagnetic depletion, according to the initially described procedure (Treleaven et al., 1984) or to our modified procedure (Favrot et al., 1986): the main modifications consisted of a ficoll separation instead of a buffy coat, a double treatment of the samples instead of a single one and the use of the new beads ME450 instead of ME330.

A cocktail of 5 monoclonal antibodies kindly provided by J. Kemshead (Institute of Child Health, London) was used: UJ13A, UJ127.11, UJ181.4, α-Thy-1 and H-11. The quality of the graft was evaluated by the total number of mononuclear cells and the number of CFU.GM (colony forming units - granulocytes monocytes) per $2 \times 10^5$ mononuclear cells before and after the purging and after the defreezing procedure when the BM is reinjected to the patient.

Hematological and Immunological Follow-up

Hematological reconstitution was surveyed by daily blood counts and BM aspirates twice a month from day 15 to discharge. Hematological reconstitution was considered achieved when granulocytes reached $500/mm^3$ and platelets were maintained at $50 \times 10^3/mm^3$ without transfusional support. CFU.GM were evaluated on each BM sample. When the number of BM cells was sufficient, CFU.GM were evaluated on the total mononuclear cell fraction and after lysis of the $CD_8+$ fraction by $CD_8$ monoclonal antibody and rabbit complement.

Immunological characteristics of BM and circulating cells were analyzed by double indirect immunofluorescence, using the following combination of markers: $CD_4$, $CD_8$-Leu$_7$, HNK$_{1a}$-$CD_2$ and HNK$_{1a}$-$CD_3$ (leu$_7$ from Becton Dickinson; HNK$_{1a}$ from Coultronics; other MoAbs were provided by one of us), and anti-mouse Igm and anti-mouse IgG subclass specific second layer coupled to TRITC and FITC (Southern Biotechnology). NK (natural killer) function was assayed against K$_{562}$ cell line using a $^{51}$Cr-release assay.

Other Laboratory Data

Patients had regular bacterial survey and viral control (serology and isolation of the virus) as well as an evaluation of kidney and liver functions. CMV serology was performed by an Elisa assay.

$CD_8$ in vivo Therapy

$CD_8$ (provided by one of us) is a mouse monoclonal antibody of IgG$_2$ subclass. 0.2 mg/kg/day were administered (with half the dose in 4 hours) by continuous infusion during 6 days. Premedication consisted of corticosteroids and antihistaminics given every day before the begining of the perfusion and 8 hours later.


RESULTS

In the group of 50 children included in our current LMCE protocol of single autograft, the median to reach 500 PN/mm³ was 25 days and 40 days to reach 50x10³ PLTS. One patient did not engraft and 4 were considered to suffer delays to engraftment since they had neither recovered PN nor PLTS at day 42. In the group of 13 patients included in the double autograft program, the median for PN recovery was 44.5 days and is was 100 days for PLTS. One patient did not engraft and 7 presented delays to engraftment. Two more delays to engraftment were recorded in children not included in either of these protocols. Other risk factors for these children are summarized in table 1. Residual BM involvement was detectable at time of BM harvesting in 6 cases. All received a BM graft pretreated in vitro by an immunomagnetic procedure. The number of reinjected CFU.GM was rather low when compared to the median in patients included in the LMCE protocol; 6 patients had liver dysfunction and 2 had a documented CMV infection.


Hematological Features

Hematological features were very similar in all patients except 2, with the appearance of a few PN (up to 0.1x10³/mm³) during the second week post-graft. From the third week post-graft, lymphocytes abnormally increased (up to 1.5x10³/mm³) whereas circulating PN disappeared. 30 to 80 % circulating lymphocytes expressed a common phenotype with a coexpression of $CD_8$ and $Leu_7$. The absolute number of these cells reached 1x10³/mm³ in half the cases. These cells expressed CD³ and $CD_{11}$ antigens but were not recogni-

TABLE 1

| BM at * harvesting | Purging** method | reinjected CFU.GM/kg | Liver functions | Documented viral infection | Protocol |
|---|---|---|---|---|---|
| (−) | modified | 1.35 x 10⁴ | hepatitis B | (−) | LMCE |
| (−) | " | 1.7 x 10⁴ | normal | (−) | " |
| (−) | " | 0.45 x 10⁴ | V O D | (−) | " |
| + | " | ? | normal | (−) | " |
| (−) | initial | 2 x 10⁴ | V O D | (−) | " |
| + | modified | 1 x 10⁴ | hepatitis B | (−) | double ABMT |
| + | initial | 1.2 x 10⁴ | − | CMV | " |
| (−) | modified | 1.9 x 10⁴ | − | (−) | " |
| + | initial | 4.2 x 10⁴ | − | (−) | " |
| + | modified | 4.5 x 10⁴ | + | CMV | " |
| (−) | non purged | 1.1 x 10⁴ | − | (−) | " |
| ? | modified | 4.8 x 10⁴ | ? | ? | " |
| + | modified | 3.37x 10⁴ | + | (−) | " |
| *** (−) | initial | 16,5x 10⁴ | + | (−) | OUT |
| *** (−) | initial | 1,7 x 10⁴ | − | CMV | OUT |

Legends

* BM was considered as positive when minimal residual involvement could be detected on one of the 4 biopsies or aspirates on the day of harvesting. Immunological staining allowed to confirm for each patient whether malignant cells were effectively present or not in the graft before and after the purging procedure.

** All patients received a BM purged by an immunomagnetic procedure. Modified and initially described purging procedures are described in the "Materials and methods" section.

*** These two patients were not included in the protocols, the first one was a stage III neuroblastoma, the second one was a stage IV neuroblastoma and received, prior to the ABMT program, high dose Melphalan without any BM rescue.

zed by $HNK_1$. The NK function against $K_{562}$ was null.

In the BM, similar subsets of cells co-expressing $CD_8$ and $Leu_7$ were observed in all patients, the percentage ranging from 20 to 70 %. On the aspirates of the 15th day post-ABMT, hematopoïetic precursors and a few CFU.GM (10 to 50 per $2x10^5$ mononuclear cells) were observed in 5 patients. In one patient, the lysis of $CD_8+$ $leu_7+$ cells markedly increased the number of CFU.GM. Further aspirates in all patients were desert.

Effect of $CD_8$ Monoclonal Antibody in vivo Therapy

Five patients were treated by $CD_8$ injection. It was remarkably tolerated and no side effect was observed.
In 2 patients, $CD_8$ induced a progressive disappearance of circulating and BM $CD_8+$ $Leu_7+$ cells from the first 24 hours of
therapy. These cells went down to 10 % under therapy and never went up again after cessation of therapy.

In one patient, $CD_8$ induced a partial disappearance of $CD_8+$ $Leu_7+$ cells which settled around 20 % under therapy. Three days after cessation of therapy, they reached the same level as before therapy. A second course of therapy with twice the dose of antibody induced an antigenic modulation with the persistance of 20 to 40 % $Leu_7+$ cells weakly expressing $CD_8$.

In the last two patients we observed this antigenic modulation after three days of therapy, with the persistance of 30 to 40 % $CD_3$, $CD_{11}$ and $Leu_7$ positive cells very weakly expressing $CD_8$, and the reappearance of more than 70 % $CD_8+$ $Leu_7+$ cells after cessation of therapy.

In the two patients for whom $CD_8$ therapy

was fully efficient, we observed the appearance of monocytes, PN and eosinophils within 72 hours of treatment; hematopoietic BM precursors and CFU.GM were observed in the aspirates 10 days after the begining of therapy and patients recovered both PN and PLTS within 20 days. In both patients, $CD_8$+ $Leu_7$+ cells remained below 10 % after cessation of therapy and the ratio $T_4/T_8$ was superior to 1. Cells with a phenotype characteristic of NK cells, ie. $HNK_1$, $CD_{11}$ positive and $CD_3$ negative, appeared within 10 days post therapy. The first patient has been followed for more than 6 months and still presents such circulating cells in the blood with a normal NK function. The $T_4/T_8$ ratio remains superior to 1 but T cell functions, as assayed by response to PHA, are very low.

The patient for whom $CD_8$ therapy was partially efficient recovered PN within 20 days but was still thrombopenic 90 days later. BM aspirates however remain very poor with low activity in culture. The $T_4/T_8$ ratio is below 1 but cells with NK phenotype appeared during the treatment and remain high after cessation of therapy.

Finally, the two patients for whom an antigenic modulation had been observed died from complications due to prolonged aplasia. Bone marrow aspirates remain desert. Both received an unsuccessful BM rescue; one was given in addition GM.CSF (granulocytes monocytes colony stimulating factor, kinkly provided by Sandoz Laboratories, Basel, Switzerland), for 5 days.

DISCUSSION

The possible suppressive effects of $CD_8$+ $Leu_7$+ cells on hematopoiesis had been previously hypothesized in patients suffering from autoimmune aplastic anaemia and severe BM aplasia (Zoumbos et al., 1985; Bagby, 1981; Torok-Storb and Hansen, 1982). Such circulating and BM cells have also been observed after an allogenic BMT,

especially in cases with severe GVHD and/or CMV
infection (Favrot et al., 1986). More recently,
this phenomenon was related to delays to
engraftment. However, experimental data remain
controversial since the in vitro lysis of $CD_8+$
BM cells has variable effects on the growth of
CFU.GM in vitro (Vinci et al., 1986; Lipton et
al., 1983; Vinci et al., 1987). In the first 2
months after ABMT, we frequently observed 5 to
10 % of these $CD_8+$ $Leu_7+$ cells in our patients,
but we very seldom found more than 10 %, apart
from the cases described above. Among the
patients autografted in our Institute for
various solid tumors, and with the exception of
the 15 cases we reported above, only three
presented more than 20 % $CD_8+$ $Leu_7+$ cells during
the first month post graft, two of them (1 child
with stage IV neuroblastoma and 1 adult with B
lymphoma) presented normal hematological reconstitution. The third one, mentioned in the introduction, presented a delay to hematological
recovery. She was a child with T lymphoma,
grafted with a T cell depleted BM (rabbit
complement lysis) and successfully treated with
$CD_8$ monoclonal antibody. Hematological and
immunological features before and after cessation of therapy were similar to those described
for the two responding neuroblastoma cases.

Various factors could be responsible for
the delay to engraftment, such as the number of
reinjected BM progenitor cells or viral infections. The most striking point is probably the
fact that 15 were neuroblastoma patients and 14
received an immunomagnetic-depleted BM. The in
vitro proliferative activity of the BM (as
assayed by CFU.GM) after the immunomagnetic
purging procedure is higher than after chemical
procedures, such as ASTA-Z 7557, and very
similar to that obtained after a rabbit complement lysis. In addition, if the procedure is
toxic, the mechanisms responsible for this
toxicity will vary from one patient to another.
Therefore, if it is certainly important to
raise the question of a possible toxicity of the
procedure, it must not be considered as fully

responsible for these observations. The role of previous chemotherapy on the BM microenvironment could be the major factor of toxicity and it should be noted that in our institute only stage IV neuroblastoma were included in a double autograft program.

Intravenous injection of $CD_8$ monoclonal antibody did not induce any side effect. Such antibody of $IgG_2$ isotype and not coupled to drug nor radiolabeled elements was indeed able to induce the disappearance of $CD_8$+ cells in the blood and the BM in 3 cases out of 6 (2 neuroblastoma cases and the T lymphoma case). The major limitation to such effect seems to be the antigenic modulation of the recognized antigen. Since the therapy was given for a short period of 6 days to very immunodeficient patients, we did not search the appearance of anti-mouse antibodies in the sera of these patients. The quick hematological reconstitution observed in the 3 patients for whom the therapy was efficient supports the hypothesis of a suppressive activity of such cells on the hematopoiesis. This hypothesis was confirmed by the observation made here and by others (Vinci et al., 1987) of an increase of CFU.GM in BM cultures after the in vitro lysis of $CD_8$+ cells by $CD_8$ monoclonal antibody and rabbit complement. Such in vitro assay will probably not have a predictive value for the efficiency of $CD_8$ monoclonal antibody given in vivo since the failures are mainly due to antigen modulation but could help to distinguish between reversible blocking of the hematopoiesis by $CD_8$+ $Leu_7$+ cells and a true non engraftment.

These preliminary results about $CD_8$ in vivo therapy are encouraging but optimal conditions of treatment remain to be determined. In the 6 patients we treated, $CD_8$+ $Leu_7$+ cells were observed from the begining of the third week post ABMT; antibodies were not injected before the fourth or the fifth week post ABMT; this relative delay to treatment could be one of the factors responsible for the 3 failures. The dose

of 0.2 mg/kg/day was somewhat arbitrarily fixed.
If the treatment is well tolerated it could be
important to increase the dose, especially in
patients for whom the antibody allows a partial
disappearance of the cells before the therapy
induces an antigenic modulation. In addition,
when antigenic modulation with $CD_8$ monoclonal
antibody is observed, the effect of a pan T
monoclonal antibody has to be tested. The
immunological follow up of such treated patients
will allow to determine whether the early
destruction of $CD_8$+ cells permits the $T_4/T_8$
lymphocyte ratio to be normal, as has been
described after allogenic BMT with T cell depleted BM (Janossy et al., 1986), and if the
percentage of circulating cells with NK function, and this NK function itself, is higher
than in the control group. Finally, it remains
to be determined whether or not this therapy
could be efficient 2 or 3 months post graft in
patients with low platelet counts but normal
granulocytes; the few patients with such hematological disorders for whom circulating lymphocytes were analyzed showed a moderate increase
of $CD_8$+ $Leu_7$+ cells ranging from 10 to 30 %.

REFERENCES

Bagby GC (1981). T lymphocytes involved in inhi
bition of granulopoïesis in two neutropenic
patients are of the cytotoxic/suppressor ($T_3$+,
$T_8$+) subset. J Clin Invest 68: 1597.
Favrot M, Janossy G, Tidman N, Blacklock H,
Lopez E, Bofill M, Lambert I, Morgenstein G,
Powles R, Prentice HG, Hoffbrand AV (1983). T
cell regeneration after allogeneic bone marrow
transplantation. Clin Exp Immunol 54: 59-72.
Favrot MC, Philip I, Combaret V, Maritaz O,
Philip T (1987). Experimental evaluation of an
immunomagnetic bone marrow purging procedure
using the Burkitt lymphoma model. Bone Marrow
Transplantation (in press).
Gorin NC, Douay L, Laporte JP, Lopez M, Mary JY,
Najman A, Salmon C, Aagerter P, Stachowiak J,
David R, Pene F, Kantor G, Deloux J, Duhamel

E, Van den Akker J, Gerota J, Parlier Y, Duhamel G (1986). Autologous bone marrow transplantation using marrow incubated with Asta Z 7557 in adult acute leukemia. Blood 67: 1367.

Janossy G, Prentice HG, Grob JP, Ivory K, Tidman N, Grundy J, Favrot M, Brenner MK, Campana D, Blacklock HA, Gilmore MJML, Patterson J, Griffiths PD, Hoffbrand AV (1986). T lympho cyte regeneration after transplantation of T cell depleted allogeneic bone marrow. Clin Exp Immunol 63: 577-586.

Lipton JM, Nadler LM, Canellos GP, Kudisch M, Reiss CS, Nathan DG (1983). Evidence for genetic restriction in the suppression of erythropoiesis by a unique subset of T lymphocytes in man. J Clin Invest 72, 694.

Philip T, Bernard JL, Zucker JM, PInkerton R, Lutz P, Bordigoni P, Plouvier E, Robert A, Carton R, Philippe N, Philip I, Chauvin F, Favrot MC (1987a). High dose chemotherapy with bone marrow transplantation as consolidation treatment in neuroblastoma: an unselected group of stage IV patients over one year of age. J Clin Oncol 5: 266-271.

Philip T, Frappaz D, Bouffet E, Farge A, Carrie C, Kremens B, Deterlizzi M, Bernard JL, Zucker JM, Favrot M, Philip I, Biron P (1987b). A pilot study of double ABMT in advanced neuro blastoma (15 patients). Accepted for the ISEH Meeting, Tokyo (Japan), august 1987.

Treleaven JG, Gibson FM, Ugelstad J, Rembaum A, Philip T, Caine GD, Kemshead JT (1984). Removal of neuroblastoma cells from bone marrow with monoclonal antibodies conjugated to magnetic microspheres. Lancet 14: 70-73.

Torok-Storb B, Hansen JA (1982). Modulation of in vitro BFU-E growth by normal Ia positive T cells is restricted by HLA-DR. Nature 298:473.

Vinci G, Vernath JP, Cordonnier C, Bracq C, Rochant H, Breton-Gorius J, Vainchenker W (1986). HLA-DR restriction in suppression of hematopoïesis by T cells from allogeneic bone marrow transplants. J Immunol 136: 3225-3230.

Vinci G, Vernant JP, Cordonnier C, Henri A, Breton-Gorius J, Rochant H, Vainchenker W

(1987). In vitro inhibition of hematopoiesis by HNK$_1$, DR-positive T cells and monocytes after allogeneic bone marrow transplantation. Exp Hematol 15: 54-64.
Zoumbos KC, Ascon P, Djeu JY, Trost SR, Young NS (1985). Circulating activated suppressor T lymphocytes in aplastic anemia. N Engl J Med 312: 257.

Advances in Neuroblastoma Research 2, pages 237–248
© 1988 Alan R. Liss, Inc.

IN VITRO TREATMENT OF AUTOLOGOUS BONE MARROW FOR NEURO-
BLASTOMA PATIENTS WITH ANTI $G_{D2}$ MONOCLONAL ANTIBODY AND
HUMAN COMPLEMENT:   A PILOT STUDY

Jerry Stein, Sarah Strandjord, Ulla Saarinen, Phyllis
Warkentin, Stanley Gerson, Hillard Lazarus, Daniel Von
Hoff, Peter Coccia, and Nai-Kong Cheung

Departments of Pediatrics and Medicine, Case Western
Reserve University, Cleveland, OH 44106 and Memorial
Sloan Kettering Cancer Center, New York, NY 10021

INTRODUCTION

       To increase the survival of children with advanced
stage neuroblastoma (NB), protocols using chemotherapeutic
agents in extremely high, or bone marrow ablative doses,
have been developed.  Infusion of allogeneic or autologous
bone marrow following supralethal chemo-radiotherapy is
essential to extend the limits of such therapy beyond the
constraints of bone marrow toxicity (August et al., 1984;
Helson, 1985; Lazarus et al., 1983).  Allogeneic transplantation is currently limited to the approximately 25% of
patients who have suitable donors.  Alternatively, a
patient's own marrow can be used for hematopoietic reconstitution following ablative chemotherapy.  However,
autologous transplantation is frequently limited by the
contamination of autologous marrow with microscopic foci of
neuroblastoma which can be detected by sensitive assays or
immunofluorescent antibody techniques.  Reinfusion of NB
contaminated marrow as part of autologous transplantation
may defeat the purpose of therapy, and increase the frequency of subsequent relapse.  In order to minimize the
tumor burden of autologous bone marrow, various techniques
have been devised to rid (purge) marrow samples of occult
NB (Reisner and Gan, 1985; Sieber et al., 1986; Reynolds et
al., 1986).

       We have previously described the use of monoclonal
antibodies (MoAb) together with human complement (C') as an
in vitro means of purging tumor cells from the bone marrow
of NB patients with no apparent detrimental effect on the

in vitro hematopoietic colony forming potential of the marrow (Saarinen et al., 1985). We have infused three patients with autologous bone marrow which had been treated with MoAb + C', in an attempt to study the immediate toxicities secondary to the purging method as well as the ability of purged marrow to reconstitute the patients'hematopoietic functions following high dose thiotepa.

MATERIALS AND METHODS

Monoclonal antibodies

Murine IgM MoAb 3G6 and $IgG_3$ 3F8 were prepared as described (Cheung et al., 1985). In brief, ascites was induced in Pristane primed mice, collected sterilely, centrifuged and filtered through glass wool to remove cellular debris. IgM antibodies were precipitated with ammonium sulfate and IgG antibodies were purified on protein-A sepharose. Both antibody preparations were dialysed against phosphate buffers. Samples were tested for the absence of bacteria, fungi, mycoplasma; and murine viruses by MAP testing, in accordance with FDA guidelines for good laboratory practices. Rabbit pyrogen test was used to rule out endotoxin contamination. Safety of the preparations was tested in mice and guinea pigs in the animal facilities of Case Western Reserve University and their pathology was reviewed by Dr. Carlos Abramowsky of University Hospitals of Cleveland.

Immunofluorescence

Aliquot samples ($10^6$ cells) of fresh and purged bone marrow from each patient were washed in ice cold, phosphate buffered saline (PBS) with 0.1% sodium azide and centrifuged at 180 x g for 5 minutes. The pellet was reacted with 100 ul of each MoAb for 20 minutes at $4^O$C. Cells were washed, underlaid with 0.5ml fetal calf serum, washed again, and then fixed with 1% formaldehyde. Cells were examined by fluorescent microscopy, and the number of fluorescent cells as a percentage of mononuclear cells was computed. Murine MoAb panel used included: 3F8 and 3G6, which were specific for ganglioside $G_{D2}$; 3E7, an $IgG_{2b}$ antibody specific for NB and nonreactive with normal bone marrow cells, and IgM antibodies specific for the ganglio-

side G$_{M2}$ (provided by Dr. P. Livingston, Memorial Sloan
Kettering Cancer Center, New York, NY).


Complement sera

ABO blood group compatible sera were obtained from
healthy family members or volunteers by allowing freshly
drawn blood to clot at 37$^{O}$C in sterile glass tubes. Serum
was passed through 0.45um followed by 0.22um filters prior
to freezing at -70$^{O}$C.


Purging procedure

10-20 ml/kg of bone marrow was harvested from patients
under general anesthesia and sterile techniques. Marrow
cells were suspended in medium premixed with heparin.
Following filtration through 0.3 mm and 0.2 mm wire mesh,
the marrow was divided into 3 equal aliquots, one of which
was cryopreserved in DMSO in liquid nitrogen, according to
the method previously described (Lazarus et al., 1983).
The other 2 aliquots were each adjusted to 1x10$^{7}$ mononuclear cells/ml with additional medium, and an equal
volume of IgM MoAb 3G6 (0.5 mg/ml in sterile PBS) was added. After incubation for one hour at room temperature with
gentle mixing, an equal volume of the previously prepared
human serum complement was incubated with the mixture for
an additional hour at 37$^{O}$C. After centrifugation at 180 x
g for 10 minutes and removal of the supernatant, the cells
were washed twice in medium and cryopreserved. Small pilot
samples were saved both before and after antibody treatment
for immunofluorescence, hematopoietic colony forming assay,
and cell viability determination by tryphan-blue exclusion.


Hematopoietic colony forming assay

Hematopoietic colony formation assays of bone marrow
samples have been previously described (Lazarus et al.,
1983; Gerson and Cooper, 1984). Cells were washed and
suspended in RPMI 1640 supplemented with 15% fetal calf
serum, to a concentration of 2x10$^{6}$ cells/mm$^{3}$. Nonadherent
cells were plated in triplicate assays using 0.3% agar
modified with 30% fetal calf serum, Iscoves modified
dubelco's medium supplemented with 2x10$^{-4}$M 2-thioglycerol,

10 mM L-asparagine, 2 mM glutamine, and 1% bovine serum albumin to a final concentration of 1 x $10^5$ cells/ml. Erythroid colony formation was stimulated with erythropoietin (Connaught Laboratories) at 0.5 U/ml, and myeloid colony formation was stimulated by 10% phytohemagglutinin: leukocyte-conditioned medium. Colonies were fixed and stained, and enumerated on day 14.

Patients

This study was carried out with the approval of the Institutional Review Board of Rainbow Babies and Childrens Hospital and Univeriːsty Hospitals of Cleveland, Cleveland, OH. Patients who were participating in a phase I study of high dose thiotepa as a single agent for the treatment of pediatric solid tumors consented to receive MoAb + C' purged autologous bone marrow infusions. All patients had relapsed NB or progressive disease while on conventional chemotherapy, which had included alkylating agents, vinka alkaloids, anthracyclines, cis-platinum, and anti-metabolites. Bone marrow was harvested at the time of minimal bone marrow disease. Although marrow purging was carried out on 7 patients, only 3 patients (patient #1-#3 in Table 1) have had their marrows reinfused at the time of this report. Surgical debulking of a large thoracic tumor was attempted in patient #3 just prior to transplantation. All three patients were prepared for marrow transplantion with thiotepa, 375 mg/m$^2$/d x 3; and following a three day rest, were infused with freshly thawed autologous marrow.

Patients received subsequent transfusions of packed red blood cells and platelets as appropriate, and were treated with intravenous hyperalimentation and antibiotics as needed. All patients received trimethoprim-sulfa during their hospital stay and for variable periods after discharge. Patient #2 received prophylactic acyclovir because of a history of recurrent herpetic infections.

Three additional patients (#4, #5, #6) with NB had received autologous bone marrow transplantation with unpurged marrow after preparation with thiotepa. Two of these patients received 375 mg/m$^2$/d x 3 of thiotepa, one received 240 mg/m$^2$/d x 3. Only patient #2 had no evidence of NB in harvested bone marrow by either conventional histochemical staining, or by immunofluorenscence with

MoAbs. Patients #1 and #5 had tumor clusters evident by light microscopy in bone marrow biopsy specimens obtained at the time of marrow harvest.


RESULTS

Table 1 summarises the results of marrow purging in 7 patients. Six patients had NB detectable by immunofluorescence in the prepurge marrows. In 5 of these patients, NB was not evident by conventional histochemical staining of either marrow aspirate or biopsy. After purging with MoAb + C, 5/6 patients had no detectable tumor by immunostaining. Patient #6 had residual tumor detected in one of the purged bags. Although none of the postpurge marrow showed colonies in the NB clonogenic assay, the number of


Table 1. Viability and immunofluorescent detection of residual NB before and after MoAb + C' purging

| Patient | % Viability (Trypan blue Exclusion) | | % Positive Cells immunofluorescence[a] | |
|---|---|---|---|---|
| | Pre-Purge | Post-Purge | Pre-Purge | Post-purge |
| #1 | 92 | 83.2 | 0.002 | negative[b] |
| #2 | 96.5 | 91.6 | negative | negative |
| #3 | 94 | 95.4 | 0.036 | negative |
| #4 | 88.9 | 84 | 0.008 | negative |
| #5 | 84.4 | 87 | 0.007 | negative |
| #6 | 96.4 | 88 | 0.013 | 0.003[c] |
| #7 | 93 | 93.5 | 0.01 | negative |

[a] 3F8, 3G6, 3E7 and anti-G$_{M2}$ antibodies were used in the MoAb panel.
[b] The limit of sensitivity in such assays averaged 0.001% when 6-8 aliquots were examined using a hemocytometer for staining with monoclonal antibodies.
[c] Only one of the 2 purged bags was positive.


colonies seen in the prepurge marrows were in general too low to be significant. Of the three patients receiving purged bone marrow transplants (#1-#3), only patient #2 had no evidence of NB in harvested bone marrow by either conventional histochemical staining or by fluorescence with monoclonal MoAbs.

The results of hematopoietic colony formation assays in conditioned medium and erythropoietin are shown in Table 2. No difference was seen when the pre- and post- purge marrow samples were compared.

Table 2. Hematopoietic colony formation of purged and unpurged bone marrow samples (Colonies/1 x $10^5$ Mononuclear Cells)

|  |  | CFU GM | BFU E | CFU MIX | TOTAL COLONIES |
|---|---|---|---|---|---|
| #1 | PURGED | 105 | 34 | 4 | 141 |
|  | PURGED | 127 | 30 | 5 | 162 |
|  | UNPURGED | 115 | 31 | 3 | 147 |
| #2 | PURGED | 76 | 8 | 2 | 101 |
|  | PURGED | 80 | 19 | 2 | 86 |
|  | UNPURGED | 85 | 14 | 2 | 101 |
| #3 | PURGED | 141 | 21 | 32 | 243 |
|  | UNPURGED | 134 | 83 | 29 | 250 |

The only untoward reaction observed during the intravenous infusion of purged bone marrow occurred in patient #3, who developed a mild urticarial eruption which responded to antihistamines.

The dose of mononuclear cells/kg, the period to engraftment, as assessed by the absolute neutrophil count and dependency on platelet transfusions are shown in Tables 3 and 4. Patients received their second high dose thiotepa 90 days after their first course.

Infectious complications among the patients receiving purged bone marrow included streptococcus viridans sepsis in patient #1 and focal subcutaneous aspergillosis in patient #3. Both infections responded to appropriate antibiotic therapy. Other complications which occurred during transplantation included severe mucositis and exfoliative

Table 3.  Time (days) required for count recovery

|  | Patient #1 | Patient #2 | Patient #3 |
|---|---|---|---|
| Number of nucleated cells infused per kg | $1.2 \times 10^8$ | $1.4 \times 10^8$ | $1.1 \times 10^8$ |
| ANC>200/mm$^3$ | 32 | 43 | 14 |
| ANC>500/mm$^3$ | 45 | 86 | 23 |
| ANC>1000/mm$^3$ | 55 | >90 | 32 |
| Duration of antibiotic therapy | 25 | 26 | 28 |
| Platelet transfusion dependency | >90 | >90 | 45 |

Table 4.  Time (days) required for count recovery

|  | Patient #1a | Patient #2a | Patient #3a |
|---|---|---|---|
| Number of nucleated cells infused per kg | $0.8 \times 10^8$ | $1.1 \times 10^8$ | $1.8 \times 10^8$ |
| ANC>200/mm$^3$ | 26 | 57 | 34 |
| ANC>500/mm$^3$ | 36 | 73 | 46 |
| ANC>1000/mm$^3$ | 53 | >90 | 60 |
| Duration of antibiotic therapy | 29 | 43 | 33 |
| Platelet transfusion dependency | 46 | 78 | >90 |

dermatitis; the extent and severity of these complications did not differ between patients who received purged or un-purged bone marrow.  After adequate count recovery, patients #1 and #2 were treated with second infusions of purged autologous bone marrow following a second course of high dose thiotepa.  All three patients subsequently re-

ceived intravenous infusions of the MoAb 3F8 in a phase II
study exploring the use of 3F8 for tumor imaging and in
vivo anti-tumor effects. The nature and severity of
allergic reactions seen during these treatments were not
different from those observed in patients who had never
received MoAb purged bone marrow infusions.


DISCUSSION

     3G6 is an IgM-kappa murine monoclonal antibody with
specificity for the cell surface disialoganglioside $G_{D2}$, an
antigen found on neuroblastoma cells and on restricted
normal tissues such as some neurons (Cheung et al., 1985).
Immunofluorescent staining with the MoAb can reliably detect occult bone marrow (BM) involvement in patients with
NB (Cheung et al., 1986).  Incubation of BM cells with MoAb
+ C' can effectively eliminate tumor cells from tumor
contaminated marrows (Saarinen et al., 1985).  The selectivity of this in vitro complement mediated cytotoxicity
is demonstrated by the preservation of hematopoietic colony
forming ability of treated marrow (Saarinen et al., 1985).
Human complement mediated cytotoxicity is regulated by
decay accelerating factor (DAF), a protein present on most
normal blood cells and epithelial tissues (Medof et al.,
1987).  The importance of DAF in protecting blood cells in
vivo is indicated by the finding that its deficiency in
patients with paroxysmal nocturnal hemoglobinuria (PNH) is
causally related to the hemolytic anemia that is characteristic of this clinical disorder.  Normal blood and marrow
elements, by virtue of possessing DAF, can thus resist
autologous complement attack.  This allows another level of
selectivity of tumor cytotoxicity by MoAb + C' in tumors
deficient in this protein, such as neuroblastoma.

     There are additional advantages of this purging
technique.  Besides effectiveness and selectivity of tumor
depletion, the use of unfractionated fresh BM in our
purging procedure eliminates the need for concentrating
mononuclear cells on density gradients, thus reducing the
loss of nucleated cells that accompanies each purification
procedure.  Moreover, human serum is the complement source
in our purging technique, and human serum is readily available and easy to prepare.  It does not contain the heterophile antibodies which have been implicated in the anti-
complementary effect observed when animal sera are used as

sources of complement in purging experiements (Martin et al., 1984).

Previous in vitro seeding experiments showed that MoAb + C' purging was effective in eliminating the clonogenic potential of NB cells in bone marrow samples. Using a panel of MoAb's directed against NB, no residual NB cells could be found by indirect immunofluorescence after BM purging. Although the expression of the G$_{D2}$ antigen is not modulated by preincubation of NB cells with specific MoAb, a small percentage (<1%) of NB cells might express low levels of G$_{D2}$ below the threshold of detection by immuno-fluorescence (Cheung et al., 1985). However, the sensi-tivity of the immunofluorescence assay is not established at extremely low concentrations of NB cells in marrow samples. At such low concentrations, clonogenic assays are also limited by their low plating efficiency of NB. In seeding experiments in which a known number of NB cells labeled with the nuclear fluorescent stain (Hoechst 33343) was added to bone marrow samples from normal donors, purging with MoAb + C' resulted in at least a 3-log tumor cell reduction in samples with high concentrations of NB cells. However, the efficiency of NB purging by MoAb + C' was nearly 100% when tumor cell burden constituted <1% of nucleated cells. As all of our patients had pre-purge BM tumor concentrations of far less than 1%, it is likely that MoAb + C' could effectively remove most if not all tumor cells from the marrow samples. In vitro hematopoietic colony forming assays showed that NB removal did not occur at the expense of hematopoietic colony forming potential. Enrichment procedures of pre- and post-purge BM samples to concentrate NB cells may allow detection of as few as 1 x $10^{-6}$ tumor cells in marrow samples, and may be a useful adjunct in monitoring the efficacy of future purging procedures (Reynolds et al., 1985).

Since in vitro hematopoietic assays may not translate in all systems to in vivo hematopoietic potentials, we have tested the ability of purged marrows to engraft in 3 patients with advanced NB. No severe immediate reactions could be attributed to the purging process. In addition, patients were able to tolerate subsequent treatment with repeated infusions of purged marrows as well as the murine IgG$_3$ antibody 3F8.

Engraftment, as defined by a return of peripheral

granulocyte counts, was similar in patients who received
purged or untreated BM following high doses thiotepa. The
overall time to engraftment was long compared to other
patients undergoing autologous transplantations. For
example, a recent report of NB patients who received autologous bone marrow transplantation using BM purged with
immunomagnetic bead techniques demonstrated recovery of
absolute neutrophil counts of >500/mm$^3$ 13-39 days after
transplantation (Philip et al., 1985). On the other hand,
the time to attain similar counts ranged from 23 to 86 days
in our patients receiving purged marrows, and from 36-73
days in patients who received untreated marrow. It is
unlikely that thiotepa directly damaged the infused marrow.
Thiotepa is an alkylating agent with an extensive tissue
distribution. However, its tissue elimination phase is
approximately one hour (Egorin et al., 1984). The three
day hiatus between the last dose of thiotepa and autologous
BM transplantation has been shown to be safe in patients
receiving drugs with substantially longer tissue half lives
than thiotepa (Eder et al., 1986) and should have been more
than adequate in our patients. Nevertheless, it is possible that the preparative regimen of high dose thiotepa
damaged the microenvironment of marrow and therefore slowed
down engraftment. The more likely explanation of delayed
engraftment in our patients is probably due to the infusion
dose of the marrow cells and the routine use of trimethoprim-sulfa in the post transplant period. A strong inverse
correlation between the infused CFU-GM and the time to
engraftment has been found by some authors (Spitzer et al.,
1980). especially when the dose of CFU-GM/kg patient body
weight was low (Hartmann et al., 1985).

In summary, we have demonstrated that bone marrow,
purged of NB cells with MoAb 3G6 + C' can be safely infused
into patients following supralethal chemotherapy. Infusion
of more BM cells and the availability of more effective
preparative regimens will make this form of therapy a
viable option for prolonging survival in patients with
refractory or relapsed NB.

ACKNOWLEDGEMENTS
    We thank Ms. Bonnie Landmeier, Ms. Cathy Gallagher and
Mr. Harvey Smith-Mensah for their excellent technical
assistance; and Ms. Elaine Halliday and Ms. Mary Ann Toth
for their secretarial assistance.

REFERENCES

August CS, Serota FT, Koch PA, Burkey E, Schlessinger H, Elkins WL, Evans AE, D'Angio GH (1984). Treatment of neuroblastoma with supralethal chemotherapy, radiation and allogeneic or autologous marrow reconstitution. J Clin Oncol 2:609-615.

Cheung NK, Saarinen UM, Neely JE, Landmeier B, Donovan D, Coccia PF (1985). Monoclonal antibodies to a glycolipid antigen on human neuroblastoma cells. Cancer Res 45: 2642-2649.

Cheung NK, Von Hoff DD, Strandjord SE, Coccia PF (1986). Detection of neuroblastoma cell bone marrow using G$_{D2}$ specific monoclonal antibodies. J Clin Oncol 4:363-369.

Eder JP, Bast RC, Peters WD, Kenner D, Sanchez E, Schryber S, Frei E, Schnipper LE (1986). Prediction of the optimal timing of bone marrow reinfusion after high dose chemotherapy. Cancer Res 46:4496-4499.

Egorin J, Akman SR, Guttierrez PL (1984). Plasma pharmacokinetics and tissue distribution of thiotepa in mice. Cancer Treatment Reports 68:1265-1268.

Gerson SL, Cooper RA (1984). Release of granulocyte-specific colony-stimulating activity by human bone marrow exposed to phorbol esters. Blood 63:878-885.

Hartmann O, Beaujean F, Bayet S, Pico JL, Tournade MF, Lemerle J, Parmentier C (1985). Hematopoetic recovery following autologous bone marrow transplantation: role of cyropreservation, number of cells infused and nature of high dose chemotherapy. Eur J Cancer Clin Oncol 21:53-60.

Helson L (1985). Autologous Bone Marrow Transplantation: A maximal therapy design for disseminated neuroblastoma. Am J Ped Hem/Oncol 7:45-50.

Lazarus HM, Herzig RH, Graham-Pole J, Wolff SN, Philips GL, Strandjord SE, Hurd D, Formon W, Gordon EM, Coccia PF, Gross S, Herzig GP (1983). Intensive melphelan chemotherapy and cryopreserved autologous bone marrow transplantation for the treatment of refractory cancer. J Clin Oncol 1:359-366.

Martin PJ, Lasner R, Hansen JA (1984). Heterophile antibodies: a possible explanation for the anti-complementary effects of human marrow monocuclear cells. Blood 64:218a.

Medof ME, Walter EI, Rutgers Jl, Knowles DM, Nussenzweig V (1987). Identification of the complement decay-accelerating factor (DAF) on epithelium and glandular cells and in body fluids. J Exp Med 165:848-864.

Philip T, Zucker JM, Favrot M, Bordigoni P, Plovier E,
Robert A, Bernard JL, Souillet G, Philip I, Lute JP, Corton
P, Kemshead J (1985). Purged autologous bone marrow
transplantation in 25 cases of very poor prognosis neuroblastoma. Lancet 576-577.
Reisner Y, Gan J (1985). Differential binding of soybean
agglutinin to human neuroblastoma cell lines: potential
applications to autologous bone marrow transplantation.
Cancer Res 45:4026-4031.
Reynolds CR, Moss TJ, Wells J, Seeger RC (1985). Sensitive
detection of neuroblastoma cells in bone marrow for
monitoring the efficacy of marrow purging procedures. In
Evans AE, D'Angio G, Seeger RC (eds): "Advances In
Neuroblastoma Research", New Yorkd: Alan R Liss, pp 425-
441.
Reynolds CP, Seeger RC, Vo DD, Black AT, Wells J, Ugelstad
J (1986). Model system for removing neuroblastoma cells
from bone marrow using monoclonal antibodies and magnetic
immunobeads. Cancer Res 46:5882-5886.
Saarinen UM, Coccia PF, Gerson SL, Pelley R, Cheung NKV
(1985). Eradication of neuroblastoma cells in vitro by
monoclonal antibody and human complement: method for
purging autologous bone marrow. Cancer Res 45:5969-5975.
Sieber F, Rao S, Rowley SD, Sieber-Blum M (1986). Dye
mediated photolysis of human neuroblastoma cells:
implication for autologous bone marrow transplantation.
Blood 68:32-36.
Spitzer G, Verna DS, Fisher R, Zonder A, Vellekoup L, Litam
J, McCredie KB, Dicke KA (1980). The myeloid progenitor
cell-its value in predicting hematopoetic recovery after
autologous bone marrow transplantation. Blood 55:317-
323.

Advances in Neuroblastoma Research 2, pages 249–262

SENSITIVE DETECTION OF RARE METASTATIC HUMAN NEUROBLASTOMA
CELLS IN BONE MARROW BY TWO-COLOR IMMUNOFLUORESCENCE AND
CELL SORTING

Christopher N. Frantz, Daniel H. Ryan, Nai-kong
V. Cheung, Reggie E. Duerst and David C. Wilbur
Departments of Pediatrics and Pathology and The
Cancer Center,University of Rochester Medical Center
Rochester, New York 14642; Department of Pediatrics,
Memorial-Sloan Kettering Cancer Institute, New
York, New York 10021

Sensitive detection of rare metastatic neuroblastoma
cells in bone marrow may predict patient outcome and be
used to determine appropriate therapy.  Detection of neuroblastoma cells in bone marrow may also be used for the study
of autologous bone marrow transplantation in the treatment
of neuroblastoma.

Immunohistochemistry has been applied to bone marrow
aspirate smears to identify metastatic neuroblastoma in bone
marrow (Moss et al., 1985).  Detection of metastatic neuroblastoma using immunofluorescent flow cytometry would also
allow the isolation of metastatic cells by cell sorting.
Isolation would aid in the biological characterization of
such cells.  However, immunofluorescent techniques tend to
identify a large number of normal bone marrow cells as
"false-positive" tumor cells.  We have devised a technique
to improve flow cytometric discrimination between neuroblastoma and normal bone marrow cells.  We describe here the use
of multiple anti-bone marrow monoclonal antibodies conjugated
to phycoerythrin in combination with an anti-tumor monoclonal
antibody conjugated to fluorescein in order to improve the
ability to detect rare metastatic neuroblastoma cells in
bone marrow.  In addition, we demonstrate that cells flow
cytometrically detected as neuroblastoma can be viably
isolated by cell sorting and that they are neuroblastoma cells
as documented by morphology, neurite extension in culture,
and binding of tetanus toxin.

MATERIALS AND METHODS

Bone marrow was collected in heparin, diluted five-fold in medium, sedimented onto a layer of Ficoll-Hypaque and washed. Residual erythrocytes were lysed by suspending the cells for 10 min at $4^{o}$C in fresh 0.16 M NH4Cl, 0.01 M K2HCO3. Cultured human neuroblastoma cells were obtained and grown as previously described (Frantz et al., 1986). All cultures were fed the day before use and were subconfluent. Antibody dependent complement mediated cytotoxicity was assayed as previously described (Duerst et al., 1986).

The 6-19 hybridoma, which produces a mouse IgG2a monoclonal antibody that binds to a cell surface antigen present on neuroblastoma but not on hematopoietic cells, was derived as previously described (Frantz, et al., 1986). The 3G6 anti-ganglioside GD2 monoclonal antibody (anti-GD2) was derived as previously described (Cheung et al., 1985). The hybridomas OKM1, MMA, GAP8.3 and R1B19 were obtained from the American Type Culture Collection, and transplantable TEPC-183 IgM myeloma from NIH. Monoclonal antibodies were purified and conjugated with fluorescein as described by Goding (1976). R-Phycoerythrin was conjugated to purified antibody as described by Molecular Probes, the manufacturer.

For direct immunofluorescent staining, the conjugated antibodies were incubated with $2 \times 10^{6}$ cells in 50 µl Puck's saline G containing 15 percent fetal calf serum and 200 mcg per ml unlabeled antibody of the same isotype at $4^{o}$C for 30 min. For incubations with 6-19 FITC the unlabeled antibody was RPC5 (IgG2a) and for anti-GD2-FITC or its control, mouse IgM-FITC (Coulter), a mixture of affinity purified mouse IgM (Cappel) and TEPC-183 mouse IgM. Bone marrow was preincubated with unlabeled antibody for 30 min at $4^{o}$C, and phycoerythrin-conjugated antibodies were then added. After an additional 30 min at $4^{o}$C, the cells were washed once and unlabeled antibody and fluorescein-conjugated antibodies added. Prior to flow cytometric examination, cells were washed three times, passed through a 20µ nylon mesh, and fixed with 1% paraformaldehyde. In some experiments, the cells were examined without fixation in the presence of 250 ng/ml propidium iodide to exclude dead cells.

Stained cells were analyzed on an Epics C flow cytometer (Coulter Epics Division, Hialeah, FL) using the 488 nm line of an argon laser at 500 mW power. Forward angle light scatter gates were set to exclude red blood cells, platelets, debris and large aggregates of cells. A total of 30,000 -

1,000,000 cells were counted per sample.  In cell sorting
experiments, fresh samples were sorted at a flow rate of 300
to 500 cells per second and a dropoff formation rate of 32kHz.
The cells were sorted into tissue culture medium containing
calf serum.  Cytocentrifuge slides were prepared and stained
with Wright-Giemsa or for tetanus toxin binding and cells
cultured as described above.

     In each experiment LA-N-1 cultured human neuroblastoma
cells or a mixture of 20% LA-N-1, 80% bone marrow were
stained identically to the bone marrow cells.  The mean
fluorescence intensity of the cultured tumor cell population
on that day was determined and used as the fluorescence
intensity above which cells in the other samples would be
counted as either true or false positive tumor cells.

     Tetanus toxin and horse anti-tetanus toxin antiserum
were the kind gift of Dr. R.O. Thompson, Wellcome Research
Laboratories.  Tetanus toxin binding was detected by sequential incubations with tetanus toxin, horse anti-tetanus toxin
(Notter and Leary, 1985; Berliner and Unsicker, 1985), affinity
purified biotinylated goat anti-horse IgG and either avidin-
FITC (Becton-Dickinson) for immunofluorescence or avidin-
peroxidase complex (Vector) for immunohistochemistry.  Cytocentrifuge slides of sorted cells were fixed for 10 min at
4°C in ethanol, quenched with 3% $H_2O_2$, and stained for tetanus
toxin binding.  Cytocentrifuge slides of normal bone marrow
and of LA-N-1 cells were stained simultaneously as negative
and positive controls.

RESULTS

Binding of Anti-Neuroblastoma Antibodies

     Binding of 6-19 and anti-GD2 monoclonal antibodies to
LA-N-1 cultured human neuroblastoma cells is depicted in
Figure 1.  Cells were incubated with 30 mcg per ml of purified
TEPC-183 IgM control (top panel), 5 mcg/ml RPC5 IgG2a control
(not shown), 5 mcg/ml 6-19 monoclonal antibody (middle panel),
or 30 mcg/ml anti-GD2 (bottom panel), washed and incubated
with fluorescein-conjugated anti-mouse Ig, and analyzed by
flow cytometry.  Much more 3G6 bound per cell than did 6-19
antibody.  Although a proportion of the cells stained with
each anti-neuroblastoma antibody fluoresced less intensely
than did cells incubated with control antibody, the distribution of fluorescence intensity for each of these antibodies

was unimodal. The distribution strongly suggests that
there is not a discrete population of antigen negative
neuroblastoma cells for these
two monoclonal antibodies.
This was confirmed by studies
using 6-19 monoclonal antibody and complement in which
99.99% of cultured neuroblastoma cells were killed with
incubation conditions that
injured less than 10% of
normal bone marrow colony-
forming cells (Duerst et al.,
1986). When studied by
immunofluorescence, the
remaining cells after complement lysis demonstrated a
fluorescence intensity similar
to the starting cell population.

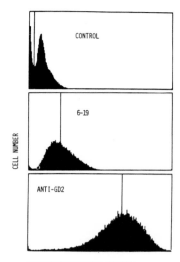

LOG GREEN FLUORESCENCE INTENSITY

Figure 1. Comparison of
binding of anti-neuroblastoma
antibodies to LA-N-1 cells.

   To confirm that essen-
tially all of the LA-N-1
cultured neuroblastoma cells
expressed GD2 ganglioside, LA-N-1 cells were incubated with
anti-GD2 antibody and complement. Greater than 99% of LA-N-1
cells were killed, and binding of anti-GD2 to the small
number of surviving LA-N-1 cells was compared to the binding
to an aliquot of LA-N-1 not treated with complement. The
distribution of fluorescence intensity was similar. Thus,
essentially all the neuroblastoma cells in this cell line
expressed the GD2 antigen. Similar unimodal distributions
of immunofluorescence intensity were obtained for both these
antibodies with the human neuroblastoma cell lines KAG,
LA-N-5, IMR-32, KCN, and KANR.

   Cultured human neuroblastoma cells also had a unimodal
distribution of tetanus toxin binding (Figure 2). LA-N-1
neuroblastoma or bone marrow cells were incubated with
(middle and bottom panels) or without (top panel) tetanus
toxin and stained with the immunodection system described
in Materials and Methods. The unimodal distribution of
antigen binding suggests that essentially all the cultured
neuroblastoma cells bind tetanus toxin. In contrast, there

is no difference in fluorescence distribution between
bone marrow cells incubated
with (bottom panel) or without (not shown) tetanus toxin.
Most importantly, fluorescence intensity clearly allows
discrimination of the majority of neuroblastoma cells
from the majority of bone
marrow cells. This difference
was even more apparent in
immunohistochemical studies,
possibly because of staining
for intracellular antigen and
the relative signal amplification due to the use of
avidin-peroxidase complex.
Four other cultured human
neuroblastoma cell lines were
examined and all demonstrated
a unimodal distribution of
tetanus toxin immunofluorescence.

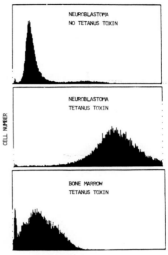

Figure 2. Binding of tetanus
toxin to LA-N-1 cells and
bone marrow.

Binding of Anti-Bone Marrow Antibodies

Four different monoclonal antibodies that bind to cell
surface antigens found on myeloid and lymphoid bone marrow
cells were purified and conjugated to phycoerythrin. Greater
than 70% of bone marrow mononuclear cells bound sufficient
antibody to result in red fluorescence intensity above auto-
fluorescence. Analysis of the $90^{\circ}$ light scatter characteristics of positive and negative staining bone marrow cells
revealed that almost all cells with high $90^{\circ}$ light scatter,
presumably monocytes and myeloid precursors that scatter
light at $90^{\circ}$ due to their granule content, were stained by
the phycoerythrin-conjugated anti-bone marrow antibody mixture (data not shown).

Quantitation of Positive and False-Positive Cells by Flow
Cytometry

In order to determine the sensitivity and quantitative

reliability of detection of neuroblastoma cells in bone
marrow, LA-N-1 cultured human neuroblastoma cells were used
as a facsimile of tumor.   In all experiments a mixture of
10-20% LA-N-1 and 80-90% normal bone marrow was stained with
a mixture of phycoerythrin conjugated anti-bone marrow
antibodies and anti-GD2-FITC.   The population of tumor cells
was obvious in comparison to normal bone marrow (Figure 3).

In the histo-
grams, bone
marrow cells
with red fluor-
escence greater
than that of
99% of the
neuroblastoma
cells are
excluded.   The
mean green
fluorescence
intensity of
the neuroblast-
oma cell popu-
lation was
determined
(vertical cur-
sor, top panel,
Figure 3).   The
number of bone
marrow cells
with higher
green fluor-
escence inten-
sity than that
mean was arbi-
trarily consid-
ered positive
or false-positive.

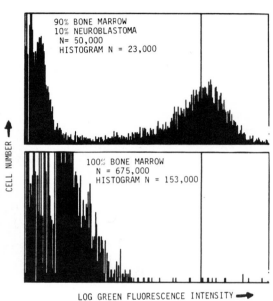

Figure 3.   Quantitation of anti-GD2-FITC
positive cells added to normal bone marrow
with exclusion of cells binding four
phycoerythrin conjugated anti-bone marrow
monoclonal antibodies.

Bone marrow from seven normal individuals
was examined in that fashion and contained between 0 and 34
positive cells per million cells counted, with a mean of
$19 \pm 11$ (S.D.).   For these studies, fresh bone marrow samples
were stained and sorted without fixation in the presence of
propidium iodide to stain dead cells red and thus allow
their exclusion.   Examination of bone marrow cells viably
frozen and then thawed on the day of analysis detected a
slightly higher number of positive normal bone marrow cells.
Similar calculations were used to quantify the detection of

cultured LA-N-1 cells added in varying proportions to normal
bone marrow cells. The number of neuroblastoma cells added
to bone marrow was very nearly the number counted (data not
shown).

Analysis of Bone Marrow Containing Metastatic Neuroblastoma

    In order to determine whether the assay as described
was applicable to patient bone marrow containing metastatic
neuroblastoma, viably frozen patient bone marrow containing
metastatic neuroblastoma was thawed and stained with the
mixture of phycoerythrin-conjugated anti-bone marrow antibodies and either anti-GD2-FITC or mouse IgM-FITC. The
histograms were superimposed and the difference between
them obtained as shown in Figure 4. Four such patient bone

marrow samples
and a mixture
of LA-N-1 and
normal bone
marrow cells
were stained
and analyzed on
the same day.
The distribu-
tions of fluor-
escence inten-
sity of the
subtraction
histograms
were all
extremely
similar, as
determined by
the standard
deviation and
coefficient
of variation.

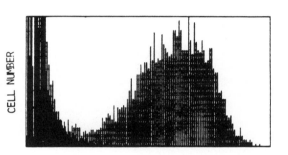

Figure 4. Subtraction histogram (spaced
vertical lines) patient bone marrow containing metastatic neuroblastoma stained
with either anti-GD2-FITC or mouse IgM-FITC.

However, the mean fluorescence intensity of
the positive tumor cell population was consistently greater
than that of LA-N-1 cultured neuroblastoma cells. Neuroblastoma in all patient bone marrows examined to date have
also shown a mean fluorescence intensity consistently greater
than that of the cultured cells. Thus, metastatic neuroblastoma cells appear to resemble cultured neuroblastoma
cells when stained with anti-GD2 FITC in terms of distribution of fluorescence intensity and fluoresce at least as

intensely as the cultured cells. This suggests that the
addition of cultured neuroblastoma cells to bone marrow
serves as a good model for metastatic neuroblastoma in bone
marrow when examined with an anti-GD2 monoclonal antibody.
In addition, detection of metastatic cells in patient marrow
should be at least as sensitive as detection of cultured
cells added to marrow.

Flow cytometric analysis of bone marrow obtained from
a patient with neuroblastoma at three different times in
his clinical course is shown in Figure 5. Analyses of these
bone marrow aspirates were performed at different times, and for each analysis, normal bone marrow cells and normal bone marrow cells mixed with cultured human neuroblastoma cells were stained and analyzed at the same time. The vertical cursors indicate the mean fluorescence intensity of the cultured human neuroblastoma cell population assayed that day. All cells with red fluorescence intensity greater than that of 99% of LA-N-1 are excluded from the histograms. At diagnosis, microscopic examination of stained bone marrow aspirates showed many tumor cells and these are apparent as a population of cells with very high

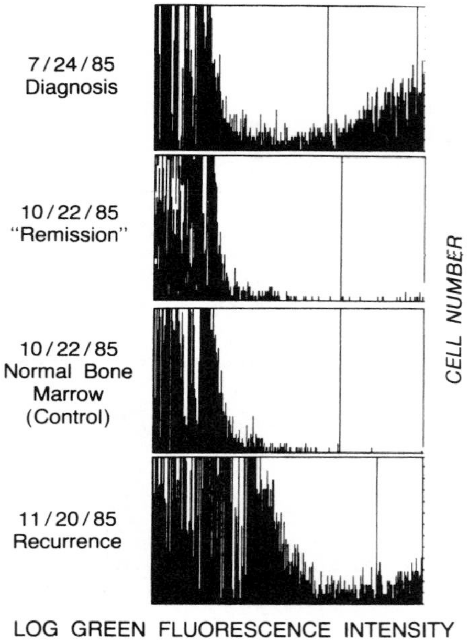

Figure 5. Flow cytometric analysis of
anti-GD2-FITC positive cell populations
in bone marrow obtained from a patient at
diagnosis, "remission," and recurrence.

green fluorescence intensity (top panel, Figure 5). Three months later there was no apparent neuroblastoma in the bone marrow aspirate on microscopic examination, but there was a small but distinct population of bright green fluorescent cells seen in the patient sample (second panel, Figure 5) but not in the control normal bone marrow (third panel, Figure 5). Examination of bone marrow from this patient one month later demonstrated the presence of neuroblastoma cells in bone marrow on routine microscopic examination, and an increase in the population of bright green fluorescent cells was once again seen (bottom panel, Figure 5).


Isolation of Neuroblastoma From Patient Bone Marrow By Cell Sorting

In order to prove that cells identified by flow cytometry were indeed neuroblastoma cells, anti–GD2–FITC–positive cells were sorted from patient bone marrow. Patient bone marrow containing metastatic neuroblastoma was stained with a mixture of monoclonal antibodies and analyzed by flow cytometry as described above (Figure 6, top left panel). Comparison with normal bone marrow stained and analyzed at the same time (Figure 6, top right panel) demonstrates the population of cells in the patient's bone marrow with bright green and low red fluorescence. Attempting to encompass the entire population of anti–GD2–FITC–positive cells, this population was visually estimated on the histogram as described by the vertical and horizontal cursor lines (top left panel, Figure 6). The population of cells described comprised 31% of the patient marrow cells but only 0.2% of the normal bone marrow cells. This population was sorted with coincidence correction and the sorted cells were analyzed by flow cytometry (bottom left panel, Figure 6). Of the cells obtained, 94% had the fluorescence characteristics of the positive cell population. Morphological analysis of a Wright's stained cytocentrifuge preparation of the sorted cells revealed that 95% of the cells had the morphology of neuroblastoma. In addition, there were aggregates of pink staining neurofibrillary material that appeared to have originated from the centers of neuroblastoma rosettes. A total of $6.9 \times 10^5$ viable cells was obtained, which was 96% of the cells with high green and low red fluorescence that were the objective of the sort. The sorted cells were also stained immunohistochemically for tetanus toxin binding, and 88% of the sorted cells were positive. Tetanus toxin did not bind to normal bone marrow cells analyzed by immunofluorescence and flow cytometry (Figure 2), and only rare cells stain by immunohistochemistry. In order to determine whether there were any tetanus toxin binding cells among the population of false-positive cells in normal bone marrow, normal bone marrow and normal bone marrow containing 10% cultured neuroblastoma cells were stained

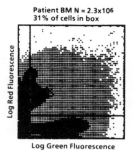

Patient BM N = 2.3x10⁶
31% of cells in box

Log Red Fluorescence

Log Green Fluorescence

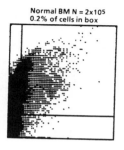

Normal BM N = 2x10⁵
0.2% of cells in box

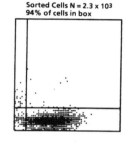

Sorted Cells N = 2.3 x 10³
94% of cells in box

SINGLE SORT RESULTS:

Yield: 6.9 X 10⁵ viable cells
    96% of cells in box

Purity: 94% by immunofluorescence

    95% by morphology
    88% by tetanus toxin
        receptor immuno-histochemistry

Viability: sustained primary culture
    with enurite extension

Figure 6. Isolation by cell sorting of neuroblastoma from patient bone marrow containing metastases apparent on light microscopic examination.

as described above. The cells from normal bone marrow that fluoresced like neuroblastoma comprised 0.005% of the normal bone marrow and were purified by serially sorting twice. A total of 5,000 cells, 86% of the population aimed for, was obtained. A cytocentrifuge preparation of these cells was stained for tetanus toxin binding, and none was seen.

DISCUSSION

This paper describes the use of two-color immunofluorescence flow cytometry to identify and enumerate human neuroblastoma cells among human bone marrow cells. The cells were stained with a mixture of fluorescein-conjugated 3G6 antibody directed against the GD2 ganglioside and four monoclonal antibodies conjugated to phycoerythrin that bind to predominately myeloid cells in bone marrow. When stained with the antibody mixture, neuroblastoma cells have green and bone marrow cells have red fluorescence. This technique appears to be highly sensitive because in normal bone marrow samples, there were fewer than 50 cells per million that stained with the characteristics of neuroblastoma. When cultured neuroblastoma cells were mixed with normal bone marrow cells and analyzed, the number detected corresponded to the number added. Thus the assay allows quantitation of cultured neuroblastoma cells added to bone marrow.

With limited analysis of clinical samples, the technique appears to detect reliably the presence of metastatic neuroblastoma in bone marrow. To date, we have examined bone marrow from nine patients containing metastatic neuroblastoma as determined by routine light microscopic examination of the aspirate. In each case, a prominent population of GD2-positive, bone marrow antigen negative cells was seen. This suggests that the assay will detect metastatic neuroblastoma in most patients when it is present, and is confirmed by the finding of GD2 antigen on most patient neuroblastomas examined (Cheung et al., 1985). Whether or not cell surface GD2 is expressed on metastatic neuroblastoma from all patients can only be determined by examination of bone marrow containing metastatic neuroblastoma from many more patients.

It has not yet been determined whether there is significant heterogeneity in GD2 ganglioside expression among metastatic neuroblastoma cells in bone marrow. This will be studied by sorting GD2 positive metastatic neuroblastoma cells from bone marrow and determining whether any neuroblastoma cells remain as assessed by tetanus toxin binding. The unimodal distribution of anti-GD2 antibody binding to cultured neuroblastoma cell lines, and the ability to kill more than 99% of cultured neuroblastoma cells with anti-GD2 monoclonal antibody and complement, demonstrates that there is not significant heterogeneity of binding of this antibody within cultured human neuroblastoma cell populations. The mean fluorescence intensity of patient tumor cells was consistently greater than that of the cultured neuroblastoma cells, and the distribution of fluorescence intensity was essentially identical. This suggests that the cultured neuroblastoma cells are a good model of metastatic neuroblastoma in terms of homogeneity of binding of antibody.

The incidence of false positive assays remains to be determined; that is, whether an increased number of cells in

bone marrow that fluoresce like neuroblastoma cells is always
due to neuroblastoma cells. However, cell sorting can be
used to demonstrate whether or not such positive cells are
indeed neuroblastoma cells. Cells with immunofluorescence
characteristics of neuroblastoma were sorted from bone marrow
containing metastatic neuroblastoma and from normal bone marrow. The cells sorted from patient bone marrow had the morphologic appearance of neuroblastoma cells and extended
neurites in culture, demonstrating that neuroblastoma cells
were present in the sorted population. The sorted neuroblastoma cells bound tetanus toxin. When false-positive cells,
i.e., cells with the immunofluorescence characteristics of
neuroblastoma, were sorted from normal bone marrow, no tetanus
toxin binding was seen. Tetanus toxin binds specifically,
with few exceptions, to central and peripheral neuronal cells.
Tetanus toxin binding has been demonstrated on 13 of 13 human
neuroblastoma tumors tested, including neuroblastomas of all
stages in both primary and metastatic disease (Berliner and
Unsicker, 1985). Thus tetanus toxin binding is a good marker
for neuroblastoma, and can be used after cell sorting to
determine whether or not flow cytometrically positive cells
in bone marrow are indeed neuroblastoma cells, and whether
all neuroblastoma cells are identified.

The flow cytometric assay might be improved by the use
of additional monoclonal antibodies that bind to neuroblastoma cell surface antigens other than ganglioside GD2. First,
if there is any significant heterogeneity of expression of
ganglioside GD2 on metastatic neuroblastoma cells in bone
marrow, those tumor cells that do not express GD2 ganglioside might express other detectable neuroblastoma-related
antigens, allowing detection of the ganglioside GD2 negative
tumor cells. Second, if any neuroblastoma tumors do not
express GD2 ganglioside at all, metastatic cells in the bone
marrow of these patients might be detected by expression of
other neuroblastoma-related antigens, allowing detection of
metastatic neuroblastoma in bone marrow from a greater proportion of patients who have metastatic disease in the bone
marrow. Finally, by producing more intense immunofluorescence of neuroblastoma cells relative to normal bone marrow
cells, discrimination of neuroblastoma cells from bone
marrow might be further improved. However, use of 6-19-FITC
and anti-GD2-FITC together in the assay was not more sensitive than the use of anti-GD2-FITC alone (data not shown).

Other possible means of further improving sensitivity

and reliability of this detection technique will require further investigation. Partial purification of neuroblastoma cells from bone marrow prior to flow cytometric analysis might further improve sensitivity. Additional anti-bone marrow phycoerythrin-conjugated antibodies that specifically identify the non-tumor positive cells in normal bone marrow might also result in a major improvement in sensitivity of the assay. The characteristics of the non-tumor positive cells have not been determined. It is possible that they express cell surface ganglioside GD2. Finally, metastatic neuroblastoma in bone marrow is typically identified because the cells are in clumps. Single cells probably also abound in many cases but these are not readily identifiable by light microscopy. It appears that most of these clumps of neuroblastoma cells are broken apart to a single cell suspension during preparation of bone marrow containing metastatic neuroblastoma for flow cytometry. It has not yet been investigated whether some clumps of cells are not broken up and are lost during sample filtration prior to flow cytometric analysis. This issue requires further investigation, including the development of techniques to dissociate clumps of neuroblastoma into viable single cells without affecting antibody binding to either neuroblastoma or bone marrow cells.

For extremely sensitive detection of very rare metastatic neuroblastoma cells in bone marrow, it may be possible to isolate from bone marrow by cell sorting those cells with the immunofluorescence characteristics of neuroblastoma. The isolated cells may then be analyzed for the binding of tetanus toxin. In this use of the flow cytometric assay, cell sorting serves as an extremely powerful "prepurification" tool to obtain cells for both confirmation of cell type and analysis of their biologic characteristics. A wide variety of biological analyses may be performed with such a purified cell population, as long as they can be performed on single cells. These include binding of antibodies, autoradiographic receptor analysis, gene expression by in situ hybridization, and in vitro investigations of metastatic neuroblastoma cells in primary culture.

ACKNOWLEDGEMENTS

This research was supported by a Research Career Development Award NS00900 from the NINCDS (CNF), a Wilmot Foundation Cancer Research Fellowship (RED), grants from the

United Cancer Council of Greater Rochester, Inc., and grants NS-22039 and RR-05403 from the Public Health Service.

REFERENCES

Berliner P, Unsicker K (1985). Tetanus toxin labeling as a novel, rapid and highly specific tool in human neuroblastoma differential diagnosis. Cancer 56:419-423.

Cheung N-KV, Saarinen UM, Neely JE, Landmeier B, Donovan D, Coccia PF (1985). Monoclonal antibodies to a glycolipid antigen on human neuroblastoma cells. Cancer Res 45:2642-2649.

Duerst RE, Ryan DH, Frantz CN (1986). Variables affecting the killing of cultured human neuroblastoma cells with monoclonal antibody and complement. Cancer Res 46:3420-3425.

Frantz CN, Duerst RE, Ryan DH, Constine LS, Gelsomino N, Rust L, Gregory P (1986). A monoclonal antibody that discriminates between human nonhematopoietic and hematopoietic cell types. Hybridoma 5:297-306.

Goding JW (1983). "Monoclonal Antibodies: Principles and Practice." New York: Academic Press, pp 208-249.

Moss TJ, Seeger RC, Kindler-Rohrborn A, Marangos PJ, Rajewsky MF, Reynolds CP (1985). Immunohistologic detection and phenotyping of neuroblastoma cells in bone marrow using cytoplasmic neuron specific enolase and cell surface antigens. In Evans AE, D'Angio GJ, Seeger RC (eds): "Advances in Neuroblastoma Research," New York: Alan R. Liss, pp 367-378.

Notter MFD, Leary JF (1985). Flow cytometric analysis of tetanus toxin binding to neuroblastoma cells. J Cell Physiol 125:476-484.

# DIFFERENTIATION AND CELL BIOLOGY

Advances in Neuroblastoma Research 2, pages 265–276
© 1988 Alan R. Liss, Inc.

# TRANSDIFFERENTIATION OF HUMAN NEUROBLASTOMA CELLS RESULTS IN COORDINATE LOSS OF NEURONAL AND MALIGNANT PROPERTIES

June L. Biedler, Barbara A. Spengler, Tien-ding Chang, and Robert A. Ross

Memorial Sloan-Kettering Cancer Center, 1275 York Avenue, New York, NY 10021 (JLB, BAS, T-dC) and Fordham University, Fordham Road, Bronx, NY 10458 (RAR)

## INTRODUCTION

Previous studies have shown that human neuroblastoma cell lines in culture often comprise two distinctly different morphological subtypes (Tumilowicz et al., 1970; Biedler et al., 1973, 1978; Ross et al., 1983). Analysis of clonal sublines of the two cell types isolated from the SK-N-SH cell line revealed that the predominant cell type, termed N, is neuroblastic and expresses enzyme activities of noradrenergic neurons (Biedler et al., 1978; Ross et al., 1983). The other variant cell type, termed S, is substrate-adherent and flattened and has biochemical properties of melanocytes or Schwann cells (Ross and Biedler, 1985a,b; DeClerck et al., 1985; Tsokos et al., 1985). Chromosomal analyses indicated that both morphological cell types were derived from a common precursor cell (Biedler et al., 1979). Experiments designed to determine directly whether N cells can convert in vitro to S cell types and vice versa demonstrated that each cell type is capable of morphological conversion and that the process is reversible, i.e., bidirectional (Ross et al., 1983). Furthermore, the change in morphology is coordinated with a switch in the neural crest differentiation program (Ross et al., 1980; Tsokos et al., 1985; Biedler et al., 1985; Ross and Biedler, 1985a,b; DeClerck et al., 1985; Ross et al., this volume), a phenomenon we have termed "transdifferentiation". A third cell type designated I has been identified recently; it is morphologically intermediate between N and S cells and may share properties with either cell type.

In order to elucidate the significance of the N⇌S transdifferentiation phenomenon in the tumor biology of neuroblastoma, we have determined the tumor-producing capacity in nude mice of N-, S-, and I-type clones isolated from three human neuroblastoma cell lines, SK-N-SH, LA-N-1, and SK-N-BE(2). In addition, we have measured anchorage independent growth capacity and expression of epidermal growth factor (EGF) receptor for the same series of clones as potentially useful independent indicators of transformation state.

MATERIALS AND METHODS

Clonal sublines of SK-N-SH and SK-N-BE(2) have been described (Biedler et al., 1973, 1978, 1979; Ross et al., 1983). Clonal sublines of the LA-N-1 neuroblastoma cell line (Seeger et al., 1977) were isolated in 96 well cluster dishes seeded at a density of 1 cell/well. All sublines are cultured in a 1:1 mixture of Eagle's Minimum Essential Medium (MEM) with non-essential amino acids and Ham's Nutrient Mixture F12 supplemented with 15% fetal bovine serum.

Cells to be tested for growth in vivo were collected in late exponential growth phase and inoculated subcutaneously into female Swiss athymic nu/nu mice at $10^7$ cells/mouse. A total of 8 to 16 mice in 3 or 4 independent experiments were used for each cloned cell line. Mice were examined periodically and tumors measured in two dimensions for assessment of growth. Anchorage-independent growth was assayed in soft agar as modified from Macpherson (1973). Cells were suspended at appropriate inocula in 1.0 ml of 0.33% Difco Bacto agar and layered above a 5 ml, 0.5% agar base in 50 mm plastic culture dishes. Colonies were counted with an inverted microscope after 14 days. Mean plating efficiency for each clone was determined from 2 to 4 independent experiments.

EGF receptor was determined in a standard binding assay (Meyers et al., 1986; Das et al., 1977). Briefly, cells growing in monolayer culture were incubated for 1 hr at 22°C in 0.1-1.0 nM $[^{125}I]$EGF in presence or absence of 100 nM unlabeled EGF, washed extensively, solubilized in 0.5N NaOH, and counted in a gamma counter. Receptor number and affinity were determined by Scatchard analysis.

RESULTS

At least three distinctive morphological cell types
have been isolated from human neuroblastoma cell lines
established in continuous culture (Figure 1). N-type
cells, presumptive neuroblasts with small round cell bodies
and multiple neurite-like processes, adhere loosely or not
at all to a plastic substrate, aggregate to form cell
clusters, and grow to a high density. S-type cells are
flattened, highly substrate adherent cells with abundant
cytoplasm; they resemble fibroblasts or epithelial cells
and grow to low density in monolayer cultures. I-type
cells are intermediate in morphology between N and S cells
and have small but flattened cell bodies and occasional
neuritic processes. Both N- and I-type cells grow readily
in culture. S-type cells, by contrast, cloned or partially purified from 7 different neuroblastoma cell lines,
generally appear to have a finite lifespan (Rettig et al.,
1987; unpublished observations). Continuously proliferating
S-type clones have been isolated from only two cell lines,
SK-N-SH and LA-N-1.

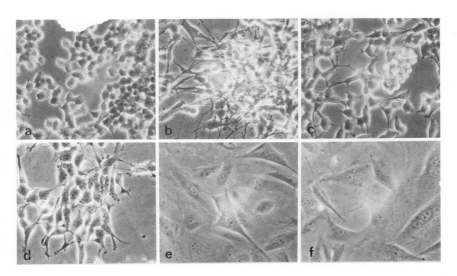

Figure 1. Phase contrast photomicrographs of N, I, and S
clones of the LA-N-1 neuroblastoma line. a, LA1-15n; b,
LA1-19n; c, LA1-21n; d, LA1-22n/i; e, LA1-5s; f, LA1-6s.
Magnification, x440.

   Confirmation of the neuronal lineage of N-type cells
has been obtained from analysis of neurotransmitter-synthesizing enzyme activities and specific uptake of norepinephrine (Figure 2; Ross et al., 1983 and Ross et al., this
volume).  All N-type cells tested have tyrosine hydroxylase
activity [as do almost all neuroblastoma cell lines assayed
to date (Ross et al., 1981)] and exhibit specific uptake of
norepinephrine (Figure 2).  Two of three I-type cell populations also have noradrenergic cell attributes, whereas
the third I-type cell, LA1-22n/i, does not (Figure 2).  By
contrast, no S-type cell clones express neuronal characteristics but all have enzyme activities typifying other
neural crest derivatives (Ross et al., this volume; Ross
and Biedler, 1985a,b).

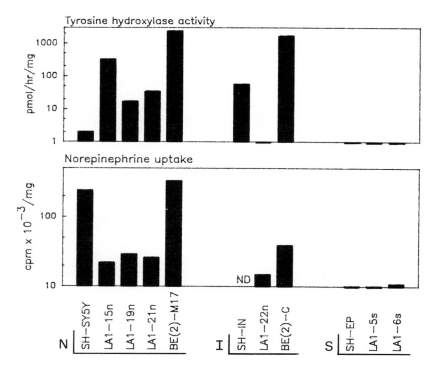

Figure 2.  Tyrosine hydroxylase activity and norepinephrine
uptake in N, S, and I clones of the SK-N-SH, LA-N-1, and
SK-N-BE(2) cell lines.  Clones are grouped by morphology.
ND, not determined.

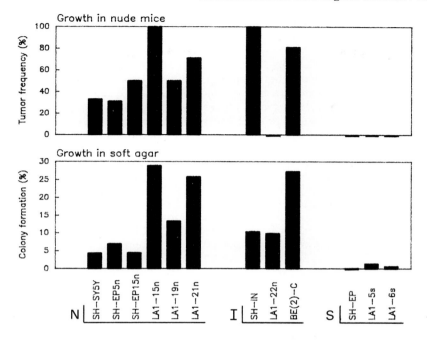

Figure 3. Frequency of tumor production in nude mice and plating efficiency in soft agar of N, S, and I clones of the SK-N-SH, LA-N-1, and SK-N-BE(2) cell lines. Clones are grouped by morphology.

## Tumor Production in Nude Mice

All N-type cell clones tested were capable of growth in vivo (Figure 3). Tumor frequency varied from 30 to 50% for N-type clones of the SK-N-SH neuroblastoma cell line and from 50 to 100% for those of LA-N-1. By contrast, S-type SH-EP, LA1-5s, and LA1-6s clones did not give rise to tumors in the 3-6 month period of observation. SH-EP was also negative when inoculated at a 5-fold higher cell number (5 x 10$^7$). Growth capacity of I-type clones varied from line to line. BE(2)-C cells were highly tumorigenic, as were early passage SH-IN cells (Figure 3), whereas LA1-22n/i, which has morphological characteristics of both N and I-type cells (Figure 1), was nontumorigenic. After prolonged cultivation in vitro, SH-IN cells appeared more flattened, i.e., more S-like, and produced tumors at a much lower frequency.

Clones with lower incidence of tumor formation were also generally characterized by slower tumor growth rates (Figure 4). Tumors formed by LA1-15n, LA1-21n, SH-IN and BE(2)-C cells, at a tumor frequency of >70%, were generally of measurable size (i.e., 5 to 10 mm in diameter) 2 to 3 weeks after inoculation and had doubled in diameter in another 2 to 3 weeks. (Assuming that the tumor is spherical and that a two-fold increase in diameter reflects an 8-fold increase in cell number, cell doubling times in vivo for these clones approximated 4 to 7 days, not unlike the 1 to 2 day doubling times observed in tissue culture.) Those cell clones with tumor frequencies of ≤50%, i.e., the SK-N-SH clones SH-SY5Y, SH-EP5n, and SH-EP15n and LA1-19n, had a markedly slower tumor growth rate and, with the exception of SH-SY5Y, a mean latent period of 2 to 4 months.

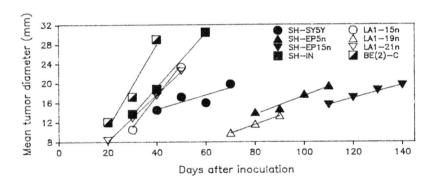

Figure 4. Tumor growth in nude mice of N- and I-type clones. Values plotted represent the mean diameter calculated from measurements of 3 to 14 tumors.

Growth in Soft Agar

The capacity for anchorage independent growth of N, I, and S cell clones in soft agar in general mirrored tumorigenic potential in nude mice (Figure 3). N-type clones of the LA-N-1 line exhibited high plating efficiencies (PE = 13 to 29%), whereas N clones of the less malignant SK-N-SH line had moderate plating efficiencies of 4 to 7%. SH-IN

and BE(2)-C, tumorigenic I clones, plated with an efficiency resembling that of the N-type clones of LA-N-1. By
contrast, nontumorigenic S cells had plating efficiencies
of 0.1 to 1.4%. A marked exception to the positive
correlation between tumorigenicity in nude mice and ability
to grow in soft agar (Figure 3) is the somewhat I-like
clone LA1-22n/i. These cells were nontumorigenic in nude
mice but formed colonies in soft agar at a 10% efficiency.

Expression of Epidermal Growth Factor Receptor

An important but not obligatory indicator of normal
cell growth behavior is dependence on exogenous factors for
growth. Since S cells were nontumorigenic in nude mice and
appeared to have a finite lifespan in culture, and since
Rettig et al. (1987) had observed differences between N and
S cells in cell surface reactivity with a monoclonal antibody to EGF receptor, we decided to systematically measure
EGF receptor level in N-, S-, and I-type clones. Studies of
binding of [$^{125}$I]EGF revealed a markedly higher number of
EGF receptors in S-type SH-EP, LA1-5s, and LA1-6s cells
(Table 1), as well as in I-type clones SH-IN, LA1-22n/i and
BE(2)-C cells, as compared to N-type cells. Calculation of
affinity constants from Scatchard plots indicated that the

Table 1. Binding of [$^{125}$I]EGF to Human Neuroblastoma Cell
Clones: Receptor Number and Affinity

| Cell clone | Cell type | Receptor number | $K_D$ (nM) |
|---|---|---|---|
| SH-SY5Y | N | 1,400 | 0.6 |
| SH-EP5n | N | 3,800 | 0.5 |
| SH-EP15n | N | 9,400 | 0.4 |
| SH-IN | I | 58,900 | 2.4 |
| SH-EP | S | 93,600 | 0.8 |
| LA1-15n | N | 2,900 | 1.0 |
| LA1-19n | N | 11,500 | 0.8 |
| LA1-21n | N | 6,700 | 0.8 |
| LA1-22n/i | N/I | 90,600 | 4.0 |
| LA1-5s | S | 60,600 | 1.1 |
| LA1-6s | S | 38,900 | 1.1 |
| BE(2)-C | I | 46,600 | 1.1 |

observed differences in binding of EGF between N and S morphological variants reflected differences in receptor number rather than differences in receptor affinity.


DISCUSSION

The studies reported here demonstrate that N-type cells, as well as some but not all I-type clones, isolated from three human neuroblastoma cell lines, SK-N-SH, LA-N-1, AND SK-N-BE(2), are tumorigenic in nude mice. This result is not surprising since N- and I-type cells have growth characteristics of transformed cells in culture, and, with the possible exception of the I-type SH-IN clone, are the numerically predominant cell type within each of the paren-tal tumor cell lines. [The SK-N-BE(2) cell line comprised mainly N-type, BE(2)-M17-like cells during the first year of continuous cultivation after which I-type cells like those comprising BE(2)-C gradually became predominant].

The finding of a considerably diminished or abrogated tumor potential for S-type clones is also not unexpected. These cells have proven difficult to clone, to maintain as morphologically homogeneous populations, or even to culti-vate over a long period, in a number of laboratories. S-type clones with the notable exception of the LA-N-1 series appear to have a finite lifespan in vitro. Whether this is due to the requirement by S cells for factors produced by N- or I-type cells or whether the S-type cells of a paren-tal line are constantly renewed by transdifferentiation of N cells is presently unknown.

Studies of the ability of the three morphological cell types to grow as colonies in soft agar substantiate the usefulness of this assay as an indicator of malignant potential. With one prominent exception, viz. LA1-22n/i, cell lines with plating efficiencies of 1.5% or lower were nontumorigenic, those with efficiencies between 2 and 10% were weakly tumorigenic, and those plating at efficiencies of 10% or higher were strongly tumorigenic. The 0.8 and 1.4% values obtained for the S-type clones of LA-N-1 are somewhat higher than generally reported for colony forma-tion by nontransformed cells in soft agar, consistent with their ability to proliferate indefinitely in culture and, also, as described by Michitsch et al. (this volume), to express the N-myc protooncogene.

The position of I-cells in the N⇌S transdifferentiation phenomenon is problematical. Categorized solely on
the basis of morphology, these cells, as reported here and
elsewhere (Ross et al., 1983; Ross et al., this volume),
have characteristics of both N and S cells. Whether I
cells are pluripotent stem cells that give rise to both N
and S cells or represent a transitional stage in the transdifferentiation process remains to be determined.

As reported recently, Rettig et al. (1987) examined
expression of growth factor receptors on a large series of
human neuroblastoma cell lines, including six pairs of N
and S cultures, by the mixed hemadsorption rosetting assay.
Cell surface reactivity with a monoclonal antibody to EGF
receptor was generally higher for S-type cells; the difference was even more marked for pairs of N and S clones of
the three lines studied here. This result was confirmed
and extended by the present EGF binding study as well as by
measurements of protein and mRNA levels (Ciccarone, 1987).
For example, Ciccarone (1987) demonstrated a 20-fold higher
level of EGF receptor protein, as determined by immunoblot
analysis with the monoclonal antibody 528 (Kawamoto et al.,
1983), and an 8- to 10-fold greater steady state level of
EGF receptor mRNA, detected with the cloned cDNA probe pE7
(Xu et al., 1984), in S-type SH-EP cells compared to N
counterparts. On the other hand, serological typing of the
three sets of clones for cell surface expression of nerve
growth factor (NGF) receptor showed a more than 20-fold
higher level for N-type cells as compared to S (Rettig et
al., 1987). Although the basis for the reciprocity of
expression of these two receptors can only be guessed at,
this finding, like that of the inverse relationship between
EGF receptor expression and tumorigenicity, indicates that
the N and S transdifferentiation process is an orderly one.
In support of this point of view is the demonstration by
Rettig et al. (1987), with 10 mouse antihuman monoclonal
antibodies to cell surface differentiation antigens, that N
and S cells from different cell lines have characteristic
patterns of antigen expression that distinguish one cell
type from the other. The shift in surface antigen expression, the neuronal characteristics of N-type cells, and the
expression by S-type cells of properties of other neural
crest derivatives such as melanocytic, Schwannian, or mesectodermal cells (Ross and Biedler, 1985a,b; Tsokos et al.,
1985; DeClerck et al., 1985; Ciccarone, 1987; Ross et al.,
this volume) together indicate that the N⇌S interconver-

sion process represents an ordered shift between alternative differentiation programs of the neural crest, as well as a shift between different states of malignant transformation.


ACKNOWLEDGEMENTS

The studies described here were supported in part by grants CA-31553 and CA-08748 from the National Cancer Institute and by the Kleberg Foundation.


REFERENCES

Biedler JL, Helson L, Spengler BA (1973). Morphology and growth, tumorigenicity, and cytogenetics of human neuroblastoma cells in continuous culture. Cancer Res 33:2643-2652.

Biedler JL, Roffler-Tarlov S, Schachner M, Freedman L (1978). Multiple neurotransmitter synthesis by human neuroblastoma cell lines and clones. Cancer Res 38:3751-3757.

Biedler JL, Spengler BA, Ross RA (1979). Chromosomal and biochemical properties of human neuroblastoma lines and clones in cell culture. Gaslini 11:128-139.

Biedler JL, Rozen MG, El-Badry O, Meyers MB, Melera PW, Ross RA, Spengler BA (1985). Growth stage-related synthesis and secretion of proteins by human neuroblastoma cells and their variants. In Evans AE, D'Angio GJ, Seeger RC (eds): "Advances in Neuroblastoma Research", New York: Alan R Liss, Inc, pp 209-221.

Ciccarone VC (1987). Human neuroblastoma cell transdifferentiation: Biochemical characteristics of cloned cell variants. Ph.D. thesis, Fordham University.

Das M, Miyakawa T, Fox CF, Pruso RM, Aharonov A, Herschman HR (1977). Specific radiolabeling of a cell surface receptor for epidermal growth factor. Proc Natl Acad Sci USA 74:2790-2794.

DeClerck YA, Bomann ET, Spengler BA, Biedler JL (1985). Phenotypic changes in human neuroblastoma cells correlate with biosynthesis of interstitial collagen. J Cell Biol 101:122a.

Kawamoto T, Sato JD, Le A, Polikoff J, Sato GH, Mendelsohn J (1983). Growth stimulation of A431 cells by epidermal growth factor: Identification of high-affinity receptors for epidermal growth factor by an anti-receptor antibody. Proc Natl Acad Sci USA 80:1337-1341.

Macpherson I (1973). Soft agar techniques. In Kruse Jr PF, Patterson Jr MK (eds): "Tissue Culture, Methods and Applications," New York: Academic Press, pp 276-280.

Meyers MB, Merluzzi VJ, Spengler BA, Biedler JL (1986). Epidermal growth factor receptor is increased in multidrug resistant Chinese hamster and mouse tumor cells. Proc Natl Acad Sci USA 83:5521-5525.

Michitsch RW, Biedler JL, Melera PW (this volume). Modulation of N-myc expression, but not tumorigenicity, accompanies phenotypic conversion of neuroblastoma cells in prolonged culture.

Rettig WJ, Spengler BA, Chesa PG, Old LJ, Biedler JL (1987). Coordinate changes in neuronal phenotype and surface antigen expression in human neuroblastoma cell variants. Cancer Res 47:1383-1389.

Ross RA, Biedler JL (1985a). Presence and regulation of tyrosinase activity in human neuroblastoma cell variants in vitro. Cancer Res 45:1628-1632.

Ross RA, Biedler JL (1985b). Expression of a melanocyte phenotype in human neuroblastoma cells in vitro. In Evans AE, D'Angio GJ, Seeger RC (eds): "Advances in Neuroblastoma Research", New York: Alan R Liss, Inc, pp 249-259.

Ross RA, Joh TH, Reis DJ, Spengler BA, Biedler JL (1980). Neurotransmitter-synthesizing enzymes in human neuroblastoma cells: Relationship to morphological diversity. In Evans AE (ed): "Advances in Neuroblastoma Research", New York: Raven Press, pp 151-160.

Ross RA, Biedler JL, Spengler BA, Reis DJ (1981). Neurotransmitter-synthesizing enzymes in 14 neuroblastoma cell lines. Cell Mol Neurobiol 1:301-312.

Ross RA, Spengler BA, Biedler JL (1983). Coordinate morphological and biochemical interconversion of human neuroblastoma cells. J Natl Cancer Inst 71:741-747.

Ross RA, Ciccarone V, Meyers MB, Spengler BA, Biedler JL (this volume). Differential expression of intermediate filaments and fibronection in human neuroblastoma cells.

Seeger RC, Rayner SA, Banerjee A, Chung H, Laug WE, Neustein HB, Benedict WF (1977). Morphology, growth, chromosomal pattern, and fibrinolytic activity of two new human neuroblastoma cell lines. Cancer Res 37:1364-1371.

Tsokos M, Ross RA, Triche TJ (1985). Neuronal, Schwannian, and melanocytic differentiation of human neuroblastoma cells in vitro. In Evans AE, D'Angio GJ, Seeger RC (eds):   "Advances in Neuroblastoma Research", New York: Alan R Liss, Inc, pp 55-68.

Tumilowicz JJ, Nichols WW, Cholon JJ, Greene AE (1970). Definition of a continuous human cell lilne derived from neuroblastoma.  Cancer Res 30:2110-2118.

Xu Y-h, Ishii S, Clark AJL, Sullivan M, Wilson RK, Ma DP, Roe   BA, Merlino GT, Pastan I (1984).  Human epidermal growth factor receptor cDNA overproduced in A431 carcinoma cells.  Nature 309:806-810.

Advances in Neuroblastoma Research 2, pages 277–289

# DIFFERENTIAL EXPRESSION OF INTERMEDIATE FILAMENTS AND FIBRONECTIN IN HUMAN NEUROBLASTOMA CELLS

Robert A. Ross, Valentina Ciccarone, Marian B. Meyers, Barbara A. Spengler, and June L. Biedler

Laboratory of Neurobiology (RAR, VC), Department of Biological Sciences, Fordham University, Bronx, NY 10458 and Laboratory of Cellular and Biochemical Genetics (MBM, BAS, JLB), Memorial Sloan-Kettering Cancer Center, New York, NY 10021

## INTRODUCTION

The human neuroblastoma cell line SK-N-SH comprises two predominant cell types in culture which undergo bidirectional interconversion (Biedler et al., 1973; Ross et al., 1983). One cell type (N) is neuroblastic in appearance, poorly substrate adherent, and contains enzymes for the synthesis of the neurotransmitter norepinephrine. By contrast, the other cell type (S) is large, flat, and attaches strongly to the culture dish. Biochemically, the S-type cells do not contain neurotransmitter biosynthetic enzymes but have activity for tyrosinase, the enzyme involved in melanin synthesis in melanocytes and melanoma (Ross and Biedler, 1985). This process of interconversion between two phenotypes within the neural crest repertoire is termed "transdifferentiation." A third cell type (I) has also been observed in SK-N-SH; it has a morphology intermediate between N and S cells and shares biochemical characteristics of both types of cells.

The present study was undertaken to determine whether the presence of different cellular morphologies is a common feature of neuroblastoma cell lines and whether the non-neuronal cells observed in different neuroblastoma cell lines share common biochemical characterisitcs similar to the S-type cells of the SK-N-SH cell line and consistent with a neural crest lineage.

Cells with N, S, and I morphologies were isolated either as clones or as enriched populations from six human neuroblastoma parental cell lines. Fig. 1 shows examples of the different morphological phenotypes for two cell lines [LA-N-1 and SK-N-BE(2)]. N, I, and S cell types were present in all six parental cell lines and each morphological subtype was similar between the different cell lines. Karyotype analysis confirmed the origin of the three morphologically-distinct cell types from a common precursor cell for each cell line.

Studies were then undertaken to determine the biochemical characteristics of the three different cell types. Clonal cell lines were examined for cell-specific marker enzymes, intermediate filament proteins, and fibronectin.

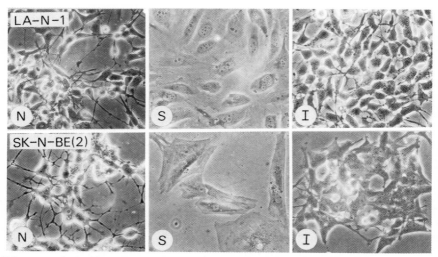

Figure 1. Phase contrast photomicrographs of clonal cell populations from human neuroblastoma cell lines LA-N-1 and SK-N-BE(2). Note the presence and similarity of the three morphological cell types. N, neuroblastic; S, substrate-adherent; I, intermediate.

PHENOTYPIC MARKER ENZYMES

Enzymes unique to a neuronal, melanocyte, or Schwann

cell phenotype were assayed as previously described (Ross
and Biedler, 1985). Tyrosine hydroxylase (TH) and dopamine-
B-hydroxylase (DBH) are specific marker enzymes for the
adrenergic neuron. In addition, the ability of the cells to
specifically take up norepinephrine was measured (Silberstein
et al., 1972). Tyrosinase activity was assayed for detection
of melanocytic properties and 2',3'-cyclic nucleotide 3'-
phosphohydrolase (CNP), an enzyme involved in the synthesis
of myelin by Schwann and glial cells, was also determined.

As shown in Fig. 2, all N clones have properties consistent with a neuroblastic phenotype, expressing activities for
TH and DBH and showing specific uptake of norepinephrine.

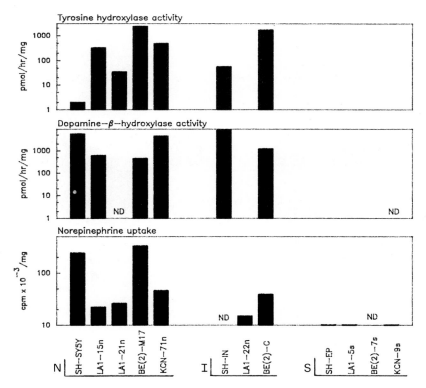

Figure 2. Tyrosine hydroxylase and dopamine-B-hydroxylase
activities and norepinephrine uptake in N, S, and I cells
from four human neuroblastoma cell lines. Each bar represents the mean value for 2-6 cultures. ND; not determined.

By contrast, S-type cells have none of these characteristics.
Of the three I-type clones studied, two [SH-IN and BE(2)-C]
expressed both TH and DBH activities.  LA1-22n showed
specific uptake of norepinephrine as did BE(2)-C.
The four clones with an S-type morphology expressed very
low (when compared to melanoma cells) but measureable levels
of tyrosinase activity whereas the N and I clones did not
(Fig. 3).  All three cell types contained comparable, low
levels of CNP activity.

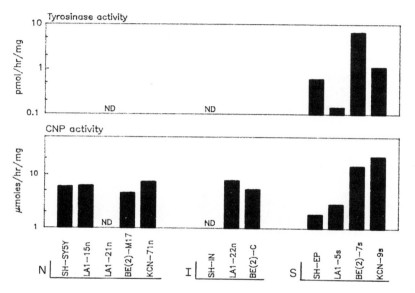

Figure 3. Expression of tyrosinase and CNP activities in N,
I, and S clones from four human neuroblastoma cell lines.
ND; not determined.


Thus, assessment of cell type-specific marker enzymes
suggests that the N-type and I-type clonal cell lines have
properties of adrenergic neuroblasts.  The clones with an
S-type morphology share properties of melanocytes.


INTERMEDIATE FILAMENT PROTEINS

Intermediate filaments are cell- and tissue-specific

components of the cytoskeleton (Lazarides, 1982; Steinert et al., 1984) and are usually retained by cells in culture (Osborn et al., 1982). Moreover, changes in the type and amount of intermediate filament have been shown to accompany cell differentiation (Franke et al., 1982; Denk et al, 1985). Thus these proteins are potentially useful in studying the process of transdifferentiation in human neuroblastoma cells. Intermediate filament proteins specific to neuroblasts (neurofilament proteins), and to Schwann, melanocyte, and mesenchymal cells (vimentin) have been well characterized.

Intermediate filament proteins were analyzed in human neuroblastoma clones by the use of Western blot procedures. Proteins in cytoskeletal-enriched fractions (Hynes and Destree, 1978) from cells with N, S, or I morphologies were separated under denaturing conditions on 7.5% polyacrylamide gels (Laemmli, 1970) and transferred to nitrocellulose (Towbin, 1979) for immunoblot analysis (Johnson et al., 1984). The following antibodies were used: rabbit polyclonal antibody to the 68K neurofilament (70-C; Dr. F. Chiu) and monoclonal antibodies to the 150K and 200K neurofilaments (NP8; Dr. P. Davies), and vimentin (Boehringer Mannheim Co.).

Neurofilament Proteins

Neurofilament proteins (NFP) are specific to neurons and neuroblasts and are composed of 3 related polypeptides with molecular weights of 68K, 150K, and 200K (Liem et al., 1978). Western blot analysis (Fig. 4) of the 68K NFP, which makes up the structural core of this intermediate filament, showed a single band of immunoreactivity in N and I clones but not in S clones. Similarly, the 150K and 200K NFP, which are attached peripherally to the core protein, were seen only in N and I cells (Fig. 5).

A summary of data obtained for clones of six neuroblastoma cell lines (Table 1) indicates that the 68K and 150K NFP are present in almost all cells with N and I morphologies. The 200K protein is present in two of the four cell lines examined [SK-N-BE(2) and IMR-32]. Since this NFP arises late in neuronal development (Shaw and Weber, 1982; Scott et al., 1985), these findings would suggest that neuroblastomas can arise at several stages of neuronal development in children.

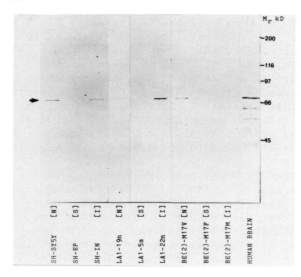

Figure 4. Immunoblot analysis of 68K neurofilament protein in N, S, and I clones from three neuroblastoma cell lines compared with human brain. N, neuroblastic; I, intermediate; S, substrate-adherent.

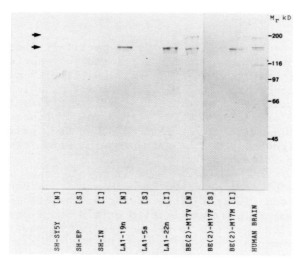

Figure 5. Immunoblot analysis of 150K and 200K neurofilament proteins in cytoskeleton from N, S, and I clones from three neuroblastoma cell lines compared with human brain. N, neuroblastic; I, intermediate; S, substrate-adherent.

Table 1. Neurofilament Proteins in Neuroblastoma Cells

| Cell type | Clone or line tested | Parent line | Neurofilament Protein | | |
|-----------|----------------------|-------------|------|------|------|
| | | | 68K | 150K | 200K |
| N | SH-SY5Y | SK-N-SH | + | + | - |
| | BE(2)-M17 | SK-N-BE(2) | + | + | + |
| | LA1-21n | LA-N-1 | + | + | - |
| | NAP(H)n | NAP | - | + | |
| | KCN-71n | SMS-KCN | | + | |
| | IMR-32 | IMR-32 | | + | + |
| I | SH-IN | SK-N-SH | + | + | - |
| | BE(2)-M17M | SK-N-BE(2) | + | + | + |
| | LA1-22n | LA-N-1 | + | + | - |
| S | SH-EP | SK-N-SH | - | - | - |
| | BE(2)-M17F | SK-N-BE(2) | - | - | - |
| | LA1-5s | LA-N-1 | - | - | - |
| | NAP(H)s | NAP | | - | |
| | KCN-9s | SMS-KCN | | - | |

N, neuroblastic; I, intermediate; S, substrate-adherent.

## Vimentin

Vimentin is an intermediate filament found in melano-cytes, Schwann cells, and mesenchymal cells (Lazarides, 1982). Thus, this protein can serve as a marker of these specific cell types. Western blot analysis of sets of N, S, and I clones from three human neuroblastoma cell lines (Fig. 6) showed that the S-type clones contained high levels of this protein. N-type cells had none or only trace amounts of vimentin. In contrast to the NFP data, I-type cells had significant amounts of vimentin compared to N-type cells. Summary of immunoblot data for vimentin expression in five human neuroblastoma cell lines (Table 2) indicates that all S-type cells expressed greater amounts of vimentin when com-pared to N-type cells which contained none or very little of this protein. I-type cells had intermediate amounts.

The presence of vimentin by itself does not definitively identify a cell's phenotype (since this protein is co-ex-pressed with other intermediate filaments by many cultured cells). However, the absence of NFP in the S cells supports the hypothesis that S cells represent melanocytes, Schwann

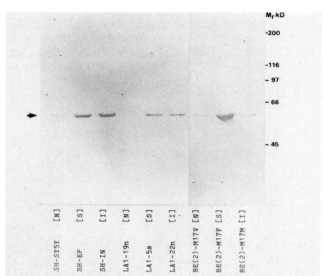

Figure 6. Immunoblot analysis of vimentin in N, S, and I cell types from three human neuroblastoma cell lines. N, neuroblastic; S, substrate-adherent; I, intermediate. Arrow indicates immunoreactivity corresponding to vimentin.

Table 2. Expression of Vimentin in Neuroblastoma Cells

| Cell type | Clone or line tested | Parent line | Vimentin |
|---|---|---|---|
| N | SH-SY5Y | SK-N-SH | +/- |
| | SK-N-BE(1)n | SK-N-BE(1) | - |
| | BE(2)-M17 | SK-N-BE(2) | +/- |
| | LA1-15n,19n | LA-N-1 | - |
| | NAP(H)n | NAP | +/- |
| I | SH-IN | SK-N-SH | ++ |
| | BE(2)-C | SK-N-BE(2) | + |
| | LA1-22n | LA-N-1 | + |
| S | SH-EP | SK-N-SH | ++ |
| | SK-N-BE(1)s | SK-N-BE(1) | ++ |
| | BE(2)-M17F | SK-N-BE(2) | ++ |
| | LA1-5s,6s | LA-N-1 | ++ |
| | NAP(H)s | NAP | ++ |

N, neuroblastic; I, intermediate; S, substrate-adherent.

cells or mesectodermal derivatives of the neural crest. Since
vimentin is also transiently expressed with NFP in neuroblasts (Bignami et al., 1982; Holtzer et al., 1982; Jacobs et
al., 1982), their combined presence in some of the neuroblastic clones may indicate that the transformation event
occurred early in neural crest differentiation.


Fibronectin

     Previous studies of N and S cells from two cell lines
have shown that the S cells produced large amounts of
stromal collagens (isotypes I and III) which are also produced by Schwann cells (DeClerck et al., 1987).  Alitalo et
al.(1981) have shown that neuroblastoma cell lines synthesize fibronectin (FN) in culture.  Since our studies raise
the possibility that these cultures contained both N and S
cells, we examined FN synthesis in N and S clones from four
human neuroblastoma cell lines.  Each cell culture with its
extracellular matrix was harvested nonenzymatically and FN
content determined by immunoblot analysis with a monoclonal
antibody from Dr. K. Lloyd (MIC-10).  Conditioned medium from
cells grown in serum-free medium for 24 hr was analyzed for
its FN content as well.  As shown in Fig. 7 and summarized in
Table 3, all of the S cells make and secrete large amounts of
FN whereas FN was not detected in N cells.  Only S cells contain FN in the extracellular matrix and in the medium. It has
previously been shown that Schwann cells, melanocytes, and
mesenchymal cells synthesize FN whereas neuroblastic cells do
not (Schachner et al., 1978; Yamada and Olden, 1978; Newgreen
and Thiery, 1980).


DISCUSSION

     The present study shows that the occurrence of distinct
N, S, and I cellular phenotypes is prevalent among neuroblastoma cell lines.  All of the N cells have properties of
neuroblastic cells, as indicated by their morphology, noradrenergic biosynthetic enzymes and norepinephrine uptake
mechanism, and expression of neurofilament proteins.  The
S cells may represent one or more of the non-neuronal neural
crest derivatives, e.g., Schwann cells, melanocytes, or mesectodermal cells.  This cell type is characterized by its
substrate-adherent morphology, lack of neuronal properties,
and expression of vimentin, fibronectin, and tyrosinase acti-

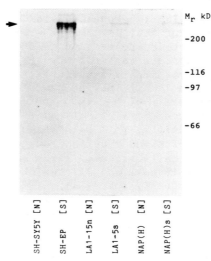

Figure 7. Immunoblot analysis of fibronectin in cells and extracellular matrix of N and S cells from three human neuroblastoma cell lines. Arrow indicates immunoreactivity corresponding to FN. N, neuroblastic; S, substrate-adherent.

Table 3. Fibronectin Synthesis in Human Neuroblastoma Cells

| Cell type | Clone or line tested | Parent line | Fibronectin | |
|-----------|---------------------|-------------|-------------|--------|
| | | | Matrix | Medium |
| N | SH-SY5Y | SK-N-SH | - | - |
| | SK-N-BE(1)n | SK-N-BE(1) | - | - |
| | LA1-15n | LA-N-1 | - | - |
| | NAP(H)n | NAP | - | |
| | | | | |
| S | SH-EP | SK-N-SH | + | + |
| | SK-N-BE(1)s | SK-N-BE(1) | + | |
| | LA1-5s | LA-N-1 | + | + |
| | NAP(H)s | NAP | + | |

N, neuroblastic; S, substrate-adherent.

vity. Of interest is the recent finding by Rettig et al. (1987) with a panel of monoclonal antibodies to cell surface antigens that S cells share some cell surface markers in common with fetal meningeal cells. Cells of both the pachymeninx and leptomeninx are derived, in part, from the neural crest (Harvey et al., 1935; LeDouarin, 1982). I cells have properties of both N and S cells. Like N cells, they contain noradrenergic biosynthetic enzymes and a specific uptake mechanism for norepinephrine as well as neurofilament proteins. Like S cells, I cells contain vimentin and fibronectin (data not shown). Thus, the I cells may be pluripotent stem cells capable of differentiating either into neuroblasts or into non-neuronal neural crest derivatives. Alternatively, I cells may represent a transitional form between N and S in the transdifferentiation process.

The specific, ordered transdifferentiation capacities observed for human neuroblastoma cells in vitro may reflect cellular changes critical for the conversion of some malignant neuroblastomas into ganglioneuromas in vivo. Thus, the presence of S cells in cultured neuroblastoma cell lines may be analogous to the occurrence of Schwann-like and mesectodermal cells seen in neuroblastoma undergoing differentiation into benign ganglioneuromas (Machin, 1982; Shimada et al., 1984). Tumor cell maturation and tumor regression may be effected in two ways: (1) Synthesis of extracellular matrix proteins or other growth regulatory factors by S cells could induce differentiation of neuroblastic cells into nonproliferating, mature neurons and/or (2) Transdifferentiation of tumorigenic N-type cells into non-malignant S-type cells (Biedler et al., this volume) could directly result in decreased malignant potential of these tumors in the patient.

ACKNOWLEDGEMENTS

Supported, in part, by grant NS-17738 (NINCDS) and grants CA-31553 and CA-08748 (NCI) from the National Institutes of Health. VC is a Shering-Plough Fellow.

REFERENCES

Alitalo K, Keski-Oja J, Vaheri A (1981). Extracellular matrix proteins characterize human tumor cell lines. Int J Cancer 27: 755-761.
Biedler JL, Spengler BA, Chang T-d, Ross, RA (this voulume). Transdifferentiation of human neuroblastoma cells results in coordinate loss of neuronal and malignant properties.
Biedler JL, Helson L, Spengler BA (1973). Morphology and growth, tumorigenicity, and cytogenetics of human neuroblastoma cell lines in continuous culture. Cancer Res 33:

2643-2652.

Bignami A, Raju T, Dahl D (1982). Localization of vimentin, the non-specific intermediate filament protein, in embryonal glia and in early differentiative neurons. Dev Biol 91: 286-295.

DeClerck YA, Bomann ET, Spengler BA, Biedler JL (1987). Correlation between phenotypic expression and collagen biosynthesis in human neuroblastoma. Manuscript in preparation.

Denk H, Weybora W, Ratschek A, Sohar R, Franke WW (1985). Distribution of vimentin, cytokeratins, and desmosomal-plaque proteins in human nephroblastomas as revealed by specific antibodies: Co-existence of cell groups of different degrees of epithelial differentiation. Differentiation 29: 88-97.

Franke WW, Schmid E, Schiller DL, Winter S, Jarasch ED, Moll R, Denk H, Jackson BW, Illmensee K (1982). Differentiation-related patterns of expression of proteins of intermediate-size filaments in tissues and cultured cells. Cold Spring Harbor Symp Quant Biol 46: 431-453.

Harvey SC, Burr HS, Van Campenhout E (1933). Development of the meninges. Further experiments. Arch Neurol Psychiatr 29: 683-690.

Holtzer H, Bennett GS, Tapscott SJ, Croop JM, Toyama Y (1982). Intermediate-size filaments: Changes in synthesis and distribution in cells of the myogenic and neurogenic lineages. Cold Spring Harbor Symp Quant Biol 46: 317-329.

Hynes RO, Destree AT (1978). 10nm filaments in normal and transformed cells. Cell 13: 151-163.

Jacobs M, Choo QL, Thomas C (1982). Vimentin and 70K neurofilament protein co-exist in embryonic neurones from spinal ganglia. J Neurochem 38: 969-977.

Johnson DA, Gautsch JW, Sportsman JR, Elder JH (1984). Improved technique utilizing nonfat dry milk for analysis of proteins and nucleic acids transferred to nitrocellulose. Gene Anal Tech 1: 3-8.

Laemmli K (1970). Cleavage of structural proteins during the assembly of the head of bacteriophage T4. Nature 227: 680-685.

Lazarides E (1982). Intermediate filaments: a chemically heterogeneous developmentally regulated class of proteins. Ann Rev Biochem 51: 219-250.

LeDouarin N (1982) "The Neural Crest." New York: Cambridge Univ Press, 260 pp.

Liem RKH, Yen SH, Salomon GD, Shelanski ML (1978). Intermediate filaments in nervous tissues. J Cell Biol 79: 637-645.

Machin GA (1982). Histogenesis and histopathology of neuroblastoma. In Pochedly C (ed): "Neuroblastoma, Clinical and
Biological Manifestations," New York: Elsevier, pp 195-231.

Newgreen D, Thiery JP (1980). Fibronectin in early embryos:
Synthesis and distribution along the migration pathways
of neural crest cells. Cell Tissue Res 211: 269-291.

Osborn M, Weber K (1982). Intermediate filaments: cell type
specific markers in differentiation and pathology. Cell
31: 303-306.

Rettig WJ, Spengler BA, Chesa PG, Old LJ, Biedler JL (1987).
Coordinate changes in neuronal phenotype and surface anti-
gen expression in human neuroblastoma cell variants.
Cancer Res 47: 1383-1389.

Ross RA, Biedler JL (1985). Presence and regulation of tyrosinase activity in human neuroblastoma cell variants in
vitro. Cancer Res 45: 1628-1632.

Ross RA, Spengler BA, Biedler JL (1983). Coordinate morphological and biochemical interconversion of human neuroblastoma cells. J Natl Cancer Inst 71: 741-747.

Schachner M, Schoonmaker G, Hynes RO (1978). Cellular and
subcellular localization of LETS protein in the nervous
system. Brain Res 158: 149-158.

Scott D, Smith KE, O'Brien BJ, Angelides KJ (1985). Characterization of mammalian neurofilament triplet proteins:
Subunit stoichiometry and morphology of native and reconstituted filaments. J Biol Chem 260: 10736-10747.

Shaw G, Weber K (1982). Differential expression of neurofilament triplet proteins in brain development. Nature
298: 277-279.

Shimada H, Chatten J, Newton Jr WA, Sachs N, Homoudi AB,
Chiba T, Marsden HB, Misugi K (1984). Histopathologic prognostic factors in neuroblastic tumors: Definition of subtypes of ganglioneuroblastoma and an age-linked classification of neuroblastomas. J Natl Cancer Inst 73: 405-416.

Silberstein SD, Johnson DF, Hanbauer I, Bloom FE, Kopin IJ
(1972). Axonal sprouting and 3H-norepinephrine uptake by
superior cervical ganglion in organ culture. Proc Natl Acad
Sci USA 69: 1450-1454.

Steinert PM, Jones JCR, Goldman RD (1984). Intermediate
filaments. J Cell Biol 99: 22s-27s.

Towbin H, Staehelin T, Gordon J (1979). Electrophoretic
transfer of proteins from polyacrylamide gels to nitrocellulose sheets: Procedure and some applications. Proc
Natl Acad Sci USA 76: 4350-4354.

Yamada KM, Olden K (1978). Fibronectins- adhesive glycoproteins of cell surface and blood. Nature 275: 179-184.

Advances in Neuroblastoma Research 2, pages 291–306

# BIOLOGICAL CLASSIFICATION OF CELL LINES DERIVED FROM HUMAN EXTRA-CRANIAL NEURAL TUMORS

C Patrick Reynolds, Mary M Tomayko, Ludvik Donner, Lawerence Helson, Robert C Seeger, Timothy J Triche, and Garrett M Brodeur

Department of Pediatrics and the Jonsson Comprehensive Cancer Center, UCLA School of Medicine, Los Angeles, CA 90024 (CPR,MMT,RCS); 50 Rockford Road, Wilmington, DE 19806 (LH); Laboratory of Pathology, National Cancer Institute, Bethesda, MD 20814 (TJT,LD); Departments of Pediatrics and Genetics, Washington University School of Medicine, St Louis, MO 63110 (GMB).

## INTRODUCTION

The diagnosis of neuroblastoma relies heavily on cellular chacteristics such as morphology, ultrastructure, catecholamine production, and various antigens which indicate a neural origin of the tumor (Reynolds and Smith, 1982; Triche 1982). Within those tumors diagnosed as neuroblastoma there is a great deal of biological heterogeneity which results in a wide variance in the clinical outcome, sometimes independent of the extent of tumor spread (Jaffe, 1976). Several prognostic indicators which help predict outcome other than the stage of disease have been identified: age at diagnosis, serum neuron specific enolase or ferritin levels, histopathology, and genomic amplification of the N-*myc* oncogene (Zeltzer et al, 1985; Hann et al, 1985; Shimada et al, 1984; Seeger et al, 1985; Evans et al, 1987).

Recent evidence indicates that there are subgroups of neural tumors that have previously been diagnosed as neuroblastoma, yet appear to be biologically distinct from "classical" neuroblastoma. These subgroups can be identified by clinical presentation and histopathology (*Askin's tumors* or *Primitive Neuroectodermal Tumors*), the presence of a specific chromosomal rearrangement (t[11;22]) and a distinctive pattern of cell surface antigens or oncogene expression (*peripheral neuroepithelioma*) (Askin et al 1979; Seemayer et al, 1975; Hashimato et al, 1983; Schmidt et al, 1985; Whang-Peng et al, 1984; Donner et al, 1985; Thiele et al, 1987). However, it is as yet unclear how each of these subgroups relate to each other in terms of biology, and which of them (if any) should be considered distinct from neuroblastoma for the purposes of prognostication and therapy.

To develop a set of markers which will provide a biologically meaningful grouping of extra-cranial neural tumors, we undertook a study 33 human cell lines derived from such tumors. Here we show that genomic amplification of N-*myc* and the pattern of cell surface antigen expression identifies groups of these cell lines that differ in tumorigenicity when xenografted into nude mice.

**MATERIALS AND METHODS**

Cell Culture

All cell lines were established in our laboratories or obtained from the originator of the cell line (Table 1). Cells were maintained *in vitro* at 37° C in a humidified 5% $CO_2$ atmosphere in RPMI 1640 with 10% fetal calf serum (FCS). All cell lines were tested by culture and Hoechst DNA staining and found to be free of mycoplasma.

Quantitation of Cell Surface Antigens

Cells were harvested from tissue culture flasks with Pucks saline A using 10 mM HEPES and 1 mM EDTA (Pucks-EDTA) (Reynolds, 1986) and pipetted into a uniform suspension with a Pasteur pipet. Viability and cell counts were determined by hemocytometer using trypan blue exclusion, and $10^6$ cells were pipetted into conical 12 x 75 mm tubes, washed x 1 with Dulbecco's Phosphate Buffered Saline without $Ca^{++}$ or $Mg^{++}$ + 5 % heat inactivated goat serum (PBS-GSAZ), and resuspended in 50 ul of PBS-GSAZ. Concentrated tissue culture supernatent (10x) from the hybridoma HSAN 1.2 (Smith and Reynolds, 1987), W6/32 (Parham et al, 1979), or a non-binding control monoclonal antibody was added (50 ul to each tube) and the tubes incubated for 30 minutes on ice after mixing. Cells were then washed x 2 with PBS–GSAZ, resuspended in 50 ul, and 50 ul of fluorescein-labeled affinity purified goat anti-mouse Ig (Kirkegaard and Perry, Gaithersburg MD) diluted 1:5 (50 ug/10$^6$ cells) in goat serum was added. After mixing, cells were incubated on ice in the dark for 30 minutes, washed once with PBS, fixed in 1% paraformaldehyde, stored at 4$^\circ$ C in the dark, and analyzed within 48 hours. Fluorescence was quantitated using an Ortho 50 H + H cytofluorograph with excitation from a 488 nm argon laser, standardized daily with fluorescent microspheres (Coulter, Hialeah, FL). Non-viable cells and debris were excluded using 90 degree vs forward angle light scatter, and 5000 cells for each sample were examined. Triplicate samples for each cell line were analyzed. Electronic gates for positive antibody binding were determined based on controls for each cell line such that controls showed 2% or less positive cells. The binding index was calculated as the % cells positive X mean fluorescence channel/100. A binding index > 10 indicates binding of the antibody was greater than controls.

## Growth of Cells in Athymic (Nude) Mice

For injection into nude mice, cultured neuroblastoma cells were removed from tissue culture flasks using Pucks EDTA, washed and resuspended in PBS. Cell clumps were dissociated by gentle pipetting with a Pasture pipette. Cell concentration and viability were determined by hemocytometer using 0.06% trypan blue, and 10$^8$ cells were injected through 22 gauge needles subcutaneously between the scapula of 6 to 12 week old Balb/c nu/nu mice (NCI Fredrick Cancer Research Facility Fredrick, MD). A minimum of 3 mice were injected for each cell line. Mice were housed in a Laminar flow caging system, (Thoren Caging Systems, Inc., Hazleton, PA), and all food, bedding, and water was autoclaved. Mice were examined weekly and the lag time to form a tumor was determined as the number of days from injection of the cell line until a palpable tumor mass was detected. Mice were terminated by cervical dislocation and the tumor was immediately dissected free of mouse skin and body tissue and touch preps made for catecholamine

294 / Reynolds et al

fluorescence.

## Catecholamine Fluorescence

The presence of catecholamines was detected histochemically in nude mouse xenografts using glyoxylic acid induced catecholamine fluorescence (Reynolds, et al 1981), as described elsewhere in this volume (Tomayko et al, 1988).

## N-*myc* Gene Copy Number

DNA was isolated from cell cultures, digested with restriction endonuclease Eco R1, fractionated on agarose gels and transferred to nitrocellulose filters. Hybridization was carried out with isotopically labeled plasmid probe pNB-1 (Brodeur et al, 1984). Equal amounts of DNA from normal leukocytes or fibroblasts were used as controls to determine the hybridization intensity of non-amplified cell lines. Quantitative determinations based on visual inspection of autoradiograms were confirmed by densitometric analysis.

## RESULTS

Each line was analyzed for the expression of the neuroblastoma-associated antigen HSAN 1.2 (antibody HSAN 1.2) and non-polymorphic class I HLA (A,B,C) antigen (antibody W6/32) using flow cytometry. Representative histograms for a neuroblastoma and a PNET cell line are shown in Figure 1. As shown in Figure 2, there was a great deal of heterogeneity of expression for both antigens. However, there was an apparent reciprocal relationship for these two antigens. Some cell lines showed high HLA expression and intermediate to low binding of HSAN 1.2, while others showed high HSAN 1.2 binding, but little or no HLA expression. In no case did a cell line show high expression of both antigens.

The gene copy number of the N-*myc* oncogene was determined by Southern analysis. As shown in Figure 3, 14 cell lines did not show N-*myc* amplification, while 19 lines had multiple copies of the N-*myc* genome, ranging from 25 to 150 copies. A comparison of Figures 2 and 3 shows an interesting relationship between the cell

Figure 1. Flow cytometry histograms of of representative N-*myc* amplified neuroblastoma (SMS-KANR) and PNET (SK-N-MC) cell lines.

SMS-KANR

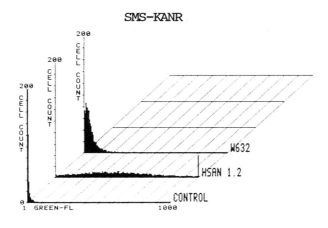

SK-N-MC

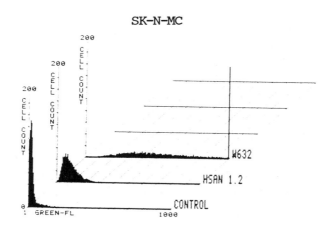

FIGURE 2. Intensity of staining with monoclonal antibodies HSAN 1.2 and W6/32 as determined by flow cytometry. Each bar represents the average binding index for 3 samples (5000 cells each).

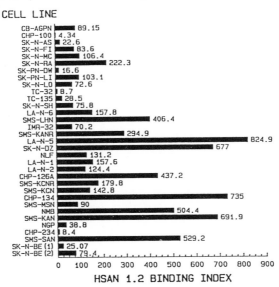

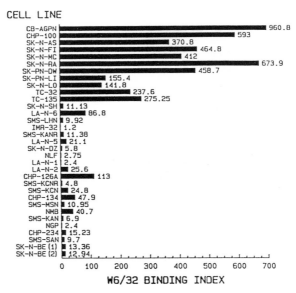

surface antigens and the N-*myc* gene copy number: no cell lines with high HLA expression (binding index > 120) demonstrated multiple copies of N-*myc*. Conversely, 13 of 19 N-*myc* amplified cell lines had high HSAN 1.2 staining (binding index > 120), and 3 of 19 showed intermediate HSAN 1.2 staining (binding index > 50 but < 120). Only one N-*myc* amplified cell line (CHP-234) showed no HSAN 1.2 reactivity. Three cell lines (SK-N-SH, LA-N-6, SMS-LHN) were unusual in that they did not have N-*myc* amplification, nor did they show high HLA expression.

As there was an inverse relationship for the expression of the HSAN 1.2 and W6/32 antigens, we calculated the ratio for the intensity of staining for W6/32 and HSAN 1.2. All N-*myc* amplified cell lines except for one (CHP-234) showed a W6/32-HSAN 1.2 ratio less than 1, as do SK-N-SH, LA-N-6, and SMS-LHN. All other non-amplified cell lines have a ratio > 1 (range 1.5 to 136).

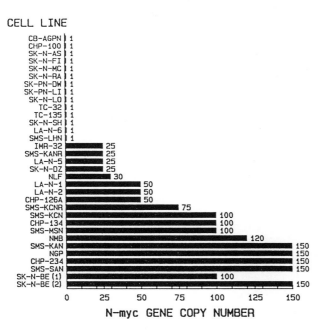

FIGURE 3. N-*myc* gene copy number of the cell lines (determined by Southern analysis).

CELL LINE

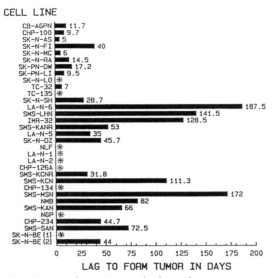

FIGURE 4. The lag time from injection to a palpable tumor in nude mice. Bars represent average values (3 to 4 mice per cell line), * = not tested.

The N-*myc* gene copy number and cell surface antigens distinguished 3 groups of cell lines. In order to determine if this grouping had biological significance, we determined the tumorigenicity of the cell lines when injected into nude mice. To decrease the number of mice needed to obtain meaningful results, mice were injected with enough cells ($100 \times 10^6$/mouse) to insure that tumors would be established in > 90% of the mice for each cell line. Tumorigenicity was then determined by measuring the time between injection until a palpable tumor was obtained (lag time). As shown in Figure 3, the average lag time for N-*myc* amplified cell lines varied from 31 to 172 days. By contrast, all of the cell lines showing high HLA expression, but lacking N-*myc* amplification, rapidly formed tumors in nude mice, most within 2 weeks. Two of the three low HLA, N-*myc* non-amplified cell lines were clearly different in tumorigenicity than the latter group, as they had very long lag times (187 days for LA-N-6 and 141 days for SMS-LHN).

The presence of catecholamines was determined for the

## TABLE 1

| CELL LINE | ORIGINAL DIAGNOSIS[*] | REFERENCE | BIOLOGICAL CLASS[**] |
|---|---|---|---|
| CB-AGPN | PNET | Reynolds (unpublished) | PNET |
| CHP-100 | NB | Schlesinger et al 1976 | PNET |
| SK-N-AS | NB | Helson (unpublished) | PNET |
| SK-N-FI | NB | Helson et al 1980 | PNET |
| SK-N-MC | NB | Biedler et al 1973 | PNET |
| SK-N-RA | NB | Helson (unpublished) | PNET |
| SK-PN-DW | PNET | Potluri et al 1987 | PNET |
| SK-PN-LI | PNET | Potluri et al 1987 | PNET |
| SK-N-LO | NB | Helson et al 1980 | PNET |
| TC-32 | NB | Whang-Peng et al 1984 | PNET |
| TC-135 | PN | ,, ,, | PNET |
| SK-N-SH | NB | Biedler et al 1973 | NB (NA) |
| LA-N-6 | NB | Wada et al 1988 | NB (NA) |
| SMS-LHN | NB | Wada et al 1988 | NB (NA) |
| IMR-32 | NB | Tumilowicz et al 1970 | NB (A) |
| SMS-KANR | NB | Reynolds et al 1986 | NB (A) |
| LA-N-5 | NB | Seeger et al 1982 | NB (A) |
| SK-N-DZ | NB | Helson et al 1980 | NB (A) |
| NLF | NB | Schwab et al 1983 | NB (A) |
| LA-N-1 | NB | Seeger et al 1977 | NB (A) |
| LA-N-2 | NB | ,, ,, | NB (A) |
| CHP-126A | NB | Schlesinger et al 1976 | NB (A) |
| SMS-KCNR | NB | Reynolds et al 1986 | NB (A) |
| SMS-KCN | NB | ,, ,, | NB (A) |
| CHP-134 | NB | Schlesinger et al 1976 | NB (A) |
| SMS-MSN | NB | Reynolds et al 1986 | NB (A) |
| NMB | NB | Brodeur et al 1977 | NB (A) |
| SMS-KAN | NB | Reynolds et al 1986 | NB (A) |
| NGP | NB | Brodeur et al 1977 | NB (A) |
| CHP-234 | NB | Schlesinger et al 1981 | NB (A) |
| SMS-SAN | NB | Reynolds et al 1986 | NB (A) |
| SK-N-BE(1) | NB | Biedler et al 1978 | NB (A) |
| SK-N-BE(2) | NB | ,, ,, | NB (A) |

* NB = neuroblastoma; PNET = Primitive neuroectodermal tumor; PN = peripheral neuroepithelioma

** Classification as determined in this study:
  NB (A)  = neuroblastoma, N-myc amplified
  NB (NA) = neuroblastoma, N-myc non-amplified
  PNET    = Primitive neuroectodermal tumor

xenografted tumors by glyoxylic acid-induced fluorescence. Except for those cell lines derived from patients who had negative urinary catecholamines (SMS-KCNR, SMS-KCN, SMS-KAN, SMS-KANR), all N-*myc* amplified cell lines that were examined showed positive catecholamine fluorescence. Of the non-amplified lines, only the three low HLA cell lines demonstrated very strong catecholamine fluorescence. Two strongly HLA-positive cell lines showed positive catecholamine fluorescence (SK-N-RA and SK-N-FI), while all other strongly HLA-positive lines were catecholamine negative.

Using a combination of N-*myc* gene copy number and cell surface antigens, we have developed a classification scheme for these cell lines:

**TABLE 2**

| Class | Neuroblastoma (A) | (NA) | PNET |
|---|---|---|---|
| # of Lines | 19 | 3 | 11 |
| N-myc amplification | 85 (25–150) | 1 | 1 |
| W6/32-HSAN 1.2 Ratio | 0.19 (0.01–1.8) | 0.24 (0.02–0.5) | 22.21 (1.5–136) |
| Catecholamine Fluorescence | + or − | + | − or + |
| Tumor growth lag in nude mice (days) | 61 (31–172) | 119.2 (29–187) | 13.4 (5–40) |

The values in Table 2 are the average values for all cell lines in each class, with the range shown under each average value. The difference in tumor growth lag was not significant between NB (A) and NB (NA) (p=0.051), but was significantly different between NB (A) and PNET (p<0.0001) and between NB (NA) and PNET (p<0.0001).

## DISCUSSION

Human neuroblastoma cell lines have been shown to express very low amounts of class I HLA antigen (Lampson et al, 1983). In a previous study, we noted that unlike most neuroblastoma cell lines, the SK-N-MC cell line (from a patient with a clinical history compatible with "Askins" tumor) expressed a high level of HLA class I antigen, as did peripheral neuroepithelioma cell lines (Donner et al, 1985). Cytogenetic studies of SK-N-MC and another "neuroblastoma" cell line with a similar clinical history (CHP-100), demonstrated the t[11;22] chromosomal rearrangement characteristic of peripheral neuro-epithelioma (Whang-Peng et al, 1986). As peripheral neuroepithelioma cell lines do not amplify N-myc (Thiele et al, 1987), it was possible that many N-myc non-amplified neuroblastoma cell lines were actually neuroepitheliomas. These observations indicated the need for a set of markers which will divide peripheral neural tumors into biologically relevant groups.

In order to develop such markers, we have undertaken a comparison of N-myc gene copy number with cell surface antigen expresion in an extensive panel of human neuroblastoma, peripheral neuroepithelioma, and PNET cell lines. Our results show that among N-myc amplified neuroblastoma cell lines there is a consistent pattern of expression of HLA class I antigen and the neuroblastoma-associated antigen HSAN 1.2 (W6/32-HSAN 1.2 ratio <1), which distinguishes them from peripheral neuroepithelioma or PNET cell lines (all of which do not show amplified N-myc and have a W6/32-HSAN 1.2 ratio > 1). We also show that 3 cell lines without N-myc amplification have CSA consistent with N-myc amplified cell lines, are strongly catecholamine positive, and are therefore classified as neuroblastoma cell lines. Other studies showing that these latter 3 lines express more N-myc protein than PNET cell lines support this conclusion (Wada et al, 1988).

There has been debate as to the appropriate terminology for neuroblastoma and related tumors (Dehner, 1986; Triche, 1986). We have chosen to designate all N-*myc* non-amplified cell lines with antigen ratios > 1 as PNET (primitive neuroectodermal tumor) lines. We use PNET (inclusive of peripheral neuroepithelioma) for these lines as they all lack N-*myc* amplification, have a common pattern of CSA expression and tumorigenicity in nude mice (Table 2), yet some do not show a t(11;22) translocation (Potluri et al, 1987). This is consistent with our classification of cell lines as neuroblastomas, most of which (but not all) show chromosome 1 deletions (Brodeur et al, 1981; Gilbert et al, 1984; Reynolds et al, 1986).

We have also chosen to classify the cell lines based on their CSA and N-*myc* amplification, without regard to their production of catecholamines. In doing so, we have placed 2 catecholamine positive cell lines in the PNET group, and 4 non-catecholamine producing lines in the neuroblastoma N-*myc* amplified group. The similar tumorigencity in nude mice of each of these 6 lines to others in their group (by our classification) supports this conclusion. Additional experiments are needed to determine if the neurotransmitter phenotype should be considered in the classification of these lines.

From the standpoint of tumor cell biology (excluding stage, age, etc.) one can segregate neuroblastoma and related tumors into N-*myc* amplified (all of which have poor clinical outcome) and N-*myc* non-amplified (which have a very heterogeneous clinical outcome). Sub-classification of the latter group is important for therapeutic decisions, and for understanding mechanisms of tumor progression other than N-*myc* amplification. The classification scheme we describe here uses cell surface antigen expression to divide N-*myc* non-amplified cell lines into two groups which differ in tumorigenicty in nude mice (Table 2). Other studies indicate that these two groups (neuroblastoma and PNET) also differ in oncogene expression (Thiele et al, 1987; Wada et al, 1988). Use of this classification scheme will aid investigators in choosing cell lines for biological and therapeutic studies, and in interpretation of their results. Further studies are needed to determine if other markers will revise the classification of some of these lines, and if the markers described here will be useful in classifying clinical tumor specimens.

## ACKNOWLEDGEMENTS

This study was supported in part by grants CA44904 (CPR); CA39771, CA01027, CA05587 (GMB); CA22794, CA16042 (RCS) from the National Cancer Institute, DHHS. LCDR Reynolds is assigned to the UCLA School of Medicine from the Department of the Navy. The views expressed in this article are those of the authors and do not reflect the official policy or position of the Department of the Navy, Department of Defense, nor the U. S. Government. We thank Dr. June Biedler for providing the SK-N-SH, SK-N-MC, SK-N-BE(1), and SK-N-BE(2) cell lines, Dr. Harvey Schlesinger and Dr. Audrey Evans for providing the CHP series of cell lines, and Donna-Maria Jones for her dedicated technical assistance.

## REFERENCES

Askin FB, Rosai J, Sibley RK, Dehner LP, McAlister WH (1979). Malignant small cell tumor of the thoracopulmonary region in childhood. A distinctive clinocopathologic entity of uncertain histogenesis. Cancer 43:2438-2451.

Biedler JL, Helson L, Spengler BA (1973). Morphology and growth, tumorigenicity, and cytogenetics of human neuroblastoma cells in continuous culture. Cancer Res 33:2643-52.

Biedler JL, Roffler-Tarlov S, Schachner M, Freedman LS (1978). Multiple neurotransmitter synthesis by human neuroblastoma cell lines and clones. Cancer Res 38:3751-7.

Brodeur GM, Seeger RC, Schwab M, Varmus HE, Bishop JM (1984). Amplification of N-myc sequences in primary human neuroblastomas Science 224:1121-1124.

Brodeur GM, Green AA, Hayes FA, Williams KJ, Williams DL, Tsiatis AA (1981). Cytogenetic features of human neuroblastomas and cell lines. Cancer Res 41:4678-4686.

Brodeur GM, Sekhon GS, Goldstein MN (1977). Chromosomal

aberrations in human neuroblastomas. Cancer 40:2256-2263.

Dehner LP (1986). Peripheral and central primitive neuroectodermal tumors. A nosologic concept seeking a consensus. Arch Pathol Lab Med 110:997-1005.

Donner L, Triche TJ, Israel MA, Seeger RC, Reynolds CP (1985). A panel of monoclonal antibodies which discriminate neuroblastoma from Ewing's sarcoma, rhabdomyosarcoma, neuroepithelioma and hematopoietic malignancies. Prog Clin Biol Res 175:347-366.

Evans AE, D'Angio GJ, Propert K, Anderson J, Hann HW (1987). Prognostic factors in neuroblastoma. Cancer 59:1853-9.

Gilbert F, Feder M, Balaban G, Brangman D, Lurie DK, Podolsky R, Rinaldt V, Vinikoor N, Weisband J (1984). Human neuroblastomas and abnormalities of chromosomes 1 and 17. Cancer Res 44:5444-5449.

Hann HW, Evans AE, Siegel SE, Wong KY, Sather H, Dalton A, Hammond D, Seeger RC (1985). Prognostic importance of serum ferritin in patients with Stages III and IV neuroblastoma: the Childrens Cancer Study Group experience. Cancer Res 45:2843-8.

Hashimoto H, Enjoji M, Nakajima T, Kiryu H, Daimaru Y (1983). Malignant neuroepithelioma (peripheral neuroblastoma). A clinicopathologic study of 15 cases. Am J Surg Pathol 7:309-18.

Helson L, Nisselbaum J, Helson C, Majeranowski A, Johnson GA (1980). Biological markers in neuroblastoma and other pediatric neoplasias. In: W. Davis, KR Harrap, G Stathopoulos (eds), "Human cancer. Its characterization and treatment," Princeton: Excerpta Medica pp. 86-94.

Jaffe N (1976). Neuroblastoma: Review of the literature and an examination of factors contributing to its enigmatic character. Cancer Treat Rev 3:61-82.

Lampson LA, Fisher CA, Whelan JP (1983). Striking paucity of HLA-A, B, C and beta 2-microglobulin on human neuroblastoma cell lines. J Immunol 130:2471-8.

Parham P, Barnstable CJ, Bodmer WF (1979). Use of a monoclonal antibody (W6/32) in structural studies of HLA-A,B,C, antigens. J Immunol 123:342-9.

Potluri VR, Gilbert F, Helson C, Helson L (1987). Primitive neuroectodermal tumor cell lines: chromosomal analysis of five cases. Cancer Genet Cytogentet 24:75-86.

Reynolds CP, German DC, Weinberg AG, Smith RG (1981).

Catecholamine fluorescence and tissue culture morphology. Technics in the diagnosis of neuroblastoma. Am J Clin Pathol 75:275–282.

Reynolds CP, Smith RG (1982). Diagnostic and biological markers for neuroblastoma. In: C Pochedly (ed) Neuroblastoma Clinical and Biological Manifestations, New York: Elsevier Biomedical, pp. 131–168.

Reynolds CP, Biedler JL, Spengler BA, Reynolds DA, Ross RA, Frenkel EP, Smith RG (1986). Characterization of human neuroblastoma cell lines established before and after therapy. JNCI 76:375–87.

Schlesinger HR, Gerson JM, Moorhead PS, Maguire H, Hummeler K (1976). Establishment and characterization of human neuroblastoma cell lines. Cancer Res 36:3094–4000.

Schlesinger HR, Rorke L, Jamieson R, Hummeler K (1981). Neuronal properties of neuroectodermal tumors in vitro. Cancer Res 41:2573–2575.

Schmidt D, Harms D, Burdach S (1985). Malignant peripheral neuroectodermal tumours of childhood and adolescence. Virchows Arch [Pathol Anat] 406:351–365.

Schwab M, Alitalo K, Klempnauer K-H, Varmus HE, Bishop JM, Gilbert F, Brodeur G, Goldstein M, Trent J. (1983). Amplified DNA with limited homology to myc cellular oncogene is shared by human neuroblastoma cell lines and a neuroblastoma tumor. Nature 305:245–248.

Seeger RC, Rayner SA, Banerjee A, Chung H, Laug WE, Neustein HB, Benedict WF (1977). Morphology, growth, chromosomal pattern, and fibrinolytic activity of two new human neuroblastoma cell lines. Cancer Res 37:1364–1371.

Seeger RC, Danon YL, Rayner SA, Hoover F (1982). Definition of a Thy-1 determinant on human neuroblastoma, glioma, sarcoma, and teratoma cells with a monoclonal antibody. J Immunol 128:983–9.

Seeger RC, Brodeur GM, Sather H, Dalton A, Siegel SE, Wong KY, Hammond D (1985). Association of multiple copies of the N-myc oncogene with rapid progression of neuroblastomas. N Engl J Med 313:1111–6.

Seemayer TA, Thelmo WL, Bolande RP, Wiglesworth FW (1975). Peripheral neuroectodermal tumors. Perspect Pediatr Pathol 2:151–172.

Shimada H, Chatten J, Newton WA Jr, Sachs N, Hamoudi AB, Chiba T, Marsden HB, Misugi K (1984). Histopathologic prognostic factors in neuroblastic tumors: definition of subtypes of ganglioneuroblastoma and an age-linked classification of neuroblastomas. J

Natl Cancer Inst 73:405-16.

Smith RG, Reynolds CP (1987). Monoclonal antibody recognizing a human neuroblastoma-associated antigen. Diag Clin Immunol 5:209-220.

Thiele CJ, McKeon C, Triche TJ, Ross RA, Reynolds CP, Israel MA (1987). Differential protooncogene expression characterizes histopathologically indistinguishable tumors of the peripheral nervous system. J Clin Invest 80:804-811.

Tomayko MM, Triche TJ, Newburgh RW, Reynolds CP (1988). Induction of catecholamine fluorescence in human neuroblastoma cell lines transplanted into nude mice. Prog Clin Biol Res, this volume, (in press).

Triche TJ (1982). Round cell tumors in childhood: the application of newer techniques to the differential diagnosis. Perspect Pediatr Pathol 7:279-322.

Triche TJ (1986). Neuroblastoma-biology confronts nosology. Arch Pathol Lab Med 110:994-996.

Tumilowicz JJ, Nichols WW, Cholon JJ, Greene AE (1970). Definition of a continuous human cell line derived from neuroblastoma. Cancer Res 30:2110-2118.

Wada R, Seeger R, Brodeur G, Slamon D, Rayner S, Tomayko M, Reynolds CP. (1988). Characterization of human neuroblastoma cell lines that lack N-myc gene amplification. Prog Clin Biol Res, this volume (in press).

Whang-Peng J, Triche TJ, Miser J, Douglass EC, Israel MA (1984). Chromosome translocation in peripheral neuroepithelialioma. New Engl J Med Aug 30:584-585.

Whang-Peng, Triche TJ, Knutsen T, Miser J, Kao-Shan S, Tsai S, Israel MA (1986). Cytogenetic characterization of selected small round cell tumors of childhood. Cancer Genet Cytogenet 21:185-208.

Zeltzer PM, Marangos PJ, Sather H, Evans A, Siegel S, Wong KY, Dalton A, Seeger R, Hammond D (1985). Prognostic importance of serum neuron specific enolase in local and widespread neuroblastoma. Prog Clin Biol Res 175:319-29.

Advances in Neuroblastoma Research 2, pages 307–316
© 1988 Alan R. Liss, Inc.

# INDUCTION OF CATECHOLAMINE FLUORESCENCE IN HUMAN NEUROBLASTOMA CELL LINES TRANSPLANTED INTO NUDE MICE.

Mary M Tomayko, Timothy J Triche, Robert W Newburgh, and C Patrick Reynolds.

Department of Pediatrics and the Jonsson Comprehensive Cancer Center, UCLA School of Medicine, Los Angeles, CA 90024 (MMT,CPR); Laboratory of Pathology, National Cancer Institute, Bethesda, MD 20814 (TJT); Office of Naval Research, Arlington, VA 22217 (RWN).

## INTRODUCTION

As most neuroblastoma tumors produce catecholamines, quantitation of catecholamines and/or their by-products in patient urine, or detection of catecholamines directly in the tumor cells, are useful tumor markers (Reynolds and Smith, 1982). Histochemical detection of the primary catecholamines, (dopamine and norepinephrine) in tumor tissue can be carried out using glyoxylic acid, which yields 2-carboxymethyl-dihydroisoquinoline derivatives that emit an intense blue-green fluorescence when viewed with a fluorescence microscope (de la Torre and Surgeon, 1976; Reynolds et al, 1981).

Although approximately 80% of human neuroblastoma tumors produce detectable levels of catecholamines in the patient (LaBrosse et al, 1980), cell lines established from such tumors fail to demonstrate catecholamine fluorescence (Reynolds et al, 1986). To determine whether the loss of catecholamine fluorescence in neuroblastoma cell lines is due directly to the *in vitro* environment or if it is due to selection of a catecholamine negative cell population by growth in culture, we studied such cell lines grown in an alternative *in vivo* environment, as xenografts in athymic (nude) mice.

**MATERIALS AND METHODS**

Cell Culture

Human neuroblastoma cell lines were established in our laboratory or obtained from the originator of the cell line (Table 1). Cells were maintained *in vitro* at 37° C in a humidified 5% $CO_2$ atmosphere in RPMI 1640 with 10% fetal calf serum (FCS). All cell lines were tested and found to be free of mycoplasma.

Nude mouse tumors of the SMS-LHN cell line that were explanted into culture were minced and cultured in tissue culture flasks in RPMI 1640 with 10% FCS and 50 ug/ml gentamicin. Cells were removed for catecholamine fluorescence after 0,1,2,3, and 5 days in culture with Pucks saline A with 1 mM EDTA and 10 mM Hepes (Pucks-EDTA) (Reynolds et al, 1986).

Catecholamine Fluorescence

The presence of catecholamines was detected histochemically using glyoxylic acid induced catecholamine fluorescence (de la Torre, 1980; Reynolds et al, 1981). A solution of Sucrose (5.1g), anhydrous $KH_2PO_4$ (2.4 g), and Glyoxylic acid (0.75 g) (SPG) (Sigma, St. Louis, MO) was dissolved in 75 ml of $H_2O$, the pH adjusted to 7.4 with 2 N NaOH, and the final SPG solution stored at -20° until use. Touch preps of freshly dissected tumor, smears of suspended cultured cells, or cytospins of cultured cells were made on glass slides and allowed to air dry. The slides were then dipped or flooded three times in the SPG solution, rapidly blown dry with compressed air, and heated for 2.5 min. on a 95° heating block. Slides were stored at 22°C in the dark until studied on a Leitz fluorescence microscope with a Ploempak 2.2 fluorescence illuminator and a "D" filter block (350 nm band pass filter and 480 nm long-pass suppression filter). Fluorescence was evaluated using a subjective scale from 0, (completely negative), to 4+, for the most intense and uniform fluorescence.

Growth of Cells in Athymic (Nude) Mice

For injection into nude mice, cultured neuroblastoma cells were removed from tissue culture flasks using Pucks-

EDTA, washed and resuspended in Dulbecco's Phosphate Buffered Saline without $Ca^{++}$ or $Mg^{++}$ (PBS). Cell clumps were dissociated by gentle pipetting with a Pasture pipette. Cell concentration and viability were determined by hemocytometer using 0.06% trypan blue, and $10^8$ cells were injected through 22 gauge needles subcutaneously between the scapula of 6 to 12 week old Balb/c nu/nu mice (NCI Fredrick Cancer Research Facility Fredrick, MD). Mice were housed in a Laminar flow caging system, (Thoren Caging Systems, Inc., Hazleton, PA), and food, bedding, and water were autoclaved. Mice were terminated by cervical dislocation and the tumor was immediately dissected free of mouse skin and body tissue. The tumor itself was incised, viable areas identified, and touch preps made on glass slides. If the tumor was to be explanted into culture, dissection was carried out under sterile conditions in a laminar flow hood.

Quantitation of Catecholamine Fluorescence

Images of representative fields from each slide were digitized into an IBM PC AT microcomputer using a Leitz Fluorescence microscope, a Dage MTI ISIT 66 intensified video camera (Dage-MTI Inc., Michigan City, IN) and an Imaging Technology frame buffer (Woburn, MA) which digitizes an image of 512 x 480 pixels with 256 gray levels (Dawson, 1986; Puls et al, 1986). The level of fluorescence intensity was determined by measuring the average pixel intensity of clusters of cells with ImagePro image processing software (Media Cybernetics, Silver Spring, MD). The system was calibrated so that the brightest fluorescence gave an average pixel intensity of 178, while background fluorescence yielded an average intensity of 78. All samples were measured on the same day.

Electron Microscopy

Growth medium in cell cultures to be fixed for electron microscopy was replaced with 2.5 % gluteraldehyde (Sigma, St Louis, MO) in PBS and fixed at $4^{\circ}C$ for 24 hrs. After washing with PBS, the cells were scraped off the flask into PBS and pipetted into Ependorf 1.5 ml centrifuge tubes, underlayered with 0.45 um filtered FCS and centrifuged to a pellet, the FCS was aspirated and replaced with 2.5% gluteraldehyde. Pellets were embedded in maraglas resin (Polysciences, Warrington, PA) and sectioned. Viable portions of nude mouse tumors approximately 2 x 2 mm were fixed in 2.5% gluteraldehyde in PBS and processed as described above.

**RESULTS**

Although cultured cells demonstrated no catecholamine fluorescence, the same lines grown as xenografts in nude mice displayed distinct catecholamine fluorescence (Table 1, Figure 1). Cell lines derived from tumors that were known to be catecholamine negative in the patient (SMS-KAN, SMS-KANR, SMS-KCN, SMS-KCNR) remained negative in the nude mice (Table 1).

To determine the time course of the loss of catecholamine fluorescence *in vitro*, a xenograft of SMS-LHN was explanted into culture. Cells and clumps of cells were removed and reacted with SPG periodically to quantitate the amount of catecholamine fluorescence decay. Although the fluorescence intensity began high, it declined to a level equal to background fluorescence by day 5 in culture (Figure 2).

We attempted to induce catecholamine fluorescence *in vitro* by supplementing the medium with catecholamine precursors or with the dopamine-B-hydroxylase co-factor, ascorbate. Cultures of SMS-SAN cells were supplemented every 48 hrs with 2 or 5 ug/ml of tyrosine, DOPA, or dopamine, or every 12 hrs with 2, 3, or 6 ug/ml of sodium ascorbate. After 1, 3, 5, and 7 days *in vitro*, cells were removed from their wells and reacted with SPG, but none demonstrated catecholamine fluorescence.

Electron microscopy of the cell lines in tissue culture showed occasional dense core (neurosecretory) granules in most of the cell lines. However, some lines showed no dense core granules *in vitro*. By contrast, dense core granules were easily seen in the same cell lines grown in nude mice, including those lines that showed no catecholamine fluorescence. Most cell lines showed more numerous neurosecretory granules *in vivo* than they did *in vitro* (Figure 3).

**TABLE 1**

| CELL LINE | MOUSE XENOGRAFT | ORIGINAL PATIENT TISSUE | ORIGIN OF CELL LINE | |
|---|---|---|---|---|
| CHP-234 | 1+ | ?* | Schlesinger et al, 1981 | |
| LA-N-5 | 4+ | ? | Seeger et al, 1982 | |
| LA-N-6 | 4+ | ?* | Wada et al, 1988 | |
| SK-N-BE(2) | 1+ | ? | Biedler et al, 1978 | |
| SK-N-DZ | 3+ | ? | Helson et al, 1980 | |
| SK-N-SH | 4+ | ?* | Biedler et al, 1973 | |
| SMS-LHN | 4+ | + | Wada et al, 1988 | |
| SMS-MSN | 4+ | + | Reynolds et al, 1986 | |
| SMS-SAN | 3+ | + | '' | '' |
| SMS-KAN | 0 | – | '' | '' |
| SMS-KANR | 0 | – | '' | '' |
| SMS-KCN | 0 | – | '' | '' |
| SMS-KCNR | 0 | – | '' | '' |

* Levels of catechols or their metabolites in the patient were elevated.

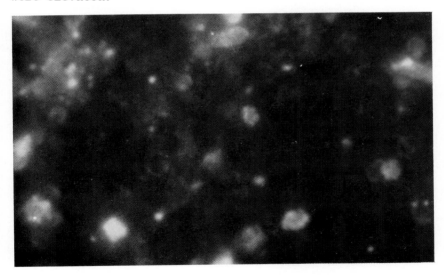

Figure 1. Glyoxylic acid induced catecholamine fluorescence of a touch prep of SMS-SAN cell line grown as a nude mouse xenograft.

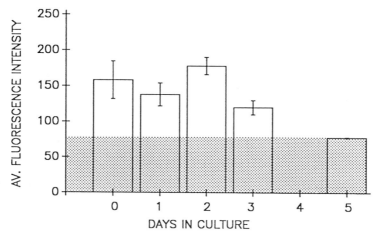

Figure 2. A catecholamine positive SMS-LHN nude mouse xenograft was explanted into tissue culture, reacted each day with SPG and fluorescence quantitated by digital image microscopy. Fluorescence decreased to the level of background (shown by stipling) after 5 days in culture.

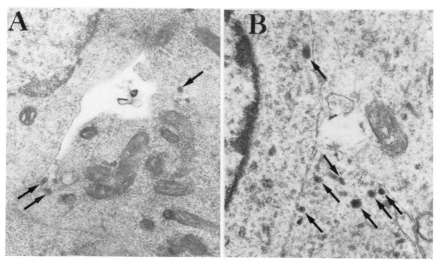

Figure 3. Electron micrographs of SMS-SAN cells grown *in vitro* (A) or in a nude mouse (B), showing the paucity of dense core (neurosecretory) granules (marked by arrows) in the cultured cells as compared to the nude mouse tumor tissue.

# DISCUSSION

Cell lines established from tumors that were catecholamine positive in the patient fail to show catecholamine fluorescence *in vitro* (Reynolds et al, 1986). Here we demonstrate that the lack of catecholamine fluorescence in the cultured cells is not a permanent change caused by the selection of a catecholamine negative cell population, as cell cultures originating from patients with elevated catecholamine levels produced catecholamine positive nude mouse xenografts.

It is possible that factor(s) present *in vivo* but not in tissue culture are necessary for catecholamine synthesis and/or storage. As human neuroblastoma cell lines contain relatively high levels of neurotransmitter synthetic enzymes (Biedler et al, 1978; Ross et al, 1981; Reynolds et al, 1986), a lack of these enzymes is unlikely to be the cause of this phenomenon. We attempted to enhance catecholamine synthesis by supplementing the medium with tyrosine, DOPA, or dopamine, or with ascorbate (a cofactor of dopamine-B-hydroxylase), all known to enhance catecholamine synthesis *in vitro* (Mains and Patterson, 1973). However, these did not induce catecholamine fluorescence in neuroblastoma cell lines *in vitro*. Although these experiments were inconclusive, they suggest that alterations in catecholamine synthetic pathways may not be related to the loss of catecholamine fluorescence *in vitro*.

The paucity of neurosecretory granules in the cells grown *in vitro* compared to the higher density of them in nude mouse tumor tissue suggests that a defect in catecholamine storage could be the reason cell cultures are negative for catecholamine fluorescence. Perhaps factors that are present *in vivo* but not present *in vitro* are necessary for the production and/or storage of neurosecretory granules.

Human neuroblastoma cell lines have been proposed as ideal *in vitro* neuronal models (Perez-Polo et al, 1982). In addition neuroblastoma cultures are being used to study some types of therapy, such as [125]I-MIBG or six-hydroxydopamine, which are dependent upon catecholamine synthesis, storage, and uptake (Reynolds et al, 1982;

Treuner et al, 1986). The observation that the storage and/or synthesis of catecholamines in human neuroblastoma cell lines in culture differs substantially from that of the same cells *in vivo* suggests that better defined *in vitro* conditions are needed for such model studies.

**ACKNOWLEDGEMENTS**

This study was supported in part by grant CA44904 from the National Cancer Institute, DHHS, and by the Office of Naval Research. LCDR Reynolds is assigned to the UCLA School of Medicine from the Department of the Navy. The views expressed in this article are those of the authors and do not reflect the official policy or position of the Department of the Navy, Department of Defense, nor the U. S. Government. We thank Dr. June Biedler, Dr. Lawerence Helson, and Dr. Robert Seeger for providing cell lines.

**REFERENCES**

Biedler JL, Helson L, Spengler BA (1973). Morphology and growth, tumorigenicity, and cytogenetics of human neuroblastoma cells in continuous culture. Cancer Res 33:2643-52.
Biedler JL, Roffler-Tarlov S, Schachner M, Freedman LS (1978). Multiple neurotransmitter synthesis by human neuroblastoma cell lines and clones. Cancer Res 38:3751-3757.
Dawson B (1986). PC transformed into image processor. Digital Design 16(3):63-73.
Helson L, Nisselbaum J, Helson C, Majeranowski A, Johnson GA (1980). Biological markers in neuroblastoma and other pediatric neoplasias. In: W. Davis, KR Harrap, G Stathopoulos (eds) Human Cancer. Its Characterization and Treatment, Princeton: Excerpta Medica, pp. 87-94.
LaBrosse J, Com-Nougue C, Zucker J, et al (1980). Urinary excretion of 3-methly-4-hydroxymandelic acid and 3-methoxy-r-hydroxyphenylacetic acid by 288 patients with neuroblastoma and related neural crest tumors. Cancer Res 40:1995-2001.
Mains RE, Patterson PH (1973). Primary cultures of

dissociated sympathetic neurons. II. Initial studies on catecholamine metabolism. J Cell Biol 59:346-360.

Perez-Polo JR, Reynolds CP, Tiffany-Castiglioni E, Ziegler M, Schulze I, Werrback-Perez K (1982). NGF effects on human neuroblastoma lines: a model system. Prog Clin Biol Res 79:285-299.

Puls JH, Bibbo M, Dytch HE, Bartels PH, Wied GL (1986). The design of an inexpensive video-based microphotometer/computer system for DNA ploidy studies. Anal Quan Cytol Hist 8:1-7.

Reynolds CP, German DC, Weinberg AG, Smith RG (1981). Catecholamine fluorescence and tissue culture morphology. Technics in the diagnosis of neuroblastoma. Am J Clin Pathol 75:275-282.

Reynolds CP, Smith RG (1982). Diagnostic and biological markers for neuroblastoma. In: C Pochedly (ed) Neuroblastoma Clinical and Biological Manifestations, New York: Elsevier Biomedical, pp. 131-168.

Reynolds CP, Biedler JL, Spengler BA, Reynolds DA, Ross RA, Frenkel EP, Smith RG (1986). Characterization of human neuroblastoma cell lines established before and after therapy. J Natl Cancer Inst 76:375-87.

Ross R, Biedler J, Spengler B, Reis D (1981). Neurotransmitter-synthesizing enzymes in 14 human neuroblastoma cell lines. Cell Molecular Neurobiol 1:301-312.

Schlesinger HR, Rorke L, Jamieson R, Hummeler K (1976). Neuronal properties of neuroectodermal tumors in vitro. Cancer Res 41:2573-2575.

Seeger RC, Danon YL, Rayner SA, Hoover F (1982). Definition of a Thy-1 determinant on human neuroblastoma, glioma, sarcoma, and teratoma cells with a monoclonal antibody. J Immunol 128:983-989.

de la Torre JC (1980). An improved approach to histofluorescence using the SPG method for tissue momoamines. J Neurosci Method 3:1-5.

de la Torre JC, Surgeon JW (1976). A methodological approach to rapid and sensitive monoamine histofluorescence using a modified glyoxylic acid technique: the SPG method. Histochem 49:81-93.

Treuner J, Feine U, Buck J, Bruchelt G, Dopfer R, Gigert R, Muller-Schauenburg W, Meinke J, Kaiser W, Niethammer D (1986). Clinical experiences in the treatment of neuroblastoma with [131]I-metaiodobenzylguanidine. Pediatric Hematol Oncol 3:205-216.

Wada RK, Seeger RC, Brodeur GM, Slamon DJ, Rayner SA, Tomayko MM, Reynolds CP (1988). Characterization of human neuroblastoma cell lines that lack N-*myc* gene amplification. Prog Clin Biol Res, this volume, (in press).

Advances in Neuroblastoma Research 2, pages 317–326
© 1988 Alan R. Liss, Inc.

# "In Situ" Modulation of Murine Neuroblastoma Growth and Biochemical Differentiation by the Adrenergic Nervous System and Nerve Growth Factor

Bernard L. Mirkin, Donald W. Fink, Jr., Robert F. O'Dea
Division of Clinical Pharmacology
Departments of Pediatrics and Pharmacology,
University of Minnesota Health Sciences Center,
Minneapolis, Minnesota 55455

## INTRODUCTION

Recent studies have suggested an intriguing interaction between host age, functional integrity of the adrenergic nervous system and murine neuroblastoma (MNB) growth (Chelmicka-Schorr et al, 1985; Fink and Mirkin, 1987a,b). It has been proposed that this relationship is dependent on endogenous polypeptides such as nerve growth factor (NGF). This factor not only modulates the maturation of adrenergic nerve fibers but may also regulate the growth and differentiation of MNB.

Studies of mice inoculated with MNB cells at different postnatal ages suggest that environmental changes occurring in the maturing host can influence tumor cell expression. Thus, cell replication as determined by time to onset of palpable tumor, was delayed in animals implanted with MNB cells 24 to 48 hours after birth (Schengruend et al, 1979). An inhibitory effect of host age on MNB tumor growth rate was not observed in animals implanted with MNB cells at 7, 14, 21 or 28 days postnatally (Fink and Mirkin, 1987a). Experiments in which MNB cells were injected into mouse embryos also support the view that biologically immature tissues can exert profound effects on the phenotypic expression of other cells (Pierce, 1983).

The influence of the adrenergic nervous system on MNB tumor growth has been evaluated in murine models using pharmacological agents that ablate or prevent development

Partially supported by grants from the USPHS (NS-17194) and Pharmaceutical Manufacturers Association Foundation.

of the adrenergic nervous system. Chlorisondamine, a
ganglionic blocking agent, has been administered to
neonatal mice causing maturational arrest of the adrenergic
nervous system and subsequent attenuation of MNB tumor
growth in this model (Chelmicka-Schorr and Aranson, 1979).
Chemical sympathectomy induced by treatment of mice with
6-hydroxydopamine (6HD) also has been reported to suppress
MNB tumor growth in both neonatal and adult mice
(Chelmicka-Schorr and Arnason, 1976; Fink and Mirkin,
1987b). It has been recently demonstrated that chemical
sympathectomy decreases the concentration of nerve growth
factor (NGF) in sympathetic ganglia and increases it in
sympathetically innervated organs such as the heart,
submandibular gland and iris (Korsching and Thoenen, 1985).
　　The present investigation has confirmed the inhibitory
effect of chemical sympathectomy on MNB growth in 30 day-
old mice that were denervated within the first week of
life. In contrast to previous studies, these data failed
to demonstrate a similar response in animals
sympathectomized during adult life. The suppression of MNB
tumor growth in neonatally sympathectomized mice may result
from the inhibitory effect of sympathectomy on NGF
secretion, since exogenous NGF reverses this effect.

## METHODS

　　__Animals__: A/J mice obtained from the Jackson Laboratory
(Bar Harbor, Maine) were mated and litters reared from this
breeding. Each litter was housed in individual cages and
pups remained with lactating mothers until weaned at
approximately four weeks of age. Mice were fed standard
mouse laboratory chow and provided with water __ad libitum__.
　　__"In Situ" Murine Neuroblastoma (MNB) Tumor Model__:
C-1300 MNB was originally provided by the Mason Research
Institute, Worcester, Mass. This tumor line has been
maintained by implantation into adult male A/J mice for
more than 100 tumor generations, each approximately 21 days
in duration. Tumors are implanted by injection of
disaggregated tumor cell suspensions ($10^6$ MNB cells/0.1 ml)
prepared by mincing the tumor in sterile 0.9% NaCl
solution. Tumor cell viability was determined by trypan
blue dye exclusion.
　　__Chemical Sympathectomy by 6-Hydroxydopamine (6HD)__:
Neonatal A/J mice were treated with 6HD (100 μg/g body
weight s.c.) on postnatal days 4, 6, 8 and 10 (see Figure
1). Vehicle treated animals received injections of a

solution consisting of 0.9% NaCl and 1.0 mg/ml ascorbic acid (used as an antioxidant). Destruction of adrenergic neurones was verified by analysis of catecholamine concentrations in sympathetic target organs (e.g., heart and spleen). This regimen caused a significant depletion of norepinephrine in the heart and spleen that persisted for at least seven weeks after the final 6HD injection.

Adult A/J mice, postnatal age 58 days, were administered five injections of 6HD (100 µg/g body weight) at intervals of 48 hours (see Figure 1).

NEONATAL

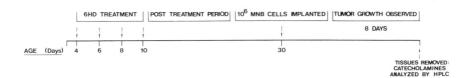

ADULT

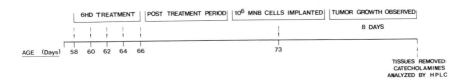

Figure 1.  Experimental Design and Dosing Schedule for 6-HD in Neonatal and Adult Mice.

**Nerve Growth Factor (NGF):** Submandibular glands were excised from male mice and NGF isolated by the method of Bocchini and Angeletti (1969).

**Analysis of Catecholamines:** High pressure liquid chromatography coupled with electrochemical detection was used to determine norepinephrine (NE), dopamine (DA), and epinephrine (EPI) concentrations in tissues. Tissues were homogenized in 0.1 M perchloric acid and catecholamines adsorbed onto alumina at alkaline pH followed by elution

with acid.  Methyldopamine was used as the internal
standard.  An aliquot of the acid eluate was injected onto
a cationic exchange column packed with corasil C/X (Water
Associates Inc., Milford, Mass) and catecholamine
concentrations determined by reference to standard curves.

Experimental Design (Figure 1):  All animals were
inoculated with $10^6$ MNB cells three weeks (neonates) or
one week (adult) after completion of 6HD administration.
Each animal was examined daily to determine the time to
palpation of a tumor mass.  The transverse diameter of
each tumor was recorded for a period of eight days after
initial palpation and the animal killed by cervical
dislocation at this time.  The brain, heart, spleen and
tumor were carefully dissected, frozen on dry ice, weighed
and stored at -80°C until assayed.

Statistics:  All data were evaluated by use of the
unpaired Student's t-test for equal and unequal variances.
Differences between the experimental groups were considered
to be significant at the p<0.05 level.

RESULTS

Effect of Chemical Sympathectomy on MNB Tumor Growth:
Host Age Dependency

The growth of MNB "in situ" was determined by the
following independent parameters:
1.    Transverse tumor diameter measured over an eight
day period starting at the time of initial palpation.  The
time-growth curves generated from measurement of transverse
tumor diameter over a fixed time interval demonstrated a
significant inhibition of MNB growth in neonatally
sympathectomized mice.  No changes in growth were observed
in animals that had been sympathectomized as adults (Figure
2).  The mean tumor diameter of neonatally sympathectomized
mice on day eight was 25% less than those of controls.  In
contrast, tumors in the sympathectomized adult animals were
slightly, but not significantly, larger than control.
2.    Tumor weight eight days after initial palpation.
In mice treated with 6HD during neonatal and adult life,
respectively, tumor weights on day eight were as follows:
(Mean ± S.E.) Neonates:  vehicle -1.87 ± 0.07 g; 6HD -0.89
± 0.08 g, and Adults:  vehicle -2.05 ± 0.19 g; 6HD -2.64 ±
0.35 g.  The mean tumor weights in neonatally
sympathectomized mice were 47% of vehicle-treated controls
and this difference was highly significant (p<0.0005).  The

mean weight of tumors excised from both groups of adult animals did not differ significantly.

    3.  <u>**Ratio of tumor weight to body weight.**</u>  This parameter of MNB growth was established in order to

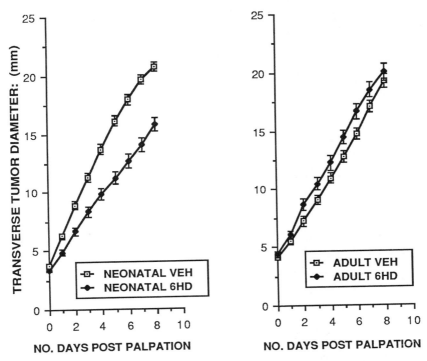

Figure 2.  Effect of chemical sympathectomy on transverse tumor diameter of neonatal and adult mice.

minimize the possible influence of lower body weight in sympathectomized animals upon tumor mass. It also confirmed that the effects of sympathectomy upon "in situ" tumor cell replication rate were host age dependent. Tumor to body weight ratios of adult animals were $10.0 \pm 1.0\%$ and $13.7 \pm 2.1\%$ in the vehicle-treated and sympathectomized animals, respectively. Comparable ratios in neonatally sympathectomized animals were $13.2 \pm 0.5\%$ for the vehicle-treated group and $8.2 \pm 0.7\%$ for the 6HD-treated group; this decrease in tumor body weight ratio was highly significant (Figure 3).

### Nerve Growth Factor (NGF) Induced Stimulation of Murine Neuroblastoma (MNB) Tumor Growth in Neonatally Sympathectomized Mice.

The hypothesis that suppression of MNB tumor growth in neonatally sympathectomized animals reflected a decrease in NGF titre was tested. NGF (12.5 μg/day i. p.) was administered to mice at the time of MNB implantation and continued through the entire experimental period. Tumor weights determined eight days after initial palpation of the tumor were as follows in each of the experimental groups (Mean ± S.E.): vehicle 2.0 ± 0.11 g; vehicle + NGF 2.06 ± 0.11 g; 6HD 0.96 ± 0.09 g; 6HD + NGF 1.6 ± 0.1 g. NGF significantly enhanced tumor growth in the neonatally sympathectomized animals, even though tumor weight was only restored to 80% of controls.

The effect of NGF on MNB growth was more dramatically observed when tumor to body weight ratios were compared. This parameter demonstrated a complete restoration of tumor growth in neonatally sympathectomized mice that had been treated with NGF (Figure 3).

### Effect of Neonatal Sympathectomy and Nerve Growth Factor (NGF) on Catecholamine Content of Murine Neuroblastoma (MNB) Tumors.

Norepinephrine (NE) and dopamine (DA) were assayed in tumors that had been excised for the study described above. Neonatally sympathectomized animals exhibited a significant increase in both NE and DA concentrations. The elevation of DA was 3.1-fold and of NE, 3.6-fold above values obtained in vehicle treated control animals. In contrast, the NE and DA concentration of tumors obtained from adult mice treated with 6HD did not differ significantly from their respective controls (Table 1). The administration of NGF to sympathectomized animals caused a pronounced decrease in the concentration of DA and NE.

## DISCUSSION

The relationship between the adrenergic nervous system, nerve growth factor (NGF) and neuroblastoma growth and differentiation has been investigated using a murine "in

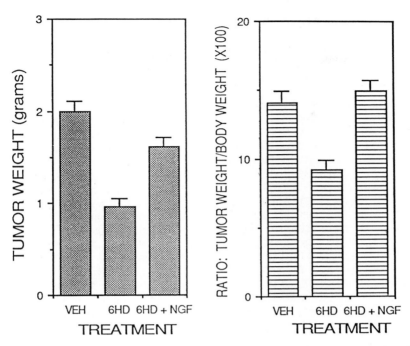

**Figure 3.** Effect of NGF on tumor weight and tumor weight/
body weight ratio of neonatally sympathectomized
mice.

TABLE 1

Catecholamine Content of Murine Neuroblastoma Tumors[†]

| Treatment | Norepinephrine[*] | Dopamine |
|---|---|---|
| Vehicle | 20.9 ± 2.5 | 16.6 ± 3.4 |
| Vehicle + NGF | 21.3 ± 3.4 | 14.0 ± 2.5 |
| 6HD | 61.4 ± 11.2 | 60.0 ± 2.7 |
| 6HD + NGF | 28.1 ± 3.2 | 21.8 ± 2.6 |

NGF  -   Nerve Growth Factor; 6HD - 6-hydroxydopamine.
  [†]-  Tumors excised 8 days after initial palpation.
  [*] -  All data expressed as ng/g tissue (wet weight);
      Mean ± S.E.

situ" model. Neonatal sympathectomy caused a significant reduction in MNB tumor growth when these animals were implanted with MNB cells 20 days later; whereas, no suppression of tumor growth was observed when mature animals were sympathectomized. In addition, the catecholamine content (norepinephrine and dopamine) of MNB tumors was significantly increased in the tumors of neonatally sympathectomized mice. Murine NGF, administered at the time of MNB cell implantation, reversed the inhibitory effect of neonatal sympathectomy on MNB growth and also decreased tumor catecholamine concentration.

The influence of somatic denervation on neuroblastoma cell growth was originally demonstrated by Batkin et al (1970), who sectioned the femoral and sciatic nerves of mouse gastrocnemius muscle and observed retardation of MNB growth. Ablation of the sympathetic nervous system by 6HD was reported to inhibit MNB tumor growth in both neonatal (Chelmicka-Schorr and Arnason, 1978) and adult mice (Chelmicka-Schorr and Arnason, 1976). These findings contrast with the present investigation in that a suppressive effect on tumor growth was observed only in animals that had been sympathectomized during neonatal life and not as adults. The reason for this significant difference is not apparent.

The mechanism(s) by which sympathectomy produces its effects on tumor growth are not well defined. Recent studies of the neurotrophic peptide, nerve growth factor (NGF), suggest it may play some role in this process. NGF has been shown to exert a differentiating action on human neuroblastoma cells in tissue culture (Sonnefeld and Ishii, 1982) and also acts as a survival factor for these cell lines (Tischler et al, 1984). If NGF is required for MNB cell replication, a decrease in circulating NGF may occur after sympathectomy and thereby suppress MNB growth "in situ". Our demonstration that exogenous murine NGF can restore tumor growth to that observed in vehicle treated controls supports this hypothesis.

Sympathectomy of the neonatal animal also appears to cause biochemical differentiation, at least as expressed via catecholamine biosynthesis. Those animals in which MNB growth was suppressed had significant increases in the tumor concentration of both norepinephrine and dopamine. It is interesting to note that the catecholamine concentration of MNB in NGF treated, neonatally sympathectomized animals decreased and approximated that of vehicle treated controls (Table 1).

This investigation has confirmed previous reports suggesting that the sympathetic nervous system exerts a modulating action on MNB tumor growth "in situ". The primary effects of sympathetic denervation appear to be suppression of tumor growth rate and enhancement of catecholamine biosynthesis and/or storage in MNB tumors. Both phenomena were host age dependent and observed only in animals that had been sympathectomized during the neonatal period (4 to 7 days postnatal age). The mechanism through which sympathectomy exerts its suppressive effect on MNB growth may be via a reduction in circulating neurotrophic polypeptide, since exogenous murine NGF restores MNB growth.

## REFERENCES

Batkin S, Piette LH, Wildman E (1970). Effect of muscle denervation on growth of transplanted tumor in mice. Proc Natl Acad Sci 67: 1521-1527.

Bocchini U, Angeletti PU (1969). The nerve growth factor: Purification as a 30,000 molecular-weight protein. Proc Natl Acad Sci. 64: 787-794.

Chelmicka-Schorr E, Arnason BG (1976). Effect of 6-hydroxydopamine on tumor growth. Cancer Res 36: 2382-2384.

Chelmicka-Schorr E, Arnason BG (1978). Modulatory effect of the sympathetic nervous system on neuroblastoma tumor growth. Cancer Res. 38: 1374-1375.

Chelmicka-Schorr E, Arnason BG (1979). Suppression of growth of mouse neuroblastoma and A10 adenocarcinoma in newborn mice treated with the ganglion-blocking agent chlorisondamine. Eur J Cancer 15: 533-535.

Chelmicka-Schorr E, Jones KH, Checinski ME, Yu RC, Arnason BG (1985). Influence of the sympathetic nervous system on the growth of neuroblastoma in vivo and in vitro. Cancer Res 45: 6213-6214.

Fink DW, Mirkin BL (1987a). Influence of host age and tumor cell burden on the growth and catecholamine content of C-1300 murine neuroblastoma in situ. J Natl Cancer Inst (in review).

Fink DW, Mirkin BL (1987b). Effects of chemical sympathectomy in neonatal and adult mice on C-1300 neuroblastoma tumor growth and catecholamine content. Cancer Res (in review).

Korsching S, Thoenen H (1985). Treatment with
6-hydroxydopamine and colchicine decreases nerve growth
factor levels in sympathetic ganglia and increases them
in the corresponding target tissues. J Neuroscience
5(4): 1058-1061.
Pierce G, Podesta A, Mullins J, Wells R (1984). The
neurula stage mouse embryo in control of neuroblastoma.
Proc Natl Acad Sci 81: 7608-7611.
Schengruend C, Repman M, Sheffler B (1979). Development
of a neonatal and metastatic murine neuroblastoma
model. Cancer Res 39: 711-713.
Sonnenfeld KH, Ishii DN (1982). Nerve growth factor
effects and receptors in cultured human neuroblastoma
cell lines. J Neurosci Res 8: 375-391.
Tischler AS, Slayton V, Costopoules DS, Leape LL, DeLellis
RA, Wolfe HJ (1981). Nerve growth factor may function
as a survival factor for human neuroblastoma in
culture. Cancer 54: 1344-1347.

Advances in Neuroblastoma Research 2, pages 327–336

5-BROMO-2'-DEOXYURIDINE INDUCES S 100 PROTEIN IN HUMAN NEUROBLASTOMA CELLS IN CULTURE

Kentaro Tsunamoto[1], Shinsaku Imashuku[2], Shigeyoshi Hibi[1], Noriko Esumi[1] and Kanefusa Kato[3]

[1]Department of Pediatrics and [2]Children's Research Hospital, Kyoto Prefectural University of Medicine, Kyoto 602 and [3]Department of Biochemistry, Institute for Developmental Research, Aichi Prefectural Colony, Aichi 480-03, Japan

INTRODUCTION

S 100 protein is an acidic, calcium-binding protein with a molecular weight of approximately 20,000, and consists of a dimer of subunits ($\alpha\alpha$, $\alpha\beta$ and $\beta\beta$ subunits) (Moore, 1965; Isobe et al, 1981). S 100 protein is localized mainly in glial and Schwann cells and regarded as one of the markers for glial and Schwann cells in the nervous system (Weiss et al, 1983). Neuron specific enolase (NSE, $\gamma\gamma$-enolase), which was demonstrated in neurons in central and peripheral nervous systems, is a glycolytic enzyme and regarded to be one of the differentiation markers of the neuronal cells (Marangos et al, 1980).

5-bromo-2'-deoxyuridine (BrdU), an analogue of thymidine, is known to affect the differentiation of several cultured cell lines after being incorporated into the cellular DNA (Ashman et al, 1980). Recently, it was demonstrated that human neuroblastoma cells possibly differentiate into glial or Schwann cells when treated by BrdU (Reynolds et al, 1985).

In this report, we describe the induction of a significantly large amount of S 100 protein in a human neuroblastoma cell line, when the growth of this cell line was suppressed by BrdU. The results indicate that neuroblastoma cells may differentiate into glial or Schwann cells and that they may be the mother cells for S 100 protein-positive cells, which were reported to be abundantly present in the well-differentiated ganglio-neuroblastoma tissues (Ishiguro et al, 1983).

## MATERIALS AND METHODS

### Cell Culture

Two human neuroblastoma cell lines, NCG and GOTO (Imashuku et al, 1985; Sekiguchi et al, 1979), were used. Cells were maintained at 37°C in RPMI 1640 medium supplemented with 10 % heat-inactivated fetal calf serum (GIBCO Laboratories, Grand Island, NY) in a humidified atmosphere of 95 % air and 5 % $CO_2$. Cells were plated at $5 \times 10^5$ per flask (25 cm², Corning Co., NY). After 48 h subculture, cells were maintained in the medium with or without 5 $\mu g/ml$ of BrdU (Sigma Chemical Co., St. Louis, MO) for 6 days with a change of medium every 48 h. During the 6 day period, the morphological changes of cells were studied under a phase-contrast microscope. On day 6 of the BrdU-treatment, cells were scraped off with a rubber policeman bar and suspended in 1-2 ml of PBS(-). The cell suspensions were centrifuged at 120xg for 5 min and the cell pellets were stored at -80°C until the assays for S $100a_0$ protein, S 100b protein and NSE. To evaluate the effect of BrdU on cell growth, $5 \times 10^4$ cells per well (24-well microplates, Corning Co., NY) were seeded and cultured with or without BrdU in the same manner as described above. On days 0, 2, 4 and 6 of the BrdU-treatment, the number of viable cells was counted by the trypan blue dye exclusion method.

As a separate experiment, a study of BrdU dose relation to cell growth inhibition in association with the induction of these proteins were performed in detail using GOTO. Cells were seeded at $5 \times 10^5$ per flask and cultured with or without BrdU. The doses of BrdU examined ranged from 0.01 to 10 $\mu g/ml$. On day 6 of the treatment, cells were harvested and subjected to the assays for S $100a_0$, S 100b protein and NSE.

### Enzyme Immunoassays for S $100a_0$ Protein (a Dimer of $\alpha\alpha$ Form), S 100b Protein ($\beta\beta$ Form) and NSE ($\gamma\gamma$ Enolase):

Cell pellets were homogenized, and the homogenates were centrifuged at 4°C at 20,000xg for 20 min. The supernatants (sup.) were subjected to enzyme immunoassays, using specific antibodies against human $\alpha$ or $\beta$ subunit of

S 100 protein and human $\gamma$ subunit of enolase. The sandwich enzyme immunoassay system (Kato et al, 1981; Kato et al, 1986), for S $100a_0$ protein was specific and showed no cross-reaction with either S 100a protein ($\alpha\beta$ subunit) or S 100b protein; however, the systems for S 100b protein and NSE showed cross-reactions, 15 % to S 100a protein and 10% to $\alpha\beta$ enolase (Kato et al, 1981; Kato et al, 1986).

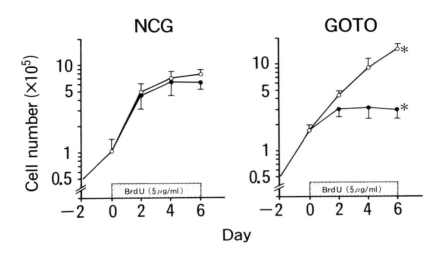

Figure 1: Effect of BrdU on the cell growth of human neuroblastoma cells in culture. After 48 h subculture, $5 \times 10^4$ cells per flask were treated with ( ● ) or without ( O ) 5 μg/ml of BrdU for 6 days. On days 0, 2, 4 and 6 of the treatment, the number of viable cells was determined by the trypan blue dye exclusion method. Values indicate mean ± SE of 4 separate experiments. Asterisk indicates the statistical significance at $p < 0.01$ by the t-test, versus control.

Others

Protein concentrations in homogenate sup. were determined with Bio-Rad Protein Assay (Bio-Rad). Statistical analysis was carried out using Student's t-test.

RESULTS

## Cell Growth and Morphology

As shown in Fig. 1, the cell growth of GOTO was significantly suppressed by treatment with BrdU. GOTO cells grew slowly from day 2 of the treatment and reaching only 14.5 % of the control growth on day 6. The morphological changes induced by BrdU were significant only in GOTO (Fig. 2). Before the treatment, GOTO cells were small and spindle-shaped. Two days after the treatment, the cells became larger and flattened-out and possessed polygonal cytoplasm which adhered firmly to the substrate of the culture flask, in association with inhibited cell growth. By contrast, NCG cells showed no morphological changes.

## Induction of S 100 Protein and NSE (Table 1)

By the BrdU-treatment, NCG cells showed no induction of S 100 protein and NSE. However, GOTO cells exhibited significant increases of S 100 protein and NSE compared to the control. The concentration of S $100a_0$ protein notably increased; 5,600-fold from 37 to 211,000 pg/mg protein after the treatment. S 100b protein and NSE in this cell line also increased from <25 to 623 pg/mg protein and from 144 to 257 ng/mg protein, respectively.

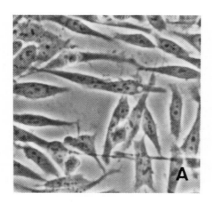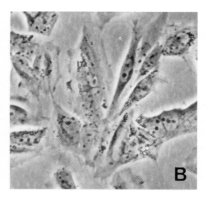

Figure 2: Phase-contrast photomicrographs of a human neuroblastoma cell line, GOTO (x300). A) Control: cells were small and spindle-shaped. B) BrdU-treatment: cells became larger, flattened and possessed polygonal cytoplasm which adhered firmly on the substrate of culture flask.

Table 1
Cellular contents of S 100 protein and NSE in neuroblastoma
cells cultured with or without 5 μg/ml BrdU for 6 days

| Cell line | S100ao protein (pg/mg protein) | S100b protein (pg/mg protein) | NSE (ng/mg protein) |
|---|---|---|---|
| NCG | | | |
| control | $230 \pm 72^a$ | <14 | $95 \pm 12$ |
| BrdU | $311 \pm 101$ | <13 | $133 \pm 25$ |
| GOTO | | | |
| control | $37 \pm 7$ | <25 | $144 \pm 20$ |
| BrdU | $211,000 \pm 82,500^b$ | $623 \pm 113^c$ | $257 \pm 34^b$ |

a. mean $\pm$ SE (n=4)
b. p<0.05 (vs. control)
c. p<0.01 (vs. control)

Dose-Relation to the BrdU-induced Increase of S 100 Protein and NSE

As shown in Fig. 3, the concentration of S 100ao protein remained very low when GOTO cells were treated by up to 0.1 μg/ml BrdU. At doses over 0.5 μg/ml, S 100ao protein increased sharply reaching at maximum 5,600 times that of the control. The concentration of S 100b protein and NSE similarly increased from undetectable (<25) to the peak value 631 pg/mg protein and from 144 to 296 ng/mg protein, respectively, corresponding to the increasing doses of BrdU, as in S 100ao protein. The cell growth inhibition of GOTO was slight at doses up to 0.1 μg/ml, however, it was significant beyond 0.5 μg/ml BrdU. The induction of S 100 proteins correlated well with the degree of cell growth inhibition (r=0.685 for S 100ao protein and r=0.711 for S 100b protein, p<0.01).

DISCUSSION

BrdU-induced growth inhibition associated with flat-type cell morphology was reported in the studies of B16 mouse melanoma cells (Wrathall et al, 1973). The growth inhibitory effect of BrdU on Friend murine erythroleukemia cells was suggested to be due to its incorporation into cellular DNA sequences during early S phase of the cell cycle, and further blocking the cells' entry into S phase (Brown et al, 1979). BrdU-induced cell differentiation was assumed to be bi-directional, i.e., exerting both differentiation and de- differentiation, indicating an "all-or-none" phenomenon (Weintraub et al, 1973). Cellular functions such as hemoglobin synthesis by Friend murine erythroleukemia cells (Brown et al, 1979) or melanine formation by $B_{16}$ mouse melanoma cells (Wrathall et al, 1973), were found to be inhibited by BrdU-treatment. In cloned rat glioma ($C_6$) cells, 5 µg/ml BrdU was reported to

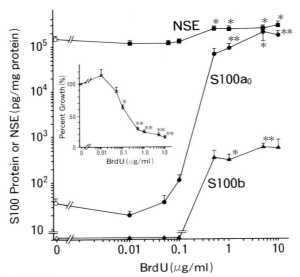

Figure 3: BrdU dose-relation to the cell growth, and the content of S 100 protein and NSE in GOTO cells. After 48 h subculture, $5 \times 10^5$ cells were treated, with various doses of BrdU (0, 0.01, 0.05, 0.1, 0.5, 1.0, 5.0, 10 µg/ml). On day 6, the number of viable cells was counted and the growth was expressed in percent against the control (no treatment). In terms of S 100 protein and NSE, the harvested cells were subjected to the enzyme immunoassay for S $100a_0$, S 100b protein and NSE as described in "Materials and Methods". Values indicate mean ± SE of 4 separate experiments. Asterisks, single and double, indicate the statistical significance at $p < 0.05$ and $p < 0.01$, respectively, by the t-test, versus control.

suppress the synthesis of S 100 protein (Kolber et al, 1978). With regard to BrdU-treated neuroblastoma cells, Schubert and Jacob (1970) first reported that murine C1300 cell line was induced to have neurite-like outgrowth of cytoplasm as a step towards neuronal differentiation. Recently, Reynolds et al (1985) observed that the human neuroblastoma cell line, SMS-KCNR, transformed into flat cells positive for myeline basic protein, one of the differentiation markers for glial and/or Schwann cells. In our present BrdU-treatment study, we found that GOTO cells showed significant cell growth inhibition in association with flat cell morphology and induction of S 100 protein. By contrast, NCG cells showed none of such changes. At the moment, the reason is unknown why the two human neuroblastoma cell lines responded quite heterogeneously to BrdU.

Our report is considered to be the first to show that neuroblastoma cells like GOTO could be stimulated to produce S 100 protein when exposed to BrdU. As shown in the Table 1, BrdU-treated GOTO cells produced significantly higher amounts of S $100a_0$, S 100b protein and NSE compared to the controls. It was also shown that 0.5 $\mu$g/ml BrdU was sufficient to obtain the maximum response. This phenomenon may indicate that S 100 protein gene(s) were activated when certain amounts of BrdU were incorporated into cellular DNA, in accordance with the report by Weintraub et al (1973) that BrdU incorporation into DNA might affect the specific target (switching loci) genes involved in hemoglobin synthesis of chick erythroblast. According to the recent study by Comi et al (1986), BrdU possibly switches the program from adult type globin to fetal type globin synthesis. The rapid induction of S 100 protein in GOTO cells between concentrations of 0.1 and 0.5 $\mu$g/ml BrdU may indicate that BrdU at this level activates the switching loci of S 100 protein gene(s) in neuroblastoma cells.

It is interesting that in BrdU-treated GOTO cells NSE also increased and among S 100 proteins, both S $100_{a0}$ and S $100_b$ increased. NSE has been regarded as one of the differentiation markers for neuronal cells, but not for glial or Schwann cells in normal nervous tissues. NSE was also demonstrated in various neoplastic nervous tissues such as glioblastomas, astrocytomas, neuroblastomas, melanomas and neuroendocrine tumors (Ishiguro et al, 1983;

Schmechel et al, 1978). On the other hand, Takahashi et al (1984) immunohistochemically demonstrated only $\alpha$ subunit of S 100 protein in neurons, both $\alpha$ and $\beta$ subunit in glial cells and only $\beta$ subunit in Schwann cells. Following the data by Takahashi et al, GOTO cells, which induced both $\alpha$ and $\beta$ subunits of S 100 protein, might be differentiated into glial cells, but not to Schwann cells. In addition, the simultaneous increase of S $100_{a0}$, S $100_b$ proteins and NSE in BrdU-treated GOTO cells may indicate that this cell line became differentiated bi-directionally to glial cells as well as neuronal cells.

Clinically, we often encounter the differentiation of neuroblastoma to ganglioneuroblastoma or ganglioneuroma, which mainly consists of ganglion cells, glial or Schwann cells and fibrous components. The glial or Schwann cell components in such tumor tissues immunohistochemically stained positive for S 100 protein (Misugi et al, 1982). To date, the exact origin of these S 100 protein- positive cells has been controversial. There are two possibilities; one is that the cells positive for S 100 protein are glial or Schwann cells which are originally located at the periphery of neuroblastoma tissues (Choi et al, 1985). These cells proliferate and migrate into the center of the tumors after the neuroblastoma cells are spontaneously or therapeutically destroyed or differentiated to ganglion cells. The other is that the glia- or Schwann-like cells are derived and differentiated from neuroblastoma cells, whether or not they remain neoplastic (Carlei et al, 1984). The evidence of induced S 100 protein in BrdU-treated GOTO cells in this report partly supports the latter theory.

With this induction system using the BrdU-treated GOTO cells, we may be able to clarify the regulatory mechanisms of S 100 protein synthesis at the gene level as well as the function of S 100 protein in the future.


REFERENCES

Ashman CR, Davidson RL (1980). Inhibition of Friend erythroleukemic cell differentiation by bromodeoxyuridine: Correlation with the amount of bromodeoxyuridine in DNA. J Cell Physiol 102: 45-50.
Brown EH, Schildkraut CL (1979). Perturbation of growth and differentiation of Friend murine erythroleukemia cells by

5-bromodeoxyuridine incorporation in early S phase. J Cell Physiol 99: 261-278.

Carlei F, Polak JM, Ceccamea A, Marangos PJ, Dahl D, Cocchia D, Michetti F, Lezoche E, Speranza V (1984). Neuronal and glial markers in tumours of neuroblastic origin. Virchows Arch 404: 313-324.

Choi HH, Anderson PJ (1985). Immunohistochemical diagnosis of olfactory neuroblastoma. J Neuropathol Exp Neurol 44: 18-31.

Comi P, Ottolenghi S, Giglioni B, Migliaccio G, Migliaccio AR, Bassano E, Amadori S, Mastroberardino G, Peschle C (1986). Bromodeoxyuridine treatment of normal adult erythroid colonies: An in vitro model for reactivation of human fetal globin genes. Blood 68: 1036-1041.

Imashuku S, Todo S, Esumi N, Hashida T, Tsunamoto K, Nakajima F (1985). Tumor differentiation - Application of prostaglandins in the treatment of neuroblastoma. In Evans AE, D'Angio GJ, Seeger RC (eds): "Advances in Neuroblastoma Research", New York: Alan R Liss, p89-98.

Ishiguro Y, Kato K, Ito T, Nagaya M (1983). Determination of three enolase isozymes and S-100 protein in various tumors in children. Cancer Res 43: 6080-6084.

Isobe T, Ishioka T, Okuyama T (1981). Structural relation of two S-100 proteins in bovine brain: Subunit composition of S-100a protein. Eur J Biochem 115: 469-474.

Kato, K, Suzuki F, Umeda Y (1981). Highly sensitive immunoassays for three forms of rat brain enolase. J Neurochem 36: 739-797.

Kato K, Kimura S, Haimoto H, Suzuki F (1986). S 100ao ($\alpha\alpha$) protein: Distribution in muscle tissues of various animals and purification from human pectoral muscle. J Neurochem 46: 1555-1560.

Kolber AR, Perumal AS, Goldstein MN, Moore BW (1978). Drug-induced differentiation of a rat glioma in vitro: II. The expression of S-100, a glial specific protein and steroid sulfatase. Brain Res 143: 513-520.

Marangos PJ, Schmechel DE, Parma AM, Goodwin FK (1980). Developmental profile of neuron-specific (NSE) and non-neuronal (NNE) enolase. Brain Res 190: 185-193.

Misugi K, Aoki I, Shimada H, Kikyo S, Sasaki Y, Tsunoda A, Nakajima T (1982). S-100 protein in neuroblastoma group tumors. Yokohama Med Bull 33: 127-131.

Moore BW (1965). A soluble protein characteristic of the nervous system. Biochem Biophys Res Commun 19: 739-744.

Reynolds CP, Maples J (1985). Modulation of cell surface

antigens accompanies morphological differentiation of human neuroblastoma cell lines. In Evans AE, D'Angio GJ, Seeger RC (eds): "Advances in Neuroblastoma Research", New York: Alan R Liss, p 13-37.

Schmechel D, Marangos PJ, Brightman M (1978). Neuron-specific enolase is a molecular marker for peripheral and central neuroendocrine cells. Nature 276: 834-836.

Schubert D. Jacob F (1970). 5-Bromodeoxyuridine-induced differentiation of a neuroblastoma. Proc Natl Acad Sci U.S.A. 67: 247-254.

Sekiguchi M, Oota T, Sakakibara K, Inui N, Fujii G (1979). Establishment and characterization of a human neuroblastoma cell line in tissue culture. Jpn J Exp Med 49: 67-83.

Takahashi K, Isobe T, Ohtsuki Y, Akagi T, Sonobe H, Okuyama T (1984). Immunohistochemical study on the distribution of $\alpha$ and $\beta$ subunits of S-100 protein in human neoplasm and normal tissues. Virchows Arch B 45: 385-396.

Weintraub H, Campbell GL, Holtzer H (1973). Differentiation in the presence of bromodeoxyuridine is "all-or-none". Nature New Biol 244: 140-142.

Weiss SW, Langloss JM, Enzinger FM (1983). Value of S-100 protein in the diagnosis of soft tissue tumors with particular reference to benign and malignant Schwann cell tumors. Lab Invest 49: 299-308.

Wrathall JR, Oliver C, Silagi S, Essner E (1973). Suppression of pigmentation in mouse melanoma cells by 5-bromodeoxyuridine: Effects on tyrosinase activity and melanosome formation. J Cell Biol 57: 406-423.

Advances in Neuroblastoma Research 2, pages 337–351
© 1988 Alan R. Liss, Inc.

NEURONAL DIFFERENTIATION OF HUMAN NEUROBLASTOMA CELLS BY A
NOVEL SYNTHETIC POLYPRENOIC ACID

Tohru Sugimoto, Tadashi Sawada, Takafumi Matsumura,
Yoshihiro Horii, Tamaki Hino, John T. Kemshead,
Yoshikazu Suzuki, Masaaki Okada and Osamu Tagaya

Children's Research Hospital (T. Su), Department of
Pediatrics (T. Sa., T. M., Y. H., T. H.), Kyoto
Prefectural University of Medicine, Kamikyo, Kyoto 602,
Eisai Co. Ltd. (Y. S., M. O., O. T.), Bunkyo, Tokyo
112, Japan; and Institute of Child Health (J. T. K.),
London WC1 1EH, England

INTRODUCTION

The prognosis of patients with advanced neuroblastoma
(NB) is still poor, despite recent progress in chemotherapy. Induction of differentiation of NB in vitro by
chemical and biological agents have been reported (Prasad
and Shinha, 1978: Sidell et al., 1981, 1984, 1985: Sugimoto
et al., 1985). In addition therapeutic trials for the
induction of differentiation in vivo by prostaglandin E2,
papaverine and nerve growth factor have been attempted
(Kumar et al., 1970: Helson et al., 1976: Imashuku et al.,
1982). These trials, however, have not proved successful.
Recently a new synthetic polyprenoic acid, E5166, which has
properties similar to retinoic acid (RA) and is less toxic
than synthetic RA, has been described (Muto and Moriwaki,
1984).

In this study two human NB cell lines, KP-N-RT(LN)
and SK-N-DZ, and 4 fresh NB samples taken from the bone
marrow of patients with advanced NB, were differentiated in
vitro with E5166. The results of these studies suggest a
possible therapeutic role for E5166 in vivo. Hopefully the
differentiation of induction of NB may lead to the total
eradication of residual NB cells after extensive
chemotherapy and surgery.

MATERIALS AND METHODS

Human NB Cell Lines and Fresh NB Tumor Cells. Two human NB cell lines, KP-N-RT(LN) and SK-N-DZ (Sugimoto et al., 1984, 1986) were cultured. Metastatic NB cells from bone marrow were aspirated from 4 patients with stage IV NB. These were partially purified by Ficoll-Hypaque discontinuous centrifugation. The presence of tumor cells in these preparations was determined by conventional morphological as well as membrane phenotypic study (Sugimoto et al., 1984, 1985, 1986).

Monoclonal Antibodies (MoAbs). For the determination of surface membrane antigen expressions, 8 MoAbs were used, and for the determination of neurofilament expression, a MoAb, recognized triplet proteins of neurofilament with MWs of 68, 160 and 200 kdal (Bio-Science, Emmenbrucke, Switzerland) were used (Table 1).

Table 1. MoAbs for Determination of Cell Surface Membrane Antigen and Neurofilament Expressions.

| MoAb | Reported specificity | References |
|------|---------------------|------------|
| Surface membrane antigens | | |
| UJ-13A | Neuroectodermal associated antigen | Sugimoto et al. 1984, 1985, 1986 |
| UJ-127-11 | Neuroectodermal associated antigen | " |
| anti-Thy-1 | Thy-1 antigen | " |
| PI 153/3 | Neural and common ALL antigen | " |
| KP-NAC 8 | "Neuroblastoma" associated antigen | Matsumura et al. 1987 |
| L 243 | HLA-DR | Watson et al. 1983 |
| B 7/21 | HLA-DP | Pesando et al. 1986, Watson et al. 1983 |
| Genox 3.53 | HLA-DQ | Pesando et al. 1986 |
| Neurofilament (68, 160, 200 kdal) | | Osborn et al. 1983 |

Indirect Immunofluorescence. For the determination of surface membrane antigen expressions, cells were stained with appropriately titrated MoAbs as previously reported (Sugimoto et al., 1984, 1985, 1986). At least 200 cells were examined and the percentage of stained cells was counted. For the determination of neurofilament expression, adherent NB cells on coverslips were fixed with 4% formaldehyde, washed and stained with appropriately titrated neurofilament MoAb.

Morphological Differentiation Induction of NB Cell

Lines  Induced by dbc AMP and E5166 in Liquid  Culture.  An
optimal  concentration of dibutyryl adenosine  3':5'-cyclic
monophosphoric  acid  (dbc AMP)  (P-L  Biochemical  Inc.,
Milwaukee,  WI), for the in vitro  induction  of  morphological differentiation, was determined as by adding this  to
cultures at concentrations ranging from 0.5 to $3.0 \times 10^{-3}$M.
E5166  (molecular weight: 302.46)(Eisai, Co.  Ltd.,  Tokyo,
Japan) (Muto and Moriwaki, 1984), whose chemical  structure
is  illustrated  in  Fig. 1  and  compared  with  all-trans
retinoic  acid  (RA), was dissolved in  dimethyl  sulfoxide
(the  final  solvent  dilution being 0.1%  by  volum).  An
optimal concentration of E5166, for the in vitro  induction
of morphological differentiation, was determined by  adding
this  to  cultures at concentrations ranging  from  0.8  to
$3.3 \times 10^{-5}$M.  Control cultures were established  containing
0.1%  solvent alone.  Medium in the cultures  was  replaced
every  4 days, and cells were maintained for a total of  12
days.

Natural Retinoid

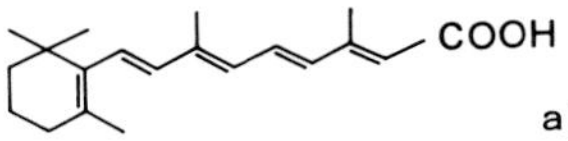

all-trans-retinoic acid
(mw. 300)

Fig. 1. Chemical
structure of all-
trans retinoic acid
and polyprenoic
acid (E5166).

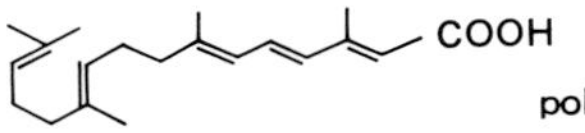

Synthetic Retinoid

polyprenoic acid (E5166)
(mw. 302)

Assessment of Morphological Differentiation in  Liqiud
Culture.  Cells  were  plated  into  60-mm  Petri  dishes
containing  10x10-mm-sized coverslips.  On day 0 of  either
dbc  AMP  or E5166 treatment, and days 2, 4, 6, 8 and  10,
coverslips were stained with May-Giemsa.  Two hundred cells
from  at least 3 different regions were examined  by  light
microscopy and scored as morphologically differentiated, if
they possessed one or more processes at least twice as long
as the soma diameter (Sugimoto et al., 1985).

Scanning  Electron  Microscopy.  Adherent NB cells  on

coverslips were fixed and observed with an Hitachi  S520-LB scanning electron microscope (Sugimoto et al., 1985, 1986).

Catecholamine,  Cyclic AMP and Neuron Specific Enolase Estimations.  Cells were harvested from culture flasks  and washed  with phosphate-buffered saline.  For  quantitative assays of catecholamines, harvested cells were homogenized, and  dopamine,  adrenaline  and  noradrenaline  levels determined by  high  performance  liquid  chromatography (1,10).  The  level  of cyclic AMP  in  treated  cells  was determined  (Honma  et al., 1977).  The  levels  of  neuron specific  enolase  in  treated  cells,  was  determined  by radioimmunoasssy  using  a  Pharmacia  kit  (Pahlman  et al.,1984).  Results are expressed as NSE levels proportional to total cellular protein levels.

N-myc Amplification  and Expression.  N-myc  amplifi- cation  was  demonstrated by Southern blot  analysis.  High molecular  weight  DNA  was cleaved  with  the  restriction enzyme EcoRI and fragments, separated by agarose (0.7%) gel electrophoresis, before transfer to nitrocellulose filters. N-myc  expression  was determined by  Northern  blotting. Total  RNA  was  extracted by  guanidine  thiocyanate  CsCl density  gradient  centrifugation,  electrophoresed  in  a formaldehyde  agarose (1.0%) gel and transfered  to  filter papers.  Filters were hybridized with $^{32}$P-labeled pNb-1 DNA in  both  Southern and Northern  blotting.  Filteres  were autoradiographed  and  quantitative  densitometry  was performed with a scanning laser densitometer.  Intensity of bands was expressed relative to that of the non-treated  NB cells  (Schwab et al., 1984: Thiele et al., 1985:  Amatruda et al., 1985).

Colony  Formation  in Soft Agar.  The ability of  NB cells  to  form colonies in soft agar in  the  presence  of E5166  was determined as previously reported (Sugimoto  et al.,1985,1986).  Ten thousand cells were suspended in 0.1ml of  0.3% Bacto-agar (Difco Lab., Detroit, MI)  in  complete medium  with  or without E5166, and seeded in 35  mm  Petri dishes  (Lux  Scientific,  Newbury  Park,  CA).  Colonies consisting of at least 20 cells were counted after 10  days with  an  inverted microscope,  and  the  colony  plating efficiency  calculated. The reduction in colony  formation in the presence of E5166 and % of neurite processes forming colonies  more than twice as long as  colony-soma  diameter was calculated.

RESULTS

Induction of Morphological Differentiation by dbc AMP and E5166 in Liquid Culture. The optimal concentration of dbc AMP that induced differentiation of KP-N-RT(LN)$_2$ cells after 10 days in culture was determined as $1.0 \times 10^{-3}$M. At this point 58 % of cells showed morphological differentiation. In contrast more cells showed a differentiated morphology treated with doses of E5166 ranging from 0.8 to $3.3 \times 10^{-5}$M. Ten days after beginning the experiment between 77 and 92% of the NB cells appeared morphologically differentiated. The dose of E5166 where optimal differentiation occcured was $1.7 \times 10^{-5}$M. In the absence of E5166 a maximum of 35% of cells appeared differentiated. With regard to SK-N-DZ cells, the maximum number of cells showing a differentiated morphology (45%) was obtained by treated cells with $1.7 \times 10^{-5}$M E5166 for day 10. Control cells treated in an identical manner apart from the omission of E5166 from the medium showed 7% of the cells with a differentiated phenotype. Only 26% of SK-N-DZ cells could be induced to differentiate upon incubation with $1.0 \times 10^{-3}$M dbc AMP. Scanning electron microscopy showed that dbc AMP and E5166 treated KP-N-RT(LN) cells formed long neurites after 4 days exposure to the agent inducing defferentiation. Following 12 day exposure to E5166, cells aggregated and formed cellular clusters that were connected with long bundled neuronal networks. In contrast, non-treated cells possessed spindle-shaped soma with short neurite processes (Fig. 2, A, B and C). After the treatment of E5166 for 12 days, SK-N-DZ cells also showed long neurite processes. However, the long bundled neural networks, observed in KP-N-RT(LN) cells, were not observed (Data not shown).

Catecholamine, Cyclic AMP and Neuron Specific Enolase Levels in Morphologically Differentiated Cells. KP-N-RT and SK-N-DZ cells were treated for 10 days with either dbc AMP or E5166. Dopamine levels in dbc AMP-treated KP-N-RT(LN) and SK-N-DZ cells and noradrenaline levels in dbc AMP-treated SK-N-DZ were significantly higher than in control non-treated cells($p < 0.05$). However no increse in dopamine, adrenaline and noradrenaline levels were noted in cells exposed to E5166 for 10 days. Similarly while cyclic AMP levels in dbc AMP-treated KP-N-RT(LN) and SK-N-DZ cells were significantly elevated as compared with non-treated cells ($p < 0.05$), exposure to E5166 did not increase cyclic

AMP levels over those of control cells. Neuron-specific
enolase activity did not increase significantly upon E5166
treatment (Table 2).

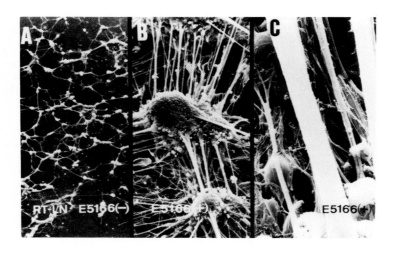

Fig. 2.A. Untreated KP-N-RT(LN) grown in culture for 12
days. NB cells with short neurite processes were seen. x250.
B and C. KP-N-RT(LN) cells after culture for 12 days in the
presence of $1.7 \times 10^{-5}$M E5166. NB cell clusters were connected
with long bundled neuronal networks. B: x250 and C: x2,000
respectively.

Table 2. Levels of Catecholamine, cyclic AMP and Neuron Specific Enolase
in dbc AMP and E5166 treated NB Cell Lines[a]

| Treatment | Catecholamine (ng/mg protein) | | | Cyclic AMP (pmol/mg protein) | Neuron Specific Enolase (ng/mg protein) |
|---|---|---|---|---|---|
| | Dopamine | Adrenaline | Noradrenaline | | |
| KP-N-RT(LN) | | | | | |
| Non-treated | $1.05 \pm 0.46^{b}$ | ND[c] | $0.10 \pm 0.03$ | $0.44 \pm 0.07^{b}$ | $319 \pm 22$ |
| dbc AMP | $2.35 \pm 0.56^{b}$ | ND | $0.74 \pm 0.24$ | $3.05 \pm 0.55^{b}$ | $322 \pm 53$ |
| E5166 | $0.68 \pm 0.20$ | ND | $0.08 \pm 0.01$ | $0.58 \pm 0.06$ | $389 \pm 30$ |
| SK-N-DZ | | | | | |
| Non-treated | $7.08 \pm 2.69^{b}$ | ND | $17.93 \pm 3.47^{b}$ | $1.16 \pm 0.32^{b}$ | $322 \pm 19$ |
| dbc AMP | $27.68 \pm 5.95^{b}$ | ND | $85.56 \pm 12.40^{b}$ | $2.39 \pm 0.29^{b}$ | $208 \pm 66$ |
| E5166 | $2.81 \pm 0.84$ | ND | $12.02 \pm 0.54$ | $1.03 \pm 0.44$ | $168 \pm 85$ |

[a] Mean ± S.E. from 5 to 6 separate experiments.
[b] Significant differences were observed ($P < 0.05$).
[c] ND = not detectable.

Altered Expression of Cell Surface Antigens by 10 Days Exposure to either dbc AMP or E5166. The percentage of cells binding a panel of MoAbs in the presence or absence of either dbc AMP or E5166 was compared by indirect immunofluorescence. Expression of the antigens recognized by UJ-13A, UJ-127-11, anti-Thy-1 and PI153 MoAbs did not change following incubation of cells for up to 10 days with either E5166 or dbc AMP. In contrast, both the overall expression and number of cells expressing the antigen recognized by MoAb KP-NAC8 increased after E5166 treatment as determined by indirect immunofluorescence ($p < 0.05$). Ninety and 89% of cells expressed this antigen after E5166 treatment as compared to 73 and 69% of control cells in KP-N-RT(LN) and SK-N-DZ cells respectively. HLA-DR, HLA-DP and HLA-DQ antigens, as defined by MoAbs L243, B7/21 and Genox3.53, were not detected on control NB cells, and the expression of these antigens was not induced by morphological differentiation with either dbc AMP or E5166 (Fig. 3).

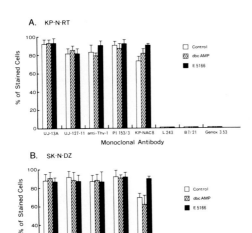

Fig. 3. Altered expression of cell surface antigens detected by indirect immunofluorescence. A. KP-N-RT(LN), B. SK-N-DZ, columns, mean % of stained cells in 4 separate experiment; bars, S.E.

Expression of Neurofilament in E5166-treated KP-N-RT (LN) Cells on Day 12. Three % of E5166 non-treated KP-N-RT (LN) cells with short neurite processes were stained with

neurofilament MoAb, whereas most of neuronal bundled
networks, induced by E5166 treatment for 12 days, were
strongly stained (Fig. 4).

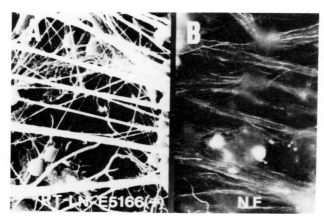

Fig. 4. Expression of neurofilament (68,160, 200 kdal) in E5166 treated KP-N-RT (LN) cells after 12 day exposure to E5166 as determined by indirect immunofluorescence. A. Scanning electron microscopy. x500. B. Neurofilament. x500.

N-myc Amplification and Expression by 10 Days
Exposure to E5166. A detectable decrease in the levels of
N-myc mRNA was observed by 24 hrs after treatment of
KP-N-RT cells with E5166. Five days after treatment, there
was a 75% decrease in the level of N-myc expression in
E5166-treated KP-N-RT cells, as compared with non-treated
cells. The expression remained at this level during the 10
day exposure to E5166. Similar decreases in N-myc
expression (75%) were observed in E5166-treated SK-N-DZ
cells after 10 days exposure. In contrast, no differences
in N-myc amplification was shown between E5166-treated and
non-treated KP-N-RT and SK-N-DZ cell lines (Fig. 5).

Dose-dependent Growth Inhibiton and Morphological
Differentiation in Soft Agar by E5166. The inhibitory
effect of E5166 on the ability of KP-N-RT(LN) cells to form
colonies in soft agar was determined. In control dishes
not-exposed to E5166, 179±12 (mean±SE in triplicate
cultures) colonies were formed, with a colony-plating
efficiency estimated to be 1.7%. A 76% of reduction in
colony numbers as compared to controls (not exposed to
E5166) was found on exposure of cells to $6.7 \times 10^{-5}$M E5166.
This reduction was dependent on the concentration of E5166
with 50% inhibition occuring at $2.0 \times 10^{-5}$M (Fig. 6). In

addition, colonies that developed in the presence of E5166 were smaller than non-treated cells and showed morphological differentiation by the criteria of expressing long bundled neurite processes. Under similar conditions control culture of SK-N-DZ cells gave 181±15 colonies with a colony-plating efficiency of 1.8%. As with KP-N-RT(LN) cells a dose-dependent growth inhibition was observed following incubation of cells with E5166. Fifty % growth inhibition occured at $0.67 \times 10^{-5}$M E5166 (Fig. 6). However under these conditons SK-N-DZ colonies were not morphologically differentiated. With regard to fresh bone marrow NB samples, a similar dose-dependent growth inhibition was observed (Fig. 6), and in 2 of 4 fresh tumor samples exposure to $1.7 \times 10^{-5}$M E5166 caused an increase in the number of colonies showing neurite formation. The percentage of colonies expressing neurites increased dose-dependently as compared to non-treated colonies (29.9 to 73.1% in KY and 24.6 to 67.5% in MO patient respectively) (data not shown) (Fig. 7). In contrast, while the number of colonies was inhibited in a dose dependent fashion in the other 2 fresh tumor samples of ST and HN patients, NB cells were not morphologically differentiated.

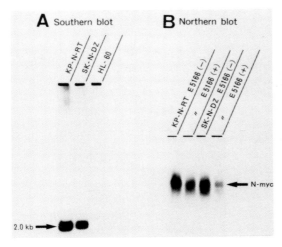

Fig. 5. N-myc amplification (A) and expression (B) in KP-N-RT(LN) and SK-N-DZ cell lines after 7 day treatment of E5166.

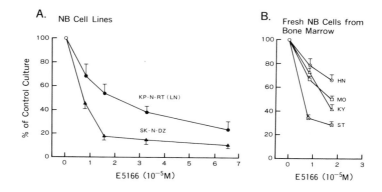

Fig. 6. Dose response curves of E5166-induced inhibition of colony formation in agar. A. KP-N-RT(LN) and SK-N-DZ cell lines. Colony-plating efficiency in KP-N-RT(LN) and SK-N-DZ cell lines were 1.7 and 1.8% respectively. B. Fresh NB cells aspirated from bone marrow of 4 patients. The % of control culture is expressed by the mean of triplicated cultures: bars. S.E.

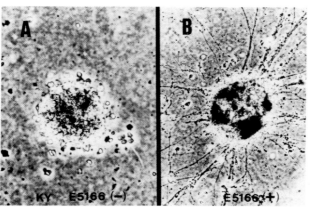

Fig. 7. Colony formation of fresh NB tumor cells aspirated from bone marrow of KY patient in agar. A. untreated colony. x200. B. Neurite process forming differentiated colony in the presence of E5166. x200.

DISCUSSION

A new synthetic polyprenoic acid, E5166, was originally discovered by Muto et al. E5166 is a derivatives of RA
that has a high binding affinity to cellular retinoic
acid-binding protein (CRABP) (Muto and Moriwaki,1984).

In the present study, two human NB cell lines, KP-N-RT
(LN) and SK-N-DZ established from one year two month and
one year old infants with stage IV NB respectively, were
induced to differentiate in liquid culture. Following 4
day exposure of KP-N-RT(LN) to E5166, the percentage of
differentiated cells gradually increased. The highest
percentage of differentiated cells (92%) was found after 10
days of exposure to $1.7 \times 10^{-5}$M E5166. A similar effect was
observed on SK-N-DZ cells (observation made on day 10).
Scanning electron microscopy showed that E5166-treated
KP-N-RT(LN) cells aggregated, forming cellular clusters
that were connected with long bundled neurite processes;
all indications of a mature "differentiated" state (Fig.2).
With regard to SK-N-DZ, E5166 induced long neurite
processes, but long bundled neural fibers, observed in
KP-N-RT(LN) cells, were not observed (Data not shown).
Transmission electron microscopy indicated the development
of Golgi apparatus, mitochondria and neural tubules,
analogous to those found in differentiated cells. However
no significant increase in dense core granules (catecholamine granules) was observed in E5166-treated cells (Data
not shown). Quantitative assays of catecholamine including
dopamine, adrenaline and noradrenaline indicated these were
not elevated in the E5166-induced KP-N-RT(LN) and SK-N-DZ
cells. However dopamine and/or noradrenaline were
significantly elevated in both SK-N-DZ and KP-N-RT(LN)
cells differentiated with dbc AMP. As no elevation of
cyclic AMP was found in either cell line treated with
E5166, this suggests the mechanism of E5166 differentiation
is not cyclic AMP dependent. Quantitative assays for
neuron specific enolase in E5166-treated KP-N-RT(LN) and
SK-N-DZ cells, showed no increase as compared with control
cells. This suggests the level of this enzyme is not be
linked to the E5166 induced differentiation of NB(Table 2).

Under the optimal condition for morphological differentiation by either dbc AMP or E5166, expressions of the
antigens defined by UJ-13A, UJ-127-11, anti-Thy-1 and
PI153/3 MoAbs were not altered by indirect membrane

immunofluorescence. In contrast, both indirect immunofluorescence and flow cytometry showed that the antigen
recognized by MoAb KP-NAC8 was significantly increased upon
treatment of KP-N-RT(LN) and SK-N-DZ with E5166. The
increased expression of the KP-NAC8 antigen may relate to
the differentiation state of NB cells, since this is
present on neoplastic neuroblast but not normal fetal
neuroblast (Matsumura et al., 1987) (Fig. 3). Neurofilament is an intermediate filament of neurons, composing
of triplet proteins of 68, 160, 200 kdal. Immature neurons
do not express these proteins, differentiated neurons
express 68 and 160 kdal proteins, and well-differentiated
neuron express all these proteins (Shaw and Weber, 1982).
The neurofilament used in this study, recognized all these
proteins, and reacted with E5166- treated KP-N-RT cells.
Therefore neuronal differentiation of this cell line by
E5166 was demonstrated (Fig. 4). The formation of NB
colonies in soft agar was inhibited by increasing
concentration of E5166 using KP-N-RT(LN) and SK-N-DZ cell
lines and 4 samples of fresh NB cells aspirated from bone
marrow (Fig. 6). Following treatment with E5166, neurite
cells with processes forming differentiated colonies were
observed in the KP-N-RT(LN) cell line and in 2 of 4 fresh
NB bone marow samples (Fig. 6 and 7).

Morphological differentiation of NB by RA (all-trans
retinoic acid) was first reported by Sidell (Sidell: 1981).
Subsequent studies demonstrated biochemical differentiation, based on the increased acetylcholinesterase
activity, and electrophysiological differentiation (Sidell
et al., 1984, 1985).

The mechanism of RA-induced differentiation of NB, is
thought to be by direct interaction with nuclear DNA via
binding to CRABP. This has been suggested as the
concentration of CRABP in the most RA responsive NB cell
line (LA-N-5) is approximately twice that in the least
responsive NB cell line (CHP 100) (Sidell et al., 1984).

Recently two independent reports, have demonstrated
decreased levels of the N-myc oncogene mRNA following
RA-induced differentiation of NB in vitro. This suggests
the regulation of N-myc mRNA could occur through the direct
action of RA, leading to a decrease in cellular proliferation and neural maturation (Thiele et al., 1985:
Amastruda et al., 1985). E5166 has a similar effect on

KP-N-RT(LN) cells which shows decreased expression of N-myc with no change in N-myc amplification (Fig. 5) (Horii et al., 1987). Further studies need to be completed to clarify the mechanism by which E5166 induces the differentiation of NB.

E5166 is one of the most potent reagents to induce morphological differentiation in various NB cell lines _in vitro_. It has equivalent differentiation activity to similar concentration of all-trans RA ($10^{-5}$M) (Matsumura _et al_ submitted), can be administerd to patients orally, and is 5 to 10 times less toxic than all-trans RA (Muto and Moriwaki, 1984). A single oral administration of 40 mg/kg body weight of E5166 to rats can achieve a level of more than $1.7 \times 10^{-5}$M E5166 (the level used for _in vitro_ differentiation) in blood, adrenal gland and most body tissues for more than 48 hrs. As much as 200 mg/kg body weight of E5166 can be administered orally to rats over a relatively long period of time (Suzuki _et al_: Unpublished observation). The clinical usefulness of E5166 in NB is suggested by the morphological differentiation and the inhibition of colony formations in soft agar in both KP-N-RT(LN) and SK-N-DZ cell lines and 4 fresh NB samples with induction of differentiation in two. The drug may be useful in advanced NB patients to eradicate residual tumor cells after surgery and chemotherapy. The effect of oral administration of E5166 on tumor growth in athymic mice bearing NB is currently underway to determine _in vivo_ efficiency.

ACKNOWLEGMENTS

Thanks are due to Dr. L. Helson for providing SK-N-DZ cell line and to Dr. H. Morioka for examining scanning electron microscopy. This work was supported in part by grants for cancer research from the Ministry of Health and Welfare of Japan.

REFERENCES

Amatruda III TT, Sidell N, Ranyard J, Koeffler HP (1985). Retinoic acid treatment of human neuroblastoma cells is associated with decreased N-myc expression. Biochem Biophys Res Commun 126: 1189-1195.

Helson L, Helson C, Peterson RF, Das SK (1976).
A rationale for the treatment of metastatic neuroblastoma. J Natl Cancer Inst 57: 727-729.

Honma M, Satoh T, Takezawa J, Ui M (1977). An ultra-
sensitive method for the simultaneous determinarion
of cyclic AMP and cyclic GMP in small volume samples
from blood and tissue. Biochem Med 18: 257-273.

Horii Y, Sugimoto T, Matsumura T, Hino T, Sawada T,
Hatanaka M (1987). Decreased N-myc expression during
morphological differentiation of human neuroblarom
cells. Igaku-no-Ayumi (in Japanese) 140: 531-532.

Imashuku S, Sugano T, Fujiwara K, Todo S, Ogita S, Goto Y
(1982). Intra-aortic prostaglandin $E_1$ infusion in
maturation of neuroblastoma. Experimentia 38: 932-933.

Kumar S, Steward JK, Waghe M, Pearson D, Edwards DC,
Fenton EL, Griffith AH (1970). The administration of
the nerve growth factor to children with widespread
neuroblastoma. J Pediatr Sugr 5: 18-22.

Matsumura M, Sugimoto T, Sawada T, Amagai T, Negoro S,
Kemshead JT (1987). A cell surface membrane antigen
present on neuroblastoma cells but not fetal neuroblasts
recognized by a monoclonal antibody (KP-NAC8).
Cancer Res In press.

Muto Y, Moriwaki H (1984). Antitumor activity of vitamin
A and its derivatives. J Natl Cancer Inst 73: 1389-1393.

Osborn M, Weber K (1983). Biology of disease, tumor
diagnosis by intermediate filament typing: a novel tool
for surgical pathology. Lab Invest 48: 372-394.

Pahlman S, Esscher T, Bergvall R, Odelstad L (1984).
Purification and characterization of human neuron-specific
enolase: radioimmunoassay development. Tumour Biol
5: 127-139.

Pesando JM, Graf L (1986). Differential expression of
HLA-DR, -DQ, and -DP antigens on malignant B cells.
J Immunol 136: 4311-4318.

Prasad KN, Shinha PK (1978). Regulation of differentiated
functions and malignancy in neuroblastoma cells in
culture. In: GF Saunders (ed.): Cell Differentiation
and Neoplasia, New York: Raven Press, pp111-141.

Schwab M, Ellison J, Busch M, Rosenau W, Varmus HE,
Bishop JM (1984). Enhanced expression of the human
gene N-myc consequent to amplification of DNA may
contribute to malignant progression of neuroblastoma.
Proc Natl Acad Sci USA 81: 4940-4944.

Shaw G, Weber K (1982). Differential expression of neurofilament triplet proteins in brain development. Nature

(Lond.) 298: 277-279.

Sidell N (1981). Retinoic acid-induced growth inhibition and morphologic differentiation of human neuroblastoma cells in vitro. J Natl Cancer Inst 68: 589-596.

Sidell N, Lucas CA, Kreutzberg GW (1984). Regulation of acetylcholinesterase activity by retinoic acid in a human neuroblastoma cell line. Exp Cell Res 155: 305-309.

Sidell N, Horn R (1985). Properties of human neuroblastoma cells following induction by retinoic acid. In: A Evans, GJ D'Angio, RC Seeger (eds.): Advances in Neuroblastoma Research, New York: Alan R Liss Inc. pp39-53.

Sugimoto T, Tatsumi E, Kemshead JT, Helson L, Green AA, Minowada, J (1984). Determination of cell surface membrane antigens common to both human neuroblastoma and leukemia-lymphoma cell lines by a panel of 38 monoclonal antibodies. J Natl Cancer Inst 73: 51-57.

Sugimoto T, Sawada T, Negoro S, Kidowaki T, Morioka H, Matsumura T, Kemshead JT, Seeger RC (1985). Altered expression of cell surface membrane antigens in a common acute lymphoblastic leukemia-associated antigen-expressing neuroblastoma cell line (SJ-N-CG) with morphological differentiation. Cancer Res 45: 358-364.

Sugimoto T, Sawada T, Matsumura T, Kemshead JT, Ishii T, Horii Y, Morioka H, Morita M, Reynolds CP (1986). Identical expression of cell surface membrane antigens on two parent and eighteen cloned cell lines derived from two different neuroblastoma metastases of the same patient. Cancer Res 46: 4765-4769.

Thiele CJ, Reynolds CP, Israel MA (1985). Decreased expression of N-myc precedes retinoic acid-induced morphological differentiation of human neuroblastoma. Nature (Lond.) 313: 404-406.

Watson AJ, DeMars R, Trowbridge IS, Bach FH (1983). Detection of a novel human class II antigen. Nature (Lond.) 304: 358-359.

Advances in Neuroblastoma Research 2, pages 353–358
© 1988 Alan R. Liss, Inc.

REMOVAL OF POLYPEPTIDES FROM HUMAN NEUROBLASTOMA ANTIGEN
DOES NOT ALTER RECOGNITION BY MONOCLONAL ANTIBODY PI 153/3

Jennifer P. Boyd and Mary Catherine Glick

Department of Pediatrics, University of Pennsylvania Medical School, Philadelphia, PA   19104

The monoclonal antibody, PI 153/3, is an IgM
antibody developed against whole human neuroblastoma
cells in mice by Kennett and Gilbert (1979). This antibody
has marked specificity for neuroblastoma tumors and cell
lines as well as retinoblastoma and glioblastoma (Kennett
and Gilbert, 1979). While it has also been shown to recognize certain leukemia cell lines (Greaves et al, 1980), it
has not been detected on any normal human adult or fetal
tissue other than fetal brain (Kennett and Gilbert, 1979).
Of clinical relevance, the PI 153/3 antibody has been used
to screen for neuroblastoma cells in the bone marrow
(Evans et al, 1985).

Momoi et al, (1980) isolated the antigen from the
human neuroblastoma cell line, IMR-32, and showed that the
epitope resided with the glycopeptide after exhaustive
digestion with Pronase. Amino acids remain attached to the
glycopeptides after Pronase treatment, therefore these
studies were extended to determine if the antigen from
human neuroblastoma cells was still recognized by the
antibody after either chemical (Samor et al, 1986) or
enzymatic (Plummer et al, 1984) removal of the
polypeptides.

An immunoaffinity column of PI 153/3 bound to anti-
IgM-Sepharose was used to directly quantitate the presence
of antigen. Binding to and elution from the antibody
column was by differential temperature of the buffer
(Lundblad et al, 1984). Glycopeptide fractions containing
the antigen were obtained by controlled trypsinization of

human neuroblastoma cells, CHP-134, which were labeled
metabolically with D-[$^3$H]glucosamine (Fig.1).

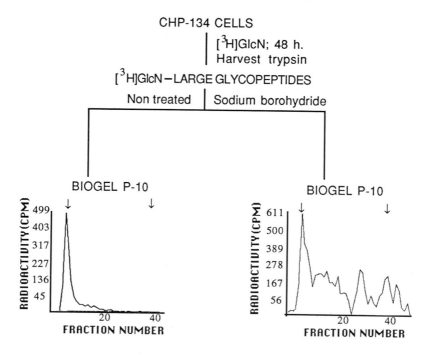

Figure 1. Chemical removal of polypeptides from PI 153/3
antigen. The large $^3$H-glycopeptides were treated or not
treated with 1 M NaBH$_4$, 0.1 M NaOH for 18 h at 37°C. The
column was calibrated with Blue Dextran 2000 and cobala-
mine, represented by the arrows left to right.

Chemical removal of polypeptides from the PI 153/3
antigen did not alter binding of the antigen to the
antibody column. (Table 1) To do these experiments, large
$^3$H-glycopeptides, $M_r > 10,000$ were treated with mild
alkaline sodium borohydride to remove the polypeptides.
Alkaline borohydride treatment removes both O-linked and
N-linked oligosaccharides from their respective polypeptides (Samor et al, 1986). The removal of the polypeptides
was verified by a reduction in size on Biogel P-10
(Fig.1). The large glycopeptides moved from the void
volume of Biogel P-10 to positions of smaller size

after NaBH$_4$ treatment. Moreover, the small fragments retained the antigenic activity.

Endoglycanase F (PNG-ase F) which cleaves between the asparagine and the core N-acetylglucosamine (Plummer et al, 1984) was also used to remove the polypeptides. After PNG-ase treatment of the large $^3$H-glycopeptides, binding to the antibody column was not impaired (Table 1) and the large glycopeptides moved to positions of smaller size on Biogel P-10.

TABLE 1. Binding to Antibody Column after Removal of Polypeptides from PI 153/3 Antigen

| $^3$H-GLYCOPEPTIDES FROM CHP-134 CELLS[c] | IMMUNOAFFINITY COLUMN | | |
|---|---|---|---|
| | Untreated | Sodium borohydride[a] | PNGase F[b] |
| | radioactivity bound[d] (cpm) | | |
| Large | 1120 | 1440 | 1248 |
| Small[e] | | | |
| Pea lectin bound[f] | 245 | 0 | |
| Pea lectin unbound | 0 | 294 | |

a. 1 M NaBH$_4$ , 0.1 M NaOH, 18 h, 37°C. See Fig. 1.
b. 0.52 units, 18 h, 25°C.
c. Obtained by controlled trypsinization of CHP-134 cells. See Fig. 1.
d. Radioactivity expressed per 10$^8$ cells.
e. Obtained by exhaustive Pronase digestion of large $^3$H-glycopeptides followed by partial purification.
f. Eluted with 0.2 M α-methyl mannoside; pea lectin requires the presence of Asn for binding.

Plant lectins are known to bind to specific oligosaccharide sequences (Lis and Sharon, 1986). Two of these lectins, lentil and pea, have similiar requirements for binding which include the presence of fucose linked α1→6 to the core N-acetylglucosamine (Kornfeld et al, 1981). However, pea lectin requires in addition the presence of asparagine on the core *N*-acetylglucosamine (Yamamoto et al, 1981). The antigen was shown to bind to both immobilized pea and lentil lectins. Therefore after removal of all the amino acids including Asn, the antigen should no longer bind to pea lectin.

To do these experiments, small $^3$H-glycopeptides were obtained by exhaustive Pronase digestion of the large $^3$H-glycopeptides. After desalting, the small $^3$H-glycopeptides were subjected to sequential Con A and lentil lectin-Sepharose chromatography (Cummings and Kornfeld, 1982). The $^3$H-glycopeptides which were unbound to Con A-Sepharose but bound to lentil-Sepharose also bound to pea agarose. After treatment with NaBH$_4$ binding to pea agarose was abolished. Nevertheless, 100% of the [$^3$H]GlcN-labeled antigen was recovered in this unbound fraction, as demonstrated by binding to the immunoaffinity column (Table 1). None of the unbound fraction of the untreated material bound to the antibody column (Table 1).

It is concluded that the epitope resides with the oligosaccharides since amino acids were not required for binding of the [$^3$H]GlcN-labeled antigen to the PI 153/3 immunoaffinity column. The exact epitope presents an intriguing problem because of its specific association with human neuroblastoma cells. Neuroblastoma glycoproteins have several unique features and one of these could be the PI 153/3 determinant. Among these unusual properties is the presence of a large amount of fucosyl residues linked α1→3 to *N*-acetylglucosamine on the oligosaccharide antennae (Santer and Glick, 1984). However, while it is a potential candidate for the epitope, the cell distribution (summarized in Foster and Glick, this volume) does not correlate completely with the antibody specificity (Kennett and Gilbert, 1979). In addition, fractionation of the antigen (unpublished observations) and distribution of the glycopeptides containing these fucosyl residues (Santer and Glick, 1984) do not completely correlate, making it unlikely that these unusual fucosyl residues, per se, are the epitope. Another unusual feature of human neuroblastoma cells is the presence of polysialic acid, recently described by Livingston et al (1987) in CHP-134 cells. Polysialic acid is a polymer of repeating α2→8 sialic acid and is associated with the neural cell adhesion molecule, N-CAM, during the migration of the neural cells (Cunningham et al, 1987).

The unusual features of neuroblastoma glycoproteins could result in unusual conformational folding of the oligosaccharides thus giving yet a third possibility for antigenic specificity. Since the PI 153/3 antibody recognizes a determinant which has been shown to reside with oligosaccharides, some of which are triantennary, it is possible that the presence of two antenna with particular folding are required for recognition, enhancing the interaction with the antibody binding site. A similar phenomenon was shown for the recognition of certain complex type oligosaccharides by the lectin, Concanavalin A (Bhattacharyya et al, 1987). Any of these possibilities would account for the restricted distribution of the PI 153/3 antigen and are being addressed.

Regardless of the exact epitope, it is clear from the experiments presented here that one of the highly specific properties of human neuroblastoma results from a post-translational modification of the glycoproteins expressed at the cell surface.

Supported by NIH PO1 CA 14489 and RO1 CA 37853.

REFERENCES

Bhattacharyya L, Haraldsson M, Brewer CF (1987). Concanavalin A interactions with asparagine-linked glycopeptides. *J Biol Chem* **262**: 1294-1299.
Cummings R, Kornfeld S (1982). Fractionation of asparagine-linked oligosaccharides by serial lectin-agarose affinity chromatography. *J Biol Chem* **257**: 11235-11240.
Cunningham BA, Hemperly JJ, Murray BA, Prediger EA, Brackenbury R, Edelman GM (1987). Neural cell adhesion molecule: Structure, immunoglobulin-like domains, cell surface modulation, and alternative RNA splicing. *Science* **236**: 799-806.
Evans AE, Griffin GC, Tartaglione M, Kennett RH (1985). A method of detecting neuroblastoma in human bone marrow by means of two monoclonal antibodies PI 153/3 and KE2. *Hybridoma* **4**: 289-293.

Greaves MF, Verbi W, Kemshead J, Kennett RH (1980).
A monoclonal antibody identifying a cell surface antigen
shared by common acute lymphoblastic leukemias and B
lineage cells. *Blood* **56:** 1141-1143.

Kennett RH, Gilbert F (1979). Hybrid myelomas producing
antibodies against a human neuroblastoma antigen present
on fetal brain. *Science* **203:** 1120-1121.

Kornfeld K, Reitman ML, Kornfeld R (1981). The carbohydrate
binding specificity of pea and lentil lectins.
*J Biol Chem* **256:** 6633-6640.

Lis H, Sharon N (1986). Lectins as molecules and as tools.
*Ann Rev Biochem* **55:** 35-67.

Livingston BD, Jacobs J, Shaw GW, Glick MC, Troy FA (1987).
Polysialic acid in human neuroblastoma cells.
*Fed Proc* **46:** 2151.

Lundblad A, Schroer K, Zopf D (1984). Affinity purification
of a glucose-containing oligosaccharide using a
monoclonal antibody. *J Immunol Methods* **68:** 227-234.

Momoi M, Kennett RH, Glick MC (1980). A membrane
glycoprotein from human neuroblastoma cells isolated
with the use of a monoclonal antibody. *J Biol Chem* **255:**
11914-11921.

Plummer TH, Jr., Elder JH, Alexander S, Phelan AW,
Tarentino AL (1984). Demonstration of peptide:
*N*-glycosidase F activity in Endo-ß-*N*-acetyl-
glucosaminidase F preparations. *J Biol Chem* **259:**
10700-10704.

Samor B, Michalski J-C, Debray H, Mazurier C, Goudemand M,
Van Halbeek H, Vliegenthart JFG, Montreuil J (1986).
Primary structure of a new tetraantennary glycan of the
*N*-acetyllactosaminic type isolated from human factor
VIII/von Willebrand factor. *Eur J Biochem* **158:**
295-298.

Yamamoto K, Tsuko T, Matsumoto I, Osawa T (1981).
Requirement of the core structure of a complex-type
glycopeptide for the binding to immobilized lentil and
pea lectins. *Biochemistry* **20:** 5894-5899.

Advances in Neuroblastoma Research 2, pages 359–375
© 1988 Alan R. Liss, Inc.

DISCUSSION

Chairmen:     J.L. Biedler and C.P. Reynolds

Discussants:  J.L. Biedler, R.A. Ross
              C.P. Reynolds, B.L. Mirkin
              K. Tsunamoto, T. Sugimoti
              J.P. Boyd

**Lipinski:** Considering the different subtypes of cells derived from the neuroblastoma cell lines, have you looked at the synthesis of NGF or EGF receptors? Also, do you think there is any type of autocrine pathway in these cells and have you looked at the presence of keratin in these different subtypes?

**Biedler:** Wolfgang Rettig has a monoclonal antibody to the NGF receptor and has found cross-reactivity with N-type cells but little or none with S-type cells. So there is an inverse correlation between NGF receptor and EGF receptor. We have not looked at either cell type for synthesis of EGF. We would like to look at the synthesis of EGF, TGF alpha, and responsiveness of cells to EGF. We have not looked at the keratins.

**Seeger:** To Dr. Ross and Dr. Biedler. These are elegant studies but I was not sure of the <u>rate</u> of bidirectional conversion. In other words, do those S-cells go back to N-cells and, if so, what is the frequency if you clone them? If the S-cell is truly a model for the ganglioneuroma, which is a benign tumor that stays benign, then I would have thought that the S-cell *in-vitro* would not have converted back to an N-cell.

**Biedler:** We have only experimentally assessed rate of conversion and demonstrated to our satisfaction that conversion is bidirectional for the SK-N-SH line. The data were published several years ago. I cannot give you a precise answer for rate. We don't believe that the S-cell is a model for ganglioneuroma but rather that the N to S cell conversion that we see *in vitro* may somehow be involved in the maturation phenomenon seen in vivo.

Seeger: If you carry one of these clones for six months, will it remain an S-cell?

Biedler: No. It is very difficult to clone these lines and maintain a clone in a homogeneous state. That is why SY5Y was subcloned three times in order to keep it as homogeneous as possible. The two morphological types are so distinct that you can see one or the other appearing in culture. The LA-N-1 clones are probably the most stable of all, but not entirely so. The proof of bidirectional interconversion was based on karyotype analysis. We showed the S-type cells derived from an N-type clone picked up a new marker chromosome. When we manipulated it in cell-culture and it went back to an N-type, it still contained that marker chromosome. The fact that, in the SK-N-SH line, the two cell-types are maintained in some sort of balance in culture suggests either that one cell type produces something that the other cell-type needs and/or that new S-type cells are generated at a constant rate during the course of cultivation.

Seeger: Have you looked at S-100? In the abstracts, Dr. Tsunamoto has S-100 evaluations. Dr. Shimada has published that the Schwann-type element of neuroblastomas are S-100 positive.

Biedler: No. We should look at that. Thank you.

Littauer: I am interested in agents that will induce transdifferentiation. For example, does demethylation affect the rate and does NGF have an effect?

Biedler: We have tried many of the agents "on the shelf". I cannot say we have looked systematically or persistently. But we have tried 5-azacytidine, BrdU, retinoic acid, dibutyrl cAMP, NGF, and EGF. That would be the prize, to experimentally make these cells convert, but we have not yet been successful in doing this.

Mirkin: Most of the compounds which seem to be extremely effective are those which are inhibitors of methylation particularly homocystine hydrolase. We found that the compounds which are the most effective are the group that we have synthesized which are adenosine anologs in which the ribose is oxidized and cleared through a periodate oxidation to a very reactive aldehye. These seem to be the most effective compounds we have encountered in doing two things: suppressing murine neuroblastoma growth in tissue culture and in the *in situ* situation. But more significantly they modify the expression in tissue culture so that there is a very sharp and profound correlation between inhibition of hydrolase activity and subsequent intracellular methylation in the neurite extensions. If this correlates with the conversion between S- and N-types, it would be very interesting because that is a potential linkage between morphological expression and biochemical intracellular events.

Littauer: Well, I was just trying to see whether we can understand the nature of this interconversion. Since the chromosome pictures are rather similar, one should look at the biochemical basis of the interconversion.

Biedler: Of course that is what we have tried to do. We have not been able to experimentally increase rate of conversion so we have been trying to understand what the consequences are and by looking at these various parameters to see whether they travel together and to try to imagine whether there are one or more controlling elements involved. Bob Ross and I would like to emphasize that these events seem to be a general phenomenon for neuroblastoma cells in culture and that is why we are willing to speculate that the N and S interconversion *in vitro* may model events occurring *in vivo*. We hope you will continue to communication your beliefs or disbeliefs to us that this may indeed occur *in vivo*.

Littauer: Yes. Am I correct in that this is not the case in the murine neuroblastoma cell lines.

Biedler: At the risk of offending the gentleman on my right (Dr. Mirkin) I will give you my view of murine neuroblstoma.

Evans: Don't tell him!

Biedler: I've done it before.

Kemshead: Could I ask about your tumor growth lag in nude mice. I think we would find the lag phase between injection and growth is extremely variable. Could you comment on the denominator (the number of animals you have in each of those groups) and the reproducibility of the finding between experiments and also whether you are passaging cell-lines actually as xenograft blocks from animal to animal.

Reynolds: In each of these cases we are looking at a minimum of three mice and in many experiments four or five mice. The standard errors were shown in the slides. There is a high degree of statistical significance between PNET's and the amplified or non-amplified neuroblastoma lines. The experiments are carried out always using the lowest passage of the cell-lines we could find. Most were below passage 20 and many below passage 12. In all data reported here we injected cell lines directly from culture. We have also done a number of serial animal passages (not reported in the data presented here) and that does produce the variability you were talking about. We chose to put in a large number of cells ($100 \times 10^6$ cells) - because we found we get a tumor with this dose in almost every single animal.

We wanted to ensure a high take rate, to minimize the number of mice needed for these experiments.

**Melera:** Dr. Reynolds - you demonstrated a correlation between N-*myc* copy number and tumor growth rate. Is that followed-up with the expression of those genes? Is the expression of N-*myc* inversely correlated as well?

**Reynolds:** We have not yet looked at expression. I think it is important to note that there is not really a simple correlation between N-*myc* copy number and growth rate. There is clearly a much more rapid growth of PNET cell-lines (which do not amplify N-*myc*, express low amounts of N-*myc*, and overexpress c-myc (Thiele et al., J Clin Invest 80:804 1987). Perhaps the high c-myc expression of the PNET lines accounts for their rapid growth. Actually, there <u>is</u> a correlation between N-*myc* copy number and growth rate in <u>neuroblastoma</u> as 2 of 3 N-*myc* non-amplified neuroblastoma lines show very long lag times compared to N-*myc* amplified lines. However, there is no correlation between copy number and growth amongst N-*myc* amplified cell lines.

**Melera:** You mean there is no positive correlation between amplified copy number and growth rate?

**Reynolds:** Right. Once you amplify, the relationship between growth rate and copy number is highly variable.

**Lipinski:** Concerning the growth rate of the different tumors, I wonder if there wouldn't be a better correlation between growth rate -- or an inverse correlation between growth rate and expression of HLA Class I antigen. It is well known that there is a high level of NK activity in nude mice and it is also well-known that N-*myc* activity has something to do with expression of Class I antigen at the level of target cells.

Reynolds: We concerned ourselves with that. I'm not sure how to explain it but there is a very rapid growth rate for anything that did express HLA Class I antigens compared to those that didn't. However, there was overlap in that there were some that expressed HLA antigens and had growth rates that were comparable to those that didn't. So, our feeling was that there was no role for the HLA antigens in terms of growth rate -- for instance in presenting an immunological target to the mouse.

Lampson: We also don't see any correlation between the Class I expression and the aggressive growth of the neuroblastoma. There is no Class I on the Stage IV and no Class I on the Stage IV-S or the Stage I. Also we have compared the growth of CHP-100 in nudes and beige nude mice and the beige nude mouse is lacking NK activity as well as T-cell activity. There is no difference between a beige nude and a nude, so we have no evidence that NK activity is important here.

Israel: Dr. Biedler, you said that under the conditions of the experiment the S-type cells did not make tumors. Does that mean that there are some conditions under which it can be made to make tumors?

Biedler: We did not generally go higher than 10 million cells. In some experiments we used 50 million cells -- but that is quite an endeavor for the flat S-type. We are not saying that if you put in 100 million cells that they wouldn't form tumors. However, we did not get tumors.

Israel: You indictated with the intermediate types that you did get some tumors. Since S doesn't seem to make tumors and N does make tumors. I was wondering about the morphology of the tumor cell that came out of the I-type cells.

Biedler: That is a good idea. We did not

look at that -- the "intermediate" classification is not a perfect one. It is based on morphology and the biochemical properties of I-type cells differ from one clone to the next. We don't know the significance of the intermediate cell. Within one individual clone there can be several varieties of so-called intermediate cells. However, we should look at the histology of the tumor.

Melera: I would just like to remind everyone of the relation with N-*myc*. Dr. Michitsch's data from yesterday indicated that N-*myc* expression levels can modulate over an order of magnitude in those cells over time, and there are still no tumors being formed. So the involvement of N-*myc* with tumorigenicity in that cell-line is questionable.

D'Angio: Two very provocative observations. I can only comment and speculate that perhaps your observations may explain the very late relapses you sometimes see in children who have either a good treatment result or even a spontaneous resolution. Several years later, when one sees a regrowth in the original site, one wonders whether what you see in the laboratory isn't happening *in vivo*.

Biedler: Thank you Dan, I'd like to comment that we in the laboratory certainly welcome some insight that you clinicians might have to be able to look at the situation *in vivo* in terms of these observations.

Cheung: Following the question by Dr. Lipinski on the establishment of tumor in nude mice. One part is the expression of HLA antigen and the other is the sensitivity of these cell lines to NK activity. Dr. Lampson pointed out that CHP-100, which is a neuroepithelioma cell line, grows well, irrespective of whether it is in NK deficient or NK intact mice. My other question is if you take a neuroblastoma and try that in an NK deficient versus an NK intact mouse, whether you would see any difference.

What you see might be explained by the fact that the neuroepithelioma cell lines are more resistant to endogenous NK activity. That's why they grow faster versus the neuroblastoma which grows a little slower.

Reynolds: We haven't done that experiment. Our feelings are that this phenomenon is due to endogenous growth rate. The growth *in vitro* parallels what we see in the mouse and there is no NK activity to affect them in the tissue culture.

Foster: One question to all of you who have been tissue-culturing and that is: have you tried growing these cells within three-dimensional cultures, for example, collagen gels, rather than in monolayer? If you have, do you then see an organization developing such as one would find within a normal tumor where these cells could arrange three-dimensional contacts and microenvironments between each other?

Ross: I can only comment that I've grown N- and S- cells on collagen and their behavior is markedly different. On plastic, N-type cells settle-down somewhat. Even though they are poorly substrate adherent they send-out processes. On collagen they sit there and don't do much, which is interesting. In contrast, S-cells on plastic grow as individual cells, become confluent, and then growth-inhibited. When grown on collagen, they become very spindle-shaped and they migrate all over the substrate. As soon as they reach a high enough cell number, they seem to revert to the flat cell type.

Foster: To follow that, I think that already we have seen, going from matrix culture *in vitro* to growing cells in nude mice, that as in many cases in which one is trying to mimic in the laboratory that which happens in normal biology, the environmental factors are enormously important to those tumors. It's the case, for example, in normal breast and breast carcinomas. Grown in monolayer culture, these cells are not responsive to many of the hormones and differentiation agents, whereas, if you put these into three-dimensional culture, in which they can arrange some sort of hierarchical organization between inside and outside, you then have an entirely different response from precisely the same cells.

Lipinski: Dr. Boyd, is your antibody an IgM?

Boyd: Yes.

Lipinski: Have you checked whether this antibody also reacts with a glycolipid containing the sugar?

Boyd: That was examined by methanol extraction and there was no reactivity of the antibody with glycolipid.

Reynolds: Dr. Sugimoto, have you compared the retinoic acid analog with retinoic acid to see if it is more potent? Does it induce more differentiation or N-myc down-regulation than normal retinoic acid?

Sugimoto: Yes. We have obtained similar results with the two in the same order of molar concentration.

Littauer: Does retinoic acid or its derivative affect phospholipase C?

Sugimoto: We haven't done that.

Reynolds: Dr. Sugimoto, with respect to the GOTO line, you see flat cells induced with BrdU and S-100 protein is increased. What is the percentage of cells you see responding to BrdU with flat cell morphology?

Sugimoto: More than 90% become flat, only 5% remain spindle.

Tsunamoto: Yes, we find almost 100% of the cells become flat.

Reynolds: When we looked at the SMS-KAN and SMS-KCNR lines with BrdU we saw about a 50-50 mixture of flat and neuronal cells, as reported at this meeting 3 years ago. What Dr. Biedler is seeing is a low level of those flat cells, without a differentiation inducer - but she has selected for and cloned these flat cells. It will be important to determine if the flat cells that appear spontaneously are the same as those induced by drugs.

Biedler: I would like to ask if you are willing to hypothesize that these neuroblastic cells are differentiating into glial cells or Schwann cells, by the chemical induction method.

Sugimoto: I think that glial differentiation in terms of expression of GFAP does not occur in our cell line. S-100 protein, especially the beta-subunit, and also CNP (which is rich in oligodendrocytes and peripheral Schwann cells), increase significantly. Such a marker study might show a similarity with ganglioneuroma. I am convinced that neuroblastoma can differentiate to a glial cell.

Bielder: When you remove BrdU, will the cells go back to a neuroblastic phenotype?

Sugimoto: I haven't tried that.

Reynolds: I'd like to comment that, in our experiments we can remove BrdU and get a long-term persistence of the combination of the flat and neuronal phenotypes, especially the flat cells. We have also seen some flat cells after treatment with retinoic acid. Did you see that in your experiment with differentiating lines?

Sugimoto: Yes, but in our case they don't show Schwannian differentiation - they don't show S-100.

Cavazzana: I am getting confused because the N-type morphology that Dr. Bielder described was more malignant in nude mice and there is a lower appearance of neuronal-type morphology in retinoic-acid induced differentiation, which is supposed to result in a less malignant phenotype. I ask the chairman to comment.

Reynolds: I think it is just a matter of terminology. What Dr. Biedler is referring to as "N-type" morphology is actually "neuroblast" morphology. When we say neuronal (ganglion cell) -like morphology we refer to larger cells with neuritic processes (a growth-arrested cell). Such cells are presumably less tumorigenic. The flat cells have been shown to have the properties of being less tumorigenic. But Dr. Biedler's neuroblast-like clones are more tumorigenic, and that would fit with what we see in patients, where a "neuroblstoma" (composed of neuroblast-like cells) is malignant, while "ganglioneuroma" (which contains a mixture of mature neuron-like cells and stroma, including glia-like cells) is benign.

Evans: I suggest following a conversation with Fred Gilbert, that there are far more cell lines being discussed and being examined by numerous investgators, than there were at our last meeting. It would now be valuable to publish as an appendix to these proceedings, a table that would include all the lines discussed together with relevant data generated.

Kemshead: There is some controversy regarding the expression of W6-32, said by some laboratories to be minimally expressed on neuroblastoma. However, in the study using coded antibodies it was found to be expressed by 50% of the lines. We are looking at quantitative differences - and it will, therefore, be very difficult to tabulate what some people see as positive and some as negative.

Evans: These differences show heterogeneity of investigators!

**Kemshead:** Could Dr. Sugimoto give any data about the comparative toxicity of retinoic acid compared to his analog in any animal model he has looked at?

**Sugimoto:** Yes. In rat and mouse, loss of body-weight and keratosis were extensively studied. The analog showed 10-20% less toxicity than retinoic acid. So, in mice, 400 mg/kg/day could be given for one month without noticeable toxicity.

**Reynolds:** Returning to the cell-line question, it is important to realize that cell lines can become contaminated with other cell-lines, they can become mislabelled in laboratories and unfortunately this cannot be prevented. Therefore, if we put together a table, we have to remember that differences in data for particular lines may reflect what someone calls 'line A' may in fact be 'line B'. Plus, selective pressure in the laboratory may change them. The most dramatic example is in the SK-N-SH line where in one lab it has one morphology and in another it has a different morphology. Dr. Biedler has demonstrated that it is able in interconvert. Therefore, when there is any discordance in data it is important to obtain cell lines from the orignator of the line, at the lowest passage number, and verify the data. For example, when we obtained CHP-126 from people other than from CHOP, it had an immunophenotype different than one would expect of neuroblastoma - suggesting that it was mixed-up with something else. We obtained a vial of CHP-126 from Philadelphia and it <u>did</u> have a neuroblastoma phenotype.

**Evans:** Most investigators' experience is that CHP-100 is a mixed line and that there are small neuroblastic cells and larger PNET - like cells. So, when someone says it is HLA-positive and someone else that it is HLA-negative, it may be due to the fact that the line is a mix of two different types of cells.

Ross: Does NSE in the GOTO line increase with BrdU treatment?

Tsunamoto: After treatment of GOTO with BrdU, NSE increases, but less than S-100 protein. Of the S-100, both alpha and beta subunits increase. Therefore, we think GOTO is probably, but not definitely, derived from Schwann cells.

Thiele: Since S-100 alpha is associated with peripheral neural cells, is it possible that what you are seeing in the BrdU-treated cultures, could indicate expression of S-100 alpha in neural cells rather than in Schwann cells? Your data seem to indicate a great increase in S-100 alpha, while only a minimal increase in S-100 beta.

Sugimoto: As you and I know, Schwann cells correspond to oligodendroglia in the CNS but Schwann cells contain only S-100 beta subunits. So, Dr. Tsunamoto's results are supporting evidence of Schwannian differentiation.

Tsunamoto: We have investigated S-100 in cultures. In the brain the main localization of S-100 alpha-beta is in glial cells. S-100 alpha-alpha is mainly localized to neurons. S-100 beta-beta is found in Schwann cells of the peripheral nervous system. In the cultures, S-100 alpha-alpha is only minimally found - only 7% using conventional antisera.

Quarlman: As a pathologist, it is interesting hearing about flat, intermediate and neuroblastic cells. There might be a biological correlate to this in human neuroblastoma biopsies. We presented a study at the Pediatric Research Meeting in Anaheim, CA. We looked at 100 neuroblastoma patients - 50 conventional and 50 in special categories with survivals ranging from 5 to 100%. We found a linear increase in S-100 positive cells in the biopsy tissues going from Stage IV to the special classes of neuroblastoma with a inverse correlation in ferritin staining within the tumors. There were three cell-types within these tumors. One was the conventional neuroblast which was ferritin positive. One was a semi-dendritic cell which was ferritin-positive and ultrastructurally looked like a perineural supportive cell. And the last was a very dendritic, S-100 positive cell which looked like a Schwann cell. The presence of the S-100 positive cell correlates with a 2-year survival of 94%. If you didn't have these cells - and only the perineural ferritin-positive cells - survival for 2 years was 29%. The correlation between these two different kinds of perineural or Schwann-like cells is very relevant to what is seen in the cultures. I would question whether this ferritin-positive perineural cells is not the intermediate cell and the more dendritic S-100 positive cell isn't the Schwann cell and that this may well be a very good biologic correlate with what is described in culture. There is also a parallel increase in lipoid aggregates from the conventional to the special stages with this increase in S-100 protein. I'm not sure what that means, but it, too, correlates with survival.

Ross: What is the karyotype of GOTO?

Brodeur: It was published in the Japanese Journal of Exp Med in 1979 (Vol 49, p67) as hypodiploid with a modal number of 44.

Sugimoto: One further comment, some neuroblastoma in patients can differentiate into Schwannian tumors.

Reynolds: I would like to ask Dr. Evans or Dr. D'Angio to comment: Spontaneous differentiation has long been seen in neuroblastoma, may be associated with spontaneous regression, and might be induced therapeutically, in some fashion. As reported here and in the last meeting both a flat cell phenotype and a neuronal-like phenotype, appear to be produced from neuroblast-like cells with differentiation. Carol Thiele has reported N-

*myc* down-regulation as an effect of differentiating agents. The comment of Dr. D'Angio that perhaps the flat cells which were reported as having high N-*myc* copy numbers, but low N-*myc* expression in culture, could explain late relapse worries me. Could it be that one can differentiatiate multi-copy cells and that they could then come back later to haunt us?

Evans: We talk a lot about differentiation in neuroblastoma - either spontaneous or treatment-induced. This is surely one of the goals of treatment. The difficulty is in treatment-induced differentiation, are you changing the cells and making them more differentiated or are you removing the neuroblast cells and leaving the stroma - which I think is more likely. I am not sure we have a lot of treatment-induced differentiation, although there are some instances where one ends up with ganglioneuromas. In the children with IV-S neuroblastoma who have a spontaneous remission, the bulk of the tumor does not differentiatiate, because if it did differentiate you would have a IV-S child with an enlarged liver filled with stroma. In those tumors you have complete disappearance of the neuroblastoma and replacement with normal liver. The only exception I would mention are those patients with skin nodules - which can appear and spontaneously disappear over a period of months. I think the skin nodules did not differentiate, because they disappeared. In one patient, over a period of 19 months, each crop of nodules was less immature and more differentiated. The first biopsy was pure neuroblastoma with primitive cells. The last biopsy we took was not even ganglioneuroma, it was neurofibroma. So, in six crops of skin nodules, each crop was more differentiated.

D'Angio: If we could get maturation by exgenous factors of whatever sort, I would say "Hurray", - because the late relapse is a rare event. Most of us can report anecdotes which particularly bear on the skin nodules. Some of these come back suddenly, and are mature ganglioneuroma. There is the rare patient who comes back with the skin nodule found to be metastatic neuroblastoma and who then died. Finally, if you can pinpoint the place where there was a skin nodule in a IV-S patient and you biopsy that area, you can find ganglion cells. So it isn't total disappearance nor is it total differentiation - maybe a mixture of both.

Reynolds: When we talk about IV-S and differentiation, we ought to keep in mind that there are probably about 1,000 neuroblasts for every neuron that makes its connection. There is an enormous turnover in development, with death of many neuroblasts. Indeed, differentiation could be a mechanism in IV-S regression in that if a cell starts to differentiate in an inappropriate environment, such as the liver, then it may simply die. Whereas, if it differentiated in another environment, such as the skin, then it can survive and form a benign tumor.

Chatten: With respect to differentiation, I can also cite the experience of the CCSG study with the Shimada classification. In stages II and IV neuroblastoma at least one third of the patients, at second look will be reclassified from unfavorable to favorable, which translated into your terms means they either become more Schwannian (we call them stroma rich), or they become more differentiated towards ganglion cells. For that one third of patients, their prognosis is not improved by the transformation.

Reynolds: But that is with cytotoxic chemotherapy. I was addressing the case of giving specific differentiation agents as opposed to cytotoxic therapy. Dr. Israel has put a lot of thought into that concept - would you please comment - is there a role for such therapy?

Israel: It is presently all speculation. I

am intrigued that these cells differentiate into neural cells and Schwann cells - not into chromaffin cells. That is something we are struggling with in the laboratory. We hope to gain understanding of molecular mechanisms. When we are able to target drugs addressed to molecular mechanisms that turn-on specific pathways, we will be able to do this. The goal will be to either change unfavorable tumors to more favorable classes that will respond to available therapies better. The goal may be to develop approaches so that people will take pills for the rest of their lives and live happily with their tumors. However, I think the relationship of what we see in the laboratory to what we observe in the histopathology is still very unclear. Nevertheless, neuroblastoma is a very provocative system.

Advances in Neuroblastoma Research 2, pages 377–394
© 1988 Alan R. Liss, Inc.

# NEUROBLASTOMA GENES IN DROSOPHILA AND HEREDITARY SUPPRESSION OF TUMOR DEVELOPMENT BY GENE TRANSFER

Bernard M. Mechler

Institute of Genetics
Johannes Gutenberg University
P.O. Box 3980
D 6500 Mainz, Fed. Rep. of Germany

## INTRODUCTION

In Drosophila the aetiology of neoplasia due to genetic mutations has been firmly established by Elisabeth Gateff who showed that mutations in a series of genes interrupt the differentiation of adult primordial cell-types and lead to an uncontrolled, invasive cell growth resulting in the premature death of the mutated animals (for review, see Gateff, 1978, 1982). These genes act as recessive determinants of cancer and their wild-type alleles can be considered as exerting a tumor suppressor function.

Similar tumor suppressor genes have been identified in familial cases of human cancer (Knudson, 1971, 1985; Murphree and Benedict, 1984; Fearon et al., 1984; Koufos et al., 1984, 1985; Orkin et al., 1984; Friend et al., 1986; Saxon et al., 1986; Weissman et al., 1987; Lee et al., 1987). During human development their normal function seems to be required for the completion of the growth and the differentiation of specific cell-types. When both alleles of these genes are inactivated, cell growth becomes unrestricted.

In Drosophila melanogaster at least 24 tumor suppressor genes have been identified which when mutated produce tissue specific tumors of either the optic adult neuroblasts, the imaginal disc cells, the blood cells or the gonial cells (Gateff, 1978; Gateff, 1982). Of these the lethal(2)giant larvae (1(2)gl) gene is the best studied. Homozygous mutations of the 1(2)gl locus are responsible for the development of a neuroblastoma of the presumptive adult

optic centers in the larval brain and a epithelioma of the
imaginal discs (Gateff and Schneiderman, 1969, 1974). Recently, we have isolated a chromosomal segment containing
a transcription unit that is structurally altered in all
l(2)gl mutant alleles (Mechler, McGinnis and Gehring, 1985)
and we have shown by gene transfer experiments that all sequences necessary for correct expression of the l(2)gl function are included within a 13.1 kb fragment of genomic DNA
(Opper et al, 1987). This DNA segment can thus fully rescue
the development of l(2)gl deficient animals which would have
normally succombed to brain and imaginal disc neoplasia. We
have furthermore sequenced the entire 13.1 kb of genomic
DNA as well as several cDNAs corresponding to the two classes of l(2)gl transcripts that are about 4.5 and 6 kb in
length (Jacob et al., 1987). Alignment of the cDNA with the
genomic sequences allowed us to define the organization of
the l(2)gl transcripts and to deduce the amino acid sequences of two l(2)gl proteins. These proteins, p127 and p78,
contain 1161 and 708 amino-acids, respectively. Using antibodies raised against a β-galactosidase / l(2)gl fusion protein we have been able to identify these two l(2)gl proteins
with the expected sizes of about 80 and 130 kd (Merz, Kissel, Friedberg and Mechler, in preparation). Further gene
transfer experiments indicated that the p78 protein is effective in controlling cell proliferation and differentiation (Jacob et al., 1987). This protein is predominantly expressed during early embryogenesis at a time when cell determination takes place. Thus, we can infer that the molecular decision towards a neoplastic development that becomes only apparent at the end of the third larval instar,
is taken very early during embryogenesis.


NEUROBLASTOMA GENES IN DROSOPHILA MELANOGASTER

     Among the 24 recessive mutations that produce tumors
in Drosophila melanogaster (Gateff, 1978, 1982), six of them
interrupt the development of the presumptive adult optic
centers of the larval brain and cause essentially an invasive proliferation of neuroblasts in the larval brain.
These genes can therefore be considered as neuroblastoma
genes although they may also primarily affect other cells
and tissues, leading either to neoplastic transformation or
cell death. The neuroblastoma genes are distributed on
three of the four Drosophila chromosomes (Table 1).

TABLE 1. Neuroblastoma Genes of Drosophila

| Neuroblastoma Genes | Number of Alleles | Chromosomal Localization | Pheno-type + | Refe-rences ++ |
|---|---|---|---|---|
| lethal(1)2 | 1 | I - n.d. | N + E | a, b |
| lethal(1)disc large-1 | 7 | I - 10B5-17 | N + E | c, d |
| lethal(2)giant larvae | 150 | II - 21A | N + E | e, f |
| lethal(2)701 | 1 | II - 59D8-9/ 59F1-60A7 | N + E | g |
| lethal(3)giant larvae | 1 | III - n.d. | N + E | a, b |
| lethal(3)brain tumor-ts | 2 | III - 97E5,6- 97F1 | N | a, b |

+ E, epithelioma; N, neuroblastoma
++ a, Gateff, 1978; b, Gateff, 1982; c, Stewart et al., 1972.
d, described as l(1)lpr-2 in Kiss et al., 1978; e, Gateff
and Schneiderman, 1969; f, Mechler, McGinnis and Gehring,
1985; g, Gateff and Phannavong, pers. comm.

All the mutants are recessive and, with the exception of
lethal(3)brain tumor-ts (l(3)bt-ts), produce malignant
transformation in two distinct presumptive adult tissues.
a.) the neuroblasts and the ganglion-mother cells of the
presumptive adult optic centers of the larval brain and
b.) the epithelial cells of the imaginal discs. In the case
of the conditional lethal temperature sensitive mutation
l(3)bt-ts, only the neuroblasts show malignant transformation at the restrictive temperature, although some other
tissues like the imaginal disc cells and the germ cells
present signs of atrophic or abnormal development (Gateff
and Löffler, pers. comm.).

The recessivity of all these mutations indicates that
the tumorous development results from a lack of gene function and, thus, stands in contrast to the dominance shown
by the viral oncogenes and cellular oncogenes (for review,
see Weinberg, 1985; Bishop, 1987; Duesberg 1985, 1987).

This lack of function is best illustrated in the case of the 1(2)gl mutations which have been molecularly characterized as chromosomal deficiencies removing part or all of the gene (Mechler, McGinnis and Gehring, 1985). However, in the case of the temperature sensitive 1(3)bt mutation, the presence of an hypomorphic or altered gene product may be envisaged and it will be of particular interest to see whether new 1(3)bt alleles resulting from chromosome deletion or gene inactivation will present also a tumorous phenotype.

## THE LETHAL(2)GIANT LARVAE GENE

Among all the Drosophila tumor suppressor genes, the 1(2)gl gene has been the best studied. 1(2)gl homozygous mutations leads to the appearance of malignant neoplasia of the imaginal discs and the presumptive adult optic centers in the larval brain (Gateff and Schneiderman, 1969, 1974). In 1(2)gl deficient animals, these malignancies first become visible at the end of the third larval instar, immediately prior to the metamorphosis of the larvae. The tumorous growth produces a complex syndrome characterized by the bloating of the larvae and the atrophy of several tissues, like the ring gland, the salivary glands and the fat bodies (for review see Hadorn, 1955). As a consequence of this bloating the 1(2)gl larvae become giant in size and die as late larvae or pseudopupae.

The imaginal discs and the brain hemispheres are not the only tissues affected. The ring gland and particularly its prothoracic portion, which is the source of ecdysone, is defective and, as a consequence, pupariation is considerably delayed. However the atrophy of the prothoracic gland is apparently not the primary defect in the mutant because neither the transplantation of a normal ring gland into 1(2)gl deficient larvae (Hadorn, 1937) nor the injection of ecdysone will fully rescue the mutant animals (Karlson and Hauser, 1952). Furthermore, ecdysone deficiency alone is not sufficient to induce neoplastic growth (Klose et al., 1980; Garen et al., 1977). The atrophy of the ring gland is probably caused by the severing of the connections between the brain neurosecretory cells and the ecdysone-producing prothoracic cells due to the growth of the malignant brain neuroblasts (Akai, 1975; Klose et al., 1980).

The first 1(2)gl mutant was discovered by Bridges in 1933 (Bridges and Brehme, 1944) and has been mapped to

position 21A at the extreme left end of the second chromosome (Lewis, 1945; Mechler et al., 1985). Subsequently, numerous spontaneous mutant alleles have been isolated from
wild populations at several locations of the Soviet Union
(Golubovsky, 1978, 1980) and in California (Green and Shepherd, 1979). Examination of wild flies revealed that about
1 % of the second chromosomes were consistently mutated at
the l(2)gl gene. The high incidence of l(2)gl mutations from
such geographically widespread wild populations suggests
that the l(2)gl gene may either be a preferred site for the
integration of a transposable element (Green and Shepherd,
1979) or may represent an unstable chromosomal region due to
its association with a telomere (Mechler et al., 1985). Thus,
the study of the l(2)gl gene presents two centers of interest: one concerns its role in the control of cell proliferation and differentiation and the other deals with its high
rate of mutability.


MOLECULAR IDENTIFICATION OF THE l(2)gl GENE

        The l(2)gl gene was isolated during a search for pole-
cell specific transcripts (Mechler et al., 1985). The pole-
cells are the first cells that arise at the posterior end
of the Drosophila embryo and become the precursor cells of
the germ line. Thus the pole cells represent one of the rare
examples of stem cells that can be identified and followed
from the time of their formation up to their terminal differentiation as gametes.

        A clone α-8 isolated from a recombinant library of
genomic Drosophila DNA and showing pole-cell specificity
was assigned by in situ hybridization to a subtelomeric
region of the left arm of chromosome 2 in the region 21A
(Mechler et al., 1985). Earlier cytogenetic mapping had
located the l(2)gl gene in the region 21A-B (Lewis, 1945)
and histological examination had revealed that the first
symptom detectable in l(2)gl animals is the atrophy and
necrosis of the male germ line in the first instar larvae
(Gloor, 1943). This faint correlation for assigning the α-8
clone to the l(2)gl locus was strengthened by hybridizing
the cloned DNA to polytene chromosomes heterozygous for the
l(2)gl mutation. A hybridization signal was only detected
over the chromosome carrying the wild-type allele (Figure
1A). Then using chromosomal walking we expanded the cloned
region to approximately 40 kb of overlapping clones. When

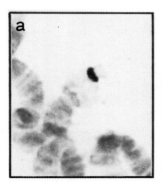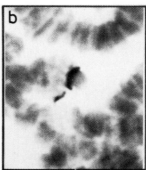

Figure 1. In situ hybridization of heterozygote 1(2)gl$^4$/+ polytene chromosomes with biotinylated ⍺-8 (a) and 8014 (b) cloned DNAs. The hybridizing site was visualized by an antibody procedure involving a final horseradish peroxidase enzyme reaction yielding dark deposits. The ⍺-8 probe hybridized only to the wild-type chromosome whereas the 8014 probe hybridized to both chromosomes indicating that the 1(2)gl$^4$ mutation is a chromosomal deletion (adapted from Mechler et al., 1985).

Figure 2. Molecular organization of the wild-type and mutant 1(2)gl region on chromosome 2L and maps of the P-element transposons containing 1(2)gl$^+$. (A) structure of 3 1(2)gl mutant alleles and (B) its corresponding wild-type allele (Mechler et al., 1985). The extent of the 1(2)gl deletions is indicated by bold lines whereas the B104 mobile element inserted in 1(2)glGB52 is shown by an open box. Above the wild-type allele map are shown an overlapping array of Drosophila inserts covering approximately 40 kb of genomic DNA. Positioned below the wild-type map are indicated the two identified 1(2)gl transcripts of 6 and 4.5 kb. (C) Diagrams of P-1(2)gl transposons (Opper et al., 1987; Jacob et al., 1987). The 1(2)gl structural gene (13.1 kb EcoR1 fragment) was inserted into the polylinker of the Carnegie 20 vector (P-1(2)gl, ry-13). In addition to P-element long terminal repeats (solid boxes), the Carnegie 20 vector carries the xanthine dehydrogenase (ry$^+$) gene. The 1(2)gl 13.1 kb fragment was also integrated into the pUChs neo vector which

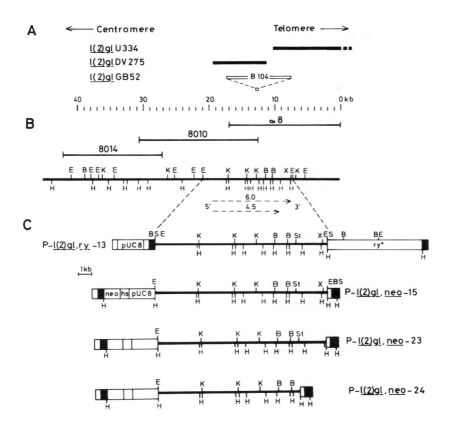

contains a bacterial neo gene attached to the Drosophila
hsp 70 heat-shock promoter and confers resistance to the
antibiotic Geneticin G418. From this transposon, P-1(2)gl,
neo-15, two further transposons, P-1(2)gl, neo-23 and 24,
were constructed by resecting the 3' extremity of the l(2)gl
13.1kb DNA fragment. All four P-1(2)gl transposons were
shown to complement l(2)gl deficiencies (Opper et al., 1987;
Jacob et al., 1987) indicating that the tumor suppressing
function is associated with the 4.5 kb transcript.

Restriction sites: B, BamH1; E, EcoR1; H, HindIII; K, Kpn1;
S, Sal1; St, Stu1; X, Xba1.

in situ hybridization was repeated with the cloned segment
8014 (Figure 2), the farthermost segment from the α-8 sequence, a hybridization signal was observed over both chromosomes (Figure 1B). This demonstrated that one of the
breakpoints of these deletions had been passed. For a more
detailed molecular study of the l(2)gl locus, the restriction pattern of the DNA from homozygous l(2)gl mutant alleles was determined by Southern genomic blotting. The analysis of more than 50 spontaneously occurring and EMS-induced
l(2)gl mutations revealed an exceptional feature of these
mutants. Almost all l(2)gl mutations consisted of large
deletions in which part or all the DNA sequence  between
the chromosomal end and the cloned region was absent.

Such terminal deficiencies did not allow a precise
molecular location of the l(2)gl gene. However, alterations
in two mutants l(2)gl GB52 and l(2)gl DV275 indicated that
the l(2)gl gene was contained in the cloned region (Figure
2). The l(2)gl DV275 mutation consists of an interstitial
deletion of about 9 kb of DNA whose breakpoints are joined
by an heterologous DNA sequence. The l(2)gl GB52 mutation
is characterized by a 10 kb insertion element which was
later identified as a transposable element on the B104 family (Lützelschwab et al., 1985).

The size of the l(2)gl gene was more precisely bracketed by analysing the RNA transcripts made from the cloned
region (Mechler et al., 1985). Northern blot analysis of
RNA isolated from sequential stages of Drosophila development revealed two transcribed regions within the cloned DNA.
The first transcription unit maps to the right of the cloned
segment and is disrupted in all l(2)gl mutant chromosomes.
This transcribed region appears to be the l(2)gl gene. The
second transcribed region is disrupted in only some l(2)gl
mutant chromosomes and lies to the left of the cloned segment.

Transcripts of the l(2)gl gene fall into two size
classes of about 6 and 4.5 kb. Both transcripts are developmentally regulated with two major periods of expression. The
most abundant expression occurs during early embryogenesis
and to a lesser degree in late third instar larvae. Although
both transcripts were detected during these two periods,
their relative proportion varies considerably. The 4.5 kb
transcript represents the major form during early embryogenesis whereas the 6 kb transcript, which is detectable

during mid and late embryogenesis constitutes the predominant RNA species during late third instar larvae.

## l(2)gl GENE TRANSFER AND RESCUE

The preceding analysis has lead to the delimitation of a transcription unit that is altered in all examined l(2)gl chromosomes and has assigned the l(2)gl gene to a 13.1 kb DNA fragment (Mechler et al., 1985). This DNA segment is small enough to test for in vivo expression with P-element mediated transformation (Spradling and Rubin, 1982; Rubin and Spradling, 1982). Using this technique, exogeneous DNA can efficiently be integrated into the DNA of germ-line chromosomes in Drosophila embryos.

For this purpose, we have constructed two different P-element transposons carrying the l(2)gl gene as shown in Figure 2. In one construct P-l(2)gl, ry-13, the 13.1 kb DNA fragment was inserted into the Carnegie 20 P-element vector (Rubin and Spradling, 1983). This vector possesses a rosy$^+$ (ry$^+$) gene which encodes xanthine dehydrogenase and is used as a selective eye color marker to assess the integration of the transposon. In the other construct, P-l(2)gl, neo-15, the 13.1 kb l(2)gl sequence was inserted into the pUChs-neo P-element-vector (Steller and Pirrotta, 1985). This vector contains a bacterial neo resistance gene that confers selective Geneticin G418 resistance to transformed Drosophila embryos and larvae.

Transformation was conducted according to the protocols as described in Figure 3. Both P-l(2)gl transposons have been successfully integrated into the germ line of heterozygous l(2)gl / + flies. In a first series of experiments 1064 embryos were injected with P-l(2)gl, ry-13 transposon and from 25 fertile adult flies, one gave rise to five ry$^+$ (cinnabar eye colored) transformed flies. These flies were then analyzed for the presence of a functional l(2)gl gene by backcrossing. As a result, progeny were obtained with white eyes and normal wings demonstrating that the l(2)gl transposon had fully rescued the development of the l(2)gl deficient animals which otherwise would have died of brain and imaginal disc neoplasia (Opper et al., 1987). A similar result was obtained with the P-l(2)gl, neo-15 transposon which was injected into 368 embryos laid by l(2)gl cn bw / In(2LR)SM1 Cy cn flies. From 40 fertile adults, two lines of transformed flies resistant to Geneticin G418 were obtained. In one line, progeny flies were recovered with normal wings and white eyes demonstrating that the integrated P-1(2)gl, neo-15 transposon can complement the 1(2)gl deficiency. In the other line, no 1(2)gl complementation was obtained and further analysis indicated that the 1(2)gl, neo transposon was associated with the In(2LR)SM1 balancer chromosome which already carries a wild-type 1(2)gl gene. Cytogenetic locations were identified by in situ hybridization. The P-1(2)gl, ry-13 transposon was inserted at 22F-23A on the left arm of chromosome 2 and the P-1(2)gl, neo-15 transposon at 15E on chromosome X. Both integrations were homozygous viable and no visible phenotype can be observed. Furthermore, genomic Southern blot experiments have shown that the 13.1 kb 1(2)gl DNA fragment has been integrated in an unrearranged form in the genome of the transformed flies.

These transformation experiments demonstrate that all the 1(2)gl genetic information is included within this 13.1 kb DNA fragment and show that the development of neuroblastomas and imaginal disc tumors results from the absence of 1(2)gl function. When this function is restored, tumor development is completely suppressed.

## STRUCTURE OF THE 1(2)gl GENE TRANSCRIPTS

Based on the results of the previous gene transfer experiments showing that the 13.1 kb DNA fragment can fully complement the 1(2)gl deficiency, we sequenced the entire DNA fragment as well as several cDNAs corresponding to the two major classes of 1(2)gl transcripts (Jacob et al., 1987).

The salient structural feature of this gene is the presence in its proximal moiety of two direct repeats, each about 2.8 kb in size (Figure 4). These repeats show a high degree (95 %) of homology. Their combined size represents almost half of the 1(2)gl gene.

We have investigated the structure of the 1(2)gl transcripts by isolating cDNA clones from 0-12 hr embryonic cDNA libraries (Poole et al., 1985) and have obtained more than 30 clones with sizeable (larger than 1 kb) 1(2)gl cDNA sequences. The longest cDNA, Ec173, 5.3 kb in length, was used for the initial alignment of the other cDNAs. Analysis of the pattern of restriction sites revealed that most of

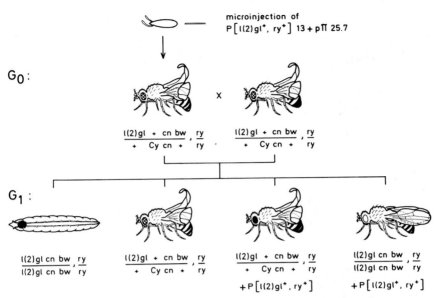

Figure 3. Selection of flies transformed to l(2)gl$^+$ (Opper et al., 1987). All the embryos produced by the first cross, the G$_0$ embryos, were injected with P-l(2)gl, ry-13 in combination with pπ 25.7wc helper P-element. Only the heterozygous embryos survived and grew to adults. These were backcrossed and the transformed progeny were identified by their phenotypes. The parent flies had curled wings (Cy) and orange eye color (crosshatched eyes) due to the combination of homozygous cn and ry. The l(2)gl mutant chromosome 2 carried the eye color marker cn and bw and was balanced by an inverted second chromosome which is homozygous lethal and contains the dominant marker Cy (curled wings) and the recessive eye color marker cn. Chromosome 3 carried the ry eye color marker. The transformed flies, heterozygous l(2)gl deficient at locus 21A, had curled wings (Cy) and bright-red (cn) eyes (black eyes). The l(2)gl rescued flies, homozygous l(2)gl deficient at locus 21A, had normal wings and white eyes due to the combination of homozygous cn and bw. G$_1$ transformed flies were further backcrossed. G$_2$ l(2)gl rescued flies were then pair crossed and lines homozygous for the insertion were established. A modified procedure was used for the selection of P-l(2)gl, neo-transformed lines. The parent stock was wild-type at the ry locus and the progeny of the G$_0$ adults were grown on food containing 1 mg/ml Geneticin G418.

the cDNA inserts were structurally identical to defined
regions of Ec173. However, two exceptions to the role was
noticed. As summarized in Figure 4, two clones Ec32 and
Ec33 presented a difference in a region adjacent to the 5'
end of Ec173 whereas another clone, Ec371, showed a divergence in the central portion of Ec173.

These structural variabilities suggested alternative
splicing of the l(2)gl exons. We have therefore determined
the sequence of these cDNAs and demonstrated that the sites
of sequence divergence in the cDNA clones corresponds to
intron-exon junctions in the genomic sequence. This sequencing revealed at least two different mechanisms of alternative splicing.One divergence occurs in the coding region of
l(2)gl and leads to the synthesis of two distinct l(2)gl
proteins whereas the other variation modifies the 5' un-
translated region and bears no consequence on the proteins.

The cDNA clone Ec173 contains 5338 nucleotides and corresponds to a nearly complete copy of the 6 kb transcript.
It extends over 10 exons as shown in Figure 4.

The sequence of the first three exons is represented
twice in the l(2)gl gene. On the basis of small nucleotide
differences, exons II and III can be shown to derive from
the second repeat. However, the sequence of exon I is identical in both repeats and thus cannot be assigned. Although
the exact 5' limit of the gene has not yet been precisely
mapped, it seems very likely that the promoter region is
duplicated so that the transcription of the l(2)gl gene can
occur simultaneously at two sites. Therefore, two primary
transcripts may be produced and the further processing of
the largest transcript containing the 5' duplication may
generate distinct patterns of splicing. Such possibility
is exemplified by the organization of the clones Ec33 and
Ec32. A distinct first exon (exon Ia) combines the sequence
of exon I, of the first intron and the proximal half of
exon II. Then the sequence of Ec33 can be directly aligned
to the beginning of exon III and is similar to the sequence
of Ec173. Because the clones Ec33 and Ec32 contain only the
proximal portion of the l(2)gl transcript, we cannot assign
then to either the 4.5 kb or 6 kb transcript.

A second difference was noticed in clone Ec371 whose
sequence of 975 nucleotides aligns within the central region of the l(2)gl gene (Figure 4). The first 190 nucleo-

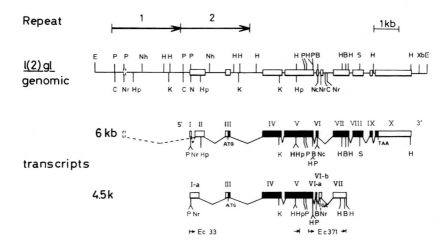

Figure 4. Map of the l(2)gl gene and transcripts (adapted from Jacob et al., 1987). Exons are drawn as boxes. The structure of the 6 kb transcript is derived from the cDNA clone Ec173 which contains 5338 nucleotides. The structure of the 4.5 kb transcript is based on the sequence analysis of the cDNA clones Ec33 and Ec371 (indicated by arrows under the 4.5 kb transcript) which showed the existence of two structural differences in the exon splicing. By comparison with the cDNA clone Ec173 the divergence occurring in the middle of Ec371 modifies the coding capacity of transcript, whereas the variation in the 5' region of the cDNA Ec33 bears no consequence on the protein structure. The 6 kb transcript encodes a putative protein of 1161 amino acids, p127 and the 4.5 kb transcript a putative protein of 708 amino acids, p78. Using antibodies raised against the N-terminal domain of    l(2)gl, two proteins with the expected sizes have been identified on Western blots of eletrophoretically separated proteins from Drosophila embryos (Merz, Kissel, Friedberg and Mechler, in preparation). The tandem duplication found in the proximal region of the l(2)gl gene is indicated by arrows 1 and 2.

Restriction sites: B, BamH1; C, Cla1; E, EcoR1; H, HindIII; Hp, Hpa1; K, Kpn1; Nc, Nco1; Nr, Nru1; P, Pvu1; S, Stu1; Xb, Xba1.

tides of Ec371 corresponds to the last 124 nucleotides of exon V and the first 66 nucleotides of exon VI. Then, by comparison to Ec173, the sequence of Ec371 is interrupted, creating a shorter exon VIa and is followed by a new exon VIb of 179 nucleotides which are found in the proximal region of the intron separated exons VI and VII. After this exon, the distal 590 nucleotides of Ec371 show a perfect alignment with Ec173 starting at the proximal boundary of exon VII and ending 6 nucleotides upstream from a putative poly (A) addition signal (ATTAAA). We presume that this cDNA corresponds to a portion of the 4.5 kb transcript because the alternative splicing of Ec371 generates a shortened 1(2)gl protein, as expected from the results of the gene transfer experiments (vide intra).


THE 1(2)gl PROTEINS

The occurence of alternative splicing leads to the prediction of at least two 1(2)gl proteins. The amino acid sequence of the 1(2)gl polypeptide encoded by the 6 kb transcript can be deduced from the Ec173 sequence. With the assumption that the first ATG codon at the 5' end of the unique large open reading frame is the initiation codon, this transcript would produce a polypeptide of 1161 amino acids in length with a relative mass of 126.905. This protein will be designated p127.

The structure of the other 1(2)gl protein can be predicted from the modification of the nucleotide sequence occurring in clone Ec371. However, because this cDNA is only a partial copy of a 1(2)gl transcript. We assume that the missing 5' translated segment is identical to the coding sequence found in the other cDNAs. We can therefore predict a polypeptide of 708 amino acids with a relative mass of 78.111. The amino acid sequence of this protein, designated as p78, is almost completely similar to the N-moiety of p127, differing only by the last amino acid, a phenylalanine residue.

The amino acid sequence of both proteins is shown in Figure 5. Using antibodies that specifically recognized a portion of the N-terminal domain common to both 1(2)gl polypeptides, we have been able to identify these two polypeptides with the expected sizes of about 80 kd and 130 kd, respectively (Merz, Kissel, Friedberg and Mechler).

```
               10         20         30         40         50         60
                |          |          |          |          |          |
    1 MLKFIRGKGQ QPSADRHRLQ KDLFAYRKTA QHGFPHKPSA LAYDPVLKLM AIGTQTGALK
   61 VFGQPGVELY GQHTLLNNSA SELNVQLLEW VYGTGRILSL TAANQLILWE PVGATLLPIK
  121 TLPFDGKLKK VSSLCCSLSK DLLWIGTEGG NIYQLDLHTF TIKEPVIYHD VVLEQVPPAY
  181 KLNPGAIESI RQLPNSPSKL LVAYNRGLCV LWDFESASVQ RAYIAPGHGQ SVGLTVNFEG
  241 SEFTWYHADG SYATWSIDNP EPPSNVNYVP YGPDPCKSIN RLYKGKRRSN DV1VFSGGMP
  301 RSAYGDHNCV SVHASDGHKV CLDFTSKVID FFVTFENNRD VAEVLVVLLE EELCAYDLTD
  361 PNICAIKAPY LHSVHASAVT CNYLASEVVQ SVYESILRAG DEQDIDYSNI SWPITGGTLP
  421 DNLEESVEED ATKLYEILLT GHEDGSVKFW DCTGVLLKPI YNFKTSSIFG SESDFRDDAA
  481 ADMSAEQVDE GEPPFRKSGL FDPYSDDPRL AVKKIAFCPK TGQLIVGGTA GQIVIADFID
  541 LPEKVSLKYI SMNLVSDRDG FVWKGHDQLN VRSNLLDGEA IPTTERGVNI SGVLQVLPPA
  601 SITCMALEAS WGLVSGGTAH GLVLFDFKNF VPVFHRCTLN PNDLTGAGEQ LSRRKSFKKS
  661 LRESFRKLRK GRSTRTNQSN QVPTTLEARP VERQIEARCA DDGLGSMF
                                                        VRC LLFAKTYVTN
  721 VNITSPTLWS ATNASTVSVF LLHLPPAQTA ATAVPSASGN APPHMPRRIS AQLAKEIQLK
  781 HRAPVVGISI FDQAGSPVDQ LNAGENGSPP HRVLIASEEQ FKVFSLPQLK PINKYKLTAN
  841 EGARIRRIHF GSFSCRISPE TLQSMHGCSP TKSTRSHGDG EADPNISGSL AVSRGDVYNE
  901 TALICLTNMG DIMVLSVPEL KRQLNAAAVR REDINGVSSL CFTNSGEALY MMSSSELQGI
  961 ALATSRVVQP TGVVPVEPLE NEESVLEEND AENNKETYAC DEVVNTYEIK NPSGISICTR
 1021 PAEENVGRNS VQQVNGVNIS NSPNQANETI SSSIGDITVD SVRDHLNMTT TTLCSINTEE
 1081 TIGRLSVLST QTNKASTTVN MSEIPNINIS NLEDLESKRN TTETSTSSVV IKSIITNISH
 1141 EKTNGDNKIG TPKTAPEESQ F
```

Figure 5. Deduced amino acid sequence of the p78 and p127 1(2)gl proteins of Drosophila melanogaster. The N-terminal segment of both 1(2)gl proteins is assumed to be identical for 707 residues. Then the putative p78 protein ends with a Phe residue provided by the first codon of exon VI-b. The putative p127 protein contains an additional C-terminal segment of 454 residues. The gene rescue experiment with the 3' resected transposon P-1(2)gl-24 suggests strongly that the p78 protein is involved in the control of cell proliferation and differentiation, whereas the p127 protein is implicated in a less vital function.
Symbols for the amino acids: A, ala; C, cys; D, asp; E, glu; F, phe; G, gly; H, his; I, ile; K, lys; M, met; N, asn; P, pro; Q, gln; R, arg; S, ser; T, thr; V, val; W, trp; Y, tyr.

## DELIMITATION OF THE TUMOR SUPPRESSING DOMAIN

To identify the functional limits of the sequence suppressing tumorigenesis within the 1(2)gl gene, we have resected both extremities of the 13.1 kb 1(2)gl DNA segment and were able to delineate the region of 1(2)gl carrying the tumor suppressing function. All tested 5' resections which removed the proximal control region of the gene resulted in the inactivation of the tumor suppressing function of 1(2)gl. In contrast, two clones in which the 3' extremity had been shortened were able to complement the 1(2)gl defi-

ciency (Figure 2). With transposon P-1(2)gl-23, this gene
complementation was expected because the 3' resection had
not removed any transcribed sequence. By contrast the tumor
suppressing activity of the transposon P-1(2)gl-24 was un-
suspected, because a larger resection of the fragment Stul-
EcoR1 had eliminated 1803 nucleotides from the 3' end of the
6 kb transcript and thus deleted 141 amino acids from the
C-terminus of the p127 protein. However, the sequence of the
4.5 kb transcript remained intact so that we can associate
the tumor suppressing activity with this transcript and,
consequently, with the p78 protein. Furthermore, these results indicate that the p127 protein plays an accessory role
during Drosophila development. Its absence leads to a phenomenon characteristic of a mutation showing incomplete pene-
trance. The animals lacking this protein are able to achieve
a complete development with no sign of neoplasia. However,
about two-thirds of them are unable to emerge from the pupal
case, and die as pharate adults. The surviving flies are
viable and fertile. This phenotype was observed in five distinct lines and thus is not caused by a genetic lesion produced by the integration of the transposon.


PROSPECTS AND CONCLUSION

       The information gained from these experiments forms
the basis for a more detailed analysis of the l(2)gl tumor
suppressing protein and the role that this protein plays
in the regulation of cell growth and differentiation. Despite
the information provided by the sequence analysis, we are
still unable to assign a precise molecular function to the
l(2)gl protein. In particular, the sequence comparison of
the l(2)gl protein with other proteins available in data-
bases has not detected any significant homology with any of
the more than 4000 published protein sequences. Furthermore,
the amino acid sequence of the l(2)gl protein has not revealed any stricking feature which would have pointed out a
functional or structural property indicating either an extracellular, transmembrane or nucleus location.

       Having defined the structure of the l(2)gl gene, we
can now move into a new phase in which mechanistic questions
can be addressed. In particular, we can now investigate (a)
the tissue distribution and the intracellular localization
of the l(2)gl proteins and (b) the critical period(s) of
development when the l(2)gl gene should be expressed to pre-

vent tumor formation. The spatial analysis of the l(2)gl tumor suppressor protein can be performed with the antibodies raised against the N-terminal portion of the l(2)gl proteins. In addition, this analysis will be carried out with the p-l(2)gl-24 rescued animals which present the advantage to synthesize exclusively the p78 protein. The critical period(s) of the l(2)gl gene expression can be studied by introducing into the fly genome inducible l(2)gl transposons which can selectively block the transcription or the translation of the l(2)gl gene and produce l(2)gl phenocopies.

Answers to these questions will provide us valuable information on the biochemical properties of the l(2)gl tumor suppressing protein and will lead us to a better understanding of the molecular basis of cancer.

## ACKNOWLEDGEMENTS

The author wishes to thank Elisabeth Gateff for continued interest and support, Mrs. H. Papadakis for excellent secretarial help in preparing this manuscript and Martin Opper, Lothar Jacob, Bernhard Metzroth and Reinhard Merz for their active collaboration. The studies reported here were supported by grants from the Deutsche Forschungsgemeinschaft SB 302 - project B20 and Me 800/1-1.

## REFERENCES

Akai H (1975). The Cell (Japan) 4:38-41.
Bishop JM (1987). Science 235:305-311.
Bridges CB, Brehme KS (1944). Carnegie Inst Wash Publ. 552.
Duesberg PH (1985). Science 228:669-677.
Duesberg PH (1987). Proc Natl Acad Sci USA 84:2117-2124.
Fearon ER, Vogelstein B, Feinberg AP (1984). Nature 318: 377-380.
Friend SH, Bernards R, Rogely S, Weinberg RA, Rapaport JM, Albert DM and Dryja TP (1986). Nature 323:643-646.
Garen A, Kauvar L, Lepesant JA (1977). Proc Natl Acad Sci USA 74:5099-5102.
Gateff E (1978). Science 200:1448-1459.
Gateff E (1982). Adv Cancer Res 37:33-74.
Gateff E, Schneiderman HA (1969). Natl Cancer Inst Monogr 31:365-397.

Gateff E, Schneiderman HA (1974). Wilhelm Roux's Arch Dev. Biol 176:23-65.
Gloor H (1943). Rev Suisse Zool 50:339-394.
Golubovsky MD (1978). Dros Inf Serv 53:179.
Golubovsky MD (1980). Genetica 52/53:139-149.
Green MM, Shepherd SHY (1979). Genetics 92:823-832.
Hadorn E (1937). Proc Natl Acad Sci USA 23:478-484.
Hadorn E (1955). In Lethalfaktoren, Thieme, Stuttgart.
Jacob L, Opper M, Metzroth B, Phannavong B, Mechler BM (1987). Cell 50: in press
Karlson P, Hauser G (1952). Z Naturforsch 7b:80-83.
Kiss I, Szabad J, Major I (1978). Molec gen Genet 164:77-83.
Klose W, Gateff E, Emmerich H. Beikirch H (1980). Wilhelm Roux's Arch Dev Biol 189:57-67.
Knudson GA (1971). Proc Natl Acad Sci USA 68: 820-823.
Knudson GA (1985). J Cancer Res 45:1437-1443.
Koufos A, Hansen MF, Lampkin BC, Workman MC, Copeland NG, Jenkins NA, Cavenee WK (1984). Nature 309:170-172.
Koufos A, Hansen MF, Copeland NG, Jenkins NA, Lampkin BC, Cavenee WK (1985). Nature 316:330-334.
Lee WH, Bookstein R, Hong F, Young LI, Shew IY, Lee EYH (1987). Science 235:1394-1399.
Lewis EB (1945). Genetics 30:137-166.
Lützelschwab R, Müller G, Wälder B, Schmidt O, Fürbass R, Mechler BM (1986). Molec gen Genet 204:58-63.
Mechler BM, McGinnis W, Gehring WJ (1985): The EMBO Journal 4:1551-1557.
Murphree AL, Benedict WF (1984). Science 223:1028-1033.
Opper M, Schuler G, Mechler BM (1987): Oncogene 1:91-96.
Orkin SH, Goldman DS, Salen SE (1984). Nature 309:172-174.
Poole SJ, Kauvar LM, Drees B, Kornberg T (1985). Cell 40: 37-43.
Rubin GM, Spradling AC (1982). Science 218:348-353.
Rubin GM, Spradling AC (1983): Nucleic Acids Res 11:6341-6351.
Saxon PJ, Srivatsam ES, Stanbridge EJ (1986). The EMBO Journal 5:3461-3466.
Spradling AC, Rubin GM (1982). Science 218:341-347.
Steller H, Pirrotta V (1985). The EMBO Journal 4:167-171
Stewart M, Murphy C, Fristrom JW (1972). Dev Biol 27:71-83.
Weinberg RA (1985). Science 230:770-776.
Weissman BE, Saxon PJ, Pasquale SR, Jones GR, Geiser AG, Stanbridge EJ (1987). Science 236:175-180.

Advances in Neuroblastoma Research 2, pages 395–407
© 1988 Alan R. Liss, Inc.

DISTINCTIVE MEMBRANE PHENOTYPES OF NEUROBLASTOMA CELLS AND
FETAL NEUROBLASTS BY A PANEL OF MONOCLONAL ANTIBODIES

Takafumi Matsumura, Tohru Sugimoto, Tadashi Sawada,
Tohru Saida, and John T. Kemshead

Department of Pediatrics (T.M., T.Su., T.Sa. ,T.Sa.)
Children's Research Hospital (T.Su.),
Kyoto Prefectural University of Medicine,
Kamikyoku, Kyoto, 602 Japan
Institute of Child Health (J.T.K.),
London WC1N 1EH, England

INTRODUCTION

Neuroblastoma(NB), the most common solid tumor in
childhood outside the brain, is thought to arise from
primitive sympathetic neuroblasts in the adrenal gland or
the sympathetic ganglion that have failed to undergo normal
differentiation. Although NB cells have been well analyzed
in immunological studies of cell surface antigens, fetal
neuroblasts, as the precursor of NB cells, have not been
studied from this aspect. Some distinctions, based on
histopathological studies (Ikeda et al 1981; Machin 1982),
between NB cells and fetal neuroblasts in the adrenal gland
have been demonstrated. However, no difference in cell
surface antigen expression has been described between these
2 cell types.

In the present paper, we examine a membrane phenotype
of fetal neuroblasts in the adrenal gland, and compare this
with that of NB cells, using a panel of 18 monoclonal
antibodies (MoAbs) including our recently developed MoAbs;
KP-NAC2, KP-NAC8, KP-NAC9 and KP-NAC10, raised against a
human NB cell line. We characterize these MoAbs and
demonstrate an immunological distinction between NB cells
and normal fetal neuroblasts.

MATERIALS AND METHODS

Cell Lines. Human tumor cell lines used in this study consisted of 17 NB lines, 25 other solid tumor lines, and 14 leukemic lines. These lines were grown in RPMI1640 with 10% heat-inactivated fetal calf serum ( Microbiological Association Bioproducts, Walkersville, MD ) containing penicillin (100 units/ml), streptomycin(100 µg/ml), and glutamine(2mM).

MoAbs. Eighteen MoAbs were used in this study; KP-NAC2, KP-NAC8 (Matsumura et al 1987), KP-NAC9, KP-NAC10, PI153/3 (Kennett et al 1979), HSAN1.2 (Reynolds et al 1980), UJ127: 11 (Kemshead et al 1983), UJ13A (Allan et al 1983), A2B5 (Eisenbarth et al 1979), ME20.4 (Ross et al 1984), anti-Thy-1 (Kemshead et al 1983), BA-1 (Abramson et al 1981), BA-2 (Kersey et al 1981), Leu-7 (Abo et al 1981), J5 (Ritz et al 1980), OKIa-1 (Reinherz et al 1979), W6/32 (Barnstable et al 1978) and Genox3.53 (Brodsky et al 1980).

Normal and Neoplastic Samples. Normal and neoplastic samples were obtained from biopsy, surgery and autopsy specimens. Tissue specimens were either frozen or minced to give single cell suspensions. Tissues for sectioning were rapidly frozen in OCT compound(Lab-Tek Products, Naperville, IL), and stored at -80°C. For single cell suspensions, tissues were minced in a stainless steel mesh and the viable cell-rich fraction was isolated by centrifugation on a Ficoll-Hypaque gradient. Mononuclear cells in either peripheral blood or bone marrow blood were prepared by gradient centrifugation. Granulocytes were obtained by a hemolytic method with $NH_4Cl$.

Immunization and Cell Fusion. 8-week-old BALB/c mice were immunized at 2-week intervals by 3 intraperitoneal injections of $1 \times 10^7$ KP-N-RT(BM) human NB cells (Sugimoto et al 1986). Three days after the final injection, the splenocytes were prepared for fusion with P3X63-Ag8.653. mouse myeloma cells (Kohler, Milstein 1975). Hybrids were selected in hypoxanthine-aminopterin-thymidine-supplemented RPMI1640 medium. Culture supernatants were screened for the presence of antibodies to KP-N-RT(BM) cells by indirect immunofluorescence. The selected hybrids were cloned by limiting dilution and their supernatants were screened for binding to NB lines, other tumor lines, fresh tumor samples, and normal cells and tissues.

Ascites Preparation. BALB/c mice were primed with 2,6, 10,14-tetramethylpentadecane ( Sigma Chemical Co., St.Louis, Mo). After 2-3 weeks, they were inoculated with $1x10^7$ hybrids. Ascitic fluid containing 0.1% sodium azide was preserved at -80°C.

Immunoglobulin Isotype. The immunoglobulin isotype of MoAb was determined by double immunodiffusion. The supernatant of the hybrid was concentrated 10-20 fold by ultrafiltration and was reacted with class specific goat anti-mouse IgG1, IgG2a, IgG2b, IgA, and IgM ( Miles Laboratories Inc., Naperville,IL ).

Indirect Immunofluorescence. For cell suspensions, cells were stained as described previously (Sugimoto et al 1984) and were observed under a BH2-RHK UV microscope (Olympus, Tokyo, Japan ). If more than 10% of all cells were stained, the reactivity was determined as positive. For frozen sections, the procedure was identical to the immunoperoxidase technique described below, except that fluorescein-labeled goat anti-mouse Ig ( Cappel ) was used as a second reagent.

Immunoperoxidase Staining. Frozen specimens in OCT compound were sectioned to 4-6μm in thickness and air-dried. Unfixed sections were incubated with horse serum to block non-specific protein binding. Sections were incubated with MoAbs, biotinylated horse anti-mouse IgG ( Vector Lab., Burlingame, CA ), and avidin-biotin-conjugated horseradish peroxidase (Vector Lab.); each step taking 30 min. Antibody binding was visualized with diaminobenzidine ( Wako Pure Chemicals, Osaka, Japan ) and $0.01\%H_2O_2$ in 0.05M Tris-HCl buffer.

Immunoprecipitation and SDS-PAGE. Immunoprecipitation was carried out as described previously (Sugimoto et al 1985). In brief, $3x10^6$ KP-N-RT(BM) cells were radiolabeled either externally with $Na^{125}I$ (New England Nuclear, Boston, MA) using 1,3,4,6-tetrachloro-3 $\alpha$-6$\alpha$ -diphenyl-glycouril (Iodo-Gen; Pierce Chemical Co., Rockford, IL), or internally with $^{35}S$-methionine (Amersham International plc Buckingham-shire, England ). Radiolabeled cells were solubilized with 2% Triton X, and the cell membrane extract was preabsorbed with fixed heat-killed Cowman I strain Staphyloccocus aureus ( Immunosorbin ; Wako ). The extract was immunoprecipitated with ascites-formed MoAb bound to Immunosorbin and the

immunoprecipitate was disrupted by boiling in electrophoresis buffer for 2 min. Radiolabeled proteins were
separated by SDS-PAGE (10% Gel). The gel was dried and autoradiographed on Kodak XAR5-X ray film.


RESULTS

Hybrids and MoAbs.    Nine hybrids were selected on the
basis of producing antibody bound to the KP-N-RT(BM) NB cell
line as determined by indirect immunofluorescence. After
screening, KP-NAC2, KP-NAC8, KP-NAC9, and KP-NAC10 were
chosen for further studies due to their apparent unique
reactivities. They were cloned by limiting dilution, and
characterized. The immunoglobulin isotypes produced by KP-
NAC2, KP-NAC8, KP-NAC9 and KP-NAC10 were determined by
immunodiffusion as IgM, IgG1, IgM and IgG3, respectively.

Characterization of Antigen. Immunoprecipitation and
SDS-PAGE demonstrated that KP-NAC2 and KP-NAC8 antibodies
bind to a Mr 66,000-68,000 and a Mr 200,000 cell surface
protein on NB cells, respectively (Fig.1). The antigens
detected by KP-NAC9 and KP-NAC10 have not yet been
characterized by these methods, and are undergoing further
analysis.

Reactivity to Human Tumor Cell Lines and Fresh tumor
Samples. Either KP-NAC2, KP-NAC8, KP-NAC9, or KP-NAC10 bound
to 14/15, 13/15, 14/15, or 13/15 NB; 1/4, 1/4, 2/4, or 0/4
rhabdomyosarcoma; 0/4, 0/4, 2/4, or 0/4 Wilms' tumor; 0/2,
1/2, 2/2, or 0/2 Ewing's sarcoma; 2/2, 0/2, 1/2, or 0/2
retinoblastoma; 3/4, 0/4, 2/4, or 0/4 glioma; 2/4, 1/4, 1/4,
or 0/4 melanoma; 2/15, 2/15, 2/15, or 8/15 leukemia cell
lines, respectively (Fig.2). Some quantitative differences
in staining among positive lines were observed. With regard
to fresh tumor samples, they all reacted with 12/12 NB, 2/2
ganglioneuroblastoma (GNB) tumor samples, and 12/12
preparation of tumor cells in bone marrow of patients with
NB or GNB (Fig.3). Ganglion cells in GNB and ganglioneuroma
(GN) tissues were reactive to KP-NAC2, KP-NAC8 and KP-NAC9.
In these instances, cytoplasmic staining was observed in
KP-NAC2 and KP-NAC8 (Fig.4). In contrast, Schwann cells in
GN tissues were reactive only to KP-NAC9. In addition, they
reacted with either 4/6, 4/6, 5/6, or 6/6 pheochromocytoma
samples, respectively. However, they did not react with
either of 2 adrenocortical adenomas. KP-NAC10 bound to 32 of

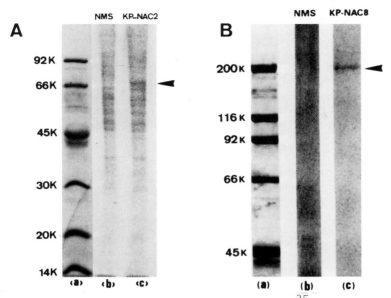

Fig.1. Autoradiography of SDS-PAGE of (A) $^{35}$S-methionine and (B) Na$^{125}$I labeled proteins from KP-N-RT(BM) cells. Cell membrane lysate was immunoprecipitated with normal mouse serum (NMS) (lane b) and KP-NAC2 or KP-NAC8 ascitic fluid (lane c). Lane (a) represents migration of standard proteins. Arrow beside lane (c) points to the Mr 66,000-68,000 (A) or Mr 200,000 (B) band specifically immuno-precipitated by KP-NAC2 or KP-NAC8.

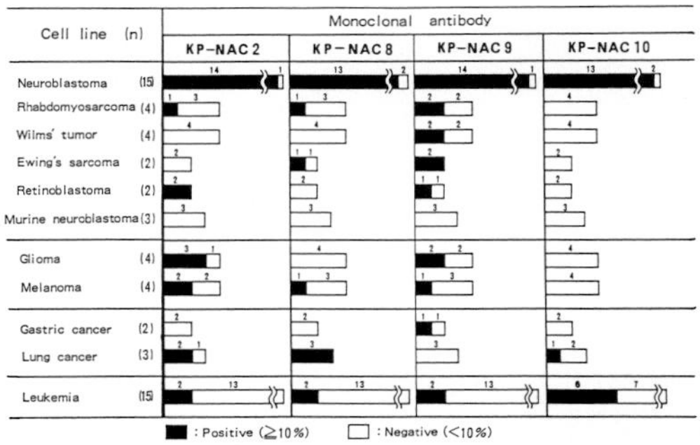

Fig.2. Reactivity of monoclonal antibodies to human tumor cell lines. Bars represent a number of cell lines tested ; closed bars indicate positive (% of stained cells>10%) and open bars indicate negative (% of stained cells<10%) lines by indirect immunofluorescence.

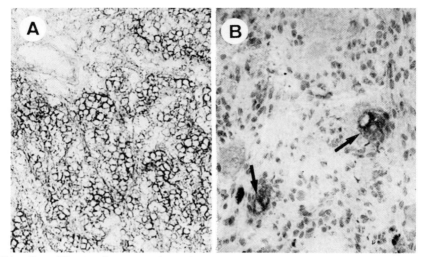

Fig.3. Photomicrograph of immunoperoxidase staining of neuroblastoma (A), and ganglioneuroma (B) tissue. Neuroblastoma cells were stained with KP-NAC8 (A). Ganglion cells (➡) showed cytoplasmic staining with KP-NAC2 (B). Counter stain used (B) was Mayer Hematoxylin. x100.

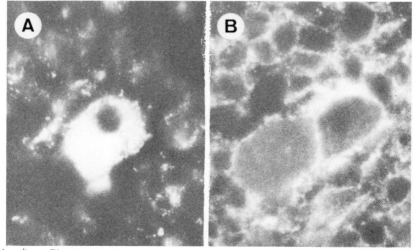

Fig.4. Photomicrograph of indirect immunofluorescence of ganglioneuroblastoma tissue. Ganglion cells showed cytoplasmic staining with KP-NAC8 (A), and surface staining with KP-NAC9 (B). Sorrounding neuroblastoma cells were also stained with KP-NAC8 (weakly) and KP-NAC9 (strongly). x400.

45 leukemia samples, all with a subtype of common ALL
(Fig.5).

    Reactivity to Normal Human Cells and Fetal Tissues. In
each of the MoAbs, cross-reactions were observed on some
normal cells (Fig.6) and fetal tissues (Fig.7). Notably,
among fetal tissues neuroblast nodules in the adrenal gland
were reactive to all 3 MoAbs but not KP-NAC8. KP-NAC8 did
not react with adrenal neuroblasts of all 5 fetuses from 12
to 21 gestational weeks. This MoAb did react with ganglion
cells but not with Schwann cells in the sympathetic
ganglion (Fig.7).

    Membrane Phenotype of Fetal Adrenal Neuroblasts and NB
cells. By using a panel of 18 MoAbs, we examined 5 fetal
adrenal glands at 12 - 21 gestational weeks and 14 NB and
GNB tissues with indirect immunofluorescence and/or immunoperoxidase staining, Fetal adrenal neuroblasts of all
samples were reactive to KP-NAC2, KP-NAC9, KP-NAC10,
PI153/3, HSAN1.2, UJ127: 11, UJ13A, A2B5, ME20.4, anti-Thy-1,
BA-1, BA-2, and Leu-7. No binding to KP-NAC8, J5, OKIa-1,
W6/32, and Genox3.53 was observed (Fig.8). While NB cells
also did not bind to J5, OKIa-1, W6/32, and Genox3.53, they
did react with all the other "anti-NB" antibodies including
KP-NAC8 (Fig.9). There were also some quantitative
differences in positive stainings.


DISCUSSION

    In this study, we reported our recently developed MoAbs
raised against a human NB cell line. These MoAbs, as well as
other MoAbs already described, are not specific for NB, and
cross-react with other tumors, normal cells, and fetal
tissues. However, the individual chracter of each MoAb was
revealed by its reactivity pattern. As KP-NAC2 bound to
several neuroectodermally derived tumors and tissues, it
might detect a neuroectodermal-related antigen (Mr 66,000-
68,000). KP-NAC8 was different from the other 3 MoAbs by the
binding to NB cells but not to fetal neuroblasts. The
antigen defined by KP-NAC8 (Mr 200,000) might be related
with either tumorigenesis or differentiation of NB cells.
KP-NAC9 revealed various cross-reactivities being identical
with those of anti-Thy-1 and ab390 antibody (Seeger et al
1982) in comparative studies (data not shown), and was
considered to detect a Thy-1 like-antigen. Alternatively,

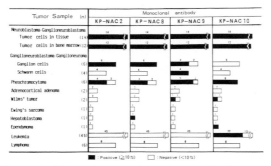

Fig.5. Reactivity of monoclonal antibodies to fresh tumor samples. Bars represent a number of samples ; closed bars indicate positive and open bars indicate negative binding as determined by indirect immunofluorescence and/or immunoperoxidase staining.

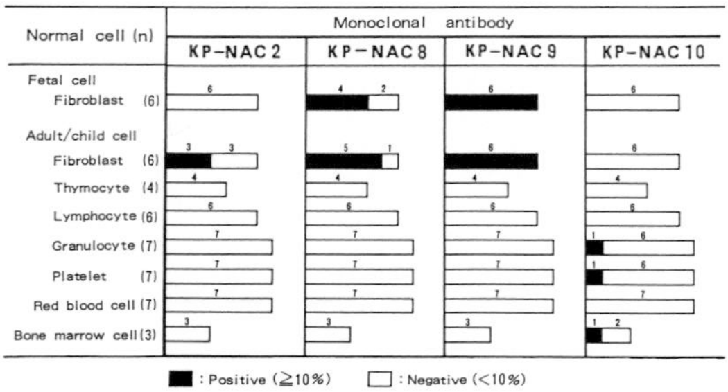

Fig.6. Reactivity of monoclonal antibodies to normal cells.

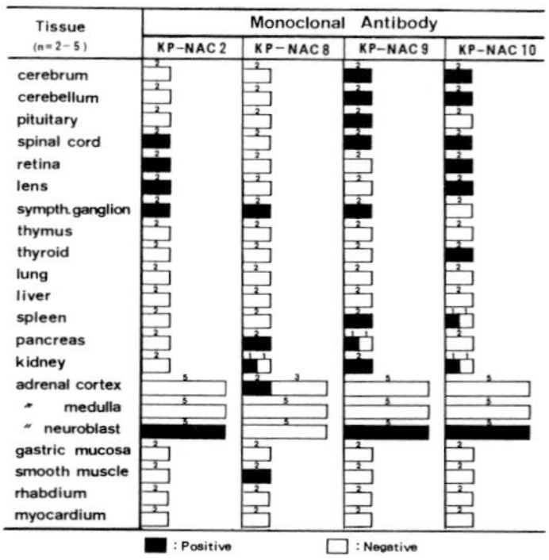

Fig.7. Reactivity of monoclonal antibodies to fetal tissues.

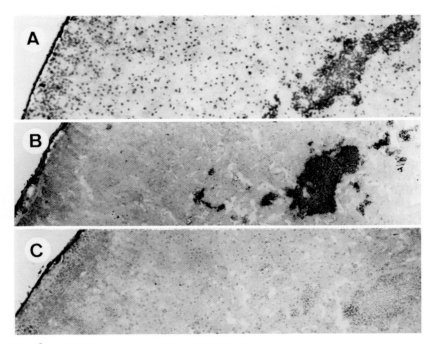

Fig.8. Photomicrographs of fetal neuroblasts nodule in the adrenal gland. (A) : Wright-Giemsa staining, (B) and (C) : immunoperoxidase staining with UJ13A (B) and KP-NAC8 (C). Fetal neuroblasts were stained with UJ13A but not with KP-NAC8. Both reagents were reactive weakly (KP-NAC8) or moderately (UJ13A) to the adrenal cortex. Counterstain used was methylgreen. x40.

| Monoclonal Antibody | Neuroblastoma Cells (n=14) Stage I—IVs | Fetal Neuroblasts (n=5) 12—21 th Week of Gestation |
|---|:---:|:---:|
| KP-NAC2 | ● | ● |
| KP-NAC8 | ● | ○ |
| KP-NAC9 | ● | ● |
| KP-NAC10 | ● | ● |
| PI153/3 | ● | ● |
| HSAN1.2 | ● | ● |
| UJ127:11 | ● | ● |
| UJ13A | ● | ● |
| A2B5 | ● | ● |
| ME20.4 | ● | ● |
| anti-Thy-1 | ● | ● |
| BA-1 | ● | ● |
| BA-2 | ● | ● |
| Leu-7 | ● | ● |
| J-5 | ○ | ○ |
| OKIa-1 | ○ | ○ |
| W6/32 | ○ | ○ |
| Genox3.53 | ○ | ○ |

● : positive    ○ : negative

Fig.9. Membrane phenotypes of neuroblastoma cells and fetal neuroblasts. Closed circles indicate positive and open circles indicate negative binding as determined by indirect immunofluorescence and/or immunoperoxidase staining.

KP-NAC10 cross-reacted with all fresh common ALL cells, as PI153/3 already described (Greaves et al 1980), and could detect a NB and common ALL-related antigen. The present results suggested that each of our developed MoAbs was not NB-specific in a strict sense, but a panel of these 4 MoAbs made it possible to distinguish NB cells from other tumor cells. Furthermore, these MoAbs should contribute to a greater understanding of the biology of NB.

In a further study, membrane phenotypes of NB cells and fetal neuroblasts were analyzed using a panel of 18 MoAbs. The comparison of the binding of MoAbs revealed that antibodies KP-NAC2, KP-NAC9, KP-NAC10, PI153/3, HSAN1.2, UJ127:11, UJ13A, A2B5, ME20.4, anti-Thy-1, BA-1, BA-2, and Leu-7 bound to both NB cells and fetal neuroblasts. Antibodies J5, OKIa-1 W6/32, and Genox3.53 did not bind to either cells. The only MoAb that could distinguish fetal neuroblasts from NB cells was KP-NAC8. The specificity of KP-NAC8 binding to NB cells but not to fetal neuroblasts should yield further information on the biological differences between NB cells and fetal neuroblasts.

NB is thought to arise from neuroblasts that have failed to undergo normal differentiation. In normal fetal development, a nodular collection of neuroblasts ( a neuroblasts nodule ) is found in the adrenal gland after the 7th week of gestation, which terminaly differentiates to chromaffin cells and disappears before full term gestation (Ikeda et al 1981; Machin 1982). Such microscopic nodules are found incidentally in the adrenal glands of autopsied infants, and are termed as NB *in situ* (Beckwith et al 1963). However, it is difficult to distinguish normal fetal neuroblasts from NB cells. Some differential features based on histopathological studies, have been described in the literature (Ikeda et al 1981; Machin 1982). Ikeda et al (1981) reported that the nuclear size of a NB cell was significantly larger (6.2±1.0 μm) than that of a fetal neuroblast (4.25±0.84 μm), and they emphasized that measurement of nuclear size might be a way of distinguishing malignant NB cells from normal fetal neuroblasts. There has, however, been no description based on immunological studies. Our report is, to the best of our knowledge, the first description of an antigen and a MoAb that can distinguish fetal neuroblasts from NB cells.

The present study demonstrates that the normal fetal

neuroblasts have a membrane phenotype different from the NB cells, and that this difference could be determined only by a different binding to KP-NAC8. As the antigen defined by KP-NAC8 is present on neoplastic neuroblasts but not on normal fetal neuroblasts, it is possible that the antigen might be the differentiation-related antigen selectively expressed on NB cells. In addition, since the antigen is present on ganglion cells but not on Schwann cells in GN tissue and fetal sympathetic ganglion, it might be related to the direction of differentiation of neuroblasts to ganglion cells. Thus, it would be very interesting to investigate this antigen expression on NB cells at various differentiation stages or clinical stages. In this regard, we are now investigating the expression of KP-NAC8 defined antigen on NB samples at various clinical stages and on NB cells chemically induced to differentiate in vitro.


ACKNOWLEDGMENTS

We gratefully thank Dr. T Amagai and Dr. S Negoro for supporting this study. We are very indebted to Dr. AA Green, Dr. L Helson, Dr. J Minowada, Dr. CP Reynolds, Dr. RC Seeger, Dr. K Sagawa, Dr. TJ Triche, Dr. AH Ross, and Dr. H Koprowski for kindly providing either cell lines or monoclonal antibodies, and to Dr. S Imashuku and many colleagues for providing clinical materials.

This work was supported in part by grants for cancer research from the Ministry of Health and Welfare, and from the Ministry of Education ( No.59480236) of Japan.


REFERENCES

Abo T, Balch CM (1981). A differentiation antigen of human NK and K cells identified by a monoclonal antibody (HNK-1) J Immunol 127: 1024-1029.
Abramson CS, Kersey JH, LeBien TW (1981). A monoclonal antibody (BA-1) reactive with cells of human B lymphocyte lineage. J Immunol 126: 83-88.
Allan PA, Garson JA, Harper EI, Asser U, Coakham HB, Brownell B, Kemshead JT (1983). Biological characterization and clinical application of a monoclonal antibody recognizing an antigen restricted to neuroectodermal

tissue. Int J Cancer 31: 591-598.

Barnstable CJ, Bodmer WF, Brown G, Galfre G, Milstein C, Williams AF, Ziegler A (1978). Production of monoclonal antibodies to group A erythrocytes, HLA and other human cell surface antigens - New tool for genetic analysis. Cell 14: 9-29.

Beckwith JB, Perrin EV (1963). *In situ* neuroblastoma : A contribution to the neural history of neural crest tumors. Am J Path 43: 1089-1104.

Brodsky FM, Parham P, Bodmer WF (1980). Monoclonal antibodies to HLA-DRw determinants. Tissue Antigens 16: 30-48.

Eisenbarth GS, Walsh FS, Nierenberg M (1979). Monoclonal antibody to plasma membrane antigen of neurons. Proc Natl Acad Sci USA 76: 4913-4917.

Greaves MF, Verbi W, Kemshead JT, Kennett RH (1980). A monoclonal antibody identifying a cell surface antigen shared by common acute lymphoblastic leukemia and B cell lineage cells. Blood 56: 1141-1144.

Ikeda Y, Lister J, Bouton JM, Buyukpamukcu M (1981). Congenital neuroblastoma, neuroblastoma *in situ*, and the normal fetal development of the adrenal. J Pediatr Surg 16: 636-644.

Kemshead JT, Goldman A, Fritschy J, Malpas JS, Prithard J (1983). Use o f panels of monoclonal antibodies in the differential diagnosis of neuroblastoma and lymphoblastic disorders. Lancet 1: 12-15.

Kemshead JT, Fritschy J, Garson JA, Allan P, Coakham H, Brown S, Asser U (1983). Monoclonal antibody UJ127: 11 detects a 220,000-240,000 kda. glycoprotein present on a subset of neuroectodermally derived cells. Int J Cancer 31: 187-195.

Kennett RH, Gilbert F (1979). Hybrid myeloma producing antibodies against a human neuroblastoma antigen present on fetal brain. Science (Wash DC) 203: 1120-1121.

Kersey JH, LeBien TW, Abramson CS, Newman R, Sutherland R, Greaves M (1981). p24 : a human leukemia associated and lymphohemopoietic progenitor cell surface structure identified with monoclonal antibody. J Exp Med 153: 726-731.

Kohler G, Milstein C (1975). Continuous cultures of fused cells secreting antibody of predefined specificity. Nature (London) 256: 495-497.

Machin GA (1982). Histogenesis and histopathology of neuroblastoma. In Pochedly C (ed): "Neuroblastoma, Clinical and Biological Manifestations." New York : Elsevier Science

Publishirg Company Inc, pp195-231.

Matsumura T, Sugimoto T, Sawada T, Amagai T, Negoro S, Kemshead JT (1987). Cell surface membrane antigen present on neuroblastoma cells but not feta l neuroblasts recognized by a monoclonal antibody (KP-NAC8). Cancer Res. (in press).

Reinherz EL, Kung PC, Pesando JM, Ritz J, Goldstein G, Schlossman SF (1979). Ia determinant on human T-cell subsets defined by monoclonal antibody. Activation stimuli required for expression. J Exp Med 150: 1472-1482.

Reynolds CP, Smith RG (1980). A sensitive immunoassay for human neuroblastoma cells. In Mitchell MS, Oettgen HF (eds) : "Hybridoma in Cancer Diagnosis and Treatment." New York : Raven Press, pp235-240.

Ritz J, Pesando JM, Notis-McConary J, Lazarus H, Schlossmann SF (1980). A monoclonal antibody to human lymphoblastic leukemia antigen. Nature (London) 283: 583-585.

Ross AH, Grob P, Bothwell M, Elder DE, Ernst CS, Marano L, Ghrist BFO, Slemp CC, Herlyn N, Atkinson BF, Koprowski H (1984). Characterization of nerve growth factor in neural crest tumors using monoclonal antibodies. Proc Natl Acad Sci USA 81: 6681-6685.

Seeger RC, Danon YL, Rayner SA, Hoover F (1982). Definition of a Thy-1 determinant on human neuroblastoma, glioma, sarcoma and teratoma cells with a monoclonal antibody. J Immunol 128: 983-989.

Sugimoto T, Sawada T, Matsumura T, Kemshead JT, Ishii T, Horii Y, Morioka H, Morita M, Reynolds CP (1986). Identical expression of cell surface membrane antigens on 2 parent and 18 clone cell lines derived from 2 different neuroblastoma metastases of the same patient. Cancer Res 46: 4765-4769.

Sugimoto T, Sawada T, Negoro S, Kidowaki T, Morioka H, Matsumura T, Kemshead JT, Seeger RC (1985). Altered expression of cell surface membrane antigens in a common acute lymphoblastic leukemia antigen-expressing neuro-blastoma cell line (SJ-N-CG) with morphological differentiation. Cancer Res 45: 358-364.

Sugimoto T, Tatsumi E, Kemshead JT, Helson L, Green AA, Minowada J (1984). Determination of cell surface membrane antigens common to both human neuroblastoma and leukemia-lymphoma cell lines by a panel of 38 monoclonal antibodies J Natl Cancer Inst 73: 51-57.

Advances in Neuroblastoma Research 2, pages 409–420
© 1988 Alan R. Liss, Inc.

BIOLOGICAL SIGNIFICANCE OF HLA-A,B,C EXPRESSION IN NEUROB-
LASTOMA AND RELATED CELL LINES

Lois A Lampson*

Children's Cancer Research Center,
Children's Hospital of Philadelphia
Philadelphia PA 19104

INTRODUCTION

It is well-established that neuroblastoma cell lines
express HLA-A,B,C weakly as compared to other cell types
(Lampson et al., '83). Yet, the molecules are under
regulatory control. HLA-A,B,C can be induced in
neuroblastoma cell lines by interferon (Lampson and Fisher, '84). The induced molecules correspond to their counterparts on control lymphoid cells in a variety of assays
(fig. 1), and express appropriate polymorphic specificities (Lampson and George, '86). In addition, HLA-A,B,C is
expressed without intentional induction in CHP-100 and
other cell lines derived from peripheral neuroectodermal
tumors (PNET) (Donner et al., '85; Lampson and George,
'86; Lampson et al. '85; Reynolds et al., '87). These tumors are closely related to neuroblastoma and, like it,
are of neural crest origin (Whang-Peng et al., '86).

Our aim has been to determine the biological significance of HLA-A,B,C modulation in these cells. First, we
have asked whether the level of HLA-A,B,C expression is
correlated with prognosis. Second, we have asked whether
increased HLA-A,B,C expression is associated with a
particular stage of differentiation of normal neurons.

Based on the evidence presented, increased HLA-A,B,C
expression does not appear to reflect direct immunological
activity, or correlate with prognosis. Nor does it appear
to reflect any stage of differentiation within the neuronal lineage. Rather, the potential for increased HLA-
A,B,C expression may reflect the cells' potential for differentiation towards a non-neuronal phenotype.

*Present address: Dr. Lois Lampson, Center for Neurologic
Diseases, Biosciences Research Building, Brigham and Wom-
en's Hospital, Boston MA 02115.

MATERIALS AND METHODS.

These are described in previous publications, as indicated
in the text.

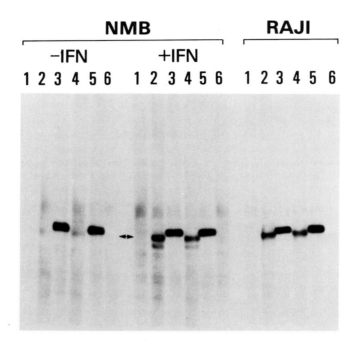

Figure 1.    Although HLA-A,B,C molecules are weakly expressed on neuroblastoma cell lines, greater expression
can be induced by interferon.    The neuroblastoma line NMB
was grown in the presence, or the absence, of gamma-interferon.    Extracts were analyzed with monoclonal antibodies
in the immunoblot assay.    Antibodies directed against the
HLA chain (lanes 2 and 4) and against actin (lanes 3 and
5), and negative controls (lanes 1 and 6) were used.  Extract from a control B cell line, RAJI, is included.    The
figure shows the increase in the HLA chain of the neuroblastoma line after interferon treatment, as compared to
the untreated control.    Detailed methods are given in
Lampson and Fisher, '84.    Additional characterization of
the induced proteins is found in Lampson and George, '86.

RESULTS

Is HLA-A,B,C Expression Correlated with Prognosis in Neuroblastoma?

In microscopic assays, HLA-A,B,C was not detected in any stage of neuroblastoma (fig. 2), including the form with a high rate of spontaneous remission, stage IV-S (Whelan et al., '85). The same lack of expression is seen in neuroblastoma-derived cell lines (Lampson et al., '83; Lampson and George, '86). These lines are derived from the most aggressive forms of the tumor, stages III and IV.

Higher levels of HLA-A,B,C are characteristic of cell lines derived from related tumors of neural crest origin. These include CHP-100 (Lampson and George, '86; Lampson et al., '85), and other lines derived from peripheral neuroectodermal tumors (PNET) (Donner et al, '85; Reynolds et al., '87). Yet these other neural crest tumors can be just as aggressive as the HLA-A,B,C-negative neuroblastomas (Whang-Peng et al., '86).

Thus, within this group of tumors, the level of HLA-A,B,C expression and prognosis appear to be independent variables. The characteristic levels of expression (low for neuroblastoma, higher for PNET) are seen in cell lines in culture, in the absence of lymphoid cells or other cell types. Thus, the levels appear to reflect intrinsic properties of the tumor or its cell of origin, rather than the direct influence of immunological activity. This led us to ask whether strong HLA-A,B,C expression might be characteristic of a particular point in the differentiation of normal neural cells.

Is Increased HLA-A,B,C Expression Associated with Any Stage of Differentiation of Normal Neurons?

Differentiating neural tissue was examined in microscopic assays, in the mouse. The expression of b2-microglobulin (b2-m), the invariant light chain of all H-2 molecules and their structural analogs, was examined. (H-2 is the murine counterpart of HLA-A,B,C.)

Regenerating neural tissue in the adult. The first developing neural tissue studied was the olfactory epithelium. This specialized neuroepithelium regenerates continuously, even in the adult. The tissue is organized into ordered layers of dividing neurons, maturing neurons,

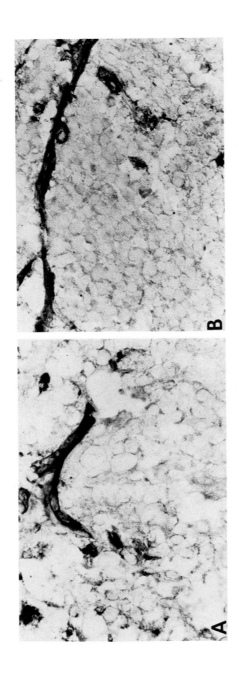

Figure 2. HLA-A,B,C is not detected in any stage of neuroblastoma in situ. Monoclonal antibodies were used to define HLA-A,B,C expression in the avidin-biotin complex (ABC) assay. This figure shows reactivity of an antiserum to b2-microglobulin, the invariant light chain of all HLA-A,B,C molecules. Frozen sections of a stage II neuroblastoma (A), and a stage IV neuroblastoma (B) are shown. Both tumors show strong antigen activity in the blood vessel walls. The tumor cells themselves are negative. Results with additional neuroblastomas and additional antibodies, and detailed methods, appear in Whelan et al, '85.

and sustentacular or supporting cells. Degenerating neurons are also present, although these cannot be identified
by location alone.

In the microscopic assay, b2-microglobulin was detected in oral and respiratory epithelium and connective
tissue, as expected. Yet b2-m was not detected in any
cell or layer of the olfactory epithelium, or the related
vomeronasal organ. Thus, increased b2-m expression was
not associated with any stage of cell death or differentiation in this special case (Whelan et al., '86b).

Neural tissue in the developing embryo. We next
examined differentiating neural tissue in the developing
mouse. Embryos were examined from gestation day 7, when
only two germ layers are present, until gestation day 14,
when the brain has begun to form. The distribution of b2-
m was determined in the microscopic assay as described
above.

In these studies, no b2-m was detected in any neural
cell of the developing neural plate, neural tube, neural
crest, spinal cord, spinal ganglia, or developing brain.
At the same time, b2-m was detected in expected non-neural
structures, including the connective tissue surrounding
the neural tube (Lampson and Whelan, '87).

Normal adult neural tissue. Preparations of adult
tissue included frozen human brain biopsies that had been
removed during therapeutic procedures, and frozen sections
of normal mouse brain. Well-fixed sections of mouse brain
from animals that had been perfused through the heart with
4% parformaldehyde/sucrose/picrate fixative were also
studied.

All of these preparations gave comparable results.
Strong expression of b2-m and, in the human tissue, HLA-
A,B,C, was detected in blood vessels within the brain, as
well as in control lymphoid tissue. Yet these antigens
were not detected in neurons, astrocytes, oligodendrocytes, or microglia in the adult brain (Lampson and
Hickey, '86; Whelan et al., '86a).

Neuroblastoma cells in tissue culture. Neuroblastoma
cell lines can assume a variety of morphological forms in
tissue culture. The cells round up during harvesting or
cell division. After a few days in culture, elongating
cells with extended processes, and also flattened cells
with fibroblast-like morphology are seen. These cultures

provide a context for examining individual cells and contacts, as a complement to the work in complex tissue.

In microscopic assays, HLA-A,B,C is not detected on most neuroblastoma cells in culture. HLA-A,B,C can be increased in neuroblastoma cell lines by adding interferon (Lampson and Fisher, '84). There also appears to be a slow rate of spontaneous modulation in the control cultures. For example, in the neuroblastoma line IMR-5, a small subpopulation (less than 1% of the cells) is b2-m and HLA-A,B,C positive even without interferon addition (fig. 3). In some cases, positive and negative cells with the appearance of mitotic sisters are seen, indicating that this is a regulatory subpopulation rather than a contaminating cell type.

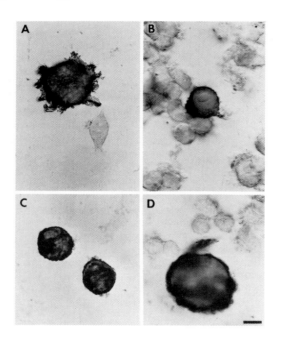

Figure 3. Some HLA-A,B,C positive cells are seen in neuroblastoma cell lines in culture. IMR-5 cells were fixed as they grew on glass coverslips, and assayed for b2-microglobulin in the peroxidase-anti-peroxidase (PAP) assay (Lampson and Siegel, '87). As the figure shows, some of the cells (less than 1%) were positive.

studies with monoclonal antibodies, In Kennett RH, Bechtol KB, McKearn TJ (eds): "Monoclonal Antibodies and Functional Cell Lines," New York: Plenum, pp 153-189.

Lampson LA (1987). Molecular bases of the immune response to neural antigens. Trends in NeuroSci 10:211-16.

Lampson LA, Fisher CA (1984). Weak HLA and b2-m expression of neuronal cell lines can be modulated by interferon. Proc Natl Acad Sci 81:6476-6480.

Lampson LA, George DL (1986). Interferon-mediated induction of class I MHC products in human neuronal cell lines: Analysis of HLA and b2-m RNA, and HLA-A and HLA-B proteins and polymorphic specificities. J Interferon Res 6:257-265.

Lampson LA, Hickey WF (1986). Monoclonal antibody analysis of MHC expression in human brain biopsies: Tissue ranging from "histologically normal" to that showing different levels of glial tumor involvement. J Immunol 136: 4054-4062.

Lampson LA, Whelan JP (1987). A role for the major histocompatibility complex in normal differentiation of non-lymphoid tissues. 19th Miami Winter Symposium: The Molecular Biology of Development. ICSU Short Reports (Cambridge University Press) 7:125.

Lampson LA, Siegel G (1987). Defining the mechanisms that govern immune acceptance or rejection of neural transplants. Progress in Brain Res: Transplantation into the Mammalian CNS, in press.

Lampson LA, Fisher CA, Whelan JP (1983). Striking paucity of HLA-A,B,C and b2-microglobulin on human neuroblastoma cell lines. J Immunol 130:2471-2478.

Lampson LA, Fisher CA, Whelan JP (1985). HLA-A,B,C and b2-microglobulin are expressed weakly by human cells of neuronal origin, but can be induced in neuroblastoma cell lines by interferon. Prog Clin Biol Res 175:379-388.

LeDouarin N (1980). Migration and diffrentiation of neural crest cells. Curr Top Dev Biol 16:31-85.

Main EK, Lampson LA, Hart MK, Kornbluth J, Wilson DB (1985). Human neuroblastoma cell lines are susceptible to lysis by natural killer cells but not by cytotoxic T lymphocytes. J Immunol 135:242-246.

Reynolds CP, Maples (1985). Modulation of cell surface antigens accompanies morphological differentiation of human neuroblastoma cell lines. Prog Clin Biol Res 175: 13-37.

Reynolds CP, Brodeur GM, Tomayko MM, Donner L, Helson, L, Seeger, RC, Triche, TJ (1987). Biological classification of cell lines derived from human extra-cranial neural tumors. THIS VOLUME.

Ross RA, Biedler JL (1985). Expression of a melanocyte phenotype in human neuroblastoma cells in vitro. Prog Clin Biol Res 175:249-259.

Ruiter, DJ, Bhan, AK, Harrist, TJ, Sober, AJ, Mihm, MC (1982). Major histocompatibility antigens and mononuclear inflammatory infiltrate in benign nevomelanocytic proliferations and malignant melanoma. J. Immunol. 129: 2808-2815.

Tsokos M, Ross, RA, Triche TJ (1985). Neuronal, Schwannian and melanocytic differentiation of human neuroblastoma cells in vitro. Prog. Clin. Biol. Res. 175: 55-68.

Whang-Peng J, Triche TJ, Knutsen T, Miser J, Kao-Shan S, Tsai S, Israel MA (1986). Cytogenetic characterization of selected small round cell tumors of childhood. Cancer Genet Cytogenet 21:185-208.

Whelan JP, Chatten J, Lampson LA (1985). HLA-A,B,C and b2-microglobulin expression in frozen and formaldehyde-fixed paraffin sections of neuroblastoma tumors. Cancer Res 45:5976-5983.

Whelan JP, Eriksson U, Lampson LA (1986a). Expression of mouse b2-microglobulin in frozen and formaldehyde-fixed central nervous tissues: Comparison of tissue behind the blood-brain barrier and tissue in a barrier-free region. J Immunol 137:2561-2566.

Whelan JP, Wysocki CJ, Lampson LA (1986b). Distribution of b2-microglobulin in olfactory epithelium: A proliferating neuroepithelium not protected by a blood-tissue barrier. J Immunol 137:2567-2571, 1986.

Advances in Neuroblastoma Research 2, pages 421–432

# MONOCLONAL ANTIBODIES AS PROBES FOR ß-D-$N$-ACETYLGLUCOS-AMINIDE α1→3FUCOSYLTRANSFERASE IN HUMAN NEUROBLASTOMA

Christopher S. Foster and Mary Catherine Glick

Joseph Stokes, Jr. Research Institute and Department of Pediatrics, University of Pennsylvania Medical School, Philadelphia, PA 19104

## INTRODUCTION

Neoplastic transformation is associated with a variety of changes in composition of cell surface carbohydrates, particularly asparagine-linked oligosaccharides (Glick et al, 1980). Fucosyl residues linked α1→3 to a branch $N$-acetylglucosamine (Fucα1→3GlcNAc) of glycoproteins or glycolipids are infrequently found in large amount in human tissues and their presence appears to be restricted to a small group of malignancies (Table 1). In human neuroblastoma, Fucα1→3GlcNAc is present on most size and charge classes of membrane glycoproteins (Santer and Glick, 1983). The presence of these specific fucosyl residues together with α1→3fucosyltransferase (Foster and Glick, 1987), the enzyme responsible for the transfer of the fucosyl residues, could represent markers for human neuroblastoma.

Fucosyltransferases comprise a diverse family of phylogenetically conserved enzymes which may be structurally related (Beyer et al, 1981). However, the characteristics of the enzymes differ in respect of fucose transfer to certain oligosaccharide substrates. For example, α1→3fucosyltransferase purified from human neuroblastoma has different substrate specificities when compared to the enzymes isolated from either human serum or from human milk (Table 2).The possibility exists, therefore, that neuroblastoma derived α1→3fucosyl-

Table 1. Expression of Fucα1→3GlcNAc in human tumors

| TUMOR | METHOD OF DETECTION | | |
|---|---|---|---|
| | α1→3FucT | α1→3 linkage | Antibody |
| NEUROBLASTOMA | | | |
| Cell lines | Foster and Glick, 1987 | Santer and Glick, 1980[a] <br> Santer et al, 1983[b] | Sakamoto et al, 1986 |
| Tumors | | Woodbury et al, 1986[a] | |
| RETINOBLASTOMA | | Santer and Glick, 1983[a] | |
| MEDULOBLASTOMA | | Santer and Glick, 1983[a] | |
| LUNG, Small cell | Holmes et al, 1985 | | Spitalnick et al,1986 <br> Sakamoto et al, 1986 |
| COLON | | Hakomori et al, 1984[b,c] | Lloyd et al, 1983 <br> Sakamoto et al, 1986 <br> Kim et al, 1986 |
| LEUKEMIA | | | |
| CGL | Johnson and Watkins, 1987 | | |
| CML | Suda et al, 1987 | | |
| T-cell | | Fukuda et al, 1986[c,d] | Sakamoto et al, 1986 |
| Erythro cell line | | | Fukuda, 1985 |
| Promyelo cell line | | Mizoguchi et al, 1984[c] | |

a) α-L-Fucosidase from almonds, specific for Fucα1→3(4)GlcNAc
b) 500-MHz $^{1}$H-NMR spectroscopy
c) Methylation
d) FAB-MS

Table 2.   Substrate requirements for α1→3fucosyl-
transferases

| Substrate | α1→3fucosyltransferases | | |
| | Human Neuroblastoma | Serum[a] | Milk[a] |
| 10 mM | Relative Activity (%) | | |
| --- | --- | --- | --- |
| Galß1→4GlcNAc | 100 | 100 | 100 |
| Galß1→3GlcNAc | 16 | 0 | 94 |
| NeuAcα2→3Galß1→4GlcNAc | NA | 170 | 106 |
| NeuAcα2→6Galß1→4GlcNAc | NA | 0 | 0 |
| Galß1→4Glc | 50 | 0 | 21 |
| NeuAcα2→3Galß1→4Glc | 0 | 3 | 30 |
| NeuAcα2→6Galß1→4Glc | 0 | 0 | 0 |
| Fucα1→2Galß1→4Glc | 15 | 1 | 74 |

a) Data from Johnson and Watkins, 1985
NA = substrate not available


transferase is intrinsically different from either of the
non tumor enzymes.

One approach to probing the specific α1→3 fucosyltransferase and investigating its role in the patho-
biology of human neuroblastoma is to generate monoclonal
antibodies in an attempt to identify a unique structural
portion of the protein. Such regions are likely to be
small and probably would not be identified by conventional
polyclonal antisera. Hitherto, no monoclonal antibodies to
α1→3fucosyltransferases from human tumors have been
reported.

Herein we describe the generation of a monoclonal
antibody to human neuroblastoma α1→3fucosyltransferase
and discuss some of the problems which may be encountered
in raising monoclonal antibodies to such enzymes.

## MATERIALS AND METHODS

*Generation of antibodies* - α1→3Fucosyltransferase was purified from human neuroblastoma cells, CHP 134 (Littauer et al, 1979) according to a recent protocol (Foster and Glick, 1987). Enzyme from three different stages of purification was employed to immunize female BALB/c mice prior to generating antibody-secreting lymphocyte hybridomas. The primary immunization was subcutaneously at multiple sites using partially purified enzyme in Freunds complete adjuvant. Thereafter, animals were boosted at 10-day intervals. On the first two occasions, a semi-purified enzyme preparation was administered intraperitoneally. Subsequently, the purified enzyme was presented as an immunogen conjugated either to Keyhole Limpet hemocyanin or to the random copolymer [D-Glu, D-Lys] using n-maleimidobenzoyl-N-hydroxy succinimide ester as coupling agent (Liu et al, 1979). Coupled enzyme was presented, intraperitoneally, on three occasions. Final immunization comprised daily intraperitoneal injections of coupled enzyme for the three days immediately prior to fusion.

Lymphocytes were prepared from the disaggregated spleen and were fused with cells of the mouse myeloma line SP-2 (Shulman et al, 1978) using poly(ethylene-glycol) according to conventional methods (Foster, 1982). The fused cells were plated in monolayer, without a feeder layer, and lymphocyte myeloma hybridomas were selectively grown using H-Y medium (Kennett et al, 1978).

*Assay for antibodies* - Mouse antibodies to the α1→3 fucosyltransferase preparation were detected in culture supernatants using a solid-phase assay (Tan et al, 1987). Hybridoma culture supernatants were incubated overnight in polystyrene centrifuge tubes precoated with donkey anti-(mouse Ig). The tubes were washed and incubated with $^{125}$I-labelled purified α1→3fucosyltransferase and bound radioactivity determined. Selected hybridomas generating monoclonal antibodies were subsequently grown as ascites fluids in Pristane-treated mice (Foster, 1982).

*Characterization of monoclonal antibodies* - The immunoglobulin class of the monoclonal antibodies contained in individual culture supernatants was

determined by immunodiffusion (Ouchterlony, 1962).
Antigens recognized by individual monoclonal antibodies
were identified by immunoprecipitation and Western blot
analysis. Each culture supernatant was incubated overnight
with $^{125}$I-labelled extract of CHP 134 cells.
Antigen-antibody complexes were precipitated with rabbit
anti-(mouse Ig) in the presence of poly-(ethylene glycol).
After washing, precipitated antigens were visualised by
autoradiography after electrophoresis on polyacrylamide
gels.

Proteins extracted from CHP 134 cells were examined
by Western blot techniques using culture supernatants or
ascites fluid of individual monoclonal antibodies. The
bound monoclonal antibodies were identified with rabbit
anti-(mouse Ig) conjugated to peroxidase and visualized
using diaminobenzidine.

The distribution of antigens identified by the
monoclonal antibodies within neuroblastoma cells was
examined by immunohistochemistry. Freshly-frozen sections
of human primary neuroblastomas were incubated with
undiluted tissue culture supernatants or with ascites
fluid of individual monoclonal antibodies. The bound
monoclonal antibodies were identified using biotin-
conjugated goat anti-(mouse Ig) and visualized with
streptavidin-Texas Red.

To immunoprecipitate enzyme activity, rabbit
anti-(mouse IgM) was conjugated to CNBr- activated
Sepharose 4B (Foster and Neville, 1987), and incubated
with monoclonal antibody ascites fluid. The immunoadsorbed
monoclonal antibodies were stabilized using
dimethylsuberimidate (Gersten and Marchalonis, 1978), and
then incubated with an extract of CHP 134 cells. After
centrifugation, the gels were assayed for $\alpha1\rightarrow3$fucosyl-
transferase using GDP-[$^{14}$C]fucose and Galß1$\rightarrow$4GlcNAc
(Foster and Glick, 1987). The reaction products were
analyzed by paper chromatography (Johnson et al, 1981).

## RESULTS

Hybridomas were visible in almost all culture wells
on Day 10 following fusion. Screening of supernatants
using a solid-phase assay (Fig. 1) initially identified 38
positive antibodies. When these hybridomas had been

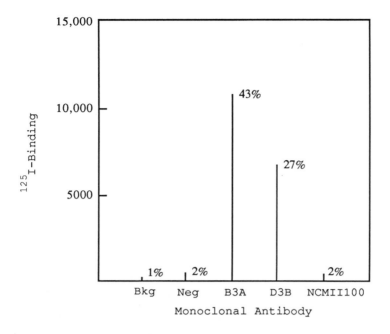

Figure 1. Solid phase assay of monoclonal antibodies
generated to α1→3fucosyltransferase preparations.
Antibody-secreting hybridomas were selected after
incubation of the culture supernatants in tubes precoated
with donkey anti-(mouse Ig) followed by binding of
purified $^{125}$I-labeled enzyme. Examples of antibodies which
were positive (B3A, D3B) and an irrelevant antibody (NCMII
100) along with controls of background (Bkg) and no
antibody (Neg) are given. Percentages of the total
$^{125}$I-enzyme bound for each antibody assay is given.

cultured for a further 10 days and rescreened by Western
blot, eight were selected for investigation. The
hybridomas producing these antibodies were transferred to
BALB/c mice and grown in ascites fluid. Immunodiffusion in
agarose revealed all eight monoclonal antibodies to be of
class IgM. Western blots of whole cell extracts showed
each monoclonal antibody to bind to a distinct spectrum of
antigens in the size range of the purified
fucosyltransferase (Fig. 2) and confirmed that the culture
supernatant and ascites fluid had the same antigenic

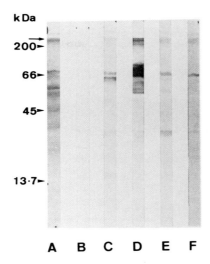

Figure 2. Western blot analysis of an extract of CHP 134 cells using monoclonal antibodies. Single arrow (→) indicates the top of the separating gel. Lane A, total protein transfered and stained with Amido black; Lane B, control with no monoclonal antibody; Monoclonal antibodies: Lane C, A10E; Lane D, D3F; Lane E, D3H; Lane F, E3G.

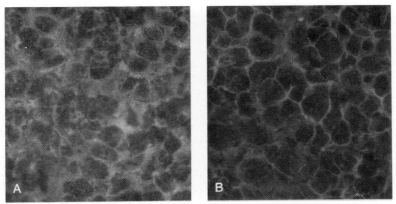

Figure 3. Immunohistochemistry of frozen sections of primary human neuroblastoma, overlayed with monoclonal antibodies and visualized using Texas Red. A) A10E showing a granular intracytoplasmic pattern; B) B3C localized to the plasma membrane.

specificity. Immunohistochemistry showed all eight monoclonal antibodies to bind to determinants within the cytoplasm of freshly frozen neuroblastoma cells, but not to the surrounding stromal connective tissue (Fig. 3). The pattern of binding within the tumor cells was slightly different for each antibody.

One antibody, A10E, was shown to immunoprecipitate $\alpha1\rightarrow3$ fucosyltransferase. Immunoprecipitation of protein from a cell extract, followed by assay for enzyme activity using $Gal\beta1\rightarrow4GlcNAc$ as substrate, showed monoclonal antibody A10E to selectively precipitate $\alpha1\rightarrow3$ fucosyl-transferase activity. The products of the enzyme reaction were separated by paper chromatography and confirmed that the major radioactive product coincided with $Gal\beta1\rightarrow4(Fuc\alpha1\rightarrow3)GlcNAc$. No active enzyme was precipitated with the other monoclonal antibodies, since chromatography of the assay mixture revealed other reaction products or only [$^{14}$C]fucose with absence of the specific product.

## DISCUSSION

The studies reported herein describe the generation and selection of mouse monoclonal antibody A10E to human $\alpha1\rightarrow3$ fucosyltransferase. The antibody is of class IgM, and does not readily immunoprecipitate by conventional methods. Nevertheless, the use of a cross-linked solid phase affinity technique has permitted isolation of enzyme activity from a whole cell extract. In assays following precipitation of activity, the specific reaction product, $Gal\beta1\rightarrow4(Fuc\alpha1\rightarrow3)GlcNAc$, was characterized by chromato-graphy. The initial studies were performed using the antibody in ascites fluid. After purification of the antibody, and further optimizing conditions for adsorbing the enzyme, selective immunoprecipitation of the enzyme was obtained.

In this study, all the selected monoclonal antibodies were of class IgM. No IgG monoclonals were identified. Unfortunately, IgM monoclonal antibodies have low affinities for the antigens containing their epitopes. To be of significant value as a probe of human neuroblastoma $\alpha1\rightarrow3$ fucosyltransferase, a monoclonal antibody with a higher affinity, IgG for example, would be preferred. Although it is common experience that IgM monoclonal antibodies are generated more frequently than IgG's (Hockfield, 1987) we attribute the absence of IgG's in this series to low levels of protein employed as an immunogen.

Glycosyltransferases may be highly conserved during evolution, and therefore non immunogenic in the mouse. It is more likely however, that two fundamental prerequisites for successful generation of monoclonal antibodies to fucosyltransferases must be followed. The first is immunization with sufficient protein presented in a manner such that it is not dissipated and destroyed before eliciting an adequate immune response. The second is a well characterized assay which is sufficiently sensitive that it is capable of identifying the required antibodies.

Monoclonal antibody, A10E will be a valuable tool in the generation of a new range of these reagents. The antibody will be administered conjointly with the enzyme protein in order to enhance the immune response to the specific antigen. In addition, the antibody will be employed to establish optimal assay conditions and hence improve detection of specific monoclonal antibodies. Thus, using this antibody, we anticipate that we will now be able to generate a new series of monoclonal antibodies with affinities necessary for purifying $\alpha1\rightarrow3$fucosyltransferase.

Supported by NIH Grants, CA 14489 and CA 38753 and M.A.R.E.F. 60870.

## REFERENCES

Beyer TA, Sadler JE, Rearick JI, Paulson JC, Hill RL (1981). Glycosyltransferases and their use in assessing oligosaccharide structure and structure-function relationships. *Meth. Enzymol* **52**: 23-175.

Foster CS (1982). Lymphocyte hybridomas. *Cancer Treatment Reviews* **9**: 59-84.

Foster CS, Glick MC (1987). *N*-Acetyl-ß-D-glucosaminide $\alpha1\rightarrow3$fucosyltransferase purified from human neuro-blastoma. *Biochem Soc Trans* **15**: 398-399.

Foster CS, Neville AM (1987). Expression of breast epithelial differentiation antigens in human primary breast cancer. *J Natl Cancer Inst*. In press.

Fukuda M (1985). Cell surface glycoconjugates as onco-differentiation markers in hematopoietic cells. *Biochem Biophys Acta* **780**: 119-150.

Fukuda M, Carlsson SR, Klock JC, Dell A (1986). Structures of *O*-linked oligosaccharides isolated from normal granulocytes, chronic myelogenous leukemia cells, and acute myelogenous leukemia cells. *J Biol Chem* **261**: 12796-12806.

Gersten DM, Marchalonis JJ (1978). A rapid, novel method for the solid-phase derivatization of IgG antibodies for immune-affinity chromatography. *J Immunol. Methods* **24**: 305-309.

Glick MC, Momoi M, Santer UV (1980). Biochemical specificities at the cell surface, in *Metastatic Tumor Growth* (Grundman, E., ed.) Cancer Verlag/Stuttgart-New York, pp. 11-19.

Hakomori S-I, Nudelman E, Levery SB, Kannagi R (1984). Novel fucolipids accumulating in human adenocarcinoma. *J Biol Chem* **259**: 4672-4680.

Hockfield S (1987). A Mab to a unique cellular neuron generated by immunosuppression and rapid immunization. *Science* **237**: 67-70.

Holmes EH, Ostrander GK, Hakomori S-I (1985). Enzymatic basis for the accumulation of glycolipids with X and dimeric X determinants in human lung cancer cells (NCI-H69). *J Biol Chem* **260**: 7619-7627.

Johnson PH, Yates AD, Watkins WM (1981). Human salivary fucosyltransferases: evidence for two distinct α-3-L-fucosyltransferase activities one of which is associated with the Lewis blood group Le gene. Biochem *Biophys Res Commun* **100**: 1611-1618.

Johnson PH, Watkins WM (1985). Acceptor substrate specificities of human α-3- and α-3/4-L-fucosyltrans-ferases. *Proc VIIIth Int Symp Glycoconjugates* **1**: 222-223.

Johnson PH, Watkins WM (1987). Sialyl compounds as acceptor substrates for fucosyltransferases in normal and leukaemic human granulocytes. *Biochem Soc Trans* **15**: 396.

Kennett RH, Denis KA, Tung AS, Klinman NR (1978). Hybrid plasmacytoma production: Fusions with adult spleen cells, monoclonal spleen fragments, neonatal spleen cells and human spleen cells. *Curr Top Microbiol Immunol* **81**: 77-94.

Kim YS, Yuan M, Itzkowitz H, Sun Q, Kaizu T, Palekar A,

Trump BF, Hakomori S-I (1986). Expression of Le$^Y$ and extended Le$^Y$ blood group-related antigens in human malignant, premalignant colonic tissues. *Cancer Res* **46**: 5985-5992.

Littauer UZ, Giovanni MY, Glick MC (1979). Differentiation of human neuroblastoma cells in culture. *Biochem Biophys Res Commun* **88**: 933-939.

Liu F-T, Zinnecker M, Hamaoka T, Katz DH (1979). New procedures for preparation and isolation of conjugates of proteins and a synthetic copolymer of D-aminoacids and immunochemical characterization of such conjugates. *Biochemistry* **18**: 690-697.

Lloyd KO, Larson G, Stromberg N, Thurin J, Karlsson KA (1983). Mouse monoclonal antibody F-3 recognizes the difucosyl type-2 blood group structure. *Immunogenetics* **17**: 537-541.

Mizoguchi A, Takasaki S, Maeda S, Kobata A (1984). Changes in asparagine-linked sugar chains of human promyelocytic leukemic cells (HL-60) during monocytoid differentiation and myeloid differentiation. *J Biol Chem* **259**: 11949-11957.

Ouchterlony O (1962). Diffusion-in-gel methods for immunological analysis II. *In: Progress in Allergy* (Kallos P & Waksman BU, Eds.) **6**: Karger, Basel, 30-154.

Sakamoto J, Furukawa K, Cordon-Cardo C, Yin BWT, Rettig WJ, Oettgen HF, Old LJ, LIoyd KO (1986). Expression of Lewis$^a$, Lewis$^b$, X, and Y blood group antigens in human colonic tumors and normal tissue and human tumor-derived cell lines. *Cancer Res* **46**: 1553-1561.

Santer UV, Glick MC (1980). An uncommon fucosyl linkage in surface membranes of human neuroblastoma cells. *Biochem Biophys Res Commun* **96**: 219-226.

Santer UV, Glick MC (1983). Presence of fucosyl residues on the oligosaccharide antennae of membrane glycopeptides of human neuroblastoma cells. *Cancer Res* **43**: 4159-4166.

Santer UV, Glick MC, Van Halbeek H, Vliegenthart JFG (1983). Characterization of the neutral glycopeptides containing the structure $\alpha$-*L*-fucopyranosyl-(1→3)-2-acetamido-2-deoxy-D-glucose from human neuroblastoma cells. *Carbohydr Res* **120**: 197-213.

Shulman M, Wilde CD, Kohler G (1978). A better cell-line for making hybridomas secreting specific antibodies. *Nature* **276**: 269-270.

Spitalnik SL, Spitalnik PF, Dubois C, Mulshine J, Magnani JL, Cuttitta F, Civin CI, Minna JD (1986). Glycolipid antigen expression in human lung cancer. *Cancer Res* **46**: 4751-4755.

Suda K, Sakamoto S, Hida K, Kano Y, Takaku F, Miura Y (1987). Electrofocusing pattern of fucosyltransferase activity in human leukemic cells. *Cancer Res* **47**: 2782-2786.

Tan KS, Foster CS, DeSilva M (1987). Human monoclonal antibodies to thyroid antigens derived by hybridization of lymphocytes from a diabetic patient. *Metabolism* **36**: 327-334.

Woodbury RA, Santer UV, Elkins WL, Glick MC (1986). Similarities in glycosylation of human neuroblastoma tumors and cell lines. *Cancer Res* **46**: 3692-3697.

Advances in Neuroblastoma Research 2, pages 433–436

DISCUSSION:

Chairmen:       U. Littauer, M.C. Glick

Discussants:    B. Mechler, T. Matsumura
                L. Lampson, C. Foster

Dr. Thiele:  Dr. Mechler, recently the sequence for the putative retinoblastoma gene was published, have you compared your sequences to this particular gene?

Dr. Mechler:  Yes, we have compared the sequences, and there is no homology.

Dr. Littauer:  What was the size of your protein?

Dr. Mechler:  It has a sequence of 708 amino acids.

Dr. Littauer:  Is the sequence similar to anything else?

Dr. Mechler:  Nothing.  The protein has no transmembrane domain nor N-terminal leader peptides and so it is presumably not a membrane protein.  It is a small protein, has at the C-terminal a large basic domain and at the N-terminal also a moderately basic domain. The rest of the protein is evenly charged.  There is no region for DNA binding.  It is a protein which is completely new. I found a cysteinehistidine repeat, which would indicate that this protein may have some relationship with nuclear alpha proteins.

Dr. Cheung:  Dr. Foster, first, does the assay you developed for screening with the anti mouse antibody have relative specificity for IgM or IgG?  Second, do you know whether your enzyme will bind to the sugar residues on your monoclonal and if so it is possible that the enzyme binds to sugar on the immunoglobulins.

Dr. Foster:  First, we use an affinity purified antibody against both IgG and IgM primary antibody.  Secondly, it is possible that the enzyme binds to the sugars present on immunoglobulins but not likely since the fucosyltransferase requires GDP-fucose to bind to its glycoprotein substrate.

Dr. Lipinski: Dr. Lampson, is the lack of expression which it has to Class I linked to the lack of expression of β2-microglobulin or is it primarily Class I which is not expressed? Do you find β2-microglobulin in brain tissue, for instance?

Dr. Lampson: No, in the human tissue we don't see either the native molecules nor the component chains. In the mouse, we have looked for the light chain, we don't see it, and we know you can't have Class I expression without the light chain. There couldn't be a heavy chain on the surface without the light chain.

Dr. Lipinski: A suggestion is to determine whether or not what happens on neuroblast cells or neuroblastoma cells is a dominant phenotype. Has anybody tried to see if this phenotype was dominant by fusing neuroblast cells with other cells that will express β2-microglobulin and HLA Class I, and see if the hybrids will then be able to express them?

Dr. Lampson: No. Relative to that is that we looked at the different messages for the heavy and light chains after we treated the cells with interferon. While before treatment both of the messages are present at low levels, after treatment both of the messages are increased. You get the same answer from Daudi as you get from a B cell that has high levels of both messages, so that the regulation at that point seems to be the same.

Dr. Littauer: Dr. Matsumara, do you know anything about the antigen to your neuron specific antibody. It is a 200k protein. Is it the sodium channel by any chance?

Dr. Kemshead (answering for Dr. Matsumura): No, they don't know what the actual biological function of the protein is. Dr. Reisfeld has an antibody called 5A7 that also recognizes a 230kb glycoprotein on the surface of neuroblastoma cells, there is a possibility that the two might be recognizing the same antigen.

Dr. Thiele: If you induce the neuroblastoma to differentiate with retinoic acid or the analog, E5166, do you see a decrease in the expression of antigen to antibody NAC8.

Dr. Matsumura: Dr. Sugimoto presented that the antigen NAC8 increased in expression after chemically-induced differentiation, and our results presented now show that antigen expression is not present in fetal neuroblasts.

Dr. Glick: Is the antigen present on mouse cells?

Dr. Sugimoto: This monoclonal does not completely react with murine neuroblastoma cells.

Dr. Kemshead: I would like to make a comment on the expression of cell surface markers on mouse neuroblastoma as compared to human neuroblastoma lines. In the comparative studies with a whole range of antibodies against human neuroblastoma, none were found to bind a mouse neuroblastoma which I find quite interesting when one considers the potential use of the mouse neuroblastoma as a model system. Dr. Mechler, have you looked with your antiserum at the antigens that you were detecting in Drosophila, to see if they are conserved in any way through any other species?

Dr. Mechler: The antibody results are quite recent, and we haven't yet performed any further experiments. We are trying not to determine the distribution of these proteins. We have looked with cDNA's to see whether we could find homologous sequences in the vertebrate genome. Using genomic DNA we find absolutely no positive signals, but, genomic DNA may have too many introns. Using a rather large piece of cDNA sequence it may well be that we were not at a sensitivity level sufficient to detect any homologous sequences. Recently, we have used a northern blot with mouse RNA probed with our cDNA's. In this case you have only about ten percent of the genome which is expressed, so you reduce the level of DJA sequences, and you also have amplification due to multiple copies of the RNA. We detect signals of about 4-6kb in brain RNA. Then we screened a grain cDNA library and unfortunately the inserts were too small. It is quite possible that the homology is not to the three prime region of the transcript but more located at the five prime region. So, we need to have a complete library and we hope that soon we are going to be able to isolate something which is homologous.

Dr. Littauer: Have you done the northern blot, fetal and adult brain, and is there a difference?

Dr. Mechler: No, we have taken only 6-7 week old mice. In retinoblastoma this gene is expressed in many tissues and not only the retinal cells, although there is a specific window during development of the retinal cells. The absence of the gene may lead to tumorogenesis, and it could be the same later on during development of the same children, that the tissues may develop sarcomas. This gene may be expressed in many different types of cells that would be found also in Drosophila, but not all of the cells are responsibe to the absence of the gene expression. So we consider this gene is really a sort of developmental gene which may give an imprint to development, and once this information is not provided the cell does not know what to do and continues to proliferate.

Advances in Neuroblastoma Research 2, pages 437–448
© 1988 Alan R. Liss, Inc.

EFFECT OF CYTOSINE ARABINOSIDE ON THE GROWTH AND PHENOTYPIC
EXPRESSION OF GI-ME-N, A NEW HUMAN NEUROBLASTOMA CELL LINE.

Ponzoni M. , Melodia A., Cirillo C., Casalaro A.
and Cornaglia-Ferraris P.
Pediatric Oncology Research Laboratory
G. Gaslini Research Children's Hospital
Via 5 Maggio 39   16148 Genoa, ITALY

SUMMARY

Cytosine-arabinoside (ARA-C) effects on a new human
neuroblastoma cell line (GI-ME-N), recently established in
our laboratory, have been extensively tested. Low doses of
ARA-C allowing virtually 100% cell viability induce morphological differentiation and growth inhibition; differentiated cells appear larger and flattened with elongated dendritic processes; such cells appeared within 48 hours after a
dose of ARA-C as low as 0.1 µg/ml. The new morphological
aspect reached the maximum expression after 5-6 days of
culture being independent   of the addition of extra drug
to the culture. A decrease in $(^3H)$-thymidine incorporation
was also observed within 48 hours being the cell growth
completely inhibited at the 6th day. Membrane immunofluorescence with specific  monoclonal antibodies showed several
dramatic changes in NB-specific antigen expression after 5
days of treatment with ARA-C. These findings suggest that
low ARA-C doses promote the differentiation of GI-ME-N
neuroblastoma cells resulting in an altered expression of
the malignant phenotype.

INTRODUCTION

The severe prognosis for the majority of children with
advanced stages of neuroblastoma (NB) highlights the need for

more effective therapies. Research on NB cell differentiation has been stimulated by two clinical peculiarities: NB has the highest overall rate of spontaneous regression of any malignant neoplasia (approximately 7% of all cases) (Evans 1980); being also capable of spontaneously differentiate or mature to a benign ganglioneuroma (Prasad, 1982). Even though such differentiation is rare, the possibility that future therapeutic strategies would include a stop of the tumor growth via differentiation, should be carefully tested.

The establishment of neuroblastoma cell lines in vitro and in nude mice has provided new interesting tools for studying the differentiation mechanism of these cells. The mouse C1300 neuroblastoma cell line (Augusti-Tocco and Sato, 1969) and its subclones have been widely used for such studies (Prasad, 1975). A variety of substances and culture conditions including dibutyryl-cAMP, nerve growth factor, dimethil sulphoxide, prostaglandin E1, sodium butyrate, 5-bromo-2'-deoxyuridine and serum free medium have been reported to induce morphological and biochemical differentiation in the C1300 cells (Ishii et al., 1978; Kimhi et al. 1976; Richelson, 1973; Simatov and Sachs, 1973; Tsumamoto, 1987; Legault-Demare et al., 1980). Moreover, several cytotoxic agents, including adriamycin, cytosine arabinoside, sulphur mustards, cisplatin and daunomycin (Bottenstein,1981; DeLatt and Van der Saag, 1982; Schengrung and Scheffler, 1982; Tonini et al., 1986; Tonini et al., in press) have proved effective inducers of both morphological and biochemical differentiation in both murine and human models; however, more experiments should be done in order to confirm it for the various human NB cell lines available.

In the present report these phenomena were tested by determining the effects of ARA-C on a new human NB cell line, GI-ME-N, established and characterized in our laboratory (Melodia et al., in press).

MATERIALS AND METHODS

Cell Cultures

Cells were maintained in the logarithmic phase of growth in 75 cm$^2$ plastic tissue culture flasks (Falcon Plastic, Oxnard, CA, USA) in RPMI 1640 medium (Flow Laboratories, Milan, ITALY) supplemented with 15% heat-inactivated fetal calf serum (FCS, Gibco Laboratories, Grand Island, NY, USA), sodium penicillin G (50 IU/ml) and streptomycin sulfate (50 ug/ml) (complete medium) at 37°C in humidified 5% $CO_2$ - 95% air. GI-ME-N cells were passaged following treatment with 0.05% trypsin and 1 mM EDTA in Kanks' salts solution (Flow Laboratories, Milan, ITALY), washed, counted and replated in fresh medium.

Assays for Inhibition of Cell Growth

Cells ($10^5$) were seeded into T-25 flasks (Falcon Plastic, Oxnard, CA, USA) with 5 ml of culture medium. One day after plating, the culture medium was replaced with medium containing ARA-C (Sigma Chemical Company, St. Louis, MO, USA) or with solvent control. The cultures were refed every 4 days with only solvent-containing fresh medium until the day of counting; at that time the cells were detached with trypsin, counted with a hemacytometer and microscopically using a Turk solution. Cell viability was determined by trypan blue exclusion test.

Assays for Inhibition of ($^3$H)-Thymidine Incorporation

Cells, $10^3$/wells, were plated in quadruplicate wells of flatbottom microtest plates (Costar, Cambridge, MA, USA). At various intervals after adding ARA-C, the plates were pulsed with 0.5 uCi ($^3$H)-thymidine/well (5 Ci/mmol, Amersham International, Buckinghamshire, UK). After 18 hours of additional incubation at 37°C, the cells were trypsinized and harvested on strips of fiberglass filter paper with the use of a multiple automated sample harvester (Flow Laboratories, Milan, ITALY) and the radioactivity associated with individual samples measured in a liquid scintillation counter

(Tri-Carb 4530, Packard Instrument Company, Downers Grove, ILL, USA).

Surface Antigens Analysis

Surface antigens were detected with indirect membrane immunofluorescence using the following monoclonal antibodies Ab 390, Ab 459, Ab 126.4, kindly provided by R. Seeger. Adherent cells were scraped off the flasks with a disposable plastic cell-scraper (Costar, Cambridge, MA, USA); 15 $\mu$l of cell suspension containing 1 x $10^6$ cells were incubated with 15 $\mu$l of the appropriately diluted monoclonal antibody for 30' at 4°C; after washing twice the reaction was developed by a second incubation with GAM-FITC (Coulter Electronics Ltd., Luton, UK) for 30' at 4°C. All reagents contained sodium azide (0.1% by volume) to prevent antigenic modulation. The cells were washed twice and observed under a microscope (Leitz Orthoplan, Leitz GmbH, Wetzlar, GERMANY) equipped with a UV 100 watt mercury bulb. At least 200 cells per sample were counted and the percentage of stained cells showing either partial or complete ring fluorescence was determined (mean +/- SD).

Neurofilaments were detected using MoAb antineurofilament 68 Kd, 160 Kd and 200 Kd (Boehringer Mannheim GmbH, Mannheim, WEST GERMANY). The cells were seeded at 25 x $10^3$/ml into multiwell slides and incubated in conditions identical to these of the assay for growth inhibition. At the defined times the slides were fixed in acetone for 10' at −20°C and incubated for 1 hour at 37°C in a umid chamber with 10 $\mu$l of the appropriately diluted monoclonal antibodies. After washing three times with PBS for 3' at room temperature, a second incubation with GAM-FITC was performed. The samples were counted as for surface antigens analysis.

Cell Morphology

GI-ME-N cells were plated and treated with ARA-C as in the cell growth inhibition assay. Starting with day 1 of ARA-C administration, 200 cells/culture from at least three

different random regions were examined daily with a phase-
contrast microscope (Olympus IMT-2, Olympus Optical Co.,
Tokyo, JAPAN). Alternatively, GI-ME-N cells ($10^3$) were plated directly on 8 well multitest slides (Flow Laboratories,
Milan, ITALY and treated with ARA-C as in the cell growth
inhibition assay. Cultures were scored for extent of morphologic differentiation after May Grünwald-Giemsa staining.

RESULTS

Dose-response Relationship of ARA-C-induced Growth Inhibition

     The dose-dependent effects of ARA-C on the prolife-
ration of GI-ME-N cells were assessed by cell counts after
8 days and by incorporation of ($^3$H)-thymidine after 6 days.
Fig. 1 and Fig. 2 show that cellular proliferation as assessed by both criteria was inhibited in a concentration-dependent manner over a range of 0.005 to 0.1 µg/ml ARA-C.

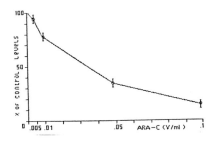 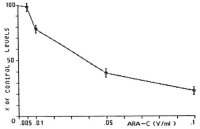

Fig.1: Dose-response curve of        Fig.2: Dose-response curve of
ARA-C induced inhibition of          ARA-C-induced inhibition of
GI-ME-N cell proliferation as        GI-ME-N cell proliferation as
assessed by viable cell counts       assessed by incorporation of
after 8 days of treatment. Va-       ($^3$H)-thymidine after 6 days of
lues are the mean +/- SD of          treatment. Values are the mean
four different experiments           +/- SD of four experiments
each done in duplicate.              each done in quadruplicate.

In these systems, about 50% inhibition of cell growth and
($^3$H)-thymidine incorporation was achieved with ARA-C concentration of 0.05 μg/ml. No decrease in the percentage of viable cells was detected in the treated cultures as compared
to that of control cultures.


Dose-response Relationship of ARA-C-induced Phenotypic
Modulation

        The dose-dependent effects of ARA-C on the phenotypic
expression were evaluated by immunofluorescence assay after
5 days of treatment. Tab. 1 shows that all 3 MoAb used to
detect NB cells were down modulated in a concentration-dependent manner over a range of 0.005 to 0.1 μg/ml ARA-C.
In contrast, the neurofilaments pattern expressed by GI-ME-N
cells did not change after ARA-C treatment (Tab. 1).

| Sample | Ab 390 | Ab 126.4 | Ab 459 | NEUROFILAMENTS | | |
|--------|--------|----------|--------|----------------|--|--|
| | | | | 68 k.d | 150 k.d | 200 k.d |
| CONTROL | 64 ± 4 | 42 ± 7 | 65 ± 5 | Neg. | Pos. | Pos. |
| ARA-C 0.005 ¥/ml | 60 ± 4 | 38 ± 3 | 60 ± 4 | Neg. | Pos. | Pos. |
| ARA-C 0.01 ¥/ml | 31 ± 6 | 13 ± 2 | 45 ± 5 | Neg. | Pos. | Pos. |
| ARA-C 0.05 ¥/ml | 19 ± 4 | 8 ± 2 | 10 ± 4 | Neg. | Pos. | Pos. |
| ARA-C 0.1 ¥/ml | 5 ± 3 | 5 ± 1 | 6 ± 5 | Neg. | Pos. | Pos. |

Tab.1: Effects of ARA-C on membrane and intracytoplasmic
markers of GI-ME-N cells.


Time-course of ARA-C-induced Growth Inhibition

        The growth curves of GI-ME-N cells in the absence and
in presence of 0.1 μg/ml ARA-C are shown in Fig. 3. The number of viable cells in both the ARA-C-treated and control
cultures were similar for 24-48 hours.

However, after 48-72 hours, cellular growth in the presence
of ARA-C was completely inhibited, with little changes in
cell count; this inhibition persisted for at least 8 days
after replacing with fresh medium, being independent from
the addition of extra drug to the culture (data not shown).
Fig. 4 shows the daily ($^3$H)-thymidine incorporation of the
ARA-C-treated and control cultures. Results were analogous
to those obtained by direct cell counts.

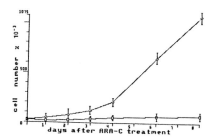

Fig.3: Time course of GI-ME-N
cell growth in the absence
(△) or presence (□) of 0.1
µg/ml ARA-C. Values are the
mean +/- SD of three different
experiments.

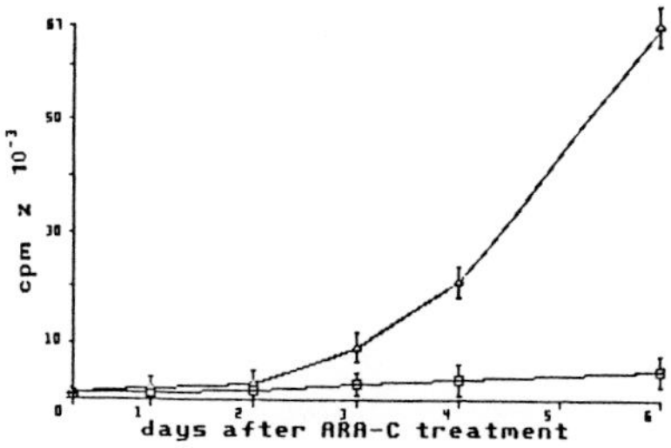

Fig.4: Time course of ($^3$H)-
thymidine incorporation by
GI-ME-N cells in the absence
(△) or presence (□) of 0.1
µg/ml ARA-C. Values are the
mean +/- SD of three different experiments.

ARA-C-induced Morphologic Differentiation

        Treatment of GI-ME-N cells with ARA-C caused a drama-
tic morphologic alteration as evidenced by formation of large flattened neuron-like cells with elongated neurite proces
ses at least twice as long the soma (Fig. 5). The ARA-C concentration causing maximum increase in the percentage of
differentiated cells ranged from 0.05 to 0.1 µg/ml. The time
course of morphologic differentiation in the absence and
presence of 0.1 µg/ml of ARA-C is shown in Fig. 5.

A significant increase in the number of differentiated cells could be detected within 48 hours (Fig. 5b); the maximum extent of differentiation occurred after approximately 5 days of treatment (Fig. 5c). The morphologic differentiation induced by ARA-C was retained by the GI-ME-N cells in the absence of the drug. When ARA-C was removed after 4 days of treatment, the large majority of the cells retained their morphologic alterations for at least 10 days (Fig. 5d).

Fig. 5

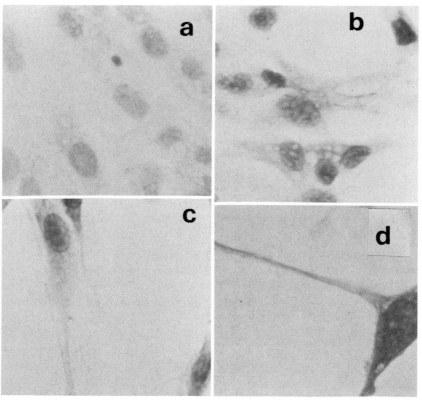

ARA-C-induced morphologic differentiation of GI-ME-N cells. (a) medium treated control; (b) cells cultured in the presence of 0.1 ug/ml ARA-C for 48 hours; (c) cells after 4 days of ARA-C treatment; (d) cells at the 10th day after the removal of the drug.

DISCUSSION

Neuroblastoma is known, in some cases, to undergo spontaneous regression in vivo (Evans et al., 1980). One mechanism for the regression has been suggested to be maturation of the tumour cells into terminally differentiated, non-proliferative, ganglion-like cells (Cushing and Wolback, 1927). In most cases, however, neuroblastoma behaves as a highly malignant tumour, insensitive to irradiation and/or chemotherapy (Evans, 1980). One attractive approach to future treatment of patients with NB would be to identify drugs inducing terminal differentiation in vivo thus arresting the tumor cells in the non-proliferative phase of the cell cycle.

The successful establishment of both mouse and human NB cell lines in vitro in recent years has made it possible to initiate studies on induced differentiation in a well-defined and well-controlled environment.

This report provides evidences for the ability of ARA-C to regulate the phenotypic expression and the morphologic differentiation of a new human NB cell line, GI-ME-N, recently established in our laboratory. The results of this study demonstrate that ARA-C induces concentration-dependent growth inhibition, morphologic alterations and membrane antigens down-modulation of the GI-ME-N cells. The fact that ARA-C treatment of GI-ME-N cells started one day after plating with no subsequent decrease in cell viability in the cultures suggests that its effects were not the result of selection of more differentiated cells by differences in plating efficiency or ARA-C cytotoxicity. This conclusion is supported by time-lapse photography, which clearly showed individual GI-ME-N cells undergoing ARA-C-induced morphologic differentiation (unpublished data). ARA-C-induced inhibition of cell growth of GI-ME-N cells could be detected after about 48 hours when assayed by incorporation of $(^3H)$-thymidine. The elapsed time before reduction of $(^3H)$-thymidine incorporation was observed corresponds to the time after ARA-C treatment before an increase was seen before the morphologic differentiation of GI-ME-N cells. This correspon

dence is consistent with the reduced rate of DNA synthesis generally associated with a differentiation process (Bottenstein, 1981) and supports the contention that true differentiation is occurring. The dose-dependent down modulation of membrane markers specific for NB cells, detected after 5 days of ARA-C treatment of GI-ME-N cells, further confirms the hypothesis that a true differentiation occurred.
In contrast, the presence of the two subclasses of neurofilaments typically expressed by more differentiated NB cells, on untreated cells leaves open the possibility that GI-ME-N are at least partially mature cells; however, studies currently in progress pertaining transmission electron microscopy and catecholamine detection seem to rule out this hypothesis.

In conclusion this report presents a new NB cell model appearing to be suitable to study the differentiating activity of antitumour drugs. This system becomes especially appealing when one considers the morphologic, biochemical and electrophysiologic modes of differentiation that might be evaluated in NB cells (Bottenstein, 1981). These findings should encourage further studies of the possible role of antitumour agents in differentiating human NB cells.

REFERENCES

- Augusti-Tocco G, Sato G (1969). Establishment of functional clonal lines of neurons from mouse neuroblastoma. Proc Natl Acad Sci 64:311.
- Bottenstein JE (1981). Differentiated properties of neuronal cell lines. In Sato GH (ed): "Functionally differentiated cell lines", New York: Alan R. Liss, p. 155.
- Cushing H, Wolbach BB (1927). The transformation of a malignant paravertebral sympathicoblastoma into a benign ganglioneuroma. Amer J Path 3:203.
- DeLatt SW, Van der Saag PT (1982). The plasma membrane as a regulatory site in growth and differentiation of neuroblastoma cells. Int Rev Cytol 74:1.
- Evans AE (1980). Natural history of neuroblastoma. In Evans AE (ed): "Advances in neuroblastoma research", New

York: Raven Press, p 3.
- Evans AE, Chatten J, D'Angio GJ, Gerson JM, Robinson J, Schnaufer L (1980). A review of 17 IV-S neuroblastoma patients at the Children's Hospital of Philadelphia. Cancer 45:833.
- Inshii DN, Fibach E, Yamasaki H, Weinstein JB (1978). Tumor promoters inhibit morphological differentiation in cultured mouse neuroblastoma cells. Science 200:556.
- Kimhi Y, Palfrey C, Spector I, Borak Y, Lstaner VZ (1976). Maturation of neuroblastoma cells in the presence of dimethyl-sulphoxide. Proc Natl Acad Sci 73:462.
- Legault-Demare L, Zeitoun Y, Laudo D, Lamands N, Grasso A, Gros F (1980). Expression of a specific neuronal protein, 14-3-2, during in vitro differentiation of neuroblastoma cells. Exp Cell Res 125:233.
- Melodia A, Cornara L, Bertelli R, Canepa G, Gimelli G, Repetto G, Cornaglia-Ferraris P (1986). Nuova linea di neuroblastoma umano derivata da midollo osseo. Patologica 78:371.
- Prasad KN (1975). Differentiation of neuroblastoma cells in culture. Biol Rev 50:129.
- Prasad KN (1982). Maturation of neuroblastoma. In Stoll BA (ed): "Prolonged arrest of cancer, new horizons in oncology", Chichester, UK: John Wiley, p 281.
- Richelston E (1973). Stimulation of tyrosine hydroxylase activity in an adrenergic clone of mouse neuroblastoma by dibutiryl cyclic-AMP. Nature New Biol 242:175.
- Schengrung CL, Scheffer BA (1982). Biochemical and morphological study of adriamycin-induced changes in murine neuroblastoma cells. Oncology 39:185.
- Simatov R, Sachs L (1973). Regulation of acetylcholine receptors in relation to acetylcholinesterase in neuroblastoma cells. Proc Natl Acad Sci 76:2779.
- Tonini GP, Parodi MT, Bologna R, Persici P, Cornaglia-Ferraris P (1986). Cisplatin induces modulation of transferrin receptor during cellular differentiation in vitro. Cancer Chemother Pharmacol 18:92.
- Tonini GP, Parodi MT, Blasi E, Gronberg A, Varesio L (in press). Daunomycin and aracytin change c-myc oncogene

transcripts in human erythroleukemic cell line during cellular differentiation. J Immunother.

- Tsumamoto K, Todo S, Imashumu S (1987). Effects of 5-bromo 2'-deoxiuridine on Arachidonic acid metabolism of neuroblastoma and leukemia cells in culture: a possible role of endogenous prostaglandins in tumor cell proliferation and differentiation. Prostaglandins Leukotrienes and Medicine 26:157.

Advances in Neuroblastoma Research 2, pages 449–461

# EVIDENCE FOR REVERSE TRANSFORMATION IN MULTIDRUG-RESISTANT HUMAN NEUROBLASTOMA CELLS.

Marian B. Meyers and June L. Biedler

Laboratory of Cellular and Biochemical Genetics, Memorial Sloan-Kettering Cancer Center, New York, NY 10021

## INTRODUCTION

Chinese hamster lung and mouse tumor cells selected for resistance to such cancer chemotherapeutic agents as vincristine and actinomycin D exhibit marked changes in in vitro growth characteristics toward a more normal phenotype and have decreased tumorigenic potential when tested in animal hosts. Together these phenotypic alterations indicated that the multidrug-resistant sublines were reverse transformed as compared to the malignant, tumorigenic drug-sensitive parental cells (Biedler et al., 1975; Biedler and Peterson, 1981; Meyers et al., 1986). How this striking transformation change correlates with the development of resistance is not known. Among the questions to be asked are whether human tumor cells undergo reverse transformation with development of this type of drug resistance and whether the normalization phenomenon, should it occur, is tissue specific.

Multidrug-resistant human neuroblastoma cell lines are currently being examined to determine whether the reverse transformation process obtains to human cells. Development of resistance to cancer chemotherapeutic agents may coincide with modification of the differentiation phenotype of neuroblastoma (or other tumor cell types), thereby influencing their malignant potential. Six cellular characteristics are being used to evaluate transformation state: tumorigenic potential in athymic mice, plating efficiency in soft agar, cell morphology, and fibronectin, epidermal growth factor receptor, and N-myc expression.

MATERIALS AND METHODS

Cell Lines

The clonally derived human neuroblastoma lines SH-SY5Y, MC-IXC, and BE(2)-C and two sublines, SH-SY5Y/VCR and MC-IXC/VCR, with high levels of resistance to vincristine (Table 1) have been described in previous reports (Biedler et al., 1973; Biedler et al., 1978; Meyers and Biedler, 1981; Biedler et al., 1983b; Meyers et al., 1985). SH-SY5Y/ACT was derived from thrice cloned SH-SY5Y by stepwise increases in concentration of actinomycin D; it is now maintained in medium containing 0.05 μg/ml of the drug. BE(2)-C/VCR was similarly selected with vincristine from cloned BE(2)-C cells to the current level of 10 μg/ml. Cells are grown as monolayer cultures in a 1:1 mixture of Eagle's Minimum Essential Medium with non-essential amino acids and Ham's F12 Medium supplemented with 15% fetal bovine serum. SH-SY5Y/ACT is EGF-dependent and is maintained in 100 ng/ml EGF.

Growth in Nude Mice and Plating Efficiency in Soft Agar

To compare oncogenic potential of drug-sensitive and -resistant cells, growth in nu/nu (nude) mice was tested. Mice were inoculated subcutaneously with $10^7$ cells into each of three weanling female Swiss background nude mice per cell line per experiment. Three separate experiments for each line were performed and tumor take determined. The soft agar technique of MacPherson (1973) was used to assay anchorage-independent growth ability.

Quantitation of mRNA

Total mRNA from cells in mid- to late-exponential growth phase was obtained by a standard guanidinium isothiocyanate procedure (Chirgwin et al., 1979). Serial dilutions of formaldehyde-denatured RNA were placed on nitrocellulose paper. Hybridization was carried out by standard procedures (Maniatis et al., 1982). The probes were a cloned rat liver fibronectin cDNA, prlf1, (Schwarzbauer et al., 1983), a cloned N-myc cDNA (clone 15-4) containing the third exon of the gene (Michitsch and

TABLE 1. Transformation characteristics of drug-sensitive and -resistant human neuroblastoma cells

| Cell line | Maintenance drug concentration (μg/ml) | Increase in resistance to selective agent | Morphology | Tumor frequency in nude mice (%) | PE in soft agar (%) |
|---|---|---|---|---|---|
| SH-SY5Y | None | 1 | | 33 | 4.3 |
| SH-SY5Y/VCR | 1.0 | 1,420 | Longer neuritic processes | 33 | 11.3 |
| SH-SY5Y/ACT | 0.05 | 30 | Flattened | 0 | ND |
| BE(2)-C | None | 1 | | 81 | 27.3 |
| BE(2)-C/VCR | 2.0 | 100 | Less flattened | ND | 43.2 |
| | 10.0 | 300 | | ND | ND |
| MC-IXC | None | 1 | | 46 | 25.8 |
| MC-IXC/VCR | 5.0 | 21,920 | Flattened, substrate-adherent | 0 | 5.7 |

PE, plating efficiency
ND, not determined

Melera, 1985), and the Cla I fragment of a cloned EGF
receptor cDNA, pE7, (Xu et al., 1984a; Merlino et al.,
1984). The probes were labeled with [α-$^{32}$P]dCTP by the
random primer labeling method (Feinberg and Vogelstein,
1984).


EGF Binding and EGF-Receptor Immunoprecipitation

Methods for measurement of binding of [$^{125}$I]EGF to
living cells in monolayer cultures have been described (Das
et al., 1977; Meyers et al., 1986). Binding was measured
after a one hour incubation at 22°C in labeled EGF in the
presence and absence of 100 nM unlabeled EGF. Immunoprecipitation of EGF receptor was accomplished with a monoclonal antibody to human receptor (mc528), a gift from
Dr. Gordon Sato (Kawamoto et al., 1983). Cells were grown
for four hours in the presence of $^{35}$S-methionine in methio-
nine-depleted medium. Washed cells were lysed in 20 mM
Hepes (pH 7.4) containing 1% glycerol and 1% Triton X-100.
Aliquots of soluble material containing 10$^6$ trichloroacetic
acid-precipitable cpm were incubated with mc528 followed by
precipitation with Protein A as described by Xu et al.
(1984b). Sodium dodecyl sulfate gel electrophoresis on
7.5% gels (0.075 x 14 x 11 cm) was used to separate the
receptor protein. Dried gels were exposed to X-ray film
for 2-3 weeks.


RESULTS

All four of the resistant sublines studied exhibit
altered morphology compared to parental cells, e.g., longer
neuritic processes or cell flattening (Table 1). Two of
the four lines tested (SH-SY5Y/ACT and MC-IXC/VCR) manifest
a decrease in tumorigenicity in nude mice and/or colony-
forming ability in soft agar (Table 1). Studies of these
characteristics in the other two (SH-SY5Y/VCR and BE(2)-
C/VCR) are incomplete but results so far suggest that these
lines have similar or increased plating efficiency in soft
agar. Tumor formation frequency of SH-SY5Y/VCR is similar
to that of SH-SY5Y.

Of the two lines tested for fibronectin expression
[SH-SY5Y/ACT and BE(2)-C/VCR], both have higher levels of
fibronectin mRNA (>100-fold and 16-fold, respectively) than

TABLE 2. Biochemical characteristics of drug-sensitive and -resistant human neuroblastoma cells

| Cell line | Increase in resistance to selective agent | Relative level of mRNA for: | | | EGF receptor number[a] |
|---|---|---|---|---|---|
| | | Fibronectin | N-myc | EGF receptor | |
| SH-SY5Y[b] | 1 | 1 | 1 | 1 | 1,400 |
| SH-SY5Y/VCR | 1,420 | ND | ND | 3[c] | 4,100 |
| SH-SY5Y/ACT | 30 | >100 | ND | 32[c] | 43,000 |
| BE(2)-C[d] | 1 | 1 | 10 | 10 | 46,600 |
| BE(2)-C/VCR ( 2.0) | 100 | ND | 10 | 10 | ND |
| (10.0) | 300 | 16 | 36 | 28 | ND |
| MC-IXC[e] | | ND | <1 | ND | 150 |
| MC-IXC/VCR | 21,920 | ND | ND | ND | 2,100 |

[a]Determined by EGF binding studies (Meyers et al., in preparation)
[b]N-ras activated
[c]Determined by hybridization analysis (Meyers et al., in preparation)
[d]N-myc amplified
[e]c-myc amplified

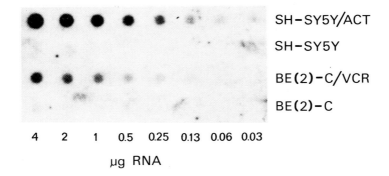

Figure 1. Dot blot analysis of steady state fibronectin
mRNA levels in two multidrug-resistant human neuroblastoma
sublines and controls. Resistant cells contain 30-60 times
more fibronectin mRNA than do parental cells.

drug-sensitive control cells (Fig. 1 and Table 2).

The three resistant sublines tested exhibit increased
levels of EGF binding (Fig. 2a). Immunoprecipitation of
[$^{35}$S]methionine-labeled receptors with monoclonal antibody
528 showed that increased binding is the result of increased receptor protein in resistant cells. Fig. 2b shows
a sample experiment of this type. There is an increased
amount of receptor protein in SH-SY5Y/VCR compared to SH-
SY5Y. By this technique SH-SY5Y/ACT and MC-IXC/VCR cells
also contain increased receptor protein (Meyers et al., in
preparation). Northern, Southern, and slot blot hybridization analyses with a cloned EGF receptor probe revealed
that the increase in protein is the result of increased
amounts of specific RNA and not gene amplification (Table
2, Fig. 3, and Meyers et al., in preparation). All resistant lines tested had increased EGF receptor mRNA compared
to controls.

Fig. 4 depicts hybridization of an N-myc probe to
total RNA of BE(2)-C and BE(2)-C/VCR cells grown at 2 and
10 µg/ml of vincristine. The already high level of N-myc
expression in BE(2)-C is unchanged in the less resistant
line but is elevated still further (2.8-fold) in BE(2)-
C/VCR cells maintained at 10 µg/ml.

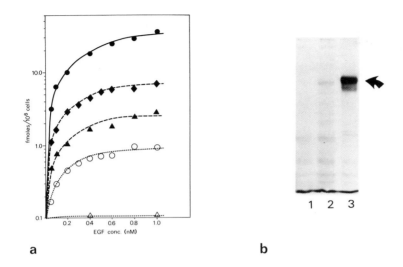

a                                    b

Figure 2a.  Binding of [¹²⁵I]EGF to drug-resistant and
-sensitive cells.  (△·····△), MC-IXC; (▲-▲), MC-IXC/VCR;
(○·····○), SH-SY5Y; (◆--◆), SH-SY5Y/VCR; (●—●), SH-SY5Y/ACT.
Figure 2b.  Immunoprecipitation of EGF receptor (arrow)
from SH-SY5Y (lane 1), SH-SY5Y/VCR (lane 2), and A431 (lane
3) control cells with monoclonal antibody 528.  A431 is a
human epidermoid carcinoma line with ~2 x 10⁶ EGF receptors
per cell.

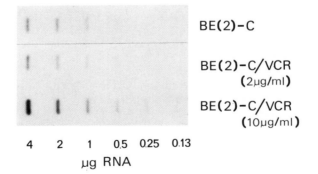

BE(2)-C

BE(2)-C/VCR
(2μg/ml)

BE(2)-C/VCR
(10μg/ml)

4    2    1    0.5  0.25  0.13

μg RNA

Figure 3.  EGF receptor mRNA steady state levels in
parental BE(2)-C cells and vincristine-resistant sublines
at different levels of resistance.

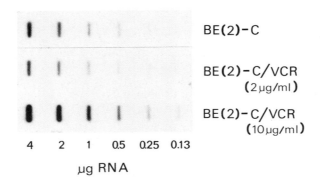

Figure 4.  Expression of N-myc mRNA in BE(2)-C and in
vincristine-resistant sublines at different levels of
resistance.

## DISCUSSION

     Two (SH-SY5Y/ACT and MC-IXC/VCR) of the four multi-
drug-resistant sublines tested, are reverse transformed by
the criteria of growth in nude mice and/or in soft agar.
Both lines have elevated EGF receptor expression compared
to controls, and SH-SY5Y/ACT synthesizes more fibronectin
than SH-SY5Y.  SH-SY5Y/VCR has elevated EGF receptor but is
not reverse transformed, by the criteria used in this
study, when compared to SH-SY5Y.  BE(2)-C/VCR has altered
morphology, increased fibronectin expression, and increased
EGF receptor mRNA as compared to BE(2)-C.  However, the
resistant cells have an even higher plating efficiency in
soft agar and elevated N-myc, suggesting that the cells are
not reverse transformed, although tumorigenic potential has
not yet been directly tested in nude mice.

     Ability of cells to grow in nude mice and, to a large
extent, ability to grow in an anchorage-independent manner
(Shin et al., 1975) are measures of cellular state of
transformation.  Changes in cell morphology and cell adhesion also correlate with malignant transformation (Folkman
and Moscona, 1978) and cellular differentiation.  These
characteristics coincide with underlying genetic (or epigenetic) properties of a cell, some of which, such as onco-

gene and growth factor receptor expression, are known to be associated with states of differentiation as well as with transformation. Three properties being investigated at this time are: EGF receptor, N-myc, and fibronectin. The relationship between growth factors, their receptors, and the malignant state of cells is a subject of intensive investigation (Stoscheck et al., 1986). In particular, EGF binding and EGF receptor modulation may be associated with state of transformation (as well as normal cell differentiation). This report reveals a correlation between low level of receptor and increased malignant potential, a correlation observed in other types of studies as well (Wakshull et al., 1985). Reduction of receptor number in malignant cells could be the result of down-regulation by TGFα, an autocrine growth factor synthesized and secreted by many neoplastic cells (Stoscheck et. al., 1986). A causal role for N-myc in the genesis and/or progression of tumors is suggested by its frequent amplification and/or overexpressison in certain tumors, particularly neuroblastoma (Brodeur et al., 1984; Rosen et. al., 1986; Small et al., 1987). N-myc is expressed at high levels in pre- and postnatal mouse brain and kidney but not in adult tissue, suggesting involvement of N-myc in the early stages of multiple differentiation pathways (Zimmerman et al., 1986). C-myc is also involved in cellular differentiation (Zimmerman et al., 1986). Decreased fibronectin synthesis is a common, though not universal, concomitant of transformation (Hynes and Yamada, 1982). Fibronectin is involved in cell adhesion, morphology, and spreading, as well as in embryonic differentiation.

The three parental neuroblastoma lines in this study may represent different stages of embryonal neuronal cell differentiation fixed at the point of malignant transformation. This idea is supported by the fact that each line contains a different activated oncogene. SH-SY5Y (atypical neuroblastoma) cells have activated N-ras (Shimizu et al., 1983), BE(2)-C ("typical" neuroblastoma) have amplified N-myc (Michitsch and Melera, 1985), and MC-IXC cells (neuro-epithelioma) have amplified c-myc (Kohl et al., 1983). Vincristine and actinomycin D are known to induce differentiation in at least one system (erythroleukemia cells) (Marks and Rifkind, 1978). These drugs could be expected to affect the differentiative pathways of the three neuroblastoma lines in different ways, and the effect could thus influence oncogenic potential in three unique modes.

It should be pointed out that a major characteristic of multidrug-resistant cells is overexpression of the plasma membrane glycoprotein gp150-180/P-glycoprotein. Indeed, amplification and overexpression of genes encoding P-glycoprotein have occurred in SH-SY5Y/VCR and MC-IXC/VCR cells (Scotto et al., 1986). In studies of multidrug-resistant Chinese hamster cells it has been estimated that as much as 3% of total membrane protein is P-glycoprotein (Safa et al., in press). The possible effect of this abundant plasma membrane protein on other membrane components and the attendant effect of the carbohydrate moieties of P-glycoprotein, in respect to the transformation or differentiation state of multidrug-resistant cells, are still to be determined. Reversion of multidrug-resistant cells to drug sensitivity is accompanied by reversion to malignant characteristics as well as by a decrease in P-glycoprotein synthesis (Biedler et al., 1983a). This suggests an epigenetic mechanism for reverse transformation and/or a role for P-glycoprotein in this phenotypic change.

These initial investigations suggest that reverse transformation, as defined in this report, may indeed be a consequence of multidrug resistance development in human tumor cells but it is not an obligatory one. Different components of the progression from malignancy to normalcy (or vice versa) may be activated in different cells. Changes in malignant potential and/or differentiation state with development of multidrug resistance may be determined by the specific tissue type or the oncogene background of the drug resistant cells. The results encourage the continued study of the characteristics described in this paper to further clarify this aspect of multidrug resistance. For that purpose a large panel of resistant neuroblastoma and carcinoma lines is being selected with different drugs to better evaluate the concordance of multidrug resistance and concomitants of progression from malignancy to normalcy.


ACKNOWLEDGMENTS

This work was supported in part by NIH grants CA-08748 and CA-28595.

REFERENCES

Biedler JL, Helson L, Spengler BA (1973). Morphology and growth, tumorigenicity, and cytogenetics of human neuroblastoma cells in continuous culture. Cancer Res 33:2643-2652.

Biedler JL, Riehm H, Peterson RHF, Spengler BA (1975). Membrane-mediated drug resistance and phenotypic reversion to normal growth behavior of Chinese hamster cells. J Natl Cancer Inst 55:671-680.

Biedler JL, Roffler-Tarlov S, Schachner M, Freedman L (1978). Multiple neurotransmitter synthesis by human neuroblastoma cell lines and clones. Cancer Res 38:3751-3757.

Biedler JL, Peterson RHF (1981). Altered plasma membrane glycoconjugates of Chinese hamster cells with acquired resistance to actinomycin D, daunorubicin, and vincristine. In Sartorelli AC, Lazo JS, Bertino JR (eds): "Molecular Actions and Targets for Cancer Chemotherapeutic Agents," Bristol-Myers Cancer Symposia, vol 2, New York: Academic Press, pp 453-482.

Biedler JL, Chang T-D, Peterson RHF, Melera PW, Meyers MB, Spengler BA (1983a). Gene amplification and phenotype instability in drug-resistant and revertant cells. In Chabner BA (ed): "Rational Basis for Chemotherapy - UCLA Symposia," vol. 4, New York: Alan R. Liss Inc, p. 71-92.

Biedler JL, Meyers MB, Spengler BA (1983b). Homogeneously staining regions and double minute chromosomes, prevalent cytogenetic abnormalities of human neuroblastoma cells. Adv Cell Neurobiol 4:267-307.

Brodeur GM, Seeger RC, Schwab M, Varmus HE, Michael BJ (1984). Amplification of N-myc in untreated neuroblastomas correlates with advanced disease stage. Science 224:1121-1124.

Chirgwin JM, Przybyla AE, MacDonald RJ, Rutter WJ (1979). Isolation of biologically active ribonucleic acid from sources enriched in ribonuclease. Biochemistry 18:5294-5299.

Das M, Miyakawa T, Fox CF, Pruso RM, Aharonov A, Herschman HR (1977). Specific radiolabeling of a cell surface receptor for epidermal growth factor. Proc Natl Acad Sci USA 74:2790-2794.

Feinberg AP, Vogelstein B (1984). A technique for radiolabeling DNA restriction endonuclease fragments to high specific activity. Anal Biochem 132:6-13.

Folkman J, Moscona A (1978). Role of cell shape in growth
control. Nature 273:345-349.
Hynes RO, Yamada KM (1982). Fibronectins: Multifunctional
modular glycoproteins. J Cell Biol 95:369-377.
Kawamoto T, Sato JD, Le A, Polikoff J, Sato GH, Mendelsohn
J (1983). Growth stimulation of A431 cells by epidermal
growth factor: Identification of high-affinity receptors
for epidermal growth factor by an anti-receptor antibody.
Proc Natl Acad Sci USA 80:1337-1341.
Kohl NE, Kanda N, Schreck RR, Bruns G, Latt SA, Gilbert F,
Alt FW (1983). Transposition and amplification of onco-
gene-related sequences in human neuroblastomas. Cell
35:359-367.
Macpherson I (1973). Soft agar techniques. In Kruse Jr
PF, Patterson Jr MK (eds): "Tissue Culture, Methods and
Applications," New York: Academic Press, pp 276-280.
Maniatis T, Fritsch EF, Sambrook J (1982). Molecular
cloning. A laboratory manual. Cold Spring Harbor
Laboratory.
Marks PA, Rifkind RA (1978). Erythroleukemia differentia-
tion. Ann Rev Biochem 47:419-448.
Merlino GT, Xu Y-h, Ishii S, Clark AJL, Semba K, Toyoshima
K, Yamamoto T, Pastan I (1984). Amplification and
enhanced expression of the epidermal growth factor
receptor gene in A431 human carcinoma cells. Science
224:417-419.
Meyers MB, Biedler JL (1981). Increased synthesis of a low
molecular weight protein in vincristine-resistant cells.
Biochem Biophys Res Commun 99:228-235.
Meyers MB, Spengler BA, Chang TD, Melera PW, Biedler JL
(1985). Gene amplification-associated cytogenetic
aberrations and protein changes in vincristine-resistant
Chinese hamster, mouse, and human cells. J Cell Biol
100:588-597.
Meyers MB, Merluzzi VJ, Spengler BA, Biedler JL (1986).
Epidermal growth factor receptor is increased in
multidrug-resistant Chinese hamster and mouse tumor
cells. Proc Natl Acad Sci USA 83:5521-5525.
Meyers MB, Shen WPV, Spengler BA, Ciccarone V, O'Brien JP,
Donner DB, Furth ME, Biedler JL. Increased epidermal
growth factor receptor in multidrug-resistant human
neuroblastoma cells. Manuscript in preparation.
Michitsch RW, Melera PW (1985). Nucleotide sequence of the
3'exon of the human N-myc gene. Nucleic Acids Res
13:2545-2558.

Rosen N, Reynolds P, Thiele CJ, Biedler JL, Israel M. (1986). Increased N-myc expression following progressive growth of human neuroblastoma. Cancer Res 46:4139-4142.

Safa AR, Glover CJ, Sewell JL, Meyers MB, Biedler JL, Felsted RL. Identification of the multidrug resistance-related membrane glycoprotein as an acceptor for calcium channel blockers. J Biol Chem. In press.

Schwarzbauer JE, Tamkun JW, Lemischka IR, Hynes RO (1983). Three different fibronectin mRNAs arise by alternative splicing within the coding region. Cell 35:421-431.

Scotto KW, Biedler JL, Melera PW (1986). Amplification and expression of genes associated with multidrug resistance in mammalian cells. Science 232:751-755.

Shimizu K, Goldfarb M, Perucho M, Wigler M (1983). Isolation and preliminary characterization of the transforming gene of a human neuroblastoma cell. Proc Natl Acad Sci USA 80:384-387.

Shin S, Freedman VH, Risser R, Pollack R (1975). Tumorigenicity of virus-transformed cells in nude mice is correlated specifically with anchorage-independent growth in vitro. Proc Natl Acad Sci USA 72:4435-4439.

Small MB, Hay N, Schwab M, Bishop JM (1987). Neoplastic transformation by the human gene N-myc. Mol Cell Biol 7:1638-1645.

Stoscheck CM, King Jr LE (1986). Role of epidermal growth factor in carcinogenesis. Cancer Res 46:1030-1037.

Wakshull E, Kraemer PM, Wharton W (1985). Multistep change in epidermal growth factor receptors during spontaneous neoplastic regression in Chinese hamster embryo fibroblasts. Cancer Res 45:2070-2075.

Xu Y-h, Ishii S, Clark AJL, Sullivan M, Wilson RK, Ma DP, Roe BA, Merlino GT, Pastan I (1984a). Human epidermal growth factor receptor cDNA overproduced in A431 carcinoma cells. Nature 309:806-810.

Xu Y-h, Richert N, Ito S, Merlino GT, Pastan I (1984b). Characterization of epidermal growth factor receptor gene expression in malignant and normal human cell lines. Proc Natl Acad Sci USA 81:7308-7312.

Zimmerman KA, Yancopoulos GD, Collum RG, Smith RK, Kohl NE, Denis KA, Nau MM, Witte ON, Toran-Allerand D, Gee DE, Minner JD, Alt FW (1986). Differential expression of myc family genes during murine development. Nature 319:780-783.

Advances in Neuroblastoma Research 2, pages 463–473
© 1988 Alan R. Liss, Inc.

OLFACTORY NEUROBLASTOMA IS NOT A NEUROBLASTOMA BUT IS
RELATED TO PRIMITIVE NEUROECTODERMAL TUMOR (PNET)

Andrea O. Cavazzana, Samuel Navarro, Rosa
Noguera, Patrick C. Reynolds, Timothy J.
Triche
Laboratory of Pathology, NCI, Bethesda
(A.O.C., S.N.,R.N., T.J.T.), and UCLA
School of Medicine, Los Angeles, CA
(P.C.R.)

# INTRODUCTION

Olfactory Neuroblastoma (ONB) is a rare tumor arising
from nasal mucosa that is generally thought to be similar
to classical neuroblastoma (NB). Despite obvious morphological similarities, ONB differs from classical NB in many
ways. First, it appears most commonly in an older group of
patients (second and third decade of life), but it can
occur in children also (Skolnik, 1966). Secondly, it is
rarely associated with catecholamine secretion (Micheau,
1975). Clinically, it is characterized by a less aggressive course than typical childhood neuroblastoma, but it is
nonetheless highly malignant (Barnes, 1985). A neural origin for this neoplasm has been assumed (as implied by both
common names, *esthesioneuroblastoma* and *olfactory neuroblastoma*) due to the presence of several neural characteristics, including an ultrastructural appearance similar to
undifferentiated neuroblastoma (Taxy, 1986) and a cytoskeleton composed of neurofilaments (Trojanowski, 1982). A
neuroendocrine origin has also been proposed, due to the
apparent presence of keratin in some ONB (Taxy, 1986).

All of the studies to date have been performed only on
excised tumor, for the lack of established olfactory neuroblastoma cell lines. This has seriously hampered efforts
to study the biology of this tumor as compared to neuroblastoma and other neural tumors. We report here the successful establishment of two such lines as well as the
first in vitro studies thereof.

## MATERIALS AND METHODS

Two ONB cell lines have been established from a metastatic chest wall lesion of a 22 yr old male (JFEN) and a
metastatic paraspinal mass in a 22 yr old female (TC-268).
Both patients originally presented with classical olfactory
mucosal tumors (fig.1A, B).  The diagnosis was confirmed
immunocytochemically (neuron specific enolase [NSE] and
neurofilament triplet protein [NFTP] positive) and
ultrastructurally  (i.e., positive for classic dense core,
neurosecretory granules, fig. 1C).

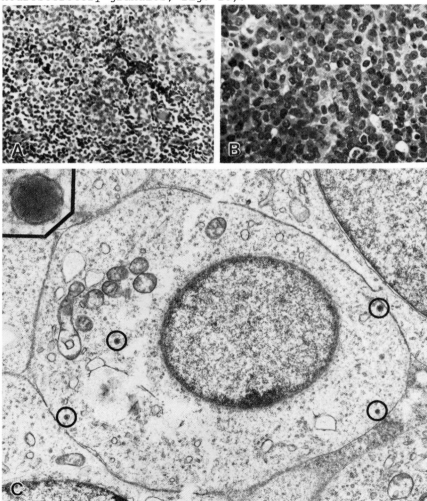

*Figure 1:* (Facing page). Microscopic appearance of the two cases of olfactory neuroblastoma studied here. Panel A is the light microscopic appearance of TC-268; panel B, the comparable appearance of JFEN, both from the original biopsy material. Panel C depicts the ultrastructural appearance of the original biopsy from TC-268. Note the 4 dense core granules (encircled).

Continuous cell lines were obtained according to the method already described (Cavazzana, 1987). Cells were grown in RPMI 1640 medium supplemented with antibiotics and L-glutamine plus 15% fetal bovine serum. In both cases, the cells grew as substrate adherent, rounded cells.

*Immunofluorescence*: Immunofluorescence studies were performed on cells plated on coverslips and fixed in cold acetone (-20 C) for 10 min. We then investigated the presence of vimentin (Dako), keratin (AE1/AE3), neurofilament (Boehringer), glial fibrillary acidic protein (Dako), chromogranin (Boehringer) and synaptophysin (Boehringer), applying the following procedure: primary antibodies were applied at optimal dilution for 1 hr at room temperature, then two washes in PBS, followed by the secondary, fluorescein-conjugated antibody (anti-mouse or anti-rabbit, as appropriate to the primary antibody) diluted 1:10 for 1/2 hr at room temperature. The coverslips were then rinsed twice in PBS and examined in a fluorescence microscope.

*Cytogenetics*: Cytogenetic analysis of tumor cell lines was carried out as already described (Whang-Peng, 1986) and metaphases were karyotyped according to the Paris Conference specifications (ISCN,1978).

*RNA Hybridization*: Northern blot analysis of total RNA was performed as described (Davis, 1986). Twenty ug of total RNA from each cell line was electrophoresed in 1% agarose and blotted by capillary action overnight to a nylon membrane (GeneSreen Plus, Dupont). The membrane was then hybridized overnight at 42 C with a $^{32}$P nick translated c-DNA probe for the third exon of c-myc and for an EcoRI-BamHI fragment of N-myc gene (Lofstrand).

*Immunologic Cell Sorter Analysis*: Acetone fixed cells from both lines were incubated with the neuroblastoma monoclonal antibody HSAN 1.2 and the HLA-I reactive monoclonal W6.32 as described elsewhere (Donner, 1986).

## RESULTS

*Cell culture*: In vitro, the tumors displayed similar
though not identical morphology.  TC-268 (fig. 2A) displayed a more epithelioid appearance, but with unmistakable
neuritic processes.  JFEN, in contrast, appeared almost
neuroblastic, with poorly substrate adherent, rounded cells
and delicate neuritic processes (fig. 2B).  The neural
character of both, however, was unmistakable.

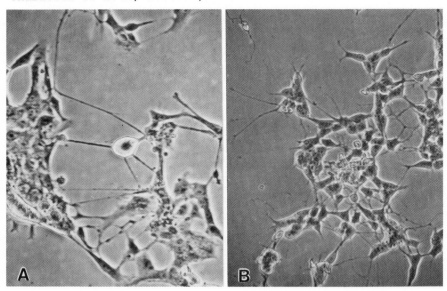

*Figure 2*:  In vitro, phase contrast appearance of the two
olfactory neuroblastoma cell lines.  A = TC-268; B = JFEN.
A neural character to both is evident, especially neurites.

The electron microscopic appearance of both cell lines
is essentially that displayed in figure 1C (from an original tumor biopsy).  There were no significant differences
between the two lines, or between the biopsy material and
the cell lines, other than a generally more primitive
appearance of the cell lines.

*Cytoskeleton*:  Three cytoskeletal proteins were identified in both cell lines by immunofluorescence.  Vimentin
(not illustrated, but positive in both lines) served only
to confirm the results with antibodies to keratin and
neurofilament triplet protein (NFTP).  Antibodies to the

160 kD subunit of NFTP were positive in both cell lines
(the result with JFEN is illustrated in figure 3A; TC-268
was less intensely positive). Surprisingly, antibodies to
keratin were also positive in both cell lines, unlike
neuroblastoma cells in culture. A typical result from
JFEN, is illustrated in figure 3B.

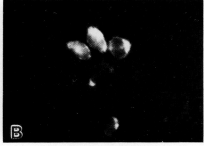

*Figure 3*: Cytoskeletal proteins in olfactory neuroblastoma. Both neurofilament (A) and keratin (B) were found in
both cell lines, as well as vimentin (not illustrated).

*Neurosecretory Proteins*: The neural character of these
tumors was further defined by analyzing their expression of
two proteins closely associated with neurosecretory granules (as observed by EM, fig. 1C). Immunocytochemical
evidence for chromogranin A expression was obtained in both
cell lines. The staining was punctate, scattered, and generally not intense (fig. 4A), but was distinctive and
reproducibly positive. Synaptophysin displayed diffuse,
intense cytoplasmic fluorescence in both lines (fig. 4B).

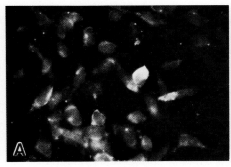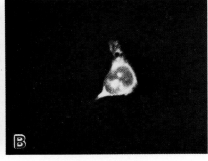

*Figure 4*: Immunodetectable chromogranin or related protein
was detected in both lines as punctate and (rarely) diffuse
staining (A); synaptophysin, in contrast, was diffusely
positive in cell cytoplasm in both lines (B).

*Cell Sorter Analysis*:   Tumor cells from both TC-268 and JFEN stained with the neuroblastoma monoclonal antibody HSAN 1.2 were moderately (but not strongly) fluorescent by cell sorter analysis (figure 5, A & B, light solid line), especially when compared to control specimens reacted with non-specific hybridoma and fluoresceinated second antibody (A & B, dotted lines).  This degree of positivity is less than that usually observed in neuroblastoma.

Reactivity with HLA-I antibody (W6/32), in contrast to HSAN 1.2, was intensely positive in both lines (fig. 5, A & B, heavy solid line).  This result has not been observed in conventional neuroblastoma (i.e., uniformly negative) in our experience.

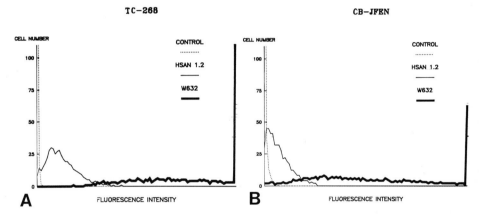

*Figure 5*:   Fluorescence activated cell sorter analysis of TC-268 (panel A) and JFEN (panel B) after reaction with control hybridoma (dotted line, each panel), HSAN 1.2 monoclonal antibody (light solid line) and HLA-I reactive monoclonal antibody (heavy solid line).  Both lines are moderately HSAN 1.2 reactive and intensely HLA-I reactive.

*Cytogenetics*:  Cytogenetic analysis of both cell lines revealed consistent abnormalities involving several chromosomes (Table 1.).  In particular, chromosome 1 displayed a 1p+ abnormality, similar to that often observed in neuroblastoma.  At the same time, however, the characteristic reciprocal chromosomal translocation (11:22) (q21:q12) previously reported in a family of neuroepithelial tumors (Ewing's sarcoma, the "Askin tumor" of chest wall (Askin,

1979) , and peripheral neuroepithelioma) was also identified in TC-268 but not JFEN. However, JFEN <u>did</u> display deletional abnormalities of chromosomes 11 and 22 (11q-, 22q-) involving the same chromosomes and same segments as the rcp(11:22) translocation found in TC-268 and the neural tumors noted above. There is thus reasonable similarity in the cytogenetic abnormalities found in both these lines. Further, this is a unique combination, combining elements of the characteristic abnormalities found in both neuroblastoma <u>and</u> peripheral neural tumors.

---

*Table 1:* Summary of Cytogenetic Abnormalities Observed in Olfactory Neuroblastoma (TC-268 and JFEN).

*JFEN*: Mode = 44 (range 26-99)

1p+, 5p+, 7q+, 8p+, 10q-, 11q-, dup14, 15-, 17-, 22q-, Xq-

*Tc-268*: Mode = 49 (range 41-51)

1p+, 8+, t(11:22)(q21:q12), 12+, 14+

---

*Oncogene Expression*: We have previously noted that neuroepithelioma, unlike all (or virtually all) cultured neuroblastomas, fails to express the N-myc oncogene in vitro (Thiele, 1987; Triche, 1987). We analyzed the two ONB lines for both N-*myc* and c-*myc* expression. Northern Blot analysis of total RNA failed to demonstrate any N-*myc* expression in either olfactory neuroblastoma (figure 6, panel B), like other peripheral neural tumors and unlike neuroblastoma.

In contrast, c-*myc* expression was striking in both ONB, even more so than for other peripheral neural tumors, and unlike neuroblastoma, which expresses no c-*myc* (panel A). This pattern is clearly that of peripheral neural tumors and unlike neuroblastoma.

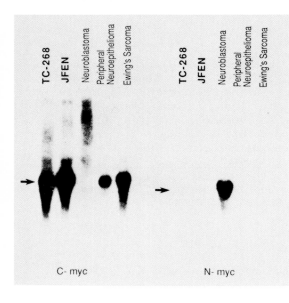

*Figure 6*: Northern analysis of *myc* oncogene expression in ONB and related tumors.

ONB (lanes 1 & 2) markedly overexpresses c-*myc* but not N-*myc* in vitro, like other peripheral neural tumors but unlike neuroblastoma.

Note that only neuroblastoma among childhood peripheral neural tumors was found to overexpress N-*myc* in this study, as in others (see text).

## DISCUSSION

Olfactory neuroblastoma (ONB) has not previously been studied in vitro, for lack of any cell line established from this tumor. Conventional studies of patient material have failed to delineate characteristics that would allow this tumor to be grouped with or distinguished from other neural tumors of children and young adults. The successful establishment of two ONB lines by the present investigators has allowed detailed biological study of this ill-understood neoplasm for the first time, and allows a far more precise categorization of this tumor in context with other neural tumors.

A neuroectodermal origin for this rare tumor has been assumed, as implied by the synonymous terms olfactory *neuroblastoma* and esthesio*neuroblastoma*. This has seemingly been confirmed by observations of NSE positivity (Taxy, 1986) and the presence of neurofilaments (Trojanoski, 1985) in this tumor in vivo. Additionally, however, the term *neuroblastoma* has also implied a close relationship with conventional neuroblastoma. Against this is the older age incidence, including adults, where neuroblastoma is vanishingly rare (Skolnik, 1966). For this is the occasional report of catecholamine positivity (Micheau, 1975), a finding not reported in peripheral neural tumors for the most part.

Our data would appear to support a largely peripheral neural character to this tumor, with one intriguing exception. Certainly the expression of proteins such as neurofilament, NSE, synaptophysin, and chromogranin provide overwhelming evidence of the neural character of this tumor. The finding of 44 kD keratin, HLA-I epitope, and c-*myc* (but not N-*myc*) expression is typical of neuroectodermal tumors but not neuroblastoma (Gould, 1986; Reynolds, 1987; Thiele, 1987). However, the presence of both chromosome 1 abnormalities (like neuroblastoma) and chromosome 11 & 22 abnormalities (like peripheral neural tumors of children) appears unique to this tumor. We have not previously seen this cytogenetic pattern among childhood neural tumors.

The biological parameters studied and discussed here serve to both confirm the neural character of this tumor and to set it apart from conventional neuroblastoma. They fail to establish whether ONB is truly a unique tumor. Most of the features are those of peripheral neural tumors, not neuroblastoma (thus suggesting that olfactory neuroblastoma is a poor choice of names), yet at least one feature, the 1p+ chromosome abnormality found in both cases here, invokes comparison with neuroblastoma. However, most neuroblastomas with 1p abnormalities likewise show rearrangement and/or amplification of N-*myc* oncogene, with concomitant over-expression. That was not found here. Does this suggest a new category, tumor heterogeneity, or an "exception to the rule?" Several PNETs have been described recently that lack the 11:22 translocation (Helson, 1987), suggesting that cytogenetic abnormalities per se may not be reliable markers for inclusion or exclusion within a given category.

On balance, it appears premature to draw firm conclusions as to the proper categorization of this tumor. Certainly, though, it is not typical neuroblastoma, and it is rather closely related to the Askin tumor, peripheral neural tumors, and Ewing's sarcoma, albeit with at least one or two differences. We view ONB as a unique form of peripheral neural tumor.

# REFERENCES

Askin FB, Rosai J, Sibley RK, et al (1979). Malignant small cell tumor of the thoracopulmonary region in childhood. Cancer 43:2438-24551.

Barnes L, Peel RL, Verbin RS (1985). Surgical Pathology of the head and neck. New York, Marcel Dekker, Inc, pp: 680-682

Cavazzana AO, Magnani JL, Ross R, Triche TJ (1987). Ewing's sarcoma is an undifferentiated neuroectodermal tumor. Prog Clin Biol Res (in press, this volume).

Davis LG, Dibner MD, Battey JF (1986). Basic Methods in Molecular Biology. Elsevier, pp 41-336

Donner L, Triche TJ, Israel MA, Seeger RC, Reynolds CP (1985). A panel of monoclonal antibodies which discriminate neuroblastoma from Ewing's sarcoma, rhabdomyosarcoma, neuroepithelioma, and hematopoietic malignancies. Prog Clin Biol Res 175:347-366.

ISCN (1978). Paris conference on chromosomes

Micheau C, Guerinot F, Bohuon C, Brugere J (1975). Dopamine beta-hydroxylase and catecholamines in a olfactory esthesioneuroma. Cancer 35:1309-1312

Potluri VR, Gilbert F, Helsen C, Helson, L (1987). Primitive neuroectodermal tumor cell lines: Chromosomal analysis of five cases. Cancer Genet Cytogenet 24:75-86.

Reynolds CP, Brodeur GM, Tomayko MM, Donner L, Helson L, Seeger RC, Triche TJ (1987). Biological classification of cell lines derived from human extra-cranial neural tumors. Prog Clin Biol Res (in press, this volume).

Skolnik EM, Massari FS, Tenta LT (1966). Olfactory neuroepithelioma; review of the world literature and presentation of two cases. Arch Otolaryngol 84:644

Taxy JB, Bharani NK, Mills SE, Frierson HF, Gould VE (1986). The spectrum of olfactory neural tumors. A light-microscopic immunohistochemical and ultrastructural analysis. Am J Surg Pathol 10:687-695.

Thiele CJ, McKeon C, Triche TJ, Ross RA, Reynolds CP, Israel MA (1987). Differential Proto-oncogene expression characterizes histopathologically indistinguishable tumors of the peripheral nervous system. J Clin Invest (submitted).

Triche TJ, Cavazzana AO, Navarro S, Reynolds CP, Slamon DJ, Seeger RC (1987). N-*myc* protein expression in small round cell tumors. Prog Clin Biol Res (this volume).

Trojanowski JQ, Lee V, Pillsbury N, Lee S (1982). Neuronal

origin of human esthesioneuroblastoma demonstrated with anti-neurofilament monoclonal antibodies. N Engl J Med 307:159-161.

Whang-Peng J, Triche TJ, Knutsen T, Miser J, Kao-Shan S, Tsai S, Israel MA (1986). Cytogenetic characterization of selected small round cell tumor of childhood. Cancer Genet Cytogenet 21:185-208

Wiedenmann B, Franke WW, Kuhn C, Moll R, Gould VE (1986). Synaptophysin: A marker for neuroendocrine cells and neoplasms. Proc Natl Acad Sci USA 83:3500-3504.

Advances in Neuroblastoma Research 2, pages 475–485
© 1988 Alan R. Liss, Inc.

N-*myc* PROTEIN EXPRESSION IN SMALL ROUND CELL TUMORS

Timothy J. Triche, A.O. Cavazzana, S. Navarro,
C.P. Reynolds, D.J. Slamon, and R.E. Seeger
*Laboratory of Pathology, NCI, Bethesda, MD
(T.J.T., A.O.C., and S.N.), and UCLA School of
Medicine, Los Angeles, CA (C.P.R., D.J.S., and
R.E.S.)*

# INTRODUCTION

N-*myc* is an oncogene first identified in and now
closely associated with childhood neuroblastoma (Schwab et
al, 1983). Amplification and/or overexpression of the
N-*myc* oncogene has been implicated in clinically aggressive
(stage III-IV) neuroblastoma (NB) (Brodeur et al, 1984;
Seeger et al, 1985). Identification of N-myc amplification
has so far been by Southern analysis of extracted DNA using
an N-*myc* specific probe. Attempts to identify N-*myc*
amplification in individual tumor cells have so far utilized this same radiolabelled probe on tumor sections by *in
situ* hybridization (Schwab et al, 1984; Grady-Leopardi et
al, 1986). This approach is defective in two respects: 1)
tumor cell morphology is poorly preserved by current *in
situ* methodology, and little useful information regarding
tumor cell cytology and tumor heterogeneity is thereby
obtained, and 2), distinctions between N-*myc* amplification
versus expression (as mRNA) are not possible.

Since N-*myc* <u>expression</u> is the most biologically relevant correlate, a method that reflects relative amounts of
N-*myc* oncogene expression, in tumor sections, while adequately preserving tumor morphology, would be most useful.
Immunocytochemistry, employing anti-oncogene antibodies, is
a promising method to address these problems. Recently, an
N-*myc* specific rabbit polyclonal antibody raised against
N-*myc* recombinant oligopeptides that can be used in conventional immunocytochemistry has been described (Slamon et
al, 1986).

We have employed that antibody and method to determine whether N-*myc* protein expression (as detected by tumor section immunocytochemistry) correlates with N-*myc* DNA amplification (as determined by Southern analysis), RNA expression (by Northern analysis), or protein expression (by Western analysis) among the so-called small, round, blue cell tumors of childhood. In this study, that group includes neuroblastoma (both N-*myc* amplified and un-amplified), other peripheral neural tumors, Ewing's sarcoma, rhabdomyosarcoma, and lymphoma.

# MATERIALS AND METHODS

Clinical Material: Twenty eight cases of childhood tumors were studied. The diagnostic grouping, based on antecedent pathologic studies that included routine light and electron microscopy and immunocytochemistry, is as follows:

| | |
|---|---|
| Neuroblastoma: | 7 cases, 1 relapse |
| Peripheral Neuroepithelioma | 6 cases |
| Esthesioneuroblastoma | 2 cases |
| Ewing's sarcoma | 5 cases |
| Rhabdomyosarcoma | 4 cases |
| Lymphoma | 3 cases |

In addition, tumor cell lines were established from 12 of the cases, and xenograft tumors were utilized in parallel when this possibility existed.

In all cases, fresh tumor tissue was surgically excised, placed in an aqueous cryoprotective embedding medium (OCT compound), sectioned (ca. 7 micron sections) in a cryostat at -40 degrees Celsius, mounted on glass slides, air dried, re-hydrated after varying periods of time with phosphate buffered saline, pH 7.4, pre-incubated in methanol and $H_2O_2$ (0.1 %), rinsed, pre-incubated in 1% goat serum in PBS, rinsed, incubated with primary antiserum (see below) for 4 hours at room temperature, rinsed X 3, incubated with biotinylated anti-rabbit antibody, rinsed, incubated·with avidin/peroxidase complexes, rinsed, developed in DAB (diaminobenzidine) with 0.03% $H_2O_2$, and the reaction product intensified by nickel chloride enhancement. Finally, the slides were lightly counterstained with nuclear fast green. Slides were dehydrated and mounted in non-aqueous mounting medium.

Hind III Digest, 15 ug DNA / lane

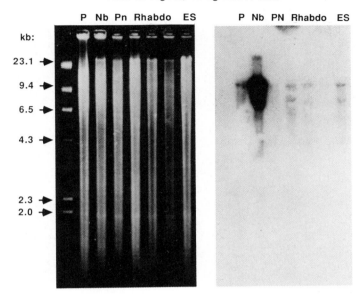

*Figure 3.* Southern analysis of N-*myc* gene copy number in a number of childhood round cell tumors. Panel A), total DNA per lane, by ethidium bromide UV fluorescence. Panel B), same gel, blotted and hybridized with N-*myc* probe. Only neuroblastoma displays increased copy number.

Because the N-*myc* oncogene has been reported expressed in the absence of gene amplification, we also assessed the extent of N-*myc* gene expression as mRNA by Northern analysis. The results are depicted in figure 4. Panel A depicts the results when hybridized with the N-*myc* probe, and panel B, the same gel hybridized with the c-*myc* probe. In this case, the two neuroblastomas that stained with N-*myc* antibody are seen in lanes 1 and 2; both show marked expression of mRNA for N-*myc*. No other tumor does so, including 2 peripheral neuroepitheliomas (PN), two esthesion-euroblastomas (EN), 3 rhabdomyosarcomas (Rhabdo), an additional PN (not included in this study), and 2 Ewing's sarcomas. By way of control (and contrast), panel B demonstrates that undegraded RNA was present in all lanes, since the c-*myc* probe hybridized to all other tumors.

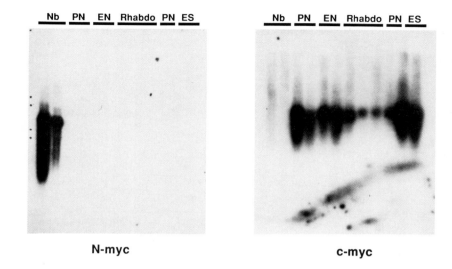

**N-myc**                **c-myc**

*Figure 4.* Northern analysis of a panel of round cell tumors of childhood. N-*myc* expression was found only in N-*myc* amplified neuroblastoma; all others were negative (panel A). All samples were undegraded and present in relatively equal amounts, as seen in panel B.

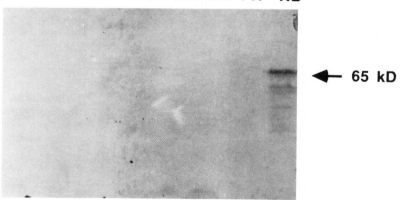

*Figure 5.* Western Analysis of a similar panel of tumors as figure 4. Only the N-*myc* amplified neuroblastoma (NB) shows evidence of N-*myc* protein production.

In view of these results, it would appear that high expression of N-*myc* protein will be limited to N-*myc* amplified neuroblastomas. Nonetheless, to verify this, we performed the analogous experiment for N-*myc* protein synthesis. The results are illustrated in figure 5. Here, the approximately 64-62 kD N-*myc* protein is identified only in association with neuroblastoma; all other tumors do not have detectable N-*myc* protein. These results are consistent with both the molecular genetic and immunocytochemical results reported above.

## DISCUSSION

The results depicted above provide compelling evidence for the close association between N-*myc* oncogene amplification and its expression. Among this group of "round cell" tumors, including both amplified and unamplified neuroblastoma, other neural tumors, Ewing's sarcoma, rhabdomyosarcoma, and lymphoma, we detected no instance of N-*myc* expression or N-*myc* protein accumulation in the absence of N-*myc* gene amplification.

The results reported here are based on a limited sample (28 cases) of a wide variety of undifferentiated childhood tumors. We are aware of a number of reports of N-*myc* expression (as mRNA) in a number of other tumors (retinoblastoma, Lee et al, 1984; astrocytoma and rhabdomyosarcoma, Garson et al, 1985, 1986; Wilms tumor, Nisen et al, 1986; rhabdomyosarcoma, Garvin et al, 1987). In particular, two separate reports have documented N-*myc* amplification in rhabdomyosarcoma (Garson, 1986; Garvin, 1987). We have found no such N-*myc* amplification, expression, or protein synthesis in our panel of tumors. This may well be due to the limitations of sample size, but other factors, such as diagnosis, may also be relevant. Larger studies of well characterized tumors with highly sensitive immunohistologic and immunoblotting techniques will be required to clarify this discrepancy.

One goal of this study was to determine whether N-*myc* protein detection would be limited to neuroblastoma, and therefore prove a useful criterion for the differential diagnosis of undifferentiated "round cell" tumors of children. The results unequivocally support the notion that among this group of tumors, the detection of N-*myc* protein is tantamount to a diagnosis of neuroblastoma. Conversely,

<u>failure</u> to detect the protein does not preclude a diagnosis
of neuroblastoma. Nonetheless, the simplicity and reliability of the technique (when used in parallel with known
positive and negative control specimens) is a viable alternative to in situ hybridization, the only other tissue sec-
tion-based method for N-*myc* detection. The results are at
least as reliable, the morphology is superior, and the
method is simpler. For diagnostic and other purposes, this
approach appears superior.

# REFERENCES

Brodeur GM, Seeger RC, Schwab M, Varmus HE, Bishop JM
(1984). Amplification of N-*myc* in Untreated Human Neuroblastomas Correlates with Advanced Disease Stage.
Science 224:1121-1124.

Davis LG, Dibner MD, Battey JF (1986). "Basic Methods in
Molecular Biology." Elsevier, pp. 41-336.

Garson JA, McIntyre PG, Kemshead JT (1985). N-*myc* Amplification in Malignant Astrocytoma. Lancet 2:718-719.

Garson JA, Clayton J, McIntyre P, Kemshead JT (1986).
N-*myc* Oncogene Amplification in Rhabdomyosarcoma at
Release. Lancet 1:1496.

Garvin AJ, Sens DA (1987). The In Vitro Growth and Differentiation of a Human Rhabdomyosarcoma Cell Line. Lab
Invest 56:26A.

Grady-Leopardi EF, Schwab M, Ablin AR, Rosenau W (1986).
Detection of N-*myc* Oncogene Expression in Human Neuroblastoma by *in Situ* Hybridization and Blot Analysis:
Relationship to Clinical Outcome. Cancer Res 46:
3196-3199.

Lee W, Murphree AL, Benedict WF (1984). Expression and
Amplification of the N-*myc* Gene in Primary Retinoblastoma. Nature 309: 458-460.

Nisen PD, Zimmerman KA, Cotter SV, Gilbert F, Alt FW
(1986). Enhanced Expression of the N-*myc* Gene in Wilms'
Tumors. Cancer Res 46:6217-6222.

Schwab M, Alitalo K, Klempnauer K-H, Varmus HE, Bishop JM,
Gilbert F, Brodeur G, Goldstein M, Trent J (1983).
Amplified DNA with limited homology to *myc* cellular
oncogene is shared by human neuroblastoma cell lines and
an neuroblastoma tumour. Nature 305:245-248.

supernatant of homogenized cells as follow: tyrosine hydroxylase by modification (Joh et al, 1973) of the method of Coyle(1972), and choline acetyltransferase (CAT) according to the method of Fonnum (1969) .

*Cytoskeleton extraction and Western Blot analysis*:
Cytoskeleton proteins were extracted as previously described (Osborn, 1977). The final detergent insoluble pellet was resuspended in sample buffer and electrophoresed in 10% SDS polyacrylamide gels. The proteins were blotted on nitrocellulose paper overnight at 4 C as described (Towbin, 1979). After blotting, the filter was soaked for 1 hr at room temperature in 5% FBS/PBS, then the first antibody at optimal dilution was added in to a sealing bag and rotated for 2 hrs at RT.

After a double washing in PBS, the filter was sealed in a new bag with the secondary antibody (peroxidase- conjugated) for 1 hr at RT. After a final extensive wash, the reaction was developed using 4-chloro-1 naphtol as reagent.

*Lipid Extraction and TLC analysis*: Total lipids were extracted by a modification of a previously described method (Kannagi, 1982). Cells are homogenized in 3 volumes of 0.4 M ammonium bicarbonate on ice. Isopropanol (8.25 volumes) was added followed by 3.75 volumes of hexane. After shaking for 30 min. at room temperature, the extract is centrifuged at 2000 rpm for 10 min. The extraction is repeated on the pellet and the supernatants are combined and evaporated under $N^2$. The dried lipid extract is then resuspended in 5 volumes of chloroform/methanol. Glycolipid extract equivalent to 2 mg packed cells is chromatographed on thin layer cromatograms for each cell line. Glycolipid antigens are detected directly on thin layer chromatograms as previously described (Magnani, 1982).

*Northern Blot Analysis*: Total RNA from cell lines was extracted according to the guanidium/isothiocyanate method as described (Davis, 1986). Twenty ug of total RNA from each line was electrophoretically separated and blotted to nylon filter (Gene Screen Plus, Du Pont) as described (Davis, 1986). The immobilized RNA was hybridized with a nick translated P-32 labelled DNA probe corresponding to the third exon of c-myc (Lofstrand), or with an ECORI/BAM H1 fragment of N-myc gene (Lofstrand) overnight at 42 C. After washing, the filter was exposed to X-ray film overnight.

## RESULTS

*Original Tumors and Establishment of cell lines*: The
five tumor cell lines used here were established from
patients referred to NCI with a diagnosis of Ewing's sarcoma. All original tumors satisfied the most stringent
diagnostic criteria either by light microscopy (LM) or
electron microscopy (EM). They were composed of a uniform
population of round small tumor cells with the classic
biphasic cellular appearance of clear and dark cells, and
with abundant cytoplasmic glycogen demonstrable by LM and
EM (fig. 1, A-B). All cases showed a bland ultrastructural
appearance with no evidence of neural differentiation (fig.
1B) and all were negative for neuron-specific enolase (NSE)
on paraffin sections. The clinical data referring to age,
sex, site of the tumors, follow-up, and cytogenetic analysis of the patients are illustrated in table 1.

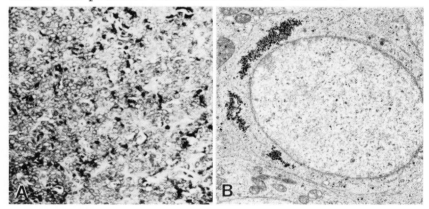

*Figure 1.* Light (A) and electron (B) microscopic appearance of Ewing's sarcoma. No differentiation of any type is
detectable by these means in any of the cases studied here.

The phase contrast appearance of the untreated tumor cell
(fig.2A ) showed a uniform population of flat, polygonal,
substratum adherent cells. Cytogenetic analysis performed
on cultured cells confirmed the presence in all five cell
lines of an 11:22 reciprocal chromosomal translocation, as
expected in bona fide Ewing's sarcoma.

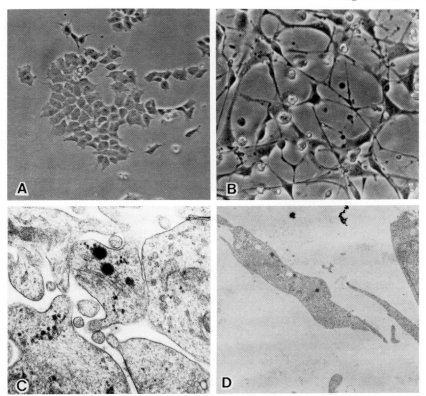

*Figure 2.* Ewing's sarcoma in vitro. Untreated cells (A) show no evidence of differentiation. After treatment with dbcAMP or TPA, neural features, especially neurites, are striking (B). By EM, neurotubules and dense core granules are readily found (C). Confirmation of the neurosecretory nature of granules is evident from uraniffin staining (D).

*Differentiation*: Since it is well known that serum inhibits the expression of a neural phenotype (Skaper et al, 1983) in many neuroectodermal derived tumor cell lines such as pheochromocytoma and neuroblastoma, we performed a first series of experiments growing cells in conditioned medium in the absence of serum. In no case were we able to demonstrate any morphological change in cultured ES cell, unlike neuroblastoma cells, which developed long neurites under such conditions.

In contrast to the above, treatment with c-AMP, TPA, or NGF produced a dramatic change in the phase contrast

appearance of cells. Treated cells significantly decreased
their growth rate, became smaller, and sprouted long cellular processes with varicosities along their course (fig.
2B), typical of the neurites seen in similarly treated
neuroblastoma cells. By EM, the processes contained neurotubules, numerous intermediate filaments, and dense core
granules (fig. 2C). The neurosecretory nature of these was
confirmed by means of the uraniffin reaction (fig 2D).

*Cytoskeleton analysis*: The intermediate filament content (vimentin, keratin, and neurofilament triplet protein)
of these tumors was investigated by indirect immunofluorescence with Western blot confirmation. Vimentin, as
expected, was always positive in all cell lines (data not
shown). Low molecular weight keratin (44 kD) was found in
3 untreated cell lines (fig 3) . Keratin-like filament
bundles had been observed by EM (3A), which prompted con-
firmatory immunologic analysis. Scattered cytoplasmic positivity for keratin was detected by immunofluorescence
(3B), and confirmed by Western analysis (3C). Thus, keratin was unequivocally expressed, even in undifferentiated
Ewing's sarcoma cells.

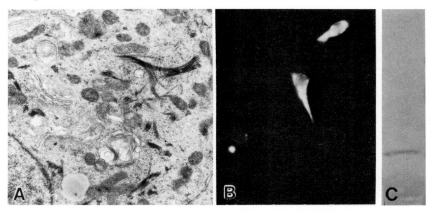

*Figure 3*. Cytoskeletal keratin. Keratin-type bundles
were occasionally found in untreated cells (A). Their
identity was confirmed by immunofluorescence with anti-
keratin antibody (B) and by Western analysis (C).

The typical neural cytoskeletal filament is neurofilament protein. We assayed the presence or absence of the
160 kD subunit of this protein similarly to keratin (vide

supra). We detected the 160 kD NFTP subunit in four out of
five untreated cell lines as weak, localized cytoplasmic
staining by immunofluorescence (fig 4A). After differentiation, intense fluorescence was noted in perinuclear
cytoplasm and along the neuritic processes described previously (fig. 4B) in all five lines. The results with NFTP
antibody were likewise confirmed by Western blot analysis
of detergent insoluble cytoskeleton. The 160 KD component
of NFTP was clearly detectable even in the four untreated
cases studied (fig. 5). The 200 KD component was present
in only one case (data not shown).

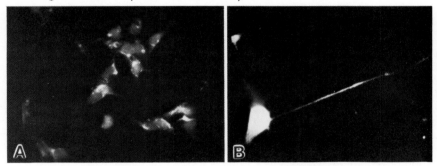

*Figure 4.* Neurofilament triplet protein as visualized
by anti-160 kD subunit specific monoclonal antibody in
undifferentiated (A) and differentiated (B) Ewing's cells.

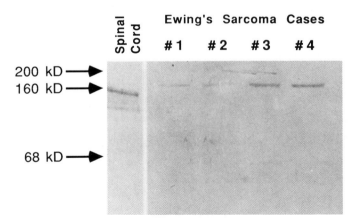

* Western Blot Analysis, anti-160 kD NFTP Monoclonal Antibody

*Figure 5.* Western analysis of NFTP in Ewing's cells.
All four lines studied for NFTP contained 160 kD subunit.

*HNK-1 epitope analysis*: HNK-1 (commercially available as Leu-7 ) is a monoclonal antibody that recognizes epitopes localized on natural killer cells and on myelin-associated glycoprotein. The latter is found on cells derived from the neural crest (Lipinski, 1986). Indirect immunofluorescence on acetone-fixed ES cells failed to demonstrate any reactivity. In contrast, when 2.5% paraformaldheyde was used as fixative, unequivocal cell surface fluorescence was detected.

The absence of staining after acetone fixation (normally used for proteinaceous antigens) but presence after formaldehyde fixation (which does not extract lipids) suggested that the detected antigen in Ewing's sarcoma cells was present in glycolipids. We therefore examined the reactivity of the HNK-1 antibody with extracted glycolipids from Ewing's sarcoma cells. Figure 6 clearly demonstrates strong reactivity with several glycolipids separated by thin layer chromatography and immunostained directly with the antibody. Quantitative staining varies, but all are reactive. Doublet bands are due to differences in ceramide composition.

GM2 → 
GM1 → 
GD1a → 
GD1b → 
GT1a → 
Origin → 

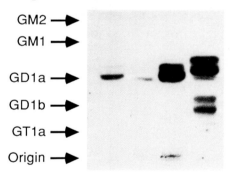

5838  71  106  4573

*Figure 6.* Immunoanalysis of extracted glycolipids separated by thin layer chromatography. All four Ewing's lines contain immunodetectable sulfate-3-glucuronyl paragloboside. A third pair of bands, from a larger glycolipid with this epitope, is present in lane 4 (line 4573).

*Neurotransmitter Enzymes:* To further confirm the neural nature of the presumed neural phenotype expressed after differentiation, we investigated the expression of neuron specific enolase (NSE), cholinesterase and chromogranin before and after treatment with differentiating agents.

In undifferentiated cells studied by immunofluorescence, little if any NSE or cholinesterase was detectable; panel 7A illustrates a typical weak positive result with anti-cholinesterase antibodies. After differentiation, in contrast, a strong fluorescence appeared localized in the cytoplasm and in processes (fig. 7B).

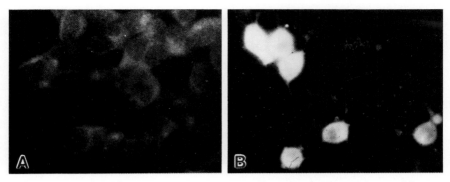

*Figure 7.* Cholinesterase content of Ewing's sarcoma cells by immunofluorescence. A, undifferentiated cells; B, after differentiation with dbcAMP.

Chromogranin, the neurosecretory granule-associated protein, was negative by immunofluorescence under all conditions. This result was confirmed by Western blot analysis of a vesicle-enriched cell fraction. Neuroblastoma cells were positive for the 68 kD protein; Ewing's sarcoma and peripheral neuroepithelioma cells were negative.

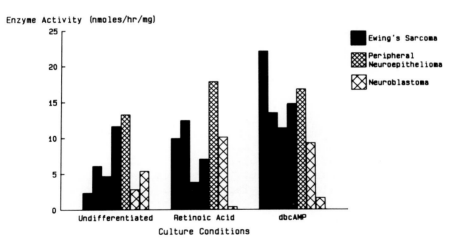

*Figure 8.* Quantitative analysis of choline acetyl transferase (CAT) activity in Ewing's sarcoma, peripheral neuroepithelioma, and neuroblastoma, before and after differentiation. Ewing's cells always contain CAT activity, which increases with neural differentiation.

Because NSE is often an unreliable index of neural character and chromogranin is still only poorly understood and evaluated in human tumors, we felt it important to verify the cholinesterase results other methods. Figure 8 is a graphic representation of the extent of neurotransmitter enzyme expression in each of the three main tumor types, under differentiating and non-differentiating conditions. It is apparent that Ewing's sarcoma (as well as other neural tumors) always expresses reasonable levels of choline acetyl transferase; these levels rise after differentiation with dbcAMP, more so than neuroblastoma or peripheral neuroepithelioma (figure 8, second and third group).

## DISCUSSION

A neural origin or character for this enigmatic tumor has been suggested by many investigators on the basis of cytogenetic analysis of tumors and cell lines (Whang-Peng et al., 1986), and as a result of immunological investigation on paraffin embedded or fresh material (Lipinski, 1986; Jaffe, 1984; Caillaud, 1984). The results presented here clearly establish that Ewing's sarcoma is indeed a neural tumor, and apparently only a neural tumor. No other type of differentiation was observed. Furthermore, this neural phenotype can be detected in some cases (neurotransmitter enzymes, neurofilament triplet protein) in undifferentiated cells as well as after differentiation.

A pluripotential character of Ewing's sarcoma has been proposed, and in fact primitive pluripotential cells such as teratocarcinoma cells can display multiple lines of differentiation in vitro (Liesi, et al, 1983). In the case of Ewing's sarcoma cells, treatment with both neural differentiating agents (such as c-AMP) as well as non-specific differentiating agents (such as TPA) seems to induce only neural differentiation. Further, even the undifferentiated tumor cells appear to display only neuroectodermal markers such as neurofilament triplet protein, an HNK-1 epitope, and cholinergic neurotransmitter enzymes (CAT). There is thus no evidence to support any other cell of origin than neuroectodermal.

The presence of simple keratin (44KD) and the expression of only cholinergic neurotransmitter enzymes is a typical phenotype observed in primitive neuroepithelia. Absence of keratin expression and acquisition of adrenergic neurotransmitter enzymes is typical of more differentiated sympathetic neural tissue and tumors (i.e., neuroblastoma).

The results reported here therefore attest to the *neural,*
but only *primitive neuroepithelial* nature of Ewing's sarcoma. This is true of a variety of neural tumors of children other than neuroblastoma, such as peripheral neuroepithelioma (Thiele, 1987), the so-called Askin tumor (Askin,
1979), and the primitive neuroectodermal tumor of bone
(Jaffe, 1984), to name only some better characterized
examples. For these, and other reasons reported elsewhere,
we interpret Ewing's sarcoma as another member of this family of non-neuroblastoma neural tumors of children and
young adults.

## REFERENCES

Askin FB, Rosai J, Sibley RK, et al (1979). Malignant
    Small Cell Tumor of the Thoracopulmonary Region. Can-
    cer 43:2438-2451.
Caillaud JM, Benjelloun S, Bosq J, Braham K, Lipinski M
    (1984). HNK-1-defined antigen detected in paraffin-
    embedded neuroectoderm tumors and those derived from
    cells of the amino precursor uptake and decarboxylation
    system. Cancer Res 44:4432-4439
Coyle JT (1972). Tyrosine hydroxylase in rat brain-cofactor
    requirements, regional and subcellular distribution.
    Biochem Pharmacol 21:1935.
Davis LG, Dibner MD, Bettey JF (1986). "Basic Methods in
    Molecular Biology." Elsevier, pp 41-336.
Dickman PS, Liotta LA, Triche TJ (1982). Ewing's sarcoma;
    Characterization in established cultures and evidence
    of its histogenesis. Lab. Invest. 47:375-382.
Fonnum F (1969). Radiochemical micro-assay for the determi-
    nation of choline acetyltransferase and acetylcholines-
    terase activities. Biochem J 115:465 Towbin (1979)
Franke W, Schimd E, Winter S, Osborn M, Weber K (1979).
    Widespread occurrence of intermediate filaments of
    vimentin-type in cultured cells from diverse verte-
    brates. Exp Cell Res 123:25-46.
Jaffe R, Santamaria M, Yunis EJ, et al (1984). The neuroec-
    todermal tumor of bone. Am J Surg Pathol 8:885-898.
Joh TH, Geghman C, Reis DJ (1973). Immunochemical demon-
    stration of increased accumulation of tyrosine hydroxy-
    lase protein in sympathetic ganglia and adrenal medulla
    elicited by reserpine. Proc Natl Acad Sci USA 70:2767
Kannagi R, Nudelman E, Levery SB, Hakomori S (1982). A
    series of human erythrocyte glycosphingolipids reacting
    to the monoclonal antibody directed to a developmen-

tally regulated antigen SSEA-1. J Biol Chem 257:14865-14874

Liesi P, Rechardt L, Wartiovaara J (1983). Nerve Growth Factor induces neuronal differentiation in F9 terato-carcinoma cells. Nature 306:265-267.

Lipinski M, Braham K, Philip I, Wiels J, Philip T, Goridis C, Lenoir GM, Tursz T (1986). Neuroectoderm-associated antigens on Ewing's sarcoma cell lines. Ca Res 47:183-187.

Magnani JL Nilsson B, Brockhaus M, Zopf D, Steplewski Z, Koprowski H, Ginsburg V (1982). A Monoclonal Antibody-defined Antigen Associated with Gastrointestinal Cancer is a Ganglioside Containing Sialylated Lacto-N-fucopentose II. J Biol Chem 257:14365-14369

Roessner A, Voss B, Rauterberger J, Immenkamp M (1980). Ewing's sarcoma: A comparative electron and immuno-fluorescence study. Thirteenth International Congress of International Academy of Pathology, Paris, September 15-19.

Skaper SD, Selak I, Varon S (1983). Serum vulnerability and time-dependent stabilization of neurites induced by Nerve Growth Factor in PC12 Pheochromocytoma cells. J Neurosc Res 10:303-315

Takahashi K, Tadashi S, Kojima M (1980). Cytological char-acterization and histogenesis of Ewing's sarcoma. Acta Pathol. Jpn. 26:167-190

Thiele CJ, McKeon C, Triche TJ, et al (1987). Differential Proto-oncogene Expression Characterizes Histopathologi-cally Indistinguishable Tumors of the Peripheral Ner-vous System. J. Clin. Invest. (submitted).

Whang-Peng J, Triche TJ, Knutsen T, Miser J, Kao-Shan S, Tsai S, Israel MA (1986). Cytogenetic characterization of selected small round cell tumor of childhood. Cancer Genet. Cytogenet. 21:185-208.

Advances in Neuroblastoma Research 2, pages 499–506
© 1988 Alan R. Liss, Inc.

DISCUSSION

Chairman:        M.C. Glick and Uriel Littauer

Discussants:     M. Ponzoni, M.B. Meyers,
                 A.O. Cavazzano, T.J.Triche

Lipinski: Dr. Cavazzano, your talk confirms some of our findings recently published. We showed that some Ewing's sarcomas produce cytokeratine and if the cells are treated with inducers of differentiation such as TPA then the small number of cells expressing cytokeratine at the start became much larger. We believe that Ewing's sarcoma cells also have the capacity to differentiate along an ectodermal pathway.

Lampson: What are the biological differences between olfactory neuroepithelioma and neuroblastoma?

Cavazzano: There are many biological differences between classical neuroblastoma and esthesioneuroblastoma. First the trimodal incidence. The different prognoses of the esthesioneuroblastoma in old age and in the second decade of life. From a strictly biological point of view, the esthesioneuroblastoma show simultaneous coexpression of neurofila and cytokeratines. This seems to indicate that there is a relationship to the primitive neural crest cell more than neuroblastoma. Neuroblastomas fail to express cytokeratines.

Glick Is esthesioneuroblastoma an earlier developmental tumor?

Cavazzano: I don't think we are at the point to say that. It is related to primitive neuroectodermal tumors which have been described in the bone or in soft tissue or related to peripheral epithelioma more than to the classical neuroblastoma.

Israel: We are particularly interested in studying esthesioneuroblastoma. While the cases you showed may be very closely related to or even the same as peripheral neuroepithelioma, I would be extremely reluctant to say that all esthesioneuroblastoma is that tumor. The literature has many cases where esthesioneuroblastoma is positive for gliol fibrillary acidic protein (GFAP). It occurs in the olfactory bulb which is very different from the neuron that we think is the neuron of origin of the PNET and there are, exactly as you pointed out, a number of gross different clinical features including prognosis, appropriate treatment and time of outset. These raise the issue that esthesioneuroblastoma is an extremely heterogeneous group of tumors and to call them PNET is not appropriate. Your other finding that was most unusual was that these tumors (esthesioneuroblastoma) were chromogranin positive. Is that right?

Cavazzano: Chromogranin expression in a neural tumor is, right now, a difficult issue to explain. We see in classical neuroblastoma, isolated positivity in single cells and all the other cells negative. In esthesioneuroblastoma isolated positivity and all other cells are negative. However, we don't rely on immunofluorescence alone. We analyze the tumors by western blotting. When we examine classical neuroblastoma, peripheral neuroblastoma, esthesioneuroblastoma and Ewing's sarcoma we find neuroblastoma is positive, esthesioneuroblastoma is slightly positive, PNET is negative and Ewing's sarcoma gives a strange cross-reaction with a protein at 58kd which we cannot yet recover. The protein we identify by this technique is 75kd on SDS-PAGE gel. This is not the real size of the molecule. The real molecular weight is 50kd. After these tumors have been injected into nude mice and subsequently cultured, neuroblastoma is still positive, esthesioneuroblastoma is still very faintly positive. For Ewing's we did not resolve the problem. By Northern hybridization, using a probe for chromogranin A, neuroblastoma is still positive, but we don't find messages in the other tumors. These experiments raise other questions: are those techniques sensitive enough to detect single cell positivity or not? What does it mean to have single-cell positivity? Is is not enough to make a similarity or a distinction between esthesioneuroblastoma and classical neuroblastoma?

Kemshead: Dr. Triche, We've looked at 12 well-characterized embryonal rhabdomyosarcomas on the basis of their clinical picture, conventional pathology, EM, immunohistology and 4 rhabdomyosarcoma cell lines. We've seen N-myc amplification in one out of the 12 of that series and that particular sample was autopsy material. In our hands we couldn't look for N-myc expression or expression of the protein product using the heteroantiserum, or antiserum raised against a synthetic peptide of the N-myc protein. Out of those 12 samples, we also have seen one that was not amplified but seemed to over-express N-myc. All the other lines we have looked at don't over-express or amplify N-myc.

Triche: Thank you, that is very encouraging. Was that the positive one you published in Lancet?

Answer: Yes.

Triche: Your results are very comparable to a further study I am researching here.

Frantz (Rochester): I am a little confused as to the differences between PNET and Ewing's sarcoma and whether it is useful trying to distinguish between them.

Triche: That is particularly important, clinically, since for some time we have had a high risk Ewing's protocol at NIH. The treatment protocol of PNET's is the same as Ewing's sarcoma for treatment. At this point, the followup is approaching 20 or 22 months. The peripheral neural tumors — and the term refers specifically to those tumors having 11-22 translocation, HLA-positive etc as we have defined it, are doing less well, although not a great deal less well. The actuarial survival projected out to 60% for the Ewing's and 50% for the primitive neuroectodermal tumors. Historically, according to the literature, treated on a less rigorous regimen, these tumors have done very poorly.

Israel: The study you have quoted contains 19 children in the Ewing's arm and 17 children in the neuroepithelioma arm and it is difficult to assess a 10% difference in outcome when these small numbers distinguish between a 50% projected actuarial outcome and a 60%! Let us say the difference in outcome is probably indicative of some biologic difference.

Brodeur: I want to ask Dr. Triche to complete the picture, could you say where the so-called Askin tumor fits into the broad umbrella of PNET? and second, have you looked at any brain tumors for N-myc expression or any other tumors particularly medulloblastomas?

Triche: The Askin tumor is more a clinico-pathological curiosity. As it turns out, they have all the same features and characteristics as the other peripheral nerve tumors and the Ewing's sarcomas. For our purposes, the only distinction I would make between so-called Askin tumors and the other peripheral neuroepitheliomas, is an anatomic location. They are only chest wall PN's in my opinion. With regard to the second question, I have virtually no access to brain tumors.

Di Bernardi (Genoa): We recently had a 17 year old boy with esthesioneuroblastoma who did not respond to therapy. He had negative MIBG scan and did not excrete catecholamines. At the same time we had a 3 year old boy with esthesioneuroblastoma who relapsed after an initial response. When he relapsed he had elevated catecholamines, MIBG positive and it clearly appeared to be a neuroblastoma. So age seems to make a difference.

Cavazzano: As far as I know, your report of the case of excretion of catecholamines by esthesioneuroblastoma is the second world report. The first being published by a French group sometime ago. There is no other evidence of catecholamine excretion by esthesioneuroblastoma. I think the second case you presented could be a classical neuroblastoma. Originally, it did not secrete catecholamines because it was localized, probably, and then when it relapsed to the bone marrow is secreted the catecholamines.

Hartmann (Villejuif): Just a word of warning - it is difficult with small children to be absolutely sure that they have esthesioneuroblastoma since it is possible to have a real neuroblastoma tumor discovered because of metastasis in this part of the skull. If you don't look carefully for the primary, you will call a tumor an esthesioneuroblastoma when it is just a metastasis from a neuroblastoma.

Kemshead (London): Dr. Cavazzano, you originally reported the cell line was positive for antigen to UJ13A and then lost expression of this antigen with respect to time. Do you have any data on the karyotypic features of this cell line that could correlate with the expression of that protein?

Cavazzano: Yes, the bone marrow that we studied and from which this cell line originated, was 95% UJ 13A positive mononuclear cells from Ficoll. After 33 passages, the cells became pseudodiploid and pseudotetrephoid with 92 chromosomes. The UJ 13A started to become lower and lower. We detected between 5 and 10% UJ 13A positive cells only after achieving 92 or 93 chromosomes, not before.

Kemshead: Is the 5% of cells which remain UJ 13A positive, stable? If you then remove them from the negative population, do you induce another population of cells that are UJ 13A positive?

Cavazzano: I've not done that.

Meyers: The multidrug resistance neuroepithelioma line MCIXC/VCR has quite different characteristics from the BE(2)-C/VCR neuroblastoma vincristine-resistant line or the SY/VCR. They fit the differences you see between different cell lines. If neuroepithelioma is not a neuroblastoma then the drugs will see these cells differently and will produce different characteristics in the resistant sublines.

Glick: Is there any similarity in your selections of cells between the multidrug studies and the Ara-C? In a way you are selecting cells when you treat them.

Cavazzano: If you increase the concentration of Ara-C you kill the cells. We chose only a very low dose which gives us 95-100% viable cells which are morphologically differentiated - but not classically drug-resistant lines.

Meyer: We may be talking about a similar type of event, but it is hard to compare an established cell line to a treated cell population.

Cavazzano: Dr. Beidler, do you observe whether the same cells having a differentiated morphology become round and reduplicate after being adherent to the plastic in culture?

Beidler: You mean the morphological transformations that were seen? Yes. If you start with a substrate-adherent population it can change gradually back to a round cell, non-substrate adherent population and that in due course may shift back again. There is no change in viability within these two cell types.

Cavazzano: If we try to separate the cells from an adherent morphology then these don't adhere any more. In a very short time we have the same kind of morphology again.

Biedler: But you are talking about a drug-treated population.

Cavazzano: It happens even if we don't treat the cells.

Biedler: To clone and maintain one of these morphological N- or S- types of clones in a pure form is something which has been rather a heroic effort over the years. I think the rate of interconnection between these two extremes vary from cell to cell.

Gilbert: Dr. Meyers, if your cells are capable of growing in soft agar, aren't they transformed? What do you mean by reverse transformed?

Meyers: Yes - when we call a cell reverse transformed as the Chinese hamster and mouse tumor cells are highly resistant to drugs, their characteristics are altered morphology, that is the resistant cells grow in a more normal fashion. They are substrate adherent, contact inhibited and when injected into animals they don't produce tumors. The neuroblastoma resistant lines have some characteristics of reverse transformation but we wouldn't call them reverse transformed unless they did not grow in nude mice and were anchorage dependent.

Gilbert: How do you postulate that the cells have lost their tumor genecity? Either a back mutation from the primary change responsible for the generation of neuroblastoma or peripheral neuroepithelioma? Or is it some new dominant mutation which affects its ability to grow?

Meyers: I believe our notion is not one of back mutation but rather one of selection of a population of resistant cells from the original total population.

Beidler: There is another process which is not genetic - except in a non-mutational process such as one can invoke for cell differentiation which will result in a marked change in phenotype and many properties but does not require mutations as DNA-sequence changes and that is what we mean by reverse transformation which is a phenotypic change. We are not laying claim to specific genetic alterations.

Gilbert: There is a paper in Science by Stanbridge who introduced normal chromosome 11 into Wilms' cells - we presume has the deleted or missing genes responsible for the tumorogenesis. There the 11+ clone was non-tumorogenic but capable of growing in soft agar. In that situation he was postulating a genetic change, but by your argument he could have been introducing something else that affected growth characteristics or differentiating phenotyped without actually reversing the primary gene change.

Biedler: We know there is a genetic change associated with the development of drug resistance and in this case is specifically the gene coding for 'P' glycoprotein. But we don't know whether that alteration in these cells has anything to do with reverse transformation process. In these drug resistance cells 3% of total membrane protein is P-glycoprotein but does this influence other membranes comparability in some way? We really don't have any evidence for a genetic alteration which results directly in reverse transformation.

Meyers: Furthermore, these cells are not normal, they may be reverse transformed by some characteristics that we define, but they are not normal cells. They are transformed cells and this goes along with the clinical observation that patients may relapse with a drug resistant tumor and they fail to live. We may not be talking about a genetic change leading to normalcy or a genetic change leading to malignancy.

Glick: Will you comment on the fact that you have reverse transformed properties and yet you increase the expression of N-myc?

Meyers: There is increased N-myc in BE(27)C/VCR cells but we haven't really studied the proper characteristics of reversed transformation. These cells were not introduced into nude mice and the preliminary study that was done on anchorage -independence in soft agar suggested increased plating efficiency. The corresponding study was done with the NNS cells. Dr. Michitsch reported this yesterday. He had S- cells - flattened cells which had elevated N-myc and these cells had elevated plating efficiency as well compared to N-cells which had a lower level of RNA for N-myc. Again, those cells hadn't been studied in nude mice. These results suggest that elevated N-myc may be concomitant

with reverse transformation in this type of study - but
we don't have the final results as yet.

# CLINICAL STUDIES
# AND INNOVATIVE THERAPIES

Advances in Neuroblastoma Research 2, pages 509–524
© 1988 Alan R. Liss, Inc.

# INTERNATIONAL CRITERIA FOR DIAGNOSIS, STAGING AND RESPONSE TO TREATMENT IN PATIENTS WITH NEUROBLASTOMA

**Chairmen and Writing Committee:** Garrett M. Brodeur, Robert C. Seeger. **Contributors:** Ann Barrett, Robert P. Castleberry, Gulio D'Angio, Bruno De Bernardi, Audrey E. Evans, Marie Favrot, Arnold I. Freeman, Gerald Haase, Olivier Hartmann, F. Ann Hayes, Larry Helson, John Kemshead, Fritz Lampert, Jacques Ninane, Thierry Philip, Jon Pritchard, Stuart Siegel, Ide E. Smith, P.A. Voute.

Washington University School of Medicine, St. Louis, MO 63110 (GMB); UCLA School of Medicine, Los Angeles, CA 90024 (RCS); Glasgow Institute of Radiotherapeutics and Oncology, Glasgow G31 4PG, Scotland (AB); University of Alabama, Birmingham, AL 35233 (RPC); Children's Hospital of Philadelphia, Philadelphia, PA 19145 (GD, AEE); Instituto Giannina Gaslini,16148 Genova, Italy (BD); Centre Leon Berard, 69373 Lyon Cedex 08, France (MF, TP), Roswell Park Memorial Institute, Buffalo, NY (AIF); Children's Hospital of Denver, Denver, CO 80218 (GH); Institut Gustave-Roussy, 94805 Villejuif Cedex, France (OH); St. Jude Children's Research Hospital, Memphis, TN 38101 (FAH); Stewart Pharmaceuticals, Wilmington, DE 19897 (LH); Institute of Child Health, London, England WC2L (JK); Leiter der Kinder-Poliklinik der Justus Liebig-Universitat, Giessen, West Germany (FL); Cliniques St. Luc, Brussels B-1200, Belgium (JN); Hospitals for Sick Children, London WC1N 3JH, England (JP); Children's Hospital of Los Angeles, Los Angeles, CA 90027 (SS); Oklahoma Children's Hospital, Oklahoma City, OK 73126 (IES); Emma Kinderziekenhuis, 1018HJ Amsterdam, Netherlands (PAV).

## INTRODUCTION

Neuroblastoma, a tumor of the peripheral nervous system, is one of the most common tumors of childhood (Young and Miller, 1975). However, there has been little improvement in the long-term survival of patients with this disease (Thomas et al, 1984), despite dramatic improvements in the survival of patients with many other pediatric malignancies, notably acute lymphoblastic leukemia and Wilms tumor. One of the obstacles to progress in treatment of this disease is the difficulty in comparing results of protocols from different centers and from different countries, largely because of a lack of uniform criteria for diagnosis, for staging, and for determining response to therapy (Ungerleider, 1981).

Neuroblastoma is a "small, round, blue cell tumor," which generaly arises in the adrenal medulla or along the sympathetic chain in a child. To confirm this diagnosis, some histologic evidence is generally required for neural origin or differentiation by light microscopy, electron microscopy or immunohistology. Alternatively, because of the frequency of involvement of the bone marrow in 50-60% of patients, some patients are considered to have neuroblastoma on the basis of "compatible cells" involving the bone marrow, with increased urinary catecholamine metabolites. A third criteria used by some is a compatible radiographic appearance with increased urinary catecholamine metabolites. Since not all groups accept all three methods of classifying a patient as having neuroblastoma, there exist some discrepancies between studies.

There are three major staging systems used for neuroblastoma throughout the world: 1) the system utilized by the Children's Cancer Study Group (CCSG), and others (Evans et al, 1971); 2) the system used by St. Jude Children's Research Hospital (SJCRH) and the Pediatric Oncology Group (POG) (Hayes et al, 1983); and 3) the TNM system proposed by the International Union Against Cancer (UICC) (AJC, 1983). Modifications of these systems are employed by the Italian Cooperative Working Group (De Bernardi et al, 1987), the Malignant Tumor Committee of the Japanese Society of Pediatric Surgeons (Sawaguchi et al, 1980), and others. In general, the various staging systems give comparable results in distinguishing low-stage, good-prognosis patients from high-stage, poor-prognosis patients. However, some of the differences between these different staging systems are substantial, particularly as applied to individual patients, and so the results of one group cannot be readily compared with another.

Points of disagreement include: 1) the prognostic significance of tumor crossing the midline, 2) the prognostic importance of ipsilateral and/or contralateral lymph node involvement, and 3) the importance of resectability of the primary tumor. Agreement on the definition of stage with regard to these and other issues would facilitate the comparison of different studies.

A variety of terms have been used to report the response of neuroblastoma patients to a given treatment protocol: complete response (CR), very good partial responses (VGPR), good partial response (GPR), partial response (PR), mixed response (MR), stable disease (SD), and progressive disease (PD). Despite the general use of these terms, the same term may have a different meaning when used by different groups. This is due in part to differences in the number and type of tests used for re-evaluation. In addition, the time at which response is evaluated often varies considerably.

A conference, sponsored by the William G. Forbeck Research Foundation, was held on 10-11 November, 1986 to begin the process of standardizing definitions for diagnosis, staging and treatment response. Individuals representing most of the major groups in the world agreed in principle on definitions and drafted documents. These documents were then circulated to participants and others not in attendance. Finally, the proposals were presented and discussed at the 4th International Symposium on Advances in Neuroblastoma Research on 14-16 May, 1987. This communication represents the conclusions reached at that meeting. A final document, which is anticipated to have few if any substantive changes from this one, will appear shortly in a peer-reviewed journal.

## DIAGNOSIS

The conferees and corresponding participants agreed on *minimum* criteria for establishing a diagnosis of neuroblastoma (Table 1):

Table 1. DIAGNOSIS OF NEUROBLASTOMA

---

A diagnosis of neuroblastoma is established if:

1. an unequivocal pathological diagnosis is made from tumor tissue by standard methods, including electron microscopy if necessary; or

2. bone marrow contains unequivocal tumor cells (e.g., syncytia) *and* urine contains increased urinary catecholamine metabolites (VMA and/or HVA > 3 SD above the mean per mg creatinine for age).

---

The above definition excludes the use of a compatible radiographic appearance and increased urinary catecholamine metabolites. One reason is that some tumors other than neuroblastoma or ganglioneuroblastoma could cause this picture (e.g., ganglioneuroma, peripheral neurepithelioma). In addition, there is increasing emphasis on biologic features of neuroblastoma cells for diagnosis or prognosis, e.g., histopathology, immunophenotype, N-*myc* gene copy number and/or expression, DNA index, etc. (Donner et al, 1985; Shimada et al, 1984; Brodeur et al, 1984; Seeger et al, 1985; Look et al, 1984). It is likely that some of these or other features will supersede the importance of some of the clinical distinctions, such as crossing the midline or lymph node involvement, as future prognostic schema or staging systems develop. In order to provide tumor tissue for these studies, it will be critical to have tissue obtained as part of the diagnostic workup.

In addition, a battery of immunologic reagents, biochemical markers and DNA probes are being developed that may allow increased specificity in making a diagnosis of neuroblastoma. It will be crucial to have tissue available for these studies as well. If surgery is necessary to obtain tissue for diagnosis (see Table 1), more definitive diagnostic and prognostic information can be obtained. This information may allow the selection of a more appropriate treatment approach and may obviate the need for subsequent, aggressive reevaluation or surgery.

## STAGING

It is clear that the primary and metastatic sites must be evaluated, but at issue is the number and type of tests used to determine the extent of disease. The proposed staging system utilizes components of previous systems (Table 2). Arabic numbers are used rather than Roman numerals or letters of the alphabet to distinguish this system from the two most widely used systems for neuroblastoma (Evans et al, 1971; Hayes et al, 1983).

Stage 1 is similar to stages I and A, and stage 4 is essentially identical to stages IV and D, respectively. We have divided stage 2 into 2A and 2B to distinguish between individuals who are classified as stage 2 based on incompletely excised tumor vs. ipsilateral lymph node involvement. There is controversy over the impact of ipsilateral vs. contralateral lymph node involvement on prognosis (Hayes et al, 1983; Rosen et al, 1985). Accordingly, it was decided to divide stage 2 into 2A and 2B, such that these patients could be analyzed separately or together. Thus, it can be determined if the behavior of the patients with

Table 2. STAGING SYSTEM FOR NEUROBLASTOMA

---

**Stage 1:** Localized tumor confined to the area of origin; complete gross excision, with or without microscopic residual disease; identifiable ipsilateral and contralateral lymph nodes negative microscopically.

**Stage 2A:** Unilateral tumor with incomplete gross excision; identifiable ipsilateral and contralateral lymph nodes negative microscopically.

**Stage 2B:** Unilateral tumor with complete or incomplete gross excision; with positive ipsilateral regional lymph nodes; identifiable contralateral lymph nodes negative microscopically.

**Stage 3:** Tumor infiltrating across the midline with or without regional lymph node involvement; or, unilateral tumor with contralateral regional lymph node involvement; or, midline tumor with bilateral regional lymph node involvement.

**Stage 4:** Dissemination of tumor to distant lymph nodes, bone, bone marrow, liver and/or other organs.

**Stage 4S:** Localized primary tumor as defined for stage 1 or 2A with dissemination limited to liver, skin or bone marrow.

---

stage 2B more closely resembles stage 2A or 3. Theoretically most stage 3 tumors will be confined to the abdomen, since tumor crossing the midline by contiguous infiltration or by lymph node involvement will be uncommon in the thorax. There is no obvious prognostic significance to the different patterns of tumor spread by which a patient is considered to have stage 3 disease, so this stage has not been subcategorized.

Stage IV-S has been retained as 4S based on the favorable outcome generally experienced with these patients (D'Angio et al, 1971; Evans et al, 1980; Nickerson et al, 1985), and because of recent biologic evidence distinguishing these patients from infants with conventional stage IV disease, such as serum ferritin, DNA index and N-*myc* copy number (Hann et al, 1981; Hann et al, 1985; Look et al, 1984; Seeger et al, 1985,).

There was some discussion concerning the issue of placing an age restriction of 1 year on Stage 4S. Some felt that the unique behavior of these patients was generally restricted to the first 6-12 months of life. Others felt that the rare patient over 1 year of age who met the criteria for stage 4S might be overtreated if assigned to Stage 4. The number of true 4S patients over 1 year of age should be very small, and it is not clear if their tumors behave in a nonaggressive manner similar to their younger counterparts, or in an aggressive manner typical of disseminated disease in older children. Since there are no age restrictions on other stages, it decided not to include an age restriction for this group of patients.

The minimum testing necessary to define these stages is presented in Table 3. Certainly, the more tests that are done, the greater the likelihood of finding disseminated disease. Uniformity with respect to minimum testing should improve the ability to compare studies, and the studies recommended can be done in most major medical centers. This is an area that is continually evolving, and recommendations undoubtedly will be made in the future that will improve determination of the extent of disease.

The specificity and sensitivity of MIBG for evaluation of bone and soft tissue involvement by neuroblastoma was discussed (Hoefnagel et al, 1985; Geatti et al 1985). Unfortunately, MIBG scintigraphy is not readily available, if at all, in most major centers in the United States as well as in some other countries. Until MIBG scintigraphy becomes more widely available, and

Table 3. MINIMUM RECOMMENDED TESTS FOR DETERMINING
EXTENT OF DISEASE

| Tumor site | Tests |
|---|---|
| Primary | CT scan, ultrasound or magnetic resonance imaging (MRI) with 3D measurements |
| Metastases | Bilateral posterior iliac bone marrow aspirates and core biopsies (4 adequate specimens necessary to exclude tumor) |
| | Bone x-rays and scintigraphy by $^{99m}Tc$-diphosphonate, and/or $^{131}I$- or $^{123}I$-meta-iodobenzylguanidine (MIBG) |
| | Abdominal and liver imaging by CT scan, ultrasound or MRI |
| | Chest x-ray (AP and lateral) and chest CT scan |
| Markers | Urinary catecholamine metabolites (VMA *and* HVA) |

Note: For evaluation of bone metastases, $^{99m}Tc$-diphosphonate scan is recommended in all patients and is essential if MIBG scan is negative in bone.

until there is more experience with its use diagnostically, $^{99m}Tc$-diphosphonate scintigraphy will remain the standard for evaluation of bone disease. It is likely that once the MIBG technique is more widely available and more experience is gained, it will be included in the routine evaluation of patients with suspected or proven neuroblastoma.

Another area of difference concerns the assessment of bone marrow disease by marrow aspirates and/or biopsy. Some centers do only a single marrow aspirate, whereas others routinely do 9 aspirates and 4 biopsies under general anesthesia. Recent studies suggest that marrow biopsies add substantially to the detection of marrow involvement by tumor. Also, it is apparent that obtaining more samples will increase the likelihood of detecting marrow involvement. However, the clinical relevance of detecting marrow involvement with additional studies if it is not detected in the first few studies is unclear. A compromise was reached to use two marrow aspirates and two biopsies from bilateral posterior iliac crests. Only a single study positive for tumor is required to document bone marrow involvement, but all four studies are required to rule it out.

The methods for detection of marrow involvement by tumor are in evolution. Many centers rely on standard cytology of marrow smears and histology of marrow biopsies, whereas others are using "neuroblastoma-specific" immunocytology (Moss et al, 1985). The latter approach is more sensitive in detecting occult disease. However, until techniques and reagents become standardized, the determination of bone marrow involvement will continue to rely on standard cytology and histopathology.

The determination of lymph node involvement has been a problem, particularly for surgeons. It is not always clear which lymph node groups need assessment if none are enlarged. In addition, the distinction between adherent, adjacent, draining, and "distant" nodes may be difficult. Any enlarged lymph nodes should be biopsied to document the presence or absence of tumor involvement, and other identifiable nodes also should be biopsied. Each lymph node that is biopsied should be labelled so that its relationship to the primary tumor is apparent. However, it is not necessary to biopsy nodes in the contralateral thorax to rule out tumor involvement if none are enlarged. A standardized approach to lymph node biopy and assessment will be formulated by surgery and pathology representatives at a later date.

## RESPONSE TO TREATMENT

Criteria for determining the response to therapy vary considerably from one institution to another, as well as the time at which the assessment of response is made. The same tests that are used for determining extent of disease (Table 3) should be used to assess response of primary and metastatic sites to treatment. Table 4 lists criteria to determine response to therapy. It is important to note that a given level of response (e.g., CR) requires that the primary and all metastatic sites fulfill CR criteria. A CR in metastatic sites and a PR in the primary tumor would be considered a PR overall. Evaluations for response for newly diagnosed patients are recommended at 3, 6, 12 and 24 months, and as indicated clinically. If a CR, VGPR or PR is achieved surgically, it should be indicated as such when reporting the response. Response must be evaluated before surgery to allow assessment of chemotherapy response as well as combined modality response.

Although examples are given for responses in organs like liver and lungs, one can evaluate other evidence of organ involvement in a similar manner. Physical examination may be informative for assessment of primary tumors in the abdomen or pelvis, as well as for assessment of metastatic disease, such as skin involvement, or other measurable lesions. This should also be included in any evaluation of response to treatment. Three-dimensional measurements should be possible for primary tumors and most metastatic lesions except bone or marrow. The response criteria are expressed as percent decreases in size and are based on the product of the greatest two diameters measurable, not on volume.

It is difficult to give a rigorous quantitative assessment to the evaluation of bone and bone marrow disease. For example, scintigraphic changes may lag behind histologic changes by weeks or months, such that an "improved" bone lesion may be free of tumor histologically but not returned to normal by scintigraphy. It would be useful to have a quantitative scintigraphic value for a bone

Table 4. Definitions of Response to Treatment

| Response[1] | Primary[2] | Metastases[2] | Markers[2] |
|---|---|---|---|
| 1) CR | No Tumor | No tumor (chest, abdomen, liver, bone, bone marrow, nodes, etc.) | HVA/VMA normal |
| 2) VGPR | Reduction >90% | No tumor (as above except bone); no new bone lesions, all pre-existing lesions improved on scan. | HVA/VMA decreased >90% |
| 3) PR | Reduction 50-90% | 50-90% reduction in measurable sites; 0-1 bone marrow samples with tumor; scan same as VGPR. | HVA/VMA decreased 50-90% |
| 4) MR | >50% reduction of any measurable lesion (primary or metastases) with <50% reduction in any other; no new lesions; <25% increase in any existing lesion (exclude bone marrow evaluation). | | |
| 5) NR | No new lesions; <50% reduction but <25% increase in any existing lesion (exclude bone marrow evaluation). | | |
| 6) PD | Any new lesion; increase of any measurable lesion by >25%; previous negative marrow positive for tumor. | | |

[1] CR = Complete Response; VGPR = Very Good Partial Response; PR = Partial Response; MR = Mixed Response; NR = No Response; PD = Progressive Disease.
[2] Evaluations of primary and metastatic disease as outlined in Table 3.

lesion at diagnosis and at re-evaluation, similar to Hounsfield units in computerized tomography. For the present, we will have to rely on more qualitative assessments until a quantitative measurement can be developed and standardized.

With respect to marrow involvement, a decrease from a packed marrow to a single clump on a single aspirate is clearly a meaningful response, although the marrow would still be viewed as "positive." Since marrow aspirates and biopsies are subject to sampling artifacts, it is difficult to be more quantitative than we have done in Table 4. Perhaps in the future, immunocytology will provide a more objective means of quantitating a percentage of marrow involvement, but the problem of sampling bias will be difficult to overcome.

## DISCUSSION

An international consensus has been reached for neuroblastoma regarding criteria for diagnosis, staging and response to treatment. These criteria do not contain any radical concepts or major changes from previous systems, but they do embody the most important features in a system that is more comprehensive and rigorously defined. The use of these criteria should facilitate greatly comparisons between clinical and laboratory studies from different institutions and different countries. As such, this represents a major milestone in international cooperation.

These criteria are a foundation upon which future modifications and improvements can be built. It is likely that advances in immunodiagnosis, molecular biology, diagnostic imaging and other areas will result in substantial changes in the above criteria. An increasing number of clinical and laboratory tests are becoming available that appear to improve diagnosis, staging, and assessment of disease status in patients with neuroblastoma.

Ultimately, it may be possible to use a combination of clinical and biological criteria to divide patients into three groups: those who require no further therapy following surgery; those who are curable with conventional therapy; and those who would fail conventional therapy and who should receive more aggressive or experimental approaches (i.e., bone marrow transplantation, new agents, differentiation therapy, immunotherapy). The international implementation of these approaches will be facilitated by the framework provided here, as well as the network of communication and cooperation that has been established.

## ACKNOWLEDGEMENTS

We wish to acknowledge the invaluable contribution of Jennifer and George Forbeck and the William Guy Forbeck Research Foundation, Hilton Head, SC, for sponsoring the initial meeting and supporting this international effort. The writing committee would like to thank the selfless efforts of all contributors from around the world who were willing to put aside personal, regional and national interests and work in a true spirit of cooperation for the sake of an international agreement on these very important issues. We also wish to thank the following individuals for helpful suggestions in the preparation of this manuscript: Frank Berthold, Julie Blatt, Christopher Fryer, Shinsaku Imashuku, Michio Kaneko, Akira Nakagawara, Mark Nesbit, Ruprecht Nitschke, Haruo Ohkawa, Teresa Vietti, K. Y. Wong.

## REFERENCES

American Joint Committee (AJC) on Cancer (1983). Neuroblastoma. In: "Manual for Staging of Cancer," 2nd ed. JB Lippincott Co, Philadelphia, pp 237-239.

Bostrom B, Nesbit ME, Brunning RD (1985). The value of bone marrow trephine biopsy in the diagnosis of metastatic neuroblastoma. Am J Ped Hematol Oncol 7: 303-305.

Brodeur GM, Seeger RC, Schwab M, Varmus HE, Bishop JM (1984). Amplification of N-*myc* in untreated human neuroblastomas correlates with advanced disease stage. Science 224: 1121-1124.

D'Angio GJ, Evans AE, Koop CE (1971). Special pattern of widespread neuroblastoma with a favorable prognosis. Lancet 1: 1046-1049.

De Bernardi B, Rogers D, Carki M, Madon E, de Laurentis T, Bagnulo S, Di Tullio MT, Paolucci G, Pastore G (1987). Localized neuroblastoma. Surgical and pathological staging. Cancer 60: 1066-1072.

Donner K, Triche TJ, Israel MA, Seeger, RC, Reynolds CP (1985). Immunohistologic detection and phenotyping of neuroblastoma cells in bone marrow using cytoplasmic neuron specific enolase and cell surface antigens. Progr Clin Biol Res 175: 367-378.

Evans AE, D'Angio GJ, Randolph JA (1971). A proposed staging for children with neuroblastoma. Children's Cancer Study Group A. Cancer 27: 374-378.

Evans AE, Chatten J, D'Angio GJ, Gerson JM, Robinson J, Schnaufer L (1980). A review of 17 IV-S neuroblastoma patients at the children's hospital of Philadelphia. Cancer 45: 833-839.

Franklin IM, Pritchard J (1983). Detection of bone marrow invasion by neuroblastoma is improved by sampling at two sites with both aspirates and trephine biopsies. J Clin Pathol 36: 1215-1218.

Geatti O, Shapiro B, Sisson JC, Hutchinson RJ, Mallette S, Eyre P, Beierwaltes WH (1985). Iodine-131 metaiodobenzylguanidine scintigraphy for the location of neuroblastoma: Preliminary experience in ten cases. J Nuc Med 26: 736-742.

Hann HWL, Evans AE, Cohen IJ, Leitmeyer JE (1981). Biologic differences between neuroblastoma stage IVS and IV, measurement of serum ferritin and E-rosette inhibition in 30 children. New Engl J Med 305: 425-429.

Hann HWL, Stahlhut MW, Evans AE (1985). Serum ferritin as a prognostic indicator in neuroblastoma: Biological effects of isoferritins. Progr Clin Biol Res 175: 331-346.

Hayes FA, Green AA, Hustu HO, Kumar M (1983).
Surgicopathologic staging of neuroblastoma:
Prognostic significance of regional lymph node
metastases. J Pediatr 102: 59-62.

Look AT, Hayes FA, Nitschke R, McWilliams NB, Green
AA (1984). Cellular DNA content aas a
predictor of response to chemotherapy in
infants with unresectable neuroblastoma. New
Engl J Med 311: 231-235.

Moss TJ, Seeger RC, Kindler-Rohrborn A, Marangos
PJ, Rajewsky MF, Reynolds CP (1985). Immunohistologic detection and phenotyping of
neuroblastoma cells in bone marrow using
cytoplasmic neuron specific enolase and cell
surface antigens. Progr Clin Biol Res        175:
367-378.

Nickersen HJ, Nesbit ME, Grosfeld JL, Baehner RL,
Sather H, Hammond D (1985). Comparison of stage
IV and IV-S neuroblastoma in the first year of
life. Med Pediatr Oncol 13: 261-268.

Rosen EM, Cassady JR, Frantz CN, Kretschmar CS,
Levey R, Sallen SE (1985). Stage IV-N: A
favorable subset of children with metastatic
neuroblastoma. Med Pediatr Oncol 13: 194-198.

Sawaguchi S. Suganuma Y, Watanabe I, Tsuchida Y,
Okabe I, Sawada T, Taguchi N, Takahashi H,
Kinumaki H, Ise T, Tsunoda A, Tsunooka H, Ueda
T, Muta H (1980). Studies of the biological and
clinical characteristics of neuroblastoma. III.
Evaluation of the survival rate in relation to
17 factors. Nippon Shoni Geka Gakkai Zasshi 16:
51-66.

Seeger RC, Brodeur GM, Sather H, Dalton A, Siegel
SE, Wong KY, Hammond D (1985). Association of
multiple copies of the N-*myc* oncogene with rapid
progression of neuroblastomas. New Engl J Med
313: 1111-1116.

Shimada H, Chatten J, Newton WA Jr, Sachs N,
Hamoudi AB, Chiba T, Marsden HB, Misugi K
(1984). Histopathologic prognostic factors in
neuroblastic tumors: Definition of subtypes of
ganglioneuroblastoma and an age-linked
classification of neuroblastomas. J Natl Cancer
Inst 73: 405-416.

Thomas PRM, Lee JY, Fineberg BB, Razek AA, Perez CA, Land VJ, Vietti TJ (1984). An analysis of neuroblastoma at a single institution. Cancer 53: 2079-2082.

Ungerleider RS (1981). Working conference on neuroblastoma treatment trials. Cancer Treat Rep 65: 719-723.

Voute PA, Hoefnagel CA, Marcuse HR, de Kraker J (1985). Detection of neuroblastoma with $^{131}$I-meta-iodobenzylguanidine. Prog Clin Biol Res, 175: 389-398.

Young JL Jr, Miller RW (1975). Incidence of malignant tumors in U.S. children. J Pediatr 86: 254-258.

Advances in Neuroblastoma Research 2, pages 525–534
© 1988 Alan R. Liss, Inc.

MASS SCREENING FOR NEUROBLASTOMA IN INFANCY.

The Japanese Mass Screening Study Group
of Neuroblastoma: T. Sawada, T. Sugimoto,
T. Matsumura, (Department of Pediatrics,
Kyoto Prefectural University of Medicine,
Kyoto, Japan. 602), A. Tunoda, T. Takeda,
K. Yamamoto, R. Koide, N. Nagahara,
Y. Hanawa, K. Nishihira, N. Sasaki,
Y. Ishiguro, N. Nakata., I. Okabe,
M. Kaneko, T. Yazawa, H. Ando.(Participating Medical and Research Institute in
Japan).

INTRODUCTION

Neuroblastoma(NB), the second most common
malignant tumor of children in Japan(Hirayama,198
1), is well known to have a poor prognosis in patients over 1 year of age and a favorable one under
1 year of age.(Breslow and McCann,1971, Sawaguchi
et al.,1979) Early diagnosis is the most important factor in its prognosis, and it is well known
that most patients with this tumor can be detected by measurement of urinary VMA(vanilmandelic acid) and HVA(homovanillic acid)(Gitlow et al.,19
70).

In 1974, an NB mass screening program,which
aims at the early detection of NB by a VMA spot
test of a urine sample at the age of 6 months, was
developed in Kyoto, Japan(Sawada et al.,1973,1978,
1982,1984). In 1981, the NB-mass screening study
group(MSSG) was organized by the Ministry of Health and Welfare to evaluate the significance of
mass screening for NB in 9 districts in Japan(Sawada et al.,1984). In 1985, according to the recommendation of the NB-MSSG, nation-wide mass screening was initiated throught the entire country.

We present Japan's NB mass screening system
and analytical studies of the 89 cases of NB

registered  by the members of MSSG by the end of
1986.

MASS SCREENING SYSTEM(Fig 1).
     In Japan, all 3-month-old infants receive
physical examinations at local Health Centers
under the Child Health Survey Program. When the
program was initiated in 1974, parents of 3-month
-old infants were given an NB screening set which
contained a small round filter paper, a return-
paid envelope and a prospectus explaining the
purpose of the screening, the method of collecting urine on the filter paper and the date the
sample should be mailed to a local institute of
public health(screening center). The mother was
asked to mail the urine sample when her infant
was 6-months old. Originally, a VMA test such as
a VMA spot test(Imashuku et al.,1967), or a VMA
dip test, was done when the sample was received
at the centers. In Sapporo(since 1981)(Sato et al
1986), Kanagawa and Kyoto(since 1985)(Yoshikawa
et al.,1987), HPLC(high power liquid chromatography), measuring urinary VMA, HVA and VLA(vanilla-
ctic acid) levels, has been used as a screening
method. When a sample is unsatisfactory--dirty
filter paper or an insufficient amount of urine--
another screening set is sent with printed information giving the reason for the retest.
     If a urine sample yields a positive VMA re-
sult, we request that the parents send two more
samples. If the infant shows VMA positive results
a second and third time, the infant is sent to a
local hospital for further examination for diagnostic physical findings, chest and abdominal X-
ray films, abdominal echogram and measurements of
urinary VMA and HVA levels.
     Our studies and the annual report of the Jap-
anese Government in 1986, showed that the incidence of NB detected by mass screening in infancy
was from 1/15,500 to 1/18,749 cases screened.

PATIENTS AND RESULTS.
     By the end of 1986, 89 cases of NB were regi-
stered by the members of NB-MSSG.
     We show their clinical findings.
1. Sex. M:F=49:40=1.23:1(Table 1).

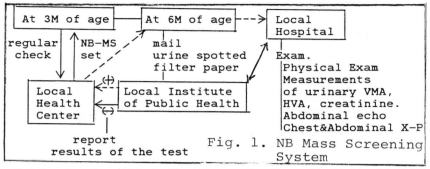

Fig. 1. NB Mass Screening System

Table 1. Age Distribution at Diagnosis.

| Age | No.of Cases |
|------|-------------|
| 6-7mo | 41(46%) |
| 8 | 25(28%) |
| 9 | 15(15%) |
| >10 | 8( 9%) |
| Total | 89(100%) |

2. Age distribution at diagnosis

As the screening test is first conducted on 6-month old infants, most patients (74%) were diagnosed with NB before they were 8 months old. It takes 1-2 months after the first screening test to get an accurate diagnosis. It is inevitable that a few mothers forget to send the urine samples of their infants at 6 months of age.

3. Symptomatology and physical findings(Table 2).
86 of these cases(96.6%) were asymptomatic and only 3 cases were symptomatic: one suffered from a urinary tract infection, with fever and anemia at further examination;the remaining 2 cases only had sweating. At the time of initial physical examination, 55(69%) of the 80 patients with abdominal NB were found to have an abdomi-

Table 2.Symptoms and physical Findings.
Symptoms: (-) 86 cases(96.6%)
           (+) 3 cases(3.4%)  1.Fever and anemia
                              2.sweating
                              3.sweating and
                                poor weight gain
Physical Examination
  80 Abdominal NB: 55(69%) were noticed
                            abdominal mass.
                  23(31%) were not detected.
   9 Mediastinal NB: No particular findings.

nal mass..Abdominal masses could not be detected
in the remaining 25 cases(31%) by physician, who
had been informed how patients demonstrating increased urinary VMA excretion should be examined
for NB. The other 9  cases, which had mediastinal
NB, did not have any pathologic findings at the
time of physical examination.
     It is  important to know  that many of the
patients with NB detected by mass screening had
no symptoms and no pathologic findings at their
physical examination.

4. Urinary VMA, HVA and other biochemical markers
     (Table 3).
     Urinary VMA levels of the 87 cases ranged
from 25.1-655 µg/mg creatinine. The normal level
in infants is under 25 µg/mg creat.. The HVA levels in these patients were 15.8-688 µg/mg creàt.. As the normal level of HVA is under 3 µg/mg creat., 77 cases(89%) showed a significantly high HVA excretion.

| Table3. Urinary VMA and HVA and Other Markers. | | |
|---|---|---|
| VMA(µg/mg creatinine) | | |
| 25.1-665: 87 cases. | | |
| HVA( " ) | | |
| 15.8-688: 87 cases | | |
| <35 | 9(11%) | |
| ≥35 | 77(89%) | |
| Serum LDH(87) | <500IU | 53(61%) |
| | ≥500 | 34(39%) |
| NSE(46) | <15ng/ml | 19(41%) |
| | ≥15 | 27(59%) |
| ferritin(31) | normal | 29(94%) |
| | high | 2( 6%) |

Other serum biochemical markers such as LDH, NSE
and ferritin were not significantly elevated in
NB infants.

5. Primary Sites of the 89 cases(Table 5).
     There were 80 cases(90%) with tumors locat-
ed in the abdomen: 51 adrenal, 23 retroperitone-
al, 4 pelvic and 2 òthers. Mediastinal tumors
accounted for 9 cases(10%). The pattern of distribution was the same as in earlier Japanese
(Registry of childhood malignacies of Japanese
Pediatric Surgeon,1979) and USA(Pochedly,1976)
reports.
     52 of the primary masses(58%) had no local
invasion. 22 cases had a unilateral extension of

Table 4. Primary Sites of NBs.

| Primary Sites | MSSG (1987) | Registry of Jap Ped Surg (1971-1975) | From Textbook of NB (C.Pochedly) (1976) |
|---|---|---|---|
| Mediastinal | 9(10%) | 60(12%) | (15%) |
| Abdominal | 80(90%) | 403(82%) | (70%) |
|   Adrenal | 51(57%) | 238(48%) | >(66%) |
|   Retroperit. | 23(26%) | 113(23%) | |
|   Pelvic | 4( 5%) | 20( 4%) | ( 4%) |
|   Others | 2(2%) | 32( 7%) | |
| Others | 0 | 12( 2%) | ( 3%) |
| Unknown | 0 | 20( 4%) | (12%) |
| Total | 89 (100%) | 495(100%) | 1,303(100%) |

the tumor mass and 12 cases had a bilateral extension.

Weights of primary masses ranged from 4.3g to 260g with a median 50g. There were 42 cases with promary tumors under 50g. There were no masses over 300g, the largest one being 269g.

Histological findings were the same as in earlier Japanese reports: there were 57 neuroblastoma cases(64%) and 26 ganglioneuroblastoma cases(29%).

6. Stage(Table 5).
The stage of the disease was evaluated for

Table 5. Distribution of stages.

| Stage | MSSG (1987) | Registry of Jap Ped Surg (1971-1976) | CCSGA (1971) |
|---|---|---|---|
| I | 19(21%) | 42( 9%) | 21( 9%) |
| II | 39(44%) | 52(11%) | 35(14%) |
| IVs | 8( 9%) | 38( 8%) | 27(11%) |
| III | 11(12%) | 83(17%) | 27(11%) |
| IV | 12(16%) | 267(55%) | 136(55%) |
| Total | 89(100%) | 482(100%) | 246(100%) |

I+II+IVs 66(74%)    132(27%)    83(34%)
each case after surgery(Evans,1980).There were 19 stage I cases(21%), 39 stage II cases(44%) and only 12 stage IV cases(14%). Stage IVs cases accounted for 8 cases(9%) in this study. It is the same percentage shown by other reports. Compared with the numbers of stage I and II cases in previous reports from CCSGA and the Japanese Pediatric Surgeon Associaton(JPSA, the occurren-

ce of stage I and II in our study was higher.
And conversely, the detection of stage IV cases
in our study(14%) had a much lower incidence than
in the CCSGA study(55%) and JPSA study(55%).

Comparing our study with the results of the
CCSGA and JPSA reports, the numbers of cases detected in the favorable stages, I, II, and IVs
clearly increased, from 34%(83/246), the figure
for the CCSGA report and 27%(132/327), the figure
for the JPSA report, to 74%(66/89) for the MSSG
study, and the number of unfavorable stage IV
cases clearly decreased fron 55%(136/246) for CC-
SGA and 55%(267/327) for JPSA to 14%(12/89) for
MSSG. It is clear that most patients were discovered at early stages.

Metastatic sites: regional lymphnodes in 42
cases, distant lymphnodes in 6 cases, bone marrow
in 13 cases, liver in 8 cases, bone in 2 cases
and metastatic lesions in other sites in 2 cases.

7. Therapy.

Total resection of the primary tumor was done
in 84 cases, partial removal in 4 and biopsy in
one case. Chemotherapy was administered in all
cases; 75 cases received vincristine and cyclophosphamide. In other cases adriamycin, cis-platin,
VM-26, and DTIC, etc. were administered.
Radiation to the tumor bed was done in 15 cases
and to bone (skull, long bones) in 2 cases.

8. Prognosis.

The median follow-up period was 1 year-8 months, and the maximum was 6 years-7 months by the
end of 1986.

87 cases(98%) are alive now: 57 cases are
off therapy and 30 cases are still in treatment.
Most of the patients can be expected to be cured.
Two cases died: one by progressive NB at 5 years
of age and another by duodenal perforation 8 days
after surgery.

DISCUSSION.

In this paper, we have analyzed the clinical
findings of the 89 patients who were discovered
through the mass screening system for NB by the
members of NB-MSSG in Japan.

Our results show that mass screening for NB at 6 months of age could detect small primary tumors in early stages in 1/15,500-1/18,749 infants screened. The prognosis of these 89 patients is remarkably favorable even in some patients with stage IV tumors.

There are still several problems associated with the screening methods, organization procedure and so on, as shown on Table 6.

Since 1985, NB-mass screening has been in effect on a nation-wide level in 81 districts in Japan under the recommendation of the Japanese Government. Most screening centers use a qualitative VMA test such as a VMA spot test or a VMA dip test for detecting NB. Screening is being done by HPLC for measurements of VMA, HVA and VLA in only 6 of the participating 81 districts.

It is well known that about 25% of NB cases do not excrete increased VMA in urine and cannot be detected by a qualitative VMA test. Furthermore, as a VMA positive or negative qualitative test is judged by the unaided eyes of an examiner, it is not always possible to get consistent results. For optimum results, the national standardization of the test system and an examiner with sufficient experience are recommended.

We think it is better to introduce the measurement of VMA and HVA by HPLC for mass screening for NB to detect the remaining 25% of NB that do not secrete VMA.

In Japan, regular checks of children's development under the Child Health Survey Program are performed at 1 month, 3 months, 1 year, 1year-6 months and 3 years of age. This program is very convenient for the mass screening of NB; however, one drawback is that the mothers receive the mass screening set when their babies are 3 months of age and must send the babies' urine samples at 6 months of age. This 3 months lag period results in a decrease in the number of infants who have urine tests returned for testing. Nearly, 70% of all infants in MSSG have received the test for NB mass screening. We have to make an even greater effort to increase the number of infants screened by increasing the effectiveness of accurate info-

rmation and education about childhood cancer.
Other problems as shown on Table 6.
The major problems that NB-MSSG faces are
the future clinical evaluation and improvement of
survival rates for NB patients.   We plan the
follow up study of patients dicovered through the
mass screening program to evaluate the usefulness
of this study.   Another important aspect that
must be considered is cost-performance.   If mass
screening is to be performed by HPLC, cost-performance has to be evaluated.

---

Table 6.Problems related to NB-Mass Screening.

1.Method.Qualitative or Quantitative.
  How much accuracy is required?
2.System.Selection of Institutes and Hospitals.
3.Age of Patients.
  Is 6-M of age suitable?
  Is it necessary to repeat the test after
  6-M of age?
4.Good public acceptance for the screening of
  childhood cancer.
5.Clinical evaluation.Follow-up is essential.
6.Re-evaluation of cost peformance.

---

REFERENCES

Breslow N, McCann B (1971). Statistical estima-
    tion of prognosis for children with neuroblast-
    oma. Cancer Res 31: 2098-2103.
Evans AE, D'Angio GJ, Randolph J (1971). A propo-
    sed staging for children with neuroblastoma.
    Cancer 27: 374-378.
Gitlow SE, Bertani LM, Rausen A et al.(1970).
    Diagnosis of neuroblastoma by qualitative and
    quantitative determination of catecholamine
    metabolites in urine. Cancer 25:1377-1383.
Hirayama T (1981). Descriptive and analytical epi-
    demiology of childhood malignancy in Japan.
    In: Kobayashi N, ed . Recent advances in mana-
    gement of children with cancer. Tokyo: Child-
    ren's Cancer Association of Japan, 27-43.
Imashuku S, Kim H, Sawada T (1967). Mass Screen-
    ing for functional neural tumors by a qualita-

tive VMA test . Jpn J Pediatr 24: 1004-1007.
Pochedly C (1976). Neuroblastoma in the Neck,
     Chest, Abdomen and Pelvis. In: Pochedly C ed.
     Neuroblastoma. Publishing Sciences Group Inc.
     Massachusettes, 59-91.
Registry of childhood malignacies of Japanese
     Pediatric Surgeon (1979). Neuroblastoma, Wilms'
     Tumor and Hepatic malignacies between 1971-
     1979. J Jpn Soc Pediatr Surg 15: 507-515.
Sato Y, Hanai J, Takasugi N et al. (1986).
     Determination of urinary vanillymandelic acid
     and homovanillic acid by high performance
     Liquid chromatography for mass screening of
     neuroblastoma. Tohoku J exp Med 150: 169-174.
Sawada T, Imashuku S, Takada H et al. (1973).
     Biochemical diagnosis of neuroblastoma. Jpn J
     Pediatr Surg Med 5:655-662.
Sawada T, Takada H, Imashuku S et al. (1978).
     Mass screening for early and immediate detect-
     ion of neuroblastoma in childhood. Acta Pediatr
     Jap 20:55-61.
Sawada T, Todo S, Fujita K et al.(1982). Mass
     screening of neuroblastoma in infancy. Am J
     Dis Child 136: 710-712.
Sawada T, Kidowaki T, Sakamoto I et al. (1984).
     Neuroblastoma: mass screening for early detect-
     ion and its prognosis. Cancer 53: 2731-2735.
Sawada T, Hirayama M, Nakata T et al. (1984).
     Mass screening for neuroblastoma in infants in
     Japan. Interim report of a Mass Screening Stu-
     dy Group. Lancet August 4: 271-273.
Sawaguchi S, Suganuma Y, Watanabe I et al. (1979).
     Studies on the biological and clinical charact-
     eristics of neuroblastoma. (I) Evaluation of
     the survival rates in relation to stage and
     age of onset. J Jpn Soc Pediatr Surg 15: 1119
     -1128.
Voorhess M. (1968). Discussion of treatment of
     neuroblastoma. J Pediatr Surg 3: 151-152.
Yoshikawa S, Okuda S, Ohe T et al. (1987). Liquid
     chromatographic determinaton of vanillylmande-
     lic acid and homovanillic acid by column swit-
     ching technique involving direct injection of
     urine. J Chromato in press.

ACKNOWLEDGMENT

This study was supported by a grant-in-aid for Research of  Mass Screening System from the Ministry of Health and Welfare of the Japanese Government.

Correspondence should be addressed to T. Sawada, Department of Pediatrics, Kyoto Prefectural University of Medicine, Kawaramachi, Kamikyoku, Kyoto, Japan 602.

Advances in Neuroblastoma Research 2, pages 535–546
© 1988 Alan R. Liss, Inc.

# MONOCLONAL ANTIBODIES TO THE SMALL ROUND CELL TUMOURS OF CHILDHOOD: AN INTERNATIONAL WORKSHOP.

J.T.Kemshead. BSc. PhD., on behalf of the Forbeck Foundation Sponsored Workshop 1.

ICRF Oncology Laboratory, Institute of Child Health, London WC2.

## INTRODUCTION.

### Study Design.

In October 1985, groups working on the small round cell tumours of childhood were contacted to determine if they wished to either submit antibodies to the study and/or take part in a screening programme. It was requested that antibodies were sent to the ICRF Oncology Laboratory in London, where their activity was checked and they were assigned a study number. Forty nine out of fifty two antibodies submitted to the study were coded and shipped to the screening centres. The three reagents lost to the study were supplied in insufficient amounts to warrant inclusion in the workshop, and delays in shipment also meant that it was not possible to readily obtain more material. Where possible individual samples of uncoded antibodies were also sent back to the centre supplying the reagents to check that activity had not been lost during shipment. No duplicates of antibodies were included in the coded antibodies supplied as two separate antibodies to the $GD_2$ ganglioside and Leu 7/HNK1 antigen were included in the reagents, as well as different antibodies to the

--------------------------

1 See Appendix.

neurofilament and desmin intermediate filament proteins.

Over a period of 4 months centres undertaking the screening were asked to test the coded reagents on a variety of tumour tissues. A list of preferences was supplied. Testing of fresh frozen biopsy material was given the highest priority followed by the screening of cell lines and normal tissues. It was left to individual centres to decide which visualization technique was used to identify antibody binding. However it was requested that pieces of biopsy material be conventionally processed so that slides could be submitted to a review panel if requested. Groups were asked to code results as positive, negative or equivocal as it was felt that attempting to grade the strength of signals observed would be too subjective on a multi-centre basis.

Results were sent to London in December and the study formally closed on 31st December 1986. Out of 13 groups supplied with antibody three failed to submit data to the study. This was despite extending the deadline for completion by a two month period. Data on a rabbit antiserum to neuron-specific enolase was insufficient to warrant inclusion in the study and this was therefore completely omitted.

## Data Analysis.

Data was processed using a relational data base (Dbase III Plus) and a Tandon AT computer (IBM Compatible). Statistical analysis of the results was undertaken using the Statgraphics programme. Full data analysis and data discs will be made available by the Forbeck Foundation in the Autumn of 1987.


## RESULTS.

### 1. Validation of Study.

It is possible to gain an idea of the accuracy of the data supplied in three different ways. Data on the specificity of coded samples

was compared with that given for uncoded
antibodies. Where sufficient data was available
for statistical analysis a correlation
coefficient and slope of the line fitting a plot
of antibody 1 v antibody 2 was obtained (Fig 1).

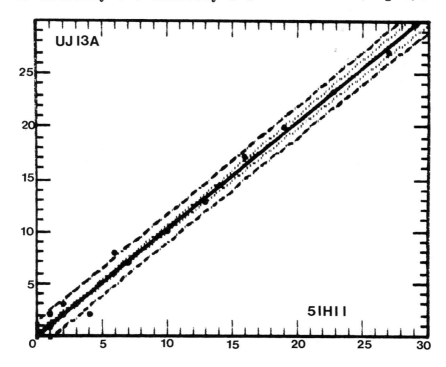

Figure 1. Correlation Coefficient and Line of
Best Fit for Two Separate Antibodies, UJ13A and
5.1.H11. A similar analysis for coded v uncoded
antibodies was undertaken ....... 95% Confidence
Limit, - - - 95% Prediction Limit.

With the exception of one result (0.538)
correlation coefficients lay in the range of
0.740 - 0.938 (n=7) with slopes of lines of best
fit ranging from 0.714 - 0.960. This data
indicates that for individual centres their
analysis was consistent for coded and non-coded
samples. Somewhat more disturbing was the
analysis of data obtained from particular cell

lines screened in different centres.  Here the
correlation coefficients lay between 0.163 and
0.938.  Obviously comparisons giving correlation
coefficients as low as 0.163 must place doubt on
the validity of the data, but it must be stressed
that the analysis is based on  relatively small
amounts of data.  Three explanations for these
result are possible.  Cell lines in different
laboratories have either drifted antigenically or
have become contaminated.  Several of the cell
lines included in this part of the study were of
myelomonocytic origin and previous leucocyte
workshops have reported similar results to  these
suggesting that these lines may be antigenically
unstable.  The third explanation of the data is
that one of the laboratories undertaking the
screening was recording data out of step with the
others.  A detailed check of the data revealed
this to be the case with results supplied from
some centres very different to those expected
from  published antibody specificities.  In spite
of this no data was excluded from the study apart
from a small number of tests undertaken on
formalin fixed material.
    The best validation of the overall accuracy
of the data comes from a comparison of the
binding of antibodies known to recognize the same
antigens.  For the two antibodies to the $GD_2$
ganglioside, the correlation coefficient was
0.980 (slope 0.973) and the Leu 7/HNK1 antigen
0.954 (slope 0.899).  Results for comparisons of
the intermediate filament proteins were not
obtained as the number of tests undertaken was
small.

2. Binding Specificities.

    In total 9118 results were reported on a
total of 31 different types of tumour material/
cell lines and normal tissues.  It is obviously
not possible to report all of these and therefore
this analysis will concentrate on neuroblastoma
as the target tissue.  For ease of analysis
antibodies were divided into groups: those raised
against neuroectodermally derived
tissues/tumours, muscle, haemopoietic tissue,
Ewing's sarcoma and Intermediate filaments.

Table 1 illustrates the binding of the group of
antibodies raised against neuroectodermal
tumours/tissues on either frozen neuroblastoma
biopsies or neuroblastoma cell lines. With the
exception of antibodies 5A7, D7 and 282/B3, all
reagents bound to more than 50% of the
tissues/lines tested. Interestingly antibody 5A7
was only reported positive on neuroblastoma
tissue from the centre supplying the reagent.
Reagents UJ13A, 3F8 and 126.4 bound to the
greatest number of cell lines and tissues tested.

Table 1. Antibody Panel Binding to Neuroblastoma
Lines and Tissues.

| Antibody | Immunogen | Lines | Tissues |
|----------|-----------|-------|---------|
| UJ13A | H.Foet.Brain | 27/28* | 30/31 |
| UJ223.8 | H.Foet.Brain | 22/28 | 26/30 |
| UJ127.11 | Gp210 HFB | 21/24 | 23/30 |
| UJ181.4 | H.Foet.Brain | 21/28 | 20/29 |
| 3.F.8. | Anti-GD2 | 26/29 | 27/30 |
| 126.4 | Anti-GD2 | 26/28 | 27/30 |
| Thy-1 | Thy.1.Ag | 24/28 | 22/29 |
| PI153/3 | IMR32 C.Line | 22/27 | 22/31 |
| 5.A.7 | LAN 1 C.Line | 8/28 | 8/29 |
| 5G3 | Gp220 Kd NBCL | 24/28 | 21/29 |
| AB459 | H.Foet.Brain | 15/24 | 17/29 |
| KPNAC2 | KP-N-RT Line | 23/27 | 20/30 |
| KPNAC8 | KP-N-RT Line | 21/29 | 17/29 |
| KPNAC9 | KP-N-RT Line | 24/29 | 22/30 |
| KPNAC10 | KP-N-RT Line | 20/29 | 10/30 |
| 1D1 | NBL Cell Line | 22/28 | 22/31 |
| 6.3 | NBL Cell Line | 28/28 | 18/30 |
| 6.19 | NBL Cell Line | 28/28 | 18/29 |
| NSE | Enolase | - | - |
| D7 | H.Symp.Ganglia. | 4/30 | 4/29 |
| 282/B3 | TE671 H.Medullo | 2/28 | 9/29 |
| 275/F2 | TE671 H.Medullo | 16/28 | 25/31 |
| 81C6 | GFAP+ve L.U251 | 21/27 | 11/29 |

* No lines tested / positive.

The results obtained using these reagents were
consistently high using either indirect
immunofluorescence or immuno-enzyme visualization
of antibody binding. This was not the case for

the other reagents where more positives were
scored using immuno-enzyme methods. One
interpretation of this is that the antigens
recognized by the latter groups of antibodies are
present in lower amounts than those recognized by
UJ13A, 3F8 and 126.4. This leads to a higher
number of negatives being reported with the less
sensitive visualization method.

Of the muscle associated antibodies 2/4
shared high levels of binding to neuroblastoma
cell lines/tissues. SOS13 bound 24/27 lines and
21/31 tissues and 5.1.H11 27/29 lines and 29/31
tissues. These reagents were raised against
muscle cell glycoproteins and skeletal muscle
cells respectively.

Of the haemopoietic group of reagents FMG25,
BA1, BA2. Leu 7 and HNK1 were found to cross
react with a high proportion of neuroblastoma
tissues/cell lines. This data is in concordance
with the known specificity of these reagents.
FMG25 is the only antibody of this group that
does not react with at least a proportion of
normal haemopoietic cell progenitors. This is
despite the immunogen used to produce this
antibody, the HUT78 T cell line. Interestingly,
despite the paucity of HLA antigens on
neuroblastoma, 40% of cell lines and 60% of
neuroblastoma biopsies were reported as binding
W6/32, recognizing a monomorphic determinant on
major histo-compatibility antigens. The cross
reactivity of this antibody with normal cells
within tumour biopsies cannot be eliminated at
this time.

The three antibodies raised against the EW1
Ewing's sarcoma cell line 11.6.2, 10.12.1, and
10.11.13, bound 18-22% of neuroblastoma cell
lines (n=27), and 43-58% of tissues tested,
(n=30/31). For the purpose of this analysis the
antibodies will not be discussed further as they
are incapable of differentiating Ewing's sarcoma
from the other small round cell tumours of
childhood.

Only two cell lines were screened with the
group of antibodies against neurofilament
proteins. Of the 7 antibodies tested on these
lines, 4 were reported as positive. In contrast
all of the anti-neurofilament antibodies bound a

proportion of fresh neuroblastoma tissues. There
was a considerable range of reactivity with
between 27.6 and 70% of the tissues reported as
positive. Presumably the variability in antibody
staining reflects the different epitopes
recognized by these reagents, although all of
them are reported to bind to the phosphorylated
form of the neurofilament protein. No cross
blocking studies have been undertaken to
determine if the reagents do recognize different
epitopes on these molecules.

In summary the analysis of the data shows
that reagents UJ13A, 3F8, 126.4, 5.1.H11, SOS13,
FMG25, BA1, BA1, BA2, Leu 7 and HNK 1 are the
reagents of choice for the recognition of the
majority of neuroblastoma cell lines/tumour
biopsies. Of these the first 4 are the only
reagent reported as recognizing (90% +) of both
lines/tissues screened.

## 3. Binding of Antibodies to Other Small Round Cell Tumours of Childhood.

None of the above selected group of
antibodies only bind to neuroblastoma tissue.
All reacted with ganglioneuroblastoma and
neuroepitheliomas, although the number of these
tumours entered into the study was small. With
the exception of FMG25 all reagents bound to the
majority of rhabdomyosarcoma biopsies screened
(Table 2).

Table 2. Antibodies Selected for their Binding
to Neuroblastoma also Cross React with other
Paediatric Solid Tumours.

| M/A. | Rhabdo | Ewing's | Lymphoma | Wilms' |
|------|--------|---------|----------|--------|
| UJ13A | 7/7 | 0/4 | 0/6 | 1/1 |
| 3F18 | 6/7 | 1/4 | 1/6* | 2/2 |
| 126.4 | 7/7 | 3/4 | 0/6 | 2/2 |
| SOS13 | 7/7 | 4/4 | 2/6 | 1/1 |
| 5.1.H11 | 7/7 | 1/4 | 0/6 | 1/1 |
| FMG25 | 0/7 | 0/3 | 0/6 | 0/1 |
| BA1 | 7/7 | 3/4 | 4/6 | 1/1 |
| BA2 | 5/6 | 4/4 | 6/6 | 1/1 |
| Leu 7 | 4/7 | 0/3 | 2/6 | 0/2 |
| HNK1 | 2/7 | 1/4 | 0/6 | 0/2 |

The data on the binding of the haemopoietic group
of antibodies is always open to doubt as the
reagents may  bind to lymphoid tissue within a
tumour.  However with the exception of the result
for BA1 data on rhabdo-cell lines agreed with
that for fresh tissue biopsies.  The binding of
many of the reagents was more restricted when
Ewing's sarcoma and lymphoma biopsies were
examined.  Whilst a general correlation was
usually achieved for data obtained on cell lines
and tissues,  Ewing's sarcoma proved the
exception to this rule.  Many of the antibodies
that were reported as negative to fresh Ewing's
sarcoma tissue bound to a small proportion of the
cell lines screened.

None of the selected group of reagents
examined were reported as negative on all the
leukaemic cell lines screened (n=21).  This is
obviously not surprising for reagents raised
against haemopoietic tissue.  It is not possible
to give a complete breakdown of the reactivity of
the other reagents, but all randomly bound a
small number of lines eg. UJ13A 3/20.  In general
more myelo-monocytic lines were reported positive
than other groups (B, T, non-B-non T, Burkitts
etc.).  These reagents were also reported as not
binding to the majority of bone marrows screened.
Occasionally however a particular antibody was
reported as binding a small number of
haemopoietic progenitors (less 1.0%) indicating
that none of the antibodies can be described as
truly negative on all types of marrow examined
(paediatric, adult, regenerating post chemotherapy).

Although not often a diagnostic problem,
Wilms' tumours were also found to bind the
majority of the selected group of antibodies.
For a more detailed breakdown of the binding of
these reagents to other tumours and normal
tissues the reader is referred to the full study
report.

## 4. Grouping of Reagents Based on a Statistical Analysis of the Binding Data.

One of the aims of this study was to attempt to identify groups of reagents for the diagnosis of neuroblastoma. An overview of the study suggests that the reagents UJ13A,and 5.1.H11, 3F8 and 126.4 have very similar binding profiles on all tumours examined. Statistical analysis of this data suggests they might bind to similar antigens or groups of antigens on the cell surface of malignant/normal tissues. Biochemical data indicates that 3.F.8 and 126.4 bind to the ganglioside $GD_2$ and UJ13A 5.1.H11 to a glycoprotein/protein associated with the cell membrane. This does not rule out the possibility of the reagents binding to shared carbohydrate determinants on the ganglioside/ glycoprotein(s) although this is unlikely.

Table 3. Statistical Analysis of Binding Profiles of Selected Antibodies in Study.

| Antibodies | Correlation Coefficient | Slope of Line |
|---|---|---|
| 3F8 v 126.4 | 0.98 | 0.973 |
| 3F8 v UJ13A | 0.965 | 1.049 |
| UJ13A v 5.1.H11 | 0.994 | 1.018 |
| UJ13A v AB459* | 0.139 | negative slope |

* Included as a control where binding profiles indicate a lack of correlation.

Repeated attempts to show UJ13A binding to $GD_2$ or other glycolipids/gangliosides have not been successful. It is also not known at this point if UJ13A and 5.1.H11 bind to the same antigen. The correlation coefficient obtained between these two antibodies is so close to unity that this is a strong possibility. However cross blocking studies indicate that neither antibody is capable of blocking the other.

Grouping of reagents to obtain dendrograms as produced in the leucocyte and small lung cell carcinoma workshops was not undertaken. This was

because, in this study, many of the antigens
recognized by the reagents were already known.
It did not seem sensible to group antibodies into
common groups if they recognize biochemically
distinct antigens. As indicated above, analysis
of data in this way would almost certainly group
anti-GD2 reagents with UJ13A and 5.1.H11, and yet
these recognize different types of membrane
components. However the option for this type of
analysis remains open if the data can be
transferred from its current format an
alternative computer programme.

## CONCLUSION.

The data presented here is not meant to
illustrate one antibody is better at identifying
neuroblastoma than another. It is meant to give
the reader an indication of the variability of
staining that can occur when coded reagents are
used in different laboratories. It is clear that
no one antibody can be used exclusively for the
identification of this malignancy. Cross
reactivity of antibodies with other small round
cell tumours of childhood is a problem that needs
to be stressed. In addition whilst screening
laboratories were asked to save biopsy material
for pathological review, this has not yet been
analyzed. There is the possibility of
misdiagnosis, particularly in the controversial
area of defining neuroblastoma from primitive
neuroepitheliomas (PNETS). The data presented
here must therefore be taken as preliminary but
the overriding conclusions about heterogeneity in
antigen expression, and the cross reactivity of
antibodies is almost certainly valid. Far more
information about the antibodies included in the
study is available, and the above should only be
taken as an outline. The full study will be
available later in the year [2].

## ACKNOWLEDGMENTS.

This work was supported by the Forbeck
Foundation, The Neuroblastoma Society and the
Imperial Cancer Research Fund.

# APPENDIX.

1). Antibodies submitted.

Dr. B.Anderton, London; 147,155,RS18,RT97,BF10.
Amersham International; Anti-Desmin, Anti-
Nfilament
Becton Dickinson, USA; Leu 7.
Dr. P. Beverley, London; 2D1.
Dr. D.Bigner, North Carolina, USA; 81C6.
Dr. W. Bodmer, London; W6/32,Tal.1B5.
Dr. Cheung, New York, US; 3F8.
Dr. C. Franz, Rochester, USA; 6.3,6.13,1D1.
Dr. N. Gross, Lausanne, Switzerland; 5A7.
Hybritech, California, USA; BA1,BA2.
Dr. J.Kemshead,London; UJ13A,UJ223.8,UJ127.11,
UJ181.4,xThy-1,FMG25,J144
Dr. R. Kennett, Philadelphia, USA; PI153/3.
Lab-Systems, Finland; Anti-Nfilament,Anti-Desmin
Dr. M. Lipinski, Paris; HNK1,11.6.2., 10.12.1,
10.11.13.
Dr.Reisfeld, La Jolla, USA; 126.4,5G3.
Dr. D.Reen, Dublin; D7.
Dr. P.Reynolds, Los Angeles, USA; HSAN1.2[*]
Dr. R.Seeger, Los Angeles, USA; 39 0[*],AB459
Drs.T.Sugimoto & Sawada, Kyoto, Japan; KPNAC2,
KPNAC8,KPNAC9,KPNAC10.
Dr. F.Walsh, London; SOS5,SOS13, 24.1.D1,
5.1.H11, A2B5[*]
Dr. P.Zeltzer, Los Angeles, USA; 282/B3,275/F2

* Antibodies supplied in insufficient amounts to
be included in the study.

II). Screening Centres.

Dr. P. Beverley, London, UK.
Dr. H. Coakham, Bristol, UK.
Dr. A. Evans & R. Kennett, Philadelphia, USA.
Dr. M. Favrot, Lyon, France.
Dr. A. Gee, Florida, USA.
Dr. N. Gross, Lausanne, Switzerland.
Dr. J. Kemshead, London, UK.
Dr. M. Lipinski, Paris, France
Dr. D. Reen, Dublin, Ireland.
Dr. P. Reynolds, Los Angeles, USA.
Drs. T. Sawada &  T. Sugimoto, Kyoto Japan.

2. Full Study Reports will be available from :

J. Forbeck
Forbeck Foundation
17 Cedar Lane
Hilton Head Island
SC29928.

Dr. J.T. Kemshead
ICRF Oncology Lab.
Institute of Child Health
30 Guilford Street,
LONDON WC2.

Advances in Neuroblastoma Research 2, pages 547–555

# BONE MARROW METASTASES IN CHILDREN'S NEUROBLASTOMA STUDIED BY MAGNETIC RESONANCE IMAGING

Dominique Couanet, Anne Geoffray,
Olivier Hartmann, Jérôme G. Leclère,
Jean D. Lumbroso

Departments of Radiology (D.C., A.G.), of
Pédiatric Oncology (O.H.) and of Nuclear
Medicine (J.G.L., J.D.L.), Institut
Gustave-Roussy, rue Camille Desmoulins
94805 Villejuif Cedex, France.

## SUMMARY

Forty-one patients (pts) presenting with a neuroblastoma underwent 52 MRI to detect bone marrow metastases. Mean age was 4 years. Acquisitions were done with a 1.5 tesla unit. T1 and T2 weighted images were obtained in coronal (legs and pelvis) and sagittal (dorso-lumbar spine) sections. In 13 cases MRI was performed for initial staging, in 30 during the follow-up. 43/52 examinations were evaluable. Out of 24 anatomically proven medullary involvment (19 pts), MRI showed focal abnormal signals in 23 (18 pts) : foci of hypersignal in T2 weighted images and hyposignal in T1 weighted images compared to the normal bone marrow (BM) and fat tissue. The lesions were more often detected in lower limbs (25) than dorso-lumbar vertebral body (15) or iliac bone (8). Nineteen examinations were performed in 15 pts with cytologically and histologically normal BM. MRI raised suspicion of BM metastases in 5 pts (7 MRI). Out of those 5 pts, 1 (2 MRI) had BM relapse 9 months later ; 1 (2 MRI) had intra cranial relapse 6 months later ; 1 (1 MRI) is disease free 1½ year later ; the follow-up is too short for 2 remaining pts (2 MRI). MRI's specificity was 88.9 % and sensitivity 84.4 %.

## INTRODUCTION

Magnetic resonance imaging (MRI) is a new

attractive modality of evaluating children with neuroblastoma because it can produce multiplanar images without radiation or invasive technique. Because of its fat content, BM gives a high signal on MRI. It seems useful to detect the modifications of BM signal intensity when the marrow cellularity changes or is infiltrated by a malignant process. Since it is well known that in the neuroblastoma, the bone marrow involment is focal ; we thought that MRI would be a good tool to explore the bone marrow without using chemical shift technique (Wismer et al., 1985).

## MATERIALS AND METHODS

41 children presenting with a neuroblastoma underwent 52 MRI. The mean age was 4 years (range from ½ year to 13 years). The acquisitions were obtained in a MRI system using a superconducting magnet operating at 1.5 tesla. Spin echo (SE) technique was used with two different pulse sequences : T1 weighted sequences having a short repetition time (TR) between 400 msec. and 600 msec. and a short echo time (TE) 20-25 msec., T2 weighted images having a long TR (1500-2000 msec.) and a long TE (80-120 msec.). The multi-slice multi-echo technique we used was very time efficient and permitted a MRI's duration of 1 hour to study the lower limbs in coronal sections as well as the iliac bones and the dorso-lumbar spine in sagittal sections. At the beginning of our study, inadequate technique, agitation or technical failure did not allow to study T1 and T2 sequences ; therefore, we had to exclude 9 MRI out of 52 on account of these problems. For the 43 remaining studies (32 pts) the legs have been explored 37 times, the iliac bones 15 times, the spine 34 times and the skull twice. Oral and rectal sedation was applied 1½ hour before the examination in children aged less than 5-7 years. MRI was performed for initial staging in 13 pts and during follow-up 30 times ; 7 children had 2 MRI, 2 children had 3 MRI.

The results of MRI's studies were compared with the medullograms (10 sternal and iliac aspirates) and 2 iliac bone marrow biopsies performed initially or during the follow-up. The time between these samplings and MRI did not exceed 15 days.

Within 10 days of the date of MRI, 32 m-I$^{123}$BG total body scintigraphy and 6 m-I$^{131}$BG therapeutic scintigraphy have been performed. The follow-up runs from 4 months to 1½ year.

## RESULTS

Abnormal foci of hypersignal in T2 weighted images and hyposignal in T1 weighted images were noted in 30 MRI (Fig. 1a - b). The comparison has been done with the feature of fat tissue and normal BM at the same level and during the same acquisition. Tibial and femoral metaphysis were more often pathological (25/37) than vertebral body (15/34) and iliac bones (8/15). Comparison between MRI's results and medullograms, including BM biopsy, are summarized in Table 1. Comparison between MRI and m-IBG scintigraphy are summarized in Table 2.

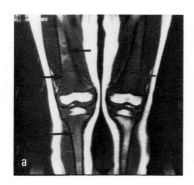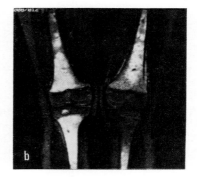

**FIG. 1 :** 2 ½ year-old child with an abdominal neuroblastoma stage IV.
Initial staging.
**a :** coronal spin echo 600/20 (TR m sec./TE m sec.) MR image demonstrates multiple lesions on both femurs and tibiae with a low signal intensity ( → ).
**b :** coronal spin echo 2000/120 MR image shows markedly strong signal intensity of the BM lesions.

We consider a true negative MRI when medullograms, BM biopsy and m-I$^{123}$BG scintigraphy are normal and the long term follow up for more than one year does not detect a medullary recurrence. We consider a true positive MRI when medullograms or BM biopsy are invaded or m-IBG uptakes are abnormal or when the follow up reveals a medullary relapse.

The specificity of MRI is 88.9 % and the sensitivity is 84.4 %. If we plan the values at the initial staging (13 MRI), there is no false negative and sensitivity is 100 % but specificity is a low 75 % because of the small number of the examinations (3 true negative results) with a false positive examination.

**TABLE 1** : Comparison between MRI and medullograms (including BM biopsy results).

|  |  | Medullograms | |
|---|---|---|---|
|  |  | Invaded | Normal |
| MRI | Abnormal | 23 | 7 |
|  | Normal | 1 | 12 |

Total 43

**TABLE 2** : Comparison between MRI and m-IBG scintigraphy

|  |  | m-IBG | |
|---|---|---|---|
|  |  | + | - |
| MRI | + | 22 (BM+) | 4 (BM-) |
|  | - | 4 (BM-) | 8 (7BM-) (1BM+) |

Total 38

BM+ : invaded bone marrow
BM- : normal medullograms and BM biopsy.

## DISCUSSION

In the literature many MRI's studies have been performed in adults to explore BM and its alterations (Olson et al., 1986). In children such studies are restricted ; MRI is not as easy to perform as in adults and such examinations are more often done to assess the extent of a solid tumor before treatment (Fletcher et al., 1985). The MR signal intensity of normal BM is related to the ratio between fat cells and hematopoïetic cells within it (Dooms et al., 1985). The normal conversion of red marrow to fat marrow during life and the multiple factors which alter the distribution of red marrow (Kricun, 1985) explain the large variability of T1 and T2 values of the BM (Bottomley et al., 1984). This explains the difficulty to detect a diffuse alteration of the MR signal intensity (Mc Kinstry et al., 1987). On the contrary, the patchy distribution of BM metastases in solid tumors, especially in neuroblastoma, allows an easier detection of these alterations. They appear with a distinct MR signal intensity compared with the normal red marrow and subcutaneous fat tissue : hyposignal in T1 weighted sequences and hypersignal in T2 weighted sequences (Fig. 2a-b).

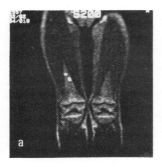 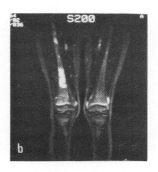

**FIG 2** : 4 year-old child resected abdominal neuroblastoma. Medullary relapse.

    **a.** coronal SE 2000/50 MR image reveals 2 foci of abnormal signal intensity on right femur.

    **b.** 5 months later ; disease progressed. Coronal SE 2000/120 MR image shows markedly increase of hypersignal sites.

We obtained a good correlation in 23 between a metastatic involvment on medullograms and pathological MRI (table 1). Out of these 23 MRI with proven involved BM, m-IBG scans were performed 21 times. In all occasions both explorations were positive (table 2). The only differences between scintigraphy and MRI were the number and the localization of the invaded regions. In one patient the scintigraphy detected foci of a lesser extent than the MRI, in two patients the vertebral bodies presented abnormal uptakes in mIBG and seemed to be normal on MRI.

In 1 patient MRI and m-I$^{123}$BG did not show the sternal residual metastase 3 years after the end of his treatment. This can be explained by the disturbances due to respiratory artifacts.

In 12 cases (10 patients), MRI and medullograms appeared normal. Out of them, 7 m-IBG scan were normal but in 4 of them mI$^{123}$BG scintigraphy showed pathological uptakes (table 2). In two of these 4 last cases the follow up showed a decrease of the pathological m-I$^{123}$BG uptake, but the current survival is short (3 months). In the third one, an increased isotope uptake was observed, MRI and medullograms will be controlled soon. MRI and medullograms became pathological 6 months after the m-I$^{123}$BG in the fourth child. We considered these 4 last cases as false negative MRI.

In 7 MRI (5 patients) medullograms were normal but MRI abnormal. The follow up revealed in 2 patients (4 MRI) a relapse 4 and 6 months later (1 with pathological medullogram, 1 intracranial metastase). 1 patient (1 MRI) is disease free 1½ years later. This patient presented at the moment of the initial staging, a solitary lesion on a vertebral body at the MRI. The lesion was very different from the initial metastatic lesions normally observed in MRI : multiple foci of abnormal MRI signal intensity more often located on femurs and tibiae than on spine. This lesion was probably due to another cause. The 2 remaining children (2 MRI) go on having negative medullograms but the follow up is short (4 and 7 months).

Post therapeutic transformations of the BM signal were noted 3 times. Vertebral fatty marrow after radiotherapy consisted in hypersignal in T1 weighted images and hyposignal in T2 weighted images, geometrically delineated.

On a post-radiotherapic vertebral boddy, a metastatic relapse modified the signal intensity which became low in SE short TR short TE sequences and strong in SE long TR long TE sequences (Fig. 3b). Medullary fibrosis appeared with a very low signal intensity in both T1 and T2 weighted images (Fig. 4a-b).

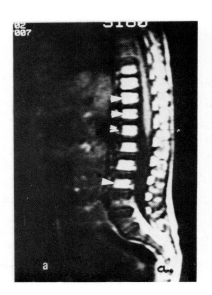 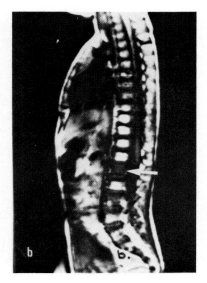

**FIG 3 :** 4 year-old child. Resected abdominal neuroblastoma, post operative radiotherapy.

**a.** sagittal SE 500/25 MR image reveals post-Rx fatty red marrow conversion on vertebral body ( ▶ ).

**b.** back pain with medullary relapse 4 months later. Sagittal SE 500/25 MR image shows a metastatic vertebral body with a low signal intensity ( ➔ ).

Our study indicates that MRI is a sensitive and non invasive technique to detect medullary metastases at the initial staging. SE 2000/120 (TR msec-TE msec) pulse sequence has a better contrast in order to differentiate metastatic regions from surrounding normal BM. In this sequence, lesions appear with a strong MR signal intensity.

One problem remains pending which is abnormal signal on MRI in otherwise remission patient. In order to differentiate a residual disease from necrosis or fibrosis, biopsy of these lesions would be a necessary investigation. The future place of MRI for assessment of bone marrow extension remains still open.

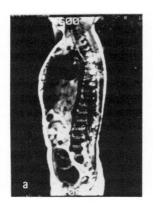 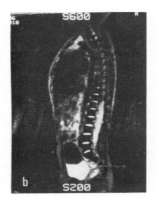

**FIG 4** : 3 year-old boy. Chemotherapy during 5 months 5 month for a stage IV abdominal neuroblastoma.
Sagittal SE 600/20 **(a)** and SE 2000/100 **(b)** MR studies : hypointense signal on lumbar vertebral bodies in both T1, and T2 weighted pulse sequences : histologically proven post-therapeutic medullary fibrosis.

# REFERENCES

Bottomley PA, Foster TH, Argersinger RE and Pfeifer ML (1984). A review of normal tissue hydrogen NMR relaxation time and relaxation mechanisms from 1-100 MHz : dependance on tissue type, NMR frequency, temperature, species, excision, and age. Med Phys 11(4) : 425-448.

Dooms GC, Fisher MR, Hricak H, Richardson M, Crooks LE, Grenant HK (1985). Bone marrow imaging : magnetic resonance studies related to age and sex. Radiology 155 : 429-432.

Fletcher BD, Kopiwoda SY, Strandjord SE, Nelson AD, Pickering SP (1985). Abdominal neuroblastoma : magnetic resonance imaging and tissue characterization. Radiology 155(3) : 699-703.

Kricun ME (1985). Red-yellow marrow conversion : its effect on the location of some solitary bone lesions. Skeletal Radiol 14 : 10-19.

Mc Kinstry CS, Steiner RE, Young AT, Jones L, Swirsky D, Aber V (1987). Bone marrow in leukemia and aplastic anemia : MR imaging before, during, and after treatment. Radiology 162 : 701-707.

Olson DO, Shields AF, Scheurich CJ, Porter BA, Moss AA (1986). Magnetic resonance imaging of the bone marrow in patients with leukemia, aplastic anemia, and lymphoma. Invest Radiol 21(7) : 540-546.

Wismer GL, Rosen BR, Buxton R, Stark DD, Brady TJ (1985). Chemical shift imaging of bone marrow : preliminary experience. AJR 145 : 1031-1037.

Advances in Neuroblastoma Research 2, pages 557–564
© 1988 Alan R. Liss, Inc.

# ELEVATION OF LUMBAR CEREBROSPINAL FLUID CATECHOLAMINE METABOLITES IN PATIENTS WITH CRANIAL AND/OR INTRACRANIAL METASTATIC NEUROBLASTOMA

BRUCE BOSTROM and BERNARD L. MIRKIN
Divisions of Clinical Pharmacology, and
Pediatric Oncology, Departments of Pediatrics
and Pharmacology, University of Minnesota
Medical School, Minneapolis, Minnesota 55455

## INTRODUCTION

The catecholamine metabolites, homovanillic acid (HVA), hydroxymethoxyphenylethyleneglycol (HMPG), and vanillylmandelic acid (VMA) are frequently elevated in the serum and urine of patients with neuroblastoma (Krivit et al, 1980). Recently, we have demonstrated elevations of HVA in the lumbar CSF of patients with intracranial tumors of neuroectodermal origin, including medulloblastomas, and retinoblastomas (Bostrom and Mirkin, 1987). Elevations in serum or urine catecholamine metabolites have not been demonstrated in intracranial tumors of neuroectodermal derivation, perhaps because of the polar nature of HVA and VMA which restrict their free movement across the blood brain barrier (Kopin, 1985).

Cranial and intracranial metastases have been reported in 25% of neuroblastoma cases (Gross et al, 1959). Most of the metastases were localized to bone, with occasional extension to the dura and leptomeninges (De La Monte et al, 1983; Alpert and Mones, 1969). Even in the presence of intracranial metastases, neuroblastoma cells are not commonly found in the CSF because invasion of the pia usually does not occur (Farr, 1972).

The objective of this study was to determine if the catecholamine metabolite concentrations in lumbar CSF would be abnormally increased in patients with cranial and/or intracranial metastatic neuroblastoma.

Supported in part by NS-17194-03 and the Childrens Cancer Research Fund.

## MATERIALS AND METHODS

<u>Patient Population</u>:  Informed consent and approval for lumbar puncture was obtained from each subject.  The study population was comprised of the following  diagnostic groups (N represents the the total number of patients in each group):
    1)  <u>Control subjects with extracranial non-neuroectodermal tumors</u>.  Control [extracranial].  This group included patients with leukemia in remission (N = 21), leukemia in marrow relapse (N = 3), lymphoma in remission (N = 6), cerebral palsy (N = 3),  Wilms tumor (N = 1), rhabdomyosarcoma (N = 1), Ewings sarcoma (N = 1) and radiculopathy (N = 1).  Leukemic patients had not received any intrathecal medication within three months and were either off systemic therapy or receiving maintenance chemotherapy, including methotrexate (20 mg/m$^2$/week).
    2)  <u>Control subjects with intracranial non-neuroectodermal tumors</u>.  Control [intracranial].  This group included patients with CNS leukemia (N =3), CNS lymphoma (N = 1), lung carcinoma with CNS metastases (N = 2), and retro-orbital rhabdomyosarcoma (N = 1).
    3)  <u>Neuroblastoma [extracranial]</u>.  This group consisted of 16 patients (1 month to 6 years of age) with extracranial neuroblastoma and no evidence of cranial or intracranial metastases. The number of patients with each clinical stage was: I (N = 3); II (N = 2); III (N = 1); IV (N = 9); IVS (N = 1).
    4)  <u>Neuroblastoma [cranial/intracranial]</u>.  This group included six patients (1 mo to 6 years of age) with stage IV disease.  These patients all had evidence of cranial and/or intracranial metastases confirmed by x-ray, bone scan, or CT (Table 1).

<u>Analytical Procedures</u>: The concentration of catecholamine metabolites, HVA, HMPG and VMA was determined in lumbar CSF by high pressure liquid chromatography [HPLC].  The HPLC system consisted of a reverse phase Bondapak $C_{18}$ column utilizing 50 mM $KH_2PO_4$ as eluent at a flow rate of 2.5 ml/min.  Vanillic acid was used as the internal standard. Vanillic acid (100 ng), 2N HCl (0.1 ml) and ethyl acetate (5.0 ml) were added to CSF (0.1 ml) and agitated on a vortex mixture for 30 seconds.  The organic phase was evaporated to dryness and redissolved in 100 µl of chromatographic eluent prior to injection.  Electrochemical detection of oxidized metabolites was performed with a

amperometric detector.   The detection threshold was 2 ng/ml for each metabolite.

Statistical Analyses:   Means and standard deviations were computed for each diagnostic group.  Intergroup comparisons were performed for HVA, HMPG,  and VMA by analysis of variance/covariance with age as the covariate to control for its effects on CSF catecholamine metabolite concentrations.

RESULTS

Neuroblastoma Patients with Cranial and/or Intracranial metastases: Cranial Imaging and Catecholamine metabolites.

   A summary of the cranial imaging studies and catecholamine metabolite concentrations in lumbar CSF are presented in Table 1.  CT scans demonstrated intracranial neuroblastoma in three patients, x-rays were positive in four patients and bone scans revealed abnormal uptake in the cranium of three patients.

### TABLE 1
### PATIENTS WITH CRANIAL AND/OR INTRACRANIAL METASTASES

| #/AGE[1] | CSF[2] | CRANIAL IMAGING[3] | | | LUMBAR CSF[4] | | | COMMENT |
|---|---|---|---|---|---|---|---|---|
| | | SCAN | XRAY | CT | HVA | HMPG | VMA | |
| 1/0.9 | − | + | + | | 93 | 90 | 95 | at diagnosis |
| 2/1.1 | − | | + | + | 22 | 5 | 0 | at diagnosis |
| 2/1.9 | + | | | + | 237 | 16 | 22 | at recurrence |
| 3/2.3 | − | − | + | | 382 | 182 | 23 | at diagnosis |
| 4/3.0 | − | + | | + | 205 | 20 | 0 | at diagnosis |
| 5/6.0 | − | | + | | 145 | 75 | 0 | at diagnosis |
| 6/18 | − | + | | − | 155 | 6 | 0 | at diagnosis |
| 6/18 | − | + | | + | 33 | 0 | 0 | after therapy |

[1]patient number and age in years
[2]CSF cytospin for tumor cells
[3]SCAN = bone scan, XRAY = skull film, CT = head CT,
 blank = test not done
[4]data expressed as ng/ml, upper limits of control
 [extracranial]:HVA = 90, HMPG = 50, VMA = 42

The middle fossa and orbits were involved with tumor at diagnosis in patient #2. The catecholamine concentrations in CSF were not elevated above control values at this time. Following recurrence of tumor in the leptomeninges the HVA concentration was markedly elevated.

A CT of the head was initially normal in patient #6, however the bone scan was abnormal. The CSF concentration of HVA was increased at this time. The patient received chemotherapy and six weeks later massive biparietal metastases to the dura were present. The HVA concentration in CSF had decreased to the normal range despite the presence of persistent intracranial disease.

All patients had elevations in the concentration of HVA in CSF at some time during the course of their disease. In addition, HMPG was elevated in three patients (#1,#3,#5) and VMA in one patient (#1).

Intergroup comparisons of catecholamine metabolite concentrations.

The mean lumbar CSF concentrations of HVA, HMPG, VMA and average patient age for each diagnostic group are presented in Table 2.

### TABLE 2
#### MEAN LUMBAR CSF CATECHOLAMINE METABOLITES

| GROUP | N | AGE[1] | HVA[2] | HMPG[2] | VMA[2] |
|-------|---|--------|--------|---------|--------|
| Control | | | | | |
|   extracranial | 37 | 17± 3 | 47± 4 | 10± 3 | 8± 2 |
|   intracranial | 7 | 33±12 | 33± 6 | 9± 5 | 6± 2 |
| | | | | | |
| Neuroblastoma | | | | | |
|   extracranial | 16 | 2± 1 | 85±12 | 12± 4 | 4± 2 |
|   cranial/intracranial | 6 | 5± 3 | 167±50 | 63±28 | 20±16 |

[1]mean age ± standard error in years
[2]mean ± standard error in ng/ml

There were no significant differences in the mean concentrations of HVA, HMPG or VMA between control subjects with either extracranial or intracranial non-neuroectodermal tumors (Table 3). In contrast, the mean values of HVA was significantly greater than control [extracranial] subjects in patients from both neuroblastoma groups. Additionally, the HVA concentration in CSF of

patients with neuroblastoma [cranial/intracranial] was also
elevated significantly above subjects with neuroblastoma
[extracranial].

The mean CSF concentration of HMPG in patients with
neuroblastoma [intracranial/cranial] was significantly
greater than that of controls [extracranial] and patients
with neuroblastoma [extracranial]. Mean VMA concentrations
differed significantly between the two neuroblastoma
groups, only.

## TABLE 3
### STATISTICAL COMPARISONS BETWEEN GROUPS P VALUE FROM ANALYSIS OF COVARIANCE[1]

| COMPARISON | HVA | HMPG | VMA |
|---|---|---|---|
| control extracranial vs neuroblastoma extracranial | .02 | NS | NS |
| control extracranial vs neuroblastoma cranial/intracranial | .0001 | .0004 | NS |
| neuroblastoma extracranial vs neuroblastoma cranial/intracranial | .05 | .006 | .04 |

[1]age was included as a covariate for all analyses of
variance, as the average age of subjects in the control
and experimental groups differed.

The concentrations of HVA and HMPG in lumbar CSF from
each patient in the neuroblastoma groups are shown in
figure 1, along with range of the control values.

## DISCUSSION

Significant elevations in the mean lumbar CSF
concentration of HVA and HMPG were observed in patients
with cranial and/or intracranial metastatic neuroblastoma
when compared to control patients [extracranial]. Patients
with neuroblastoma [extracranial] also had a significant
increase of the mean HVA concentration when compared to
controls [extracranial]. The mean concentrations of all
three metabolites were significantly greater in the lumbar
CSF of patients with neuroblastoma [cranial/intracranial]
than in patients with neuroblastoma [extracranial].

LUMBAR CSF CONCENTRATIONS OF HVA AND HMPG
IN PATIENTS WITH NEUROBLASTOMA

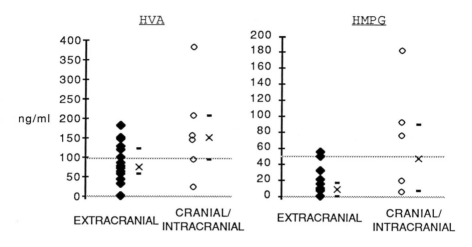

FIG 1. HVA (left graph) and HMPG (right graph)
concentrations in lumbar CSF from patients with
neuroblastoma. Individual values are plotted for
patients with extracranial metastases only (◆ )
and cranial and/or intracranial metastases (o ).
The (✕ ) represents the median, and the ( - ) 25th
and 75th percentiles. The range of control values
are designated by ( ⸺⸺⸺⸺ ).

    In previous studies,we have demonstrated elevations in
the mean concentration of HVA in lumbar CSF from patients
with primary intracranial neuroectodermally derived tumors,
including medulloblastoma and retinoblastoma (Bostrom and
Mirkin, 1987). Other investigators have reported
elevations in CSF catecholamines concentrations from
patients with primary intracerebral neuroblastoma
(Azzarelle et al, 1977; Williams et al, 1986).
    This increase in the CSF concentration of catecholamine
metabolites could result from production of catecholamines
or metabolites by the intracranial tumor or from
alterations in formation and transport of catecholamine
metabolites in the central nervous system. It is
interesting to note that patients with

non-neuroectodermally derived tumors metastatic to the CNS, did not demonstrate any elevation in the lumbar CSF concentration of catecholamine metabolites. This observation suggests that increments in CSF catecholamine metabolite concentrations do not result merely from a nonspecific effect of tumor on the CNS.

HVA or VMA produced by a tumor within the central nervous system would be expected to accumulate in the CSF as they are polar compounds which do not readily cross the blood brain barrier (Kopin, 1985). In contrast, HMPG, a neutral metabolite diffuses across the blood brain barrier and its elevation in the CSF from patients with intracranial neuroblastoma might be related to peripheral production of HMPG. Since patients with neuroblastoma and no cranial and/or intracranial metastases did not show a significant increase in the mean concentration of HMPG in CSF, it is unlikely that this is occuring.

These data suggest that the analysis of catecholamine metabolites in CSF may be useful in identifying patients with neuroblastoma who have cranial and/or intracranial metastases. Studies will be required in a larger patient population to determine the clinical utility and discriminatory threshold of this diagnostic approach as well as its value in assessing response to chemotherapy.

## REFERENCES

Alpert JN, Mones R (1969). Neurologic Manifestations of Neuroblastoma. J Mt Sinai Hospital (New York) 36:37-47.

Azzarelle B, Richards DE, Anton AH, Roessmann U (1977). Central Neuroblastoma: Electron microscopic observations and catecholamine determinations. J Neuropathol Exp Neurol 36:384-392.

Bostrom B, Mirkin BL (1987). Elevations of lumbar cerebrospinal fluid catecholamine metabolites in patients with intracranial tumors of neuroectodermal origin. J Clin Oncol (in press).

De La Monte SM, Moore GW, Hutchins GM (1983). Nonrandom Distribution of Metastasis in Neuroblastic Tumors. Cancer 52:915-925.

Farr GH, Hadju S (1972). Exfoliative cytology of metastatic neuroblastoma. Acta Cytol (Baltimore) 16:203-206.

Gross RE, Farber S, Martin LW (1959). Neuroblastoma
  Sympatheticum: A Study and Report of 217 Cases. Pediatr
  23:1179-1191.
Kopin IJ (1985). Catecholamine metabolism: Basic aspects
  and clinical significance. Pharmacological Reviews
  37:333-365.
Krivit W, Mirkin BL, Freier E, Nesbit M, Cooper MJ (1980).
  Serum catecholamine metabolites in stage IV
  neuroblastoma, in Evans AE (ed): Advances in
  Neuroblastoma Research. New York, Raven Press, pp
  33-41.
Williams DL, Faraj B, Camp M, Ragab AH (1986).
  Cerebrospinal fluid catecholamine levels in children
  with intracerebral neuroblastomas. Pediatr Res
  20:289 (abstr).

Advances in Neuroblastoma Research 2, pages 565–571
© 1988 Alan R. Liss, Inc.

DISCUSSION:

Chairman:     A.E. Evans and J. Kemshead

Discussants:  G.M. Brodeur, T. Sawada, J. Kemshead,
              D. Couanet, B. Bostrom

Lampson: The staging systems of NBL implies a passage or progression of stage in an individual with time, e.g., Stages I to IV. How often is this seen clinically?

Brodeur: Staging systems are not meant to imply a progression of disease, orderly or otherwise, in individuals. Its value lies in accurately determining extent of disease. e.g. stage, at diagnosis for two purposes:
(1) Prognosis; (2) Determine appropriate treatment and its intensity. With reference to disease progression, the majority of early stage disease patients do well with little or no treatment. There is a subset of Stage II patients who will progress and these are being identified by biological markers.

Lampson: Dr. Sawada, your program has a higher percentage of early stage patients. Is your screening picking up patients that would not progress and thus be undiagnosed or are you picking up potentially progressive cases at an early non-advanced stage?

Sawada: Prior to mass screening in Kyoto 1981, NBL presented in two age peaks: <2 years and 2-3 years. Since screening affects only those below one year the age peak remains implying one has picked up those that would have been picked up in the second 2-3 year old age peak.

Matthay: CCG data show in Stage II patients diagnosed before one year of age survival is 96-98%. Stage I have 100% survival. It is hard to believe that identifying these patients earlier would change the prognosis and I feel that your screening is only picking up good prognosis patients who would otherwise survive with little or no intervention.

Evans: Has the incidence of NBL changed since the advent of screening?

Sawada: No. The incidence of NBL under 15 years of age is the same before/after screening.

Seeger: Another way to address the question is to ask what is the frequency of Stage IV NBL over one year of age before and after the screening, for example if incidence has fallen dramatically since advent of screening, one can say you have picked them early. Otherwise, you must argue that your screening is picking up Stages I, and II patients who would not progress.

Sawada: In 1975 25% of cases of NBL were diagnosed under one year of age. In 1985 (post screen) 40% of NBL cases are diagnosed under one year of age. I do not know the proportion of Stage IV disease.

D'Angio: One way around this concern is to screen children over one year of age since these have a poorer prognosis group. This would avoid the hazard of over diagnosing and treating which is highly relevant as I notice one of the two deaths in your study was iatrogenic.

Evans: A report from Kyoto, Japan compared the outcome of two sets of NBL patients treated at the same hospital. One group was from the inner city screening program; the other group from the outlying area not screened. The latter has more advanced disease and did not do as well implying the screened population was caught earlier in the disease course with better results in the same treatment program.

Lumbroso: I feel MIBG investigation should have a pre-emminent position in your hierarchy of disease evaluation/staging. The work of Voute with many scans has shown MIBG to be useful in: (1) Evaluation of the primary tumor; (2) Evaluation of bone/bone marrow metastatic work-up as it is a specific tumor marker unlike technetium scintography which shows non-specific reactions; (3) Helps to differentiate between bone marrow and bone metastasis which can differentiate Stage IV and IVS disease. Non-specific bone scans may be falsely positive due to bone marrow disease giving non-specific critical reactions and a false impression of bone disease. This does not happen with MIBG scan; (4) Used in the definition of complete remission since CR with negative MIBG scan is <u>not</u> the same as CR with positive MIBG scans.

Brodeur: We agree MIBG is an important and powerful modality.
Would you write down your recommendations for me? The problems with MIBG are: (1) Not available in all countries, such as USA; and (2) Not as accurately standarized as other modalities. Therefore, it is hard to incorporate in a common denominator universal protocol or recommendation. It is, nonetheless, not our prerogative to say that centers comfortable and experienced in MIBG useage should not use this mode. A compromise is to use MIBG but if negative should do a Technetium Bone Scan since some NBL do not take up MIBG. I agree also, it is beneficial in assessing primary site, response to therapy and establishment of CR. It will be recommended in the future.

Lambruso: However, in your recommendations MIBG is mentioned only for assessment of metastatic bone disease.

Evans: We must make a distinction between the number and extent of testing one would do to stage a patient accurately and the number needed for staging diagnosis since expense is a big factor. One or two tests will tell you a child has Stage IV disease, the numerous tests should be limited to study protocols necessitating accurate extent of disease at diagnosis, response to therapy, and evaluation of CR.

Brodeur: (1) The Study recommendations did not imply you do all the modalities, eg CT - Bone Scan - MIBG - Skeletal Survey, etc. Do the minimum necessary to accurately stage. (2) If on a study protocol one must determine <u>all</u> sites of disease so that one can assess response.

Kemshead: The role of MIBG for diagnosis still controversial in Europe since (1) MIBG labelled with different isotopes; (2) Curving different doses; (3) Studying for different lengths of time. The whole field needs more studies.

Reynolds: Thanks Dr. Kemshead for his work in the blind screening project of NBL monoclonal antibodies. However, I have several concerns: (1) Leu7 clone is identical to HNK1 antibody; (2) 50% reactivity with W632 concerns us since we have not had this experience. Could this be due to: (a) Interpretation of positive versus negative response, (b) A large proportion of PNETs in study specimens which react differently to NBL with regard to monoclonal antibody responses/staining. We need to know how the study was done; what the tissues were that were studied, and what were the nature of the cell lines. (3) The third most disturbing concern is that many ab's submitted to the study were not included on the study.

Kemshead: (1) The HNK1 and Leu7 gave good correlation in study; (2) W632 has available binding to tissue lines. The study is preliminary. I agree with Dr. Reynold's comments in that many tissues studied may have been PNET; interpretation of positive versus negative binding needs closer evaluation. (3) Antibodies not included in study were due to lack of compliance to study guidelines or deadlines with up to three months delays.

Smith (comment): CCSG/POG surgeons met at the American Pediatric Surgical Association and discussed staging. We were pleased with (1) Criteria of resection grading from biopsy to 50%, 50-90% or complete removal. We will help recording. (2) Problems with lymph nodes: since it is hard to define lymph nodes adherent to the primary tumor. Those distant but in same cavity are easier to define.

Philip: Regarding the criteria of remission/response, we feel these concepts must be clarified clearly: (a) response to therapy (everything possible) up to surgery, (b) remission: define after surgery. (2) We feel Group II or very good partial response (VGPR) category cannot have presence of bony mets. VGPR must include no evidence of bony mets. Agree on all other response criteria as outlined by international conference.

Brodeur: This qualification of Group II responders was introduced because complete healing of bone lesions by technetium bone scan can take three to four months and up to 12 months in the face of biopsy proven negative histology at these sites. Hence, in order not to exclude these patients who may have no active disease from a good responder group the above qualification made. MIBG may eventually resolve this dilemma of differentiating between the positive technetium bone scan due to active disease or healing sterile lesions. Since this will be negative in a healing lesion.

Philip: Then we concur that in time MIBG negative patients will be classified as Group II?

Brodeur: Yes!

Philip: We must have a normal CT scan post-operatively to confirm a complete surgical excision of primary. Also for Group II responders they must become catecholamine negative post surgical excision.

Brodeur (comment): Yes, but the problem is that some tumors differentiate into benign ganglioneuromas which still secrete catecholamines. Therefore, we introduced this qualification in Group II responders so that this type of patient was not excluded. In practical experience also, the majority of patients whose tumor is reduced to ≤10% will become catecholamine negative. We can resolve this issue. We need also to differentiate between response and remission criteria. Adequate pretreatment evaluation is needed to gauge effects of chemo-radiotherapy on tumor. Patients will have unresectable masses at the primary site which become resectable, may have primary masses which remain unchanged in size but which mature and become stromal, benign ganglioneuromas. Whether these are removed surgically or unresectable but biopsy documented as being benign can be documented as presurgical or postsurgical responders or CR's.

D'Angio: I am concerned by limiting Stage IVs to those with primary IIAs. If a child has primary IIB (positive lymph node) he is classified as Stage IV with its associated poor prognosis and recommendation for intensive treatment of autologous bone marrow transplant. We believe some IVs can have positive lymph nodes, thus such patients would be grossly overtreating.

Brodeur: This was done in an endeavor to comply with the Evans and D'Angio staging system which states IVs is allowed primary I or II disease with metastatic disease confined to skin, liver and bone marrow, excluding bone and distant lymph node which would make them Stage IV.

D'Angio (comment): Our Stage IIs include tumors with unilateral lymph node involvement. I feel Stage IIA or Stage IIB with other features of Stage IVs disease should be classified accordingly to avoid overtreatment.

Graham-Pole: Could you comment on the use of the hierarchy of monoclonal antibodies for immunotherapy and data on the in vivo versus in vitro reactivity and cytotoxicity of these monoclonal antibodies?

Kemshead: The correlation of in vitro and in vivo reactivity with the majority of cell lines is good with the exception of E.S. It is probably coincidental that the two MoAbs IG $GD_2$ and UJ13A have already been explored as agents for immunotherapy and diagnosis when used with targeted radioisotopes (in our hands) and high doses of non-radio labelled MoAbs (in Dr. Cheung's hands). There are far greater problems in targeting with MoAbs other than picking the ideal one. The biggest problem is getting the antibody to the tumor site as well as specificity difficulties.

Philip: How do you separate what is bone marrow disease from bone disease on MRI?

Couanet: Bone has no signal on MRI and therefore any positivity reflects bone marrow disease.

Hartmann: What is the definition of bone lesions which allocate patients under one year as Stage IV?

Evans: Any radiographic evidence of bone lesion. Our experience is with diphosphenate scintigraphy. With regard to biological IVs disease, they have minimal bone marrow disease which probably would be negative on any scan.

Hartmann: Therefore, any positive bone scan excludes the diagnosis of Stage IVs disease.

D'Angio: One cannot "knock" success, as our experience with skeletal survey/bone scan adequately separated Stage IVS from IV. With introduction of MIBG one may be "muddying" the water as we do not know the significance of those findings currently. Therefore, Stage IVs is as defined on any visualization scans.

Brodeur: The use of MIBG scans may not differentiate focal bone marrow involvement from bone disease and, therefore, confuse Stage IVs with Stage IV disease. This is an important point to consider.

Philip: Is Stage VIs disease only in those less than one year of age?

Evans: No, it may include those over one year.

DiBernardi: Are you open for modifications on the INSS and treatment response criteria?

Brodeur: We are reluctant to change the proposal too much and feel it needs implementation as soon as possible. Modifications can be made in time but not all, especially the Italian and Japanese groups, were not represented at the conference. At present we feel only major objections will be considered to prevent the implementation of the proposal.

Advances in Neuroblastoma Research 2, pages 573–582
© 1988 Alan R. Liss, Inc.

PHASE II STUDIES OF COMBINATIONS OF DRUGS WITH HIGH DOSE CARBOPLATIN IN NEUROBLASTOMA (800 mg/m² to 1 g 250/m²) : A REPORT FROM THE LMCE GROUP.

Thierry Philip[1], Jean-Claude Gentet[2], Christian Carrie[1], Anne Farge[1], Fathia Meziane[1], Eric Bouffet[1], Jean-Michel Zucker[3], Bernard Kremens[1], Maud Brunat-Mentigny[1].

[1]: Centre Leon Berard, Pediatric Department, 28 rue Laennec, 69373 Lyon, France.
[2]: Hopital de la Timone, Service d'Oncologie 13000 Marseille, France.
[3]: Institut Curie, Paris, France.
Supported by grant INSERM 486022. LMCE is Lyon Marseille, Curie, East of France group.

Stage IV neuroblastoma in children over 1 year of age at diagnosis remains one of the major therapeutic challenges in pediatric oncology. Despite advances in conventional regimens and the recent introduction of high dose chemoradiotherapy with bone marrow rescue, the long term outcome remains questionable (Hartmann et al, 1979; Pritchard et al, 1984; Pritchard et al, 1986; Bernard et al, 1987; Philip, Bernard et al, 1987).
One of the major problem is the lack of accurate and complete assessement of response to therapy in published studies. This makes comparison between the various induction regimen virtually impossible. The Societe Française d'Oncologie Pediatrique (SFOP) group agreed in 1985 on strict criteria for response and remission which has allowed the two major french group (LMCE and Institut Gustave Roussy (IGR)) to compared easily their data. The proposed french system for the definition of response and remission will be used in this study (Philip, Helson et al, 1987).

Until recently, most chemotherapy regimens for neuroblastoma were variations of strandard sarcoma combination with adriamycin, cyclophosphamide and vincristine. The addition of cis platin (CDDP) and the epidophyllotoxins (etoposide i.e. VP16 and teniposide i.e. VM26) has had a significant impact in the initial response rate but durable remissions remain difficult to achieve (Bernard et al, 1987). To date, the most effective drugs in the treatment of neuroblastoma are cyclophosphamide, cisplatinum (CDDP), adriamycin, VP16, VM26, vincristine peptichemio and melphalan (Philip, Bernard et al, 1987). Investigators at St Jude Memphis U.S.A have clearly shown that combinations of drugs are more effective than single drugs and also that the sequence of drug administration plays a major role in the response rate (Hayes et al, 1981). The dose effect relationship has also been clearly demonstrated by a trial conducted at Villejuif, Paris, with a 2-3 fold increase in the dose of cyclophosphamide and adriamycin improving response rates from 40 to 90% (Hartmann et al, 1979; Philip and Pinkerton , 1987).

The first evidence for efficacy of CDDP in stage IV neuroblastoma was the 70% response rate in primary refractory patients reported by Hayes in 1981 (Hayes et al, 1981). Shafford and the London group with the OPEC regimen used as a front line regimen reported a 74% response rate with a combination including CDDP (Pritchard et al, 1984). Bernard and the LMCE group also had reported a 43% CR (complete response) + VGPR (very good partial response) response rate and a 94% response rate with combination of CADO (an adriamycin containing regimen) and PE (an OPEC like regimen) (Bernard et al, 1987).

The first evidence of a dose effect relationship in neuroblastoma with CDDP is found in a recent SFOP study in which 47 patients in relapse or refractory to initial therapy (including CDDP in some cases) were treated with VP16 100 mg/m² x 5 and CDDP 40 mg/m² x 5 for two successive courses. 20 had previously received CDDP and 55% of response and 22% of CR were reported (Philip, Ghalie et al, 1987). Median duration of response was 10 months and 8/47 patients are still disease free at 20 months (but they received additional therapy). Toxicity was acceptable mainly gastro intestinal, bone marrow and hearing loss.

Unpublished data from the SFOP group and the ENSG group (Hartmann, submitted) has shown that high dose VP16 CDDP and adriamycin containing regimen in alternance are able to produce 40% CR + VGPR in 3 months whereas the same alternance at conventional dose produce 43% CR + VGPR in 5 months (Bernard et al, 1987). However no treatment related deaths were reported with PE/CADO at conventional dose whereas the high dose VP16 CDDP/IVAD produced 2/20 treatment related death. Thus although CDDP is a very effective drug, toxicity is of concern.

Diaminocyclobutanedicarboxylatoplatinum (CBDCA) had the same antitumor activity as CDDP but produce less emesis, less neurotoxicity, less ototoxicity and less nephrotoxicity. CBDCA is also more easy to use with shedules of short 1 hour infusion every day (Von Hoff, 1987). Phase I and II studies have shown the feasibility of CBDCA administration in children (Hill and Whelan, 1981; Bacha, et al, 1986; Pritchard, et al 1987; Philip, Carrie, et al, 1987; Allen, et al, 1987) and also define that 800 mg/m$^2$ of CBDCA is equivalent to 200 mg/m$^2$ of CDDP. The major problem with CBDCA is myelotoxicity (Von Hoff, 1987). It was our objective in this pilot study to explore the toxicity and response of high dose CBDCA in combination for neuroblastoma patients.

## PATIENTS AND METHODS

9 patients age 2 to 8 years old, 6 having previously received cisplatinum (120 to 1200 mg/m$^2$ median 400 mg/m$^2$) entered the phase II study of VP16 - CBDCA. 7 patients were initially stage IV and entered this study when in relapse or refractory to front line therapy. 1 patient was stage III having previously received VP16 - CDDP high dose and relapsed while off therapy for 9 months. 1 patient was an intracerebral peripheral neuroectodernal tumor (PNET). 2 out of 9 were patients in relapse after bone marrow transplantation. These 9 patients are summarized in Table 1. A median of 4 evaluable targets for CBDCA response was available (range 1 to 7). These 9 patients received a combination of VP16 100 mg/m$^2$/day over 5 days CBDCA 200 mg/m$^2$/day over 5 days as detailed in Table 2.

## Table 2: CBDCA, VP16 high dose schedule

- Day 1 to day 5 included :
  - . 10 a.m. VP16 100 mg/m$^2$ in 250 cc saline solution infused during 1 hour.
  - . 05 p.m. CBDCA 200 mg/m$^2$ in a dextrose solution (250 cc) infused during one hour.
  - . Hydration is 1000 cc for 12 hours (dextrose + 2 g ClNa, 1 g ClK) for 30 kg

TABLE 1 : Age, Stage, Details and response to first line therapy, interval from diagnosis to the phase II study, status at therapy, response and duration of response for the 9 patients.

| LMCE NB | AGE AT DIAG. AND STAGE | 1st LINE TREATMENT DOSE OF CDDP (mg/m²) | INTERVAL DIAGNOSIS to VP16 CBDCA (months) | STATUS AT HIGH DOSE VP16 CBDCA | STATUS AFTER VP16 CBDCA | RESPONSE AND DURATION | MAJOR TOXICITY |
|---|---|---|---|---|---|---|---|
| 1 LA | 3 years stage IV | 400 | 8 | progressive disease (local, nodes, marrow, bones, and HVA) | Local 75% PR<br>Nodes CR<br>Marrow CR<br>Bones PR<br>HVA CR | PR 3 months (AT) | Thrombopenia Transaminases elevation |
| 2 DH | 3 years stage IV | - | 7 | primary refractory (marrow, local, bones) | Marrow PR<br>Local CR<br>Bones MR | PR 7 months + (AT BMT-> CR) | Herpes No major hematological toxicity |
| 3 BZ | 4 years stage III | 400 | 17 | nodes and mediastinum relapse off therapy | Nodes CR<br>Mediastinum CR<br>75% PR | PR 7 months + (AT BMT-> CR) | Mild transaminases elevation. No major hematological toxicity |
| 4 BK | 8 years stage IV | - | 7 | primary refractory (bones, tumor, nodes, marrow) | Bones CR<br>Tumor and Nodes PR<br>Marrow CR | PR 5 months + (AT BMT-> CR) | No major toxicity |
| 5 MM | 8 years stage IV | - | 7 | progressive disease in relapse (tumor, nodes, bones, marrow, skin, HVA, VMA) | Transient clinical improvement | PD | Thrombopenia with hemorragic cystitis |
| 6 SM | 2 years stage IV | 400 | 12 | Relapse post BMT (nodes, primary, mediastinum, skin, bones, liver, CNS) | Progressive disease | Progressive disease | Died day 33 of interstitial pneumonia while in progression |
| 7 AM | 6 years stage IV | 1200 | 16 | Progressive disease at relapse (orbit marrow, bones, initial, VMA) | Transient minor response (close to 50% at 4 weeks) | Progressive disease | Thrombopenia |
| 8 TD | 3 years intra cerebral PNET | 120 | 11 | CSF involvement and CNS disease in progression with coma | Transient clinical improvement but CT scan and CSF unchanged | Minor response | Hematological toxicity |
| 9 ML | 5 years stage IV | 600 | 25 | Relapse post ABMT Local abdominal | 50% improvement at CT scan after one course | PR 2 months+ (Radiotherapy after one course) | Hematological and platelets toxicity (excluded after 5 weeks post course 1 see text) |

AT : Additional therapy
NB : Number
DIAG. : Diagnosis

3 of these patients (2 stage IV, 1 stade III (number 2, 3 and 4 in Table 1)) subsequently received a combination of BCNU VM26 and 1 g 250/m² of CBDCA as a conditioning regimen prior to bone marrow transplantation. This regimen is detailed in Table 3.

**Table 3: Centre Leon Berard experience with high dose CBDCA as a conditioning regimen for ABMT.**

| Days | 1 | 2 | 3 | 4 | 5 | 6 | 7 | 8 |
|---|---|---|---|---|---|---|---|---|
| BCNU 300 mg/m² | X | | | | | | | |
| VM26 250 mg/m² | | X | X | X | X | | | |
| CBDCA 250 mg/m² | | X | X | X | X | X | | |
| ABMT | | | | | | | | X |

All parents were informed of the experimental aspect of the trial and gave informed consent. The protocols were reviewed and accepted by the Comite d'Ethique de l'Universite Claude Bernard et des Hospices Civils de Lyon France.

The initial targets for response were defined before the first course of CBDCA and VP16. A persistent or recurrent solid tumor was defined and measured clinically, if possible, or with a computed tomography (CT) scan or ultrasonography by measurement in three dimensions. Initial bone marrow involvement was defined by only one or two aspirates if heavily involved, and by an extensive superstaging with combination of biopsies and aspirates if moderately invaded. Bone lesions were defined with meta-iodo-benzyl-guanidine (MIBG) scanning. The levels of VMA-HVA (i.e. metabolites of catecholamines), and, if available, dopamine, were defined, compared with normal range, and considered evaluable if elevated to at least three times normal.
The response for each evaluable site was defined 30 days after the second course of VP16/CBDCA with the exception

of PD (progressive disease) after one course. CR was defined as a complete disappearance of all previously involved sites with no progression for at least 2 months. PR was defined as ≥ 50% reduction in measurable sites with no progression elsewhere. Minor response (MR) was defined as objective effect with < 50% reduction of initial evaluable disease. Non response (NR) was defined as no effect without any progression at day 30 after the second course, whereas any new involved site or progressing site was defined as PD.

Response according to these criteria for each evaluable site and overall response (CR + PR only) are shown in Table 1. For the initial solid masses, the response was defined either clinically by the same observer or with CT scann or ultrasonography measurement. For bone marrow response, CR was defined under general anesthesia as a completely cleared marrow in at least seven aspirates and two biopsies. All other bone marrow aspects including very minor persistent disease, were called NR. Bone scan response was difficult to standardize, but response was defined using the ratio between the number of involved sites before and after treatment (i.e., four sites reduced to two is 50% and thus PR). Catecholamine metabolites response was also defined according to the ratio between initial and post second course level of each metabolite. Duration of response is indicated in Table 1 which also indicates when additional therapy was used after the second course of VP16/CBDCA. Toxicity was studied before and after each course. For each courses, vomiting, weight loss, magnesium level from day 0 to day 7, and phosphate level from day 0 to day 7 were recorded. When patients were not at home between two courses, the nadirs of WBC and platelets were also recorded. Plasma creatinine levels were measured before and after each course and clearance was calculated. Audiometry was studied with pre- and post treatment audiogram when possible and by audio-evoked response for the youngest children. Parents were always asked about detectable clinical hearing loss. Any other major unexpected toxicity was also recorded and ototoxic antibiotics were not used during sepsis.

## RESULTS

Among the 9 patients receiving VP16 and CBDCA according to the regimen in Table 2, 5 PR were observed, 3 patients had progressive disease and 1 a non response. The

five response are shown in detail in Table 1. All patients
received additional therapy after response to this protocol and the duration of response is therefore difficult to
clearly assess. However all five PR were converted to CR
with additional treatment and 4 out of five are still
alive progression free 2 to 7 months after completion of
the second course of VP16 CBDCA.
Toxicity was mainly hematologic. All patients had a WBC
count less than 1000 during the post chemotherapy period.
The nadir for WBC was observed at day 15 (10-17) and the
median duration was of 8 days. The nadir of platelets was
at day 17 (10-35), with a median duration at less than
50.000 platelets/mm³ of 9 days. A median of 4 platelets
transfusions was neccessary (1-6). With the exception of
this hematological toxicity the treatment was well tolerated. Vomiting more than grade 2 (WHO) was recorded in 2
out of 14 courses whereas antibiotics were used only in 3
of 14 courses. Creatinine clearence was unchanged in all 9
patients after one or two courses. No hearing loss was recorded except for one patient who showed loss at 2000
Hertz but with no clinical deafness after two courses
(this patient had not previously received CDDP). Mild
transaminases increase was recorded in 2 cases during the
21 days after chemotherapy. One patient died of interstitial pneumonitis while in disease progression including
marrow involvement (case 6, Table 1). This pneumonitis was
related more to end stage disease than therapy. The second
course was given if there was no disease progression, and
was initiated after 4 weeks in 2 cases with normal marrow
and, after 5 weeks in 4 cases who had invaded marrow at
time of inclusion in this trial. One case in which a clear
partial response was observed after one course was withdrawn from the study 5 weeks after the first course because of severe thrombopenia and radiotherapy was begun
(this patient had relapsed post bone marrow transplantation, number 9 table 1). He is now in CR and will be included as a PR response to this protocol.

The post induction period in the 3 patients who had
received CBDCA 1 g 250/m² with BCNU and VM26 as conditioning regimen prior to transplantation was similar to 10 of
our patients previously treated with a similar regimen but
with CDDP at 200 mg/m² instead of CBDCA. However 1 developed mild erythma when vancomycin was prescribed and a second was complicated by a severe "loboster like syndrom"
when antibiotics were prescribed (ticarcillin, netromycin

and vancomycin). This patients showed a complete recovery of the skin problem at day 35 post graft. No other toxicities were of note with this combination of drugs including very high dose CBDCA.

## DISCUSSION

It is clear from this pilot study that the combination of VP16 and high dose CBDCA is effective in advanced neuroblastoma. The five partial response out of 9 evaluable cases compare favorably with our previous studies with cisplatinum (Philip and Pinkerton, 1987; Philip, Ghalie, et al, 1987). The question of whether CBDCA has cross resistance with CDDP is still an area of debate (Von Hoff, 1987). In this study among the five responders 3 had previously received CDDP (including high dose in one) whereas 2 had not. Our preliminary results clearly showed than CBDCA is less nephrotoxic less ototoxic and also causes less emesis than CDDP. However carboplatin is more myelosuppressive than CBDCA and because of this the interval between cures was about 5 weeks whereas a second course of high dose CDDP is usually feasible after 4 weeks (Philip and Pinkerton, 1987). This could be a major disadvantage for CBDCA, compared with CDDP in front line therapy for neuroblastoma. A dose effect relationship with CDDP clearly exists and also a possible time advantage (3 months to obtain the same response as after 5 months of conventional dosage (Philip and Pinkerton, 1987; and Hartmann to be published)). Carboplatin may be an adjunct to, more than a replacement for cisplatin as discussed by Von Hoff (Von Hoff, 1987). The reduction in non hematopoietic toxicity and possibly the lack of total cross resistance between the two drugs stimulates speculation at to whether CBDCA should perhaps be reserved for conditioning regimens prior to BMT (bone marrow transplantation) in neuroblastoma patients who have previously responded to a CDDP containing regimen. In this setting the two drugs could be complementary in the treatment of advanced neuroblastoma. The 3 patients having received 1 g 250 of CBDCA with high dose BCNU and VM26 are of interest and confirm recent Boston studies in adults showing than 1 g 250 oF CBDCA is tolerable in association with other drugs (K. Antmann, personal communication). However the cutaneous allergy observed in two patients including one which was life threatening is of concern and deserves carefull evaluation in further studies.

In conclusion CBDCA at high dosage is effective in advanced neuroblastoma. Because of a major hematological toxicity, this drug may not replace CDDP in induction regimens for neuroblastoma. We think, however, that CBDCA is a major drug to be used as part of conditioning regimen prior to bone marrow transplantation for these patients.

## REFERENCES

Allen JC, Walker R, Luks E, Jennings M, Barfoot S, Tan C (1987). Carboplatin and recurrent childhood brain tumors. J Clin Oncol 5:459-463.

Bacha DM, Caparros-Sison B, Allen JA, Walker R, Tan C (1986). Phase I study of Carboplatin in children with cancer. Cancer Treat Rep 70:865-869.

Bernard JL, Philip T, Zucker JM, Frappaz D, Robert A, Marguerite G, Boiletot A, Philippe N, Lutz P, Roche H, Pinkerton R (1987). Sequential cis platinum VM26 and vincristine cyclophosphamide doxorubicin in metastatic neuroblastoma : an effective alternating non cross regimen. J Clin Oncol (in press).

Hartmann O, Scopinaro M, Tournade MF, Sarazin D, Lemerle J (1979). Neuroblastomes traités à l'Institut Gustave Roussy de 1975 à 1979. Cent soixante treize cas. Arch Fr Pediatr 40:15-21.

Hayes FA, green AA, Casper J, Cornet J, Evans WE (1981). Clinical evaluation of sequentially scheduled cisplatin and VM26 in neuroblastoma : response and toxicity. Cancer 48:1715-1718.

Hill BT, Whelan RDH (1981). Assessments of the sensitivities of cultured human neuroblastoma cells to antitumour drugs. Pediatr Res 15:117-1122.

Philip T, Bernard JL, Zucher JM, Pinkerton R, Lutz P, Bordigoni P, Plouvier E, Robert A, Carton R, Philippe N, Philip I, Chauvin F, Favrot MC (1987). High dose chemoradiotherapy with bone marrow transplantation as consolidation treatment in neuroblastoma : an unselected group of stage IV patients over one year of age. J Clin Oncol 5:266-271.

Philip T, Carrie C, Brunat Mentigny M (1987). High dose carboplatin and neuroblastoma. Lancet (Submitted).

Philip T, Ghalie R, Pinkerton R, Zucker JM, Bernard JL, Leverger G, Hartmann O (1987). A phase II study of high dose cisplatin and VP16 in neuroblastoma : a report from the Société Française d'Oncologie Pediatrique. J Clin Oncol (In press).

Philip T, Helson L, Bernard JL, Zucker JM, Kremens B, Favrot MC, Hartmann O (1987) Definition of response and remission in children over one year of age with advanced neuroblastoma : a proposition for a scoring system. Pedia Hematol Oncol (in press).

Philip T, Pinkerton R (1987). Treatment directions in neuroblastoma. In Magrath Y, (ed) "New Directions in Cancer Treatment" (In press).

Pritchard J, Whelan R, Hill BT (1984). Sequential cis platinum and VM26 in neuroblastoma (OPEC regimen) : laboratory and clinical studies. In Evans AE, D'Angio GD, Seeger RC (eds) "Advances in neuroblastoma research", Prog Clin Biol Res, 175 pp 545-555.

Pritchard J, Germond S, Jones D, Dekraker J, Love S (1986). Is high dose Melphalan of value in treatment of advanced neuroblastoma ? Preliminary results of a randomised trial by the European Neuroblastoma Study Group. Proc Am Soc Clin Oncol, 5:205.

Pritchard J, Hill BT, Kellie S, Whelan RDH (1987). Carboplatin and neuroblastoma. Lancet, January 24, 112.

Von Hoff DD (1987) Whether carboplatin ? A replacement for or an alternative to cisplatin ? J Clin Oncol 5:169-171.

Advances in Neuroblastoma Research 2, pages 583–594
© 1988 Alan R. Liss, Inc.

# KINETICS OF VERY HIGH-DOSE CISPLATIN IN STAGE IV NEUROBLASTOMA

J.C. Gentet[1], M. Charbit[2], J.L. Bernard[1], T. Philip[3],
J.M. Zucker[4],V. Breant[2],C. Raybaud[1], J.P. Cano[2]

[1] Department of paediatric oncology, Hôpital d'Enfants de la Timone;
[2] Laboratoire Hospitalo–Universitaire–U 278–
   Faculté de pharmacie. 13385 Marseille Cedex 5.
[3] Centre Léon Bérard, Lyon.
[4] Institut Curie, Paris – FRANCE.

INTRODUCTION

High-dose cisplatinum (CP) is known to be effective in combination with etoposide in some adult cancer diseases (Ozols 1983), and in neuroblastoma (Philip 1985, 1987). Experimental (Drewinko 1973) and clinical (Lokich 1980, Salem 1984, Posner 1986) studies have intestigated standard dose CP delivered by continuous infusion, and shown this regimen to be less toxic and perhaps more efficient than bolus or rapid infusion delivery. Several workers have published kinetic data comparing various dosages, never exceeding 125 mg/m$^2$, administered by continuous or by rapid infusion schedules. They found body exposure to free platinum (FP) species, as expressed by area under the curve versus time (AUC), to be equivalent in both treatment regimen (Vermorken 1986) or greater in the continuous infusion schedule (Belliveau 1986). In this study, we examined pharmacokinetic parameters and body exposure to free and total platinum (TP) in children with stage IV neuroblastoma receiving very high-dose cisplatin, either by continuous infusion, or by fractionated rapid infusion, over five days.

PATIENTS AND METHODS

8 patients, aged 18 mth to 8 yr ( mean : 5 yr), received 1 to 3 courses of cisplatinum at a dose rate of 40 $mg/m^2/d$ for five days. A total of 16 kinetics were evaluable. A first group of 4 patients received 7 courses of CP by continuous infusion (reg. A). In this group, 3 children had been previously treated by chemotherapy and were in relapse, one had undergone a total body irradiation and had received 300 $mg/m^2$ of CP before, two patients had been nephrectomised. The other 4 children received 9 courses of CP by fractionated rapid infusions (reg. B). All of them were untreated new patients.

All children received normal NaCl with added KCl (1.5 g/l), $CaCl_2$ (10 $ml/m^2/d$) and $MgSO_4$ (5ml/$m^2$/d) at a rate of 3l/$m^2$/d . This hydration began with infusion in regimen A , and was anticipated 24 hr before the first infusion in reg. B. It was stopped 24 hr after completion in both treatments (fig 1).

In fractionated protocol, CP was reconstituted in 3% NaCl, as described by Ozols, and infused within an hour between 9 and 10 A.M..

In continuous regimen, the daily dose was delivered through a central catheter, by means of an electric syringe.

Sampling procedure was heavy because we wanted to explore the late elimination phase, but it was facilitated by using peripheral microcatheters which were rinced and left in place after each taking of blood. Samples were drawn at 12, 24, 48, 72, 96, 120 hr during infusion in regimen A, and before, at the end, and 2 hr after each infusion in regimen B. On the last day of treatment, the following times were drawn in both regimen, after the end of infusion : 30, 60, 90, 120, 180, 240 min, 6, 12, 24, 48, 96, 144 hr, and 10, 14, 21, 28 days.

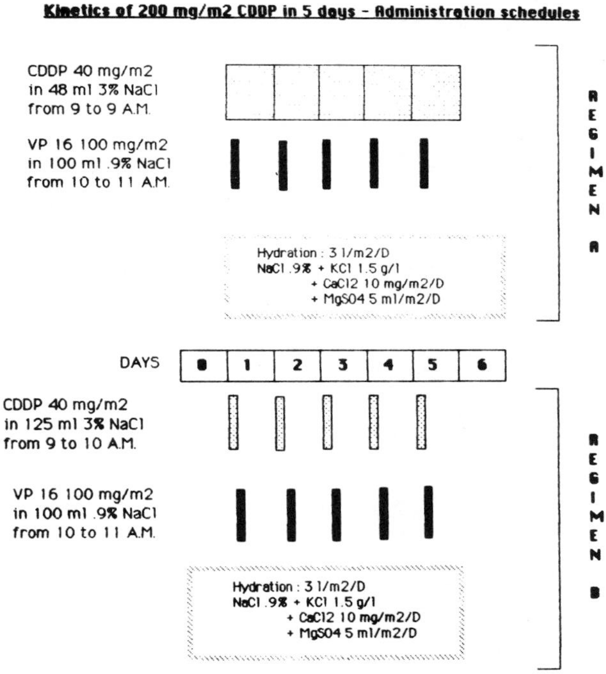

**Kinetics of 200 mg/m2 CDDP in 5 days - Administration schedules**

Figure 1

Samples were immediately centrifuged and the plasma was removed. Plasmas ultrafiltrates were obtained by using Micropartition systems MPS-1 (Amicon) centrifuged at

2000 g for 15 mn. All separations were completed within 30 mins after taking of blood. Samples were stored at -20° C until analysis. In the two groups of children, during at least one of the courses of treatment, urine samples were collected, as voided for 2 patients and during 12 hr intervals in 3 patient. The concentrations of TP and FP were performed by means of flameless atomic absorption spectroscopy, with a detection limit of 0.010 µg/ml (Cano 1982).

RESULTS

After 5-day infusion of high-dose CP, the maximum plasma TP concentration at the end of infusion ranged from 1.78 to 3.575 µg/ml in regimen A and from 1.91 to 4.10 in regimen B. TP levels recorded in reg. A during the administration showed that the steady-state concentration had not been achieved at the end of infusion (fig. 2). After cessation, the mean terminal T1/2 values varied from 155.5 to 418 hr in reg. A and from 208 to 335 hr in reg. B. Total plasma corrected TP clearances ranged from 0.179 to 0.306 l/h/1.73 $m^2$ after continuous infusion and from 0.231 to 0.443 after fractionated infusion.
Plasma FP levels before and after each daily infusion in regimen B are summarised in table 1.
During continuous infusion, FP levels were about 10 to 20 times lower than TP levels (fig. 2). By contrast, FP levels after 1 hr infusion corresponded closely to TP peak plasma levels (fig 3).

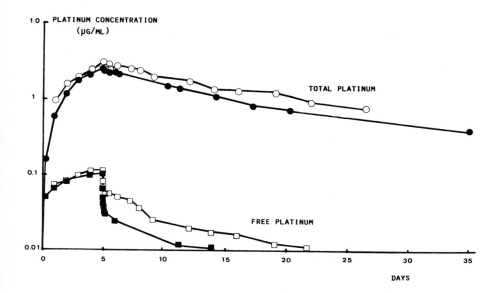

Figure 2

The decrease in FP levels, after the end of infusion, seemed to follow a biexponential kinetic pattern, with a prolonged elimination half-life from 69 to 157 hr (mean : 102.6 ± 38.5) in regimen A and from 76.5 to 151.2 hr (mean 108.25 ± 35.46) in regimen B (fig 4). FP was still detectable in the plasma 10 days after the end of infusion, with levels above 0.010 µg/ml. FP AUC (0-2 hr and 0-∞) were determined in order to know the total amount of FP available to the tissues during and after infusion. The mean AUC determined after continuous infusion were 769 ± 328 µg.min/ml (range : 529 – 1486) at 2 hr and 1094 ± 513 µg.min/ml (range : 771 – 2339) at ∞. In regimen B, mean AUC were 516 ± 135 µg.min/ml (range : 358 – 803.5) at 2 hr and 1078 ± 273.5 (range : 665.5 – 1671.5).

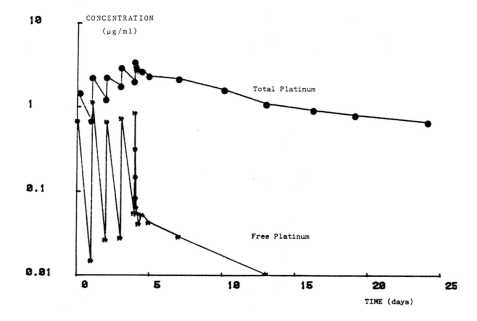

Figure 3

If inter-individual differences were observed, there was no intra-individual differences in AUC values, except for the youngest patient in reg. A who showed signs of hydro-electrolytic disturbance during the first course.

The maximum urinary concentrations of platinum (pt) attained during the 5 days of administration in urine voided varied between 7.66 and 15.2 mg/l ( A ) and between 17.7 and 27.76 ( B ). The maximum urinary excretion rate ranged from 0.35 to 0.40 mg/hr (A) and from 3.35 to 3.61 (B). 27 to 31% (A) and 36.7 to 52% (B) of the administered dose was eliminated within the 5 days of infusion (table 2).

A good clinical comparison is not possible in this study, as the two groups are differents. Nevertheless, vomitings were less important with regimen A (no grade 2 emesis versus 6/9 courses in reg. B). No neurotoxicity was associated to these high-dose treatments.

For all the patients a good partial response or a complete remission was obtained.

DISCUSSION

In this study, two groups of 4 children received 200 mg/m$^2$/day in 5 days, by continuous or fractionated infusion. Plasma levels, pharmacokinetic parameters and urine concentrations were examined.

If we first consider plasma free platinum levels in fractionated regimen, we see that peaks of short duration recorded each day have similar values. Those very high levels, which correspond closely to total platinum levels, are in relation to the rate of drug delivery. However, the residual values grow each day, showing a progressive accumulation of the drug (table 1). If we look at the continuous regimen, it appears that free platinum levels remains ten to twenty times lower than total platinum during the 5 days. After the end of infusion, in both cases, FP levels are detectable above 10 ng/ml up to 10 days. This finding should be taken into account when cisplatinum is included in massive therapies before bone marrow transplantations.

Concerning kinetic parameters, one can see that half-lives, clearances and distribution volume are within the same range in the two protocols. We have to note that terminal half-life is high, in the order of three to six days, and corroborate other reports (De Gregorio 1985).

**5-DAY FRACTIONATED INFUSION**

| Patient & course N° | Dose cisplatin (mg) | Maximum plasma concentration of free platinum after each infusion (ng/ml) | | | | |
|---|---|---|---|---|---|---|
| | | 1st dose | 2nd dose | 3rd dose | 4th dose | 5th dose |
| -1 | 25 x 5 | 705.5 | 675.5 | 971 | 925.5 | 613 |
| 1 -2 | 25 x 5 | 940 | 626.5 | 710 | 843 | 599 |
| -3 | 24 x 5 | 707.5 | 1068 | 1081 | 1106 | 1325 |
| -1 | 31 x 5 | 685.5 | 1142.5 | 672 | 740.5 | 857 |
| 2 -2 | 31 x 5 | 1030 | 763 | 1063 | 1208 | 945 |
| -1 | 23 x 5 | 1007 | 1184 | 890.5 | 1108 | 1255 |
| 3 -2 | 23 x 5 | 984 | 1318 | 1430 | 1510 | 1453 |
| -3 | 22 x 5 | 1100 | 947 | 1103 | 650 | 814 |
| 4 - 2 | 30 x 5 | 1247 | 1140 | 1305 | 1148 | 685 |
| Mean : | | 934 | 985 | 1025 | 1026 | 949.5 |
| Standard deviation : | | 196 | 245.5 | 249.5 | 265 | 320.5 |

| Patient & course N° | Dose cisplatin (mg) | Plasma concentration of free platinum before each infusion (ng/ml) | | | | |
|---|---|---|---|---|---|---|
| | | 1st dose | 2nd dose | 3rd dose | 4th dose | 5th dose |
| -1 | 25 x 5 | - | 7 | 16 | 26 | 27 |
| 1 -2 | 25 x 5 | - | 18.5 | 21 | 33 | 63 |
| -3 | 24 x 5 | - | 9.5 | 27 | 31 | 47 |
| -1 | 31 x 5 | - | 15.5 | 27.5 | 29 | 56.5 |
| 2 -2 | 31 x 5 | - | 19 | 37.5 | 51 | 68 |
| -1 | 23 x 5 | - | 8.5 | 15 | 20 | 25.5 |
| 3 -2 | 23 x 5 | - | 11 | 23.5 | 33.5 | 44 |
| -3 | 22 x 5 | - | 14 | 24.5 | 31.5 | 32 |
| 4 - 2 | 30 x 5 | - | 19 | 27 | 37.5 | 40.5 |
| Mean : | | - | 13.5 | 24.5 | 32.5 | 44.8 |
| Standard deviation : | | - | 4.75 | 6.75 | 8.5 | 15.5 |

Table 1

FP AUC versus time is a measure of the overall availability of ultrafilterable species which is the component responsible for cytotoxicity ( Holdener 1983).

We determined AUC up to two hours after infusion, since a convergence between intact CP and ultrafilterable pt has been shown 3 years ago (Sternson 1984) . This value reflect the total amount of drug available to the tissues during and after infusion. After two hours, CP metabolites appears, and several workers have suggested that these

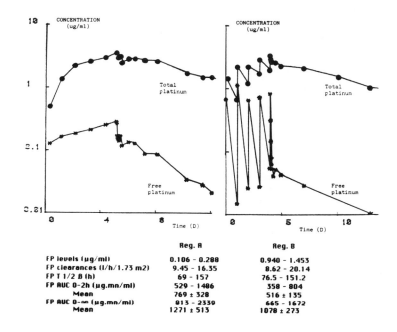

| | Reg. A | Reg. B |
|---|---|---|
| FP levels (µg/ml) | 0.106 - 0.288 | 0.940 - 1.453 |
| FP clearances (l/h/1.73 m2) | 9.45 - 16.35 | 8.62 - 20.14 |
| FP T 1/2 β (h) | 69 - 157 | 76.5 - 151.2 |
| FP AUC 0-2h (µg.mn/ml) | 529 - 1406 | 358 - 804 |
| Mean | 769 ± 328 | 516 ± 135 |
| FP AUC 0-∞ (µg.mn/ml) | 813 - 2330 | 665 - 1672 |
| Mean | 1271 ± 513 | 1078 ± 273 |

## Figure 4

ultrafilterable species, which are probably less effective, could play a role in the development of oto and neprotoxicity (Daley-Yates 1982, Earhart 1983, Daley-Yates 1984).
CP exposure was at least as important in continuous regimen (fig 4).
Data concerning urines allows to find the expression of differences observed in free platinum plasma levels, as higher platinum concentration and excretion rate are recorded in urine voided when cisplatin dose is fractionated. Indeed, these differences are less important if one consider urines collected by twelve hours interval. In regimen A, these values are lower, and similar to those

| | Reg. A | Reg. B |
|---|---|---|
| TP levels (µg/ml) | 1.78 - 3.575 | 1.91 - 4.10 |
| TP clearances (l/h/1.73 m2) | 0.142 - 0.306 | 0.231 - 0.443 |
| TP T1/2 β (h) | 155.5 - 418 | 208 - 335 |
| Max. urin. excretion rate (mg/h) | | |
|     urine voided | 0.36 - 0.40 | 3.35 - 3.61 |
|     12 h interval | 0.205 - 0.50 | 0.46 - 1.055 |
| Max. urine concentration (mg/l) | | |
|     urine voided | 7.66 - 15.2 | 17.7 - 27.76 |
|     12 h interval | 4.12 - 5.46 | 5.395 - 13.635 |
| % administerded dose excreted (5 D.) | 27 - 31 | 36.7 - 52 |

Reg. A = 5-day continuous infusion
Reg. B = 5-day fractionated infusion

Table 2

obtained with the same schedule at the dose of 100 mg/m$^2$ (Bues-Charbit 1982). So continuous infusion reduces urinary concentration of pt which is probably the best way to reduce nephrotoxicity (Corden 1985).

In high-dose treatments body exposure to intact cisplatin is at least identical in 5 days continuous regimen when compared to daily fractionated one hour infusion. Continuous infusion clearly prevent peak plasma and urine levels recorded daily in fractionated regimen ; so, it could provide identical efficiency, with less oto and nephrotoxicity. Continuous infusion of high dose cisplatinum is warranted for phase II and III studies.

SUPPORTED IN PARTS BY INSERM GRANT 486022 AND BY LIGUE NATIONALE POUR LA LUTTE CONTRE LE CANCER.

# REFERENCES

Belliveau JF et al. (1986). Cisplatin administered as a continuous 5-day infusion : Plasma platinum levels and urine platinum excretion. Cancer Treatment Report, 70 (10), 1215-1217.

Bues-Charbit et al. (1982) Pharmacokinetic study of Cis-dichlorodiammine platinum II (CDDP) administered as a constant 5-day infusion. 8th Annual Meeting of European Society for Medical Oncology. Nice, December 1982. Cancer Chemother. Pharmacol. , 9 Supp., 8 .

Cano JP et al. (1982). Platinum determination in plasma and urine by flameless atomic absorption spectrophotometry. J. App. Toxicol. , 2, 33-38.

CORDEN BJ (1985). Clinical pharmacology of high-dose cisplatin. Cancer Chemother. Pharmacol., 14, 38-41.

Daley-yates PT and Mc Brien DCH (1982) The inhibition of renal ATPase by cisplatin and some biotransformation products. Chem. Biol. Interactions , 40, 325-334 .

Daley-yates PT and Mc Brien DCH (1984). Cisplatin metabolites in plasma, a study of their pharmacokinetics and importance in the nephrotoxic and antitumor activity of cisplatin. Biochem. Pharmacol. , 33, 3063-3070.

De Gregorio MW et al. (1985) Concerning the paper Clinical pharmacology of high-dose cisplatin by Corden et al. Cancer Chemother. Pharmacol. , 15, 183-184.

Drewinko B et al. (1973). The effect of cis-diamminedichloroplatinum (II) on cultured human lymphoma cells and its therapeutic implications. Cancer Res. , 33, 3091-3095.

Earhart RH et al. (1983) Improvement in the therapeutic index of cisplatin (NSC 119875) by pharmacologicaly induced chloruresis in the rat. Cancer Res 43, 1187-1194.

Holdener EE et al. (1983). Effect of mannitol and plasma on the cytotoxicity of cisplatin. Eur. J. Clin. Oncol. , 19, 515-518.

Lokich JJ (1980) Phase I study of cis-diamminedichloroplatinum (II) administered as a constant 5-day infusion. Cancer Treat. Rep. , 64, 905-908.

Ozols RF et al. (1983) Treatment of poor prognosis nonseminomatous testicular cancer with a "high-dose" platinum combination chemotherapy regimen. Cancer , 51,1803-1807.

Philip T. et al.(1985) Etoposide and very high dose cisplatin : salvage therapy for patients with advanced neuroblastoma, XVIIth S.I.O.P. Meeting, Venice, abstracts 246-247.

Philip T. et al. (1987). Very high-dose VP 16- cisplatinum in refractory neuroblastoma, Journal of Clinical Oncology, in press.

Salem P et al. (1984). Cis-diamminedichloro- platinum (II) by 5-day continuous infusion. A new dose schedule with minimal toxicity. Cancer , 53, 837-840.

Sternson LA et al. (1984). Disposition of cisplatin versus total platinum in animals and man. In : Hacker MP, Douple EB, Krakoff IH, eds, Platinum Coordination Complexes in Cancer Chemotherapy. Martinus Nijhoff, Boston, 126-137.

Vermorken JB et al. (1986). Pharmacokinetics of free and total platinum species after rapid and prolonged infusions of cisplatin. Clin. Pharmacol. Ther. , 39, 136-144 .

Advances in Neuroblastoma Research 2, pages 595–604
© 1988 Alan R. Liss, Inc.

IODINE 131 LABELED G$_{D2}$ MONOCLONAL ANTIBODY IN THE DIAGNOSIS
AND THERAPY OF HUMAN NEUROBLASTOMA

Nai-Kong V. Cheung and Floro D. Miraldi

Department of Pediatrics, Memorial Sloan Kettering
  Cancer Center, New York, NY 10021 and
Departments of Pediatrics and Radiology, Case Western
  Reserve University , Cleveland, OH 44106

INTRODUCTION

High dose marrow ablative therapy followed by autologous bone marrow transplantation (ABMT) has prolonged
survival in patients with neuroblastoma (Pritchard et al.,
1982; August et al., 1984; Philip et al., 1985; Seeger et
al., 1987). Total body and focal irradiation play an
integral role in the overall treatment of this disease.
The biological basis for radiation is the radiosensitivity
and the lack of sublethal repair in neuroblastoma cells
(Deacon et al., 1985). However, radiation therapy has not
by itself been adequate because of the usual widespread
nature of neuroblastoma and the inability to achieve
selective tumor versus normal tissue delivery, especially
at multiple tumor sites. Monoclonal antibodies are agents
selected for their specificity for human tumors. In vivo
they have the ability of targeting selectively to occult
metastases. The availability of radioisotopes and the
development of conjugation chemistries have greatly
expanded the potentials of these antibodies. The limiting
factor has been the identification of antigen systems that
are optimal for tumor targeting. The ganglioside G$_{D2}$ is an
oncofetal antigen expressed in many human tumors (Cahan et
al., 1982; Schultz at al.,; Cheung et al., 1985). It has
been demonstrated to be an ideal tumor antigen for
targeting to human neuroblastoma. Since this ganglioside
is present on other human tumors, findings in neuroblastoma
targeting studies may have general applications to these
other malignancies.

GANGLIOSIDE $G_{D2}$ AND MONOCLONAL ANTIBODIES

Chemical analysis has shown that the ganglioside $G_{D2}$ is densely expressed in human neuroblastoma at an average of 10 million molecules per cell (Wu et al., 1986). Using monoclonal antibodies to $G_{D2}$, immunostaining of human tissue sections suggested that most of the $G_{D2}$ is present on the cell surface. Most, if not all, neuroblastoma tumors screened possessed this ganglioside and >95% of tumor cells were consistently positive. Some neuroepithelioma cell lines were shown to be negative or poorly reactive with these $G_{D2}$ antibodies. The ganglioside $G_{D2}$ does not modulate after binding to monoclonal antibodies in vitro. This is important for tumor targeting, given the difficulty encountered with glycoproteins and protein antigens in previous studies.

Its distribution in normal tissues has been found to be highly restricted. Biochemical analyses have shown that $G_{D2}$ is a minor ganglioside in the human brain. It is present on neurons and neuropil (Cordon-Cardo, 1987). This degree of cross-reactivity with the human nervous system would have prohibited the in vivo use of these antibodies, if not for the fact that monoclonal antibodies in general do not penetrate the intact blood brain barrier. Minor stainings of other normal tissues have also been noted. These include cytoplasmic staining of some connective tissues around the renal glomerulus, some stromal cells in the testes and ovary, myometrium, selective cells in the basal layer of the epidermis, as well as the adnexus, sensory pain fibers and lymphoid follicles in the spleen. The ganglioside $G_{D2}$ is also detectable in serum of neuroblastoma patients. Although the amount of circulating $G_{D2}$ antigen can be high (Schultz et al., 1985; Cheung et al., 1987a), it is probably not antigenically accessible to ganglioside $G_{D2}$ specific antibodies since it has not interfered with in vivo imaging studies in patients. A number of monoclonal antibodies to ganglioside $G_{D2}$ has been reported. 3F8 is one of the murine $IgG_3$'s (Cheung et al., 1985; Mujoo et al., 1987) which was selected for in vivo studies. The dissociation constant (Kd) of 3F8 is 1 nM on Scatchard analyses and the estimated antibody binding sites on human neuroblastoma averaged 5-10 million molecules per cell. These characteristics are largely responsible for the initial successes in the radiotargeting to this tumor antigen system in human neuroblastoma.

PRECLINICAL STUDIES OF RADIO-TARGETING IN XENOGRAFTED MICE

Human neuroblastoma and other G$_{D2}$ positive tumors were passaged in athymic nude mice. Previous studies have shown that after intravenous injection of iodine-131 radiolabeled monoclonal antibody 3F8 (I-131-3F8), selective uptake of antibody could be detected in human neuroblastoma, in contrast to control IgG$_3$ antibody against sheep red cells (N-S.7) and G$_{D2}$ negative tumors like Hela (Table 1) (Cheung et al., 1987b). The percent uptake per gram averaged between

Table 1.  Tumor specificity of 3F8 biodistribution

TUMOR TO NONTUMOR RATIOS

| TISSUE | NB | | HELA | | EWING'S | |
|---|---|---|---|---|---|---|
| | 3F8 | N-S.7 | 3F8 | N-S.7 | 3F8 | N-S.7 |
| Blood | 27.6* | 0.5 | 1.4 | 0.6 | 1.4 | 0.3 |
| Lung | 27.1 | 0.9 | 2.0 | 1.5 | 3.1 | 0.8 |
| Skin | 28.0 | 1.1 | 1.6 | 1.7 | 3.5 | 0.9 |
| Kidney | 39.1 | 1.4 | 3.0 | 2.0 | 4.7 | 1.1 |
| Heart | 64.9 | 1.6 | 4.1 | 2.8 | 4.8 | 1.1 |
| Stomach | 39.6 | 2.5 | 2.2 | 3.1 | 7.1 | 2.3 |
| Spleen | 24.2 | 2.3 | 1.3 | 1.9 | 5.7 | 1.6 |
| Liver | 59.0 | 2.0 | 2.7 | 1.7 | 7.8 | 1.8 |
| S Bowel | 79.7 | 2.8 | 2.8 | 3.5 | 9.4 | 2.9 |
| Bone | 121.0 | 4.0 | 3.9 | 3.8 | 11.6 | 2.9 |
| Muscle | 130.0 | 4.4 | 7.4 | 5.5 | 14.1 | 2.9 |
| L Bowel | 28.3 | 3.2 | 5.8 | 5.2 | 18.0 | 5.5 |
| Brain | 403.0 | 12.3 | 26.7 | 16.0 | 36.2 | 14.8 |

*
Arithmetic means of tumor to nontumor ratios.  n = 5 for NB line IMR-6, n = 4 for Hela and n = 8 for Ewing's tumors.

20 to 40% depending on the size of the tumor. Larger tumors tended to have lower percentages probably because of the uneven penetration of the antibody 3F8 as well as the presence of areas of nonviable tumor. Since the percent per gram uptake is dependent on the relative amount of normal tissue versus tumor, these calculated percentages cannot be easily extrapolated to human patients. Nevertheless, if one assumes that a 25 kg patient has 10$^3$-fold

more normal tissues to compete with each gram of tumor for binding, a 40% per gram uptake in mice translates into 0.04 percent per gram uptake in patients.

Initial therapeutic experiments using nude mice xenografts have shown that established tumors can be ablated completely with 0.5 mCi of I-131-3F8 (Cheung et al., 1986). In addition, these treated mice sustained no detectable radiation damage to bone marrow or the lymphoid tissues. When the radiation dose delivered by radiolabeled 3F8 was analyzed, only those tumors that received more than 4,000 rads were ablated without recurrence at follow-up.

BIODISTRIBUTION OF I-131-3F8 IN PATIENTS WITH NEUROBLASTOMA

Based on the estimations from nude mice xenograft biodistribution and therapeutic studies, a phase I biodistribution study was carried out in patients with widespread neuroblastoma (Miraldi et al., 1986). The antibody was radiolabeled with iodine 131 using chloramine T method, and between 2 to 5 mCi was injected into patients with neuroblastoma. Nuclear imaging was done using a LFOV set at a 364 MeV window. Mutiple views (anterior, posterior, and lateral) were taken. Scintigraphic studies were carried out for up to seven days. Radiolocalization was demonstrated in human neuroblastoma irrespective of sites. These included primary tumors in the mediastinum, the abdomen, metastatic disease to the lymph nodes, bone marrow, and bone (both axial and apendicular). Figure 1 shows gamma images of a patient with metastatic neuroblastoma. Focal uptake was seen in multiple sites of suspected disease. Such focal uptakes correlated with lesions found by conventional studies: CT scans of the chest and abdomen, bone scans, as well as MRI scans. However, there were sites detected with I-131-3F8 that were not obvious or detectable on conventional bone scans. This was probably secondary to the fact that bone marrow disease was not easily evident on conventional bone scans unless there was bone erosion or reactive bone formation. From these serial scintigraphic studies, radiation dose delivered to the tumors was calculated. Tumor sizes were estimated from CT and other conventional scans. The radioactivity in mCi per cc was calculated for selected tumor sites as well as normal tissues. The estimated radiation dose delivered was based on these kinetic studies. In patients who had tumors

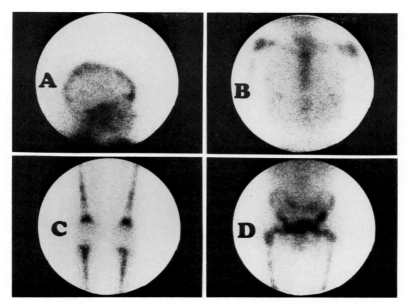

Figure 1. Gamma images 20 hours after intravenous injection of I-131-3F8 in a patient with metastatic neuroblastoma. a. Right lateral skull; b. Anterior chest; c. Knees; d. Anterior pelvis. Abnormal areas of uptake were seen in the skull, sternum, pelvis and long bones. This patient also had an upper anterior mediastinal mass. No abnormal uptake was seen in the liver or spleen.

removed at surgery within five days after radioimaging, the tissues were counted and correlated with the dosimetry estimations. Agreements between the measured tissue radioactivities and dose estimations based on planar scintigraphy have validated the dosimetry calculations. The estimated percent uptake of radioactivity per gram as well as the calculated radiation doses to tissues are tabulated in Table 2 (Miraldi et al., 1986). A therapeutic dose (>4,000 rads) of radiation to tumor is possible with all other normal tissues tested receiving less than 400 rads. There is however, a significant radiation dose in the blood, which could harm the patient's bone marrow.

Table 2.   Approximate I-131-3F8 concentrations and radiation dose

| | 24 hr after MoAB injection | |
|---|---|---|
| Tissue | Percent administered I-131-3F8 dose/ml | Average I-131 Radiation Dose (rad/mCi) |
| Tumor | 80 x $10^{-3}$ | 36.6 |
| Blood | 21 x $10^{-3}$ | 3.4-5.2 |
| Brain | 2.2 x $10^{-3}$ | 0.6 |
| Liver | 7.5 x $10^{-3}$ | 2.1 |
| Lung | 5.7 x $10^{-3}$ | 1.5 |
| Kidney | 10.0 x $10^{-3}$ | 3.3 |
| Muscle | 7.7 x $10^{-3}$ | 2.0 |

THERAPEUTIC STUDIES USING 131-IODINE-3F8 IN PATIENTS WITH METASTATIC NEUROBLASTOMA

In a pilot study three patients with metastatic neuroblastoma were studied (Cheung et al., 1987a). They all had refractory disease despite combined chemotherapy and local radiation. All three had bone and bone marrow disease. One patient (see figure 1) had an anterior mediastinal mass and another patient had a right adrenal mass. After a single intravenous dose of 100 mCi I-131-3F8, all three patients had subjective responses with resolution of bone pain and a sense of well being. They all showed decreased tumor on repeat bone marrow biopsies within one month after the antibody treatment. One patient normalized his bone scan and another patient showed less than partial reduction in size (with calcifications) of his mediastinal tumor. Although pain, hypertension and urticaria were severe in patients receiving the nonradioactive 3F8 antibody (Cheung et al., 1987c), such side effects were not signifcant in patients receiving >10 mg/m$^2$ of I-131-3F8. In vitro studies showed that radiolabeled 3F8, although retaining immunoreactivity, has markedly decreased ability to mediate human complement dependent or cell dependent cytotoxicities. This loss of Fc effector function may explain the relative absence of acute side effects during the radiolabeled antibody infusion. Although there was measurable response of the tumors in the bone marrow within the first 2 weeks of therapy, all three

patients had marked cytopenia requiring transfusions.
Figure 2 depicts the blood counts after exposure to I-131-
3F8 in one patient. Although none of the patients required
hospitalization secondary to complications from low blood
counts, bone marrow radiation damage was evident based on
these preliminary studies. All of these patients had bone
marrow involvement by neuroblastoma at the time of treatment with I-131-3F8. The selectivity was nevertheless not
adequate to avoid bone marrow damage. Even though they all
had both subjective and objective responses, the duration
of response was short.

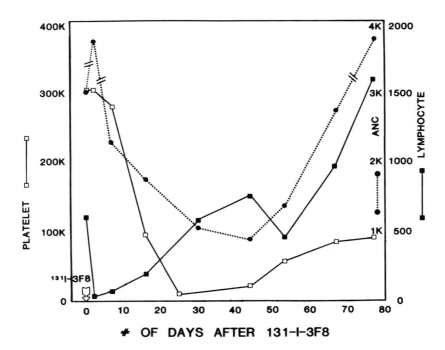

Figure 2. Blood counts after a single injection of 100 mCi
of I-131-3F8 administered on day 0. ANC = absolute
neutrophil count.


FUTURE APPLICATIONS OF RADIOLABELED 3F8

Bone marrow suppression is currently the major limiting
toxicity for the use of I-131-3F8 in patients with meta-

static neuroblastoma. It is likely that patients with less
advanced bone marrow disease will have less myelo-
suppression. Further improvements in biodistribution of
I-131-3F8 may also reduce marrow toxicity. Preliminary
studies in nude mice xenografts suggested that the
injection of a second antibody specific for $IgG_3$ could
clear the blood radioactivity and potentially reduce the
blood dose, as well as increase the overall tumor to
nontumor ratios. The recent development of genetically
engineered human hematopoietic colony-stimulating factors
may also be useful in accelerating marrow recovery after
such radiation damage (Clark et al., 1987). In addition,
bone marrow can now be harvested and purged (Treleaven et
al., 1984; Reynolds et al., 1986) before cryopreservation.
Thus, targeted radiotherapy utilizing I-131-3F8 can be
escalated to realize its anti-tumor potential beyond the
constraints of bone marrow toxicity. It may also be useful
as part of the preparative regimen before autologous bone
marrow transplantation.

ACKNOWLEDGEMENTS

This work was supported in part by grants from the
American Cancer Society (CDA85-7, RD-226), NIH (CA-39320),
and the Ireland Cancer Center, Cleveland, OH.
We want to thank Dr. P.F. Coccia, Dr. S. Strandjord,
Dr. P. Warkentin, Dr. S. Susan, Dr. M. Gordon, Dr. B.
Gordon, Dr. J. Stein, Ms. N. Albanese and nurses, and
residents of Rainbow Babies and Childrens Hospital,
Cleveland, OH for taking care of the patients in these
studies.
We are grateful for the technical assistance of Ms. B.
Landmeier, Mr. D. Donovan, and Mr. W. Smith-Mensah and the
dosimetry measurements by Dr. D. Nelson.

REFERENCES

August CS, Serota FT, Koch PA, Burkey E, Schlessinger H,
    Elkins WL, Evans AE, D'Angio GH (1984). Treatment of
    neuroblastoma with supralethal chemotherapy, radiation
    and allogeneic or autologous marrow reconstitution. J
    Clin Oncol 2:609-615.
Cahan LD, Irie RF, Singh R, Cassidenti A and Paulson JC
    (1982). Identification of a human neuroectodermal tumor

antigen (OFA-2) as ganglioside $G_{D2}$. Proc Natl Acad Sci USA 79: 7629-7633.

Cheung N-KV, Saarinen UM, Neely JE, Landmeier B, Donovan D, Coccia PF (1985). Monoclonal antibodies to a glycolipid antigen on human neuroblastoma cells. Cancer Research 45: 2642-2649.

Cheung N-KV, Landmeier B, Neely J, Nelson D, Abramowsky C, Ellery S, Adams RB, Miraldi FD (1986). Complete tumor ablation with iodine 131-radiolabeled disialoganglioside $G_{D2}$ specific monoclonal antibody against human neuroblastoma xenografted in nude mice. J Natl Can Inst 77: 739-745.

Cheung N-KV, Miraldi FD (1987a). Ganglioside $G_{D2}$ specific antibodies in the diagnosis and therapy of human neuroblastoma. In Kemshead JT (ed): "Monoclonal Antibodies in the Diagnosis of Childhood Solid Tumors", Florida: CRC Press, (in press).

Cheung N-KV, Neely JE, Landmeier B, Nelson D, Miraldi F (1987b). Targeting of ganglioside $G_{D2}$ monoclonal antibody to neuroblastoma. J Nucl Med (in press).

Cheung N-KV, Lazarus H, Miraldi F, Abramowsky C, Kallick S, Saarinen S, Spitzer T, Strandjord S, Coccia P, Berger N (1987c). Ganglioside $G_{D2}$ specific monoclonal antibody 3F8: a phase I study in patients with neuroblastoma and malignant melanoma. J Clin Oncol (in press).

Clark SC, Kamen R (1987). The human hematopoietic colony-stimulating factors. Science 236: 1229-1237.

Cordon-Cardo C (1987) (personal communications).

Deacon JM, Wilson PA, Peckham MJ (1985). The radiobiology of human neuroblastoma (1985). Radiotherapy and Oncology 3: 201-209.

Miraldi FD, Nelson AD, Kraly C, Ellery S, Landmeier B, Coccia PF, Strandjord SE, Cheung N-KV (1986). Diagnostic imaging of human neuroblastoma with radiolabeled antibody. Radiology 161: 413-418.

Mujoo K, Cheresh D, Yang HM, Reisfeld R (1987). Disialo-ganglioside $G_{D2}$ on human neuroblastoma cells: Target antigen for monoclonal antibody mediated cytolysis and suppression of tumor growth. Cancer Research 47: 1098-1102.

Philip T, Zucker JM, Favrot M, Bordigoni P, Plovier E, Robert A, Bernard JL, Souillet G, Philip I, Lute JP, Corton P, Kemshead J (1985). Purged autologous bone marrow transplantation in 25 cases of very poor prognosis neuroblastoma. Lancet 576-577.

Pritchard J, McElwain TJ, Graham-Pole J (1982). High dose

melphalan with autologous marrow for treatment of advanced neuroblastoma. Brit J Cancer 45:86-94.

Reynolds CR, Moss TJ, Wells J, Seeger RC (1985). Sensitive detection of neuroblastoma cells in bone marrow for monitoring the efficiency of marrow purging procedures. In Evans AE, D'Angio G, Seeger RC (eds): "Advances in Neuroblastoma Research", New York: Alan R Liss, pp 425-441.

Schultz G, Cheresh DA, Varki NM, Yu A, Staffileno LK, Reisfeld RA (1985). Detection of ganglioside $G_{D2}$ in tumor tissues and sera of neuroblastoma patients. Cancer Research 44:5914-5920.

Seeger RC, Lenarsky C, Moss T, Feig S, Selch M, Ramsey N, Harris R, Reynolds P, Siegel S, Sather H, Hammond D, Wells J (1987). Bone marrow transplantation for poor prognosis neuroblastoma. Proc ASCO (abstract).

Treleaven JG, Gibson FM, Ugelstad J, Rembaum A, Philip T, Caine GD, Kemshead JT (1984). Removal of neuroblastoma cells from bone marrow with monoclonal antibodies conjugated to magnetic microspheres. Lancet 1:70-73.

Wu ZL, Schwartz E, Seeger R, Ladisch S (1986). Expression of $G_{D2}$ ganglioside by untreated primary human neuroblastomas. Cancer Research 46:440-443.

Advances in Neuroblastoma Research 2, pages 605–617

# REPEATED EXPOSURE OF NON-HUMAN PRIMATES TO MONOCLONAL ANTIBODY AND FRAGMENTS: PHARMACOKINETIC STUDIES AND THEIR IMPLICATIONS FOR TARGETED THERAPY.

Lashford L.S. MRCP. (1,2)   Elsom G.(1)
Clarke J. MSc.(1)   Gordon I. FRCR.(2)
Kemshead J.T. PhD.(1)

(1) Imperial Cancer Research Fund,
Oncology Laboratory, Institute of Child
Health, London.
(2) The Hospital for Sick Children, Great
Ormond Street, London.

## INTRODUCTION.

The monoclonal antibody, UJ13A, recognises an antigen of pan-neuroectodermal origin and has been evaluated as both a scintigraphic agent (Goldman et al.1984) and for targeting radiotherapy in childhood neuroblastoma (Lashford et al.1987). The biodistribution of the radiolabelled antibody has been established in patients (Lashford et al. Submitted), and a phase 1 toxicity study of the 131-I labelled conjugate undertaken.

Two problems have been identified which limit the use of the antibody as an immunolocalising agent. Firstly, despite supporting evidence of immunoreactive disease, uptake of radiolabel at large tumour sites has been poor. Secondly, prior exposure to the antibody may significantly alter pharmacokinetics and hasten clearance of the conjugate.

Experience with other monoclonal antibodies suggests that the changes in pharmacokinetics may be due to the production of anti-mouse immunoglobulin (Ig) response in the patient (Schroff R. et al.1985). Human anti-mouse Ig response have been reported to both the Fc protein and the

idiotypic domains of the molecule. Which type of
response is ellicited may be dependent on the dose
and course of antibody administration. In
developing UJ13A as a radiation delivery system it
is important to determine whether rapid
elimination of therapeutic amounts of antibody is
a result of an anti-mouse Ig response, and if so
to which part of the molecule the response is
generated.

To address this question we have employed a
non human primate model, the common marmoset. In
this species, we have demonstrated that the
pharmacokinetics of antibody handling mirror those
seen in children (Jones D.et al.1987). Marmosets
have been given doses of radiolabelled antibody
(Ig and Fab) proportional (on a weight basis) to
those given to children. This strategy
circumvents the ethical problems associated with
undertaking these studies in children relapsing
with metastatic neuroblastoma. Detailed studies
have been undertaken on the biodistribution of the
conjugates by direct venous sampling and gamma
camera scintigraphy.

**METHODS.**

Protein Preparation.
A single batch of monoclonal antibody was
prepared from ascites using protein A Sepharose.
The material was concentrated to 1 mg/ml and
aliquots of 100ug were stored at $-20^{\circ}$C until
required for use.

Fab monomer was prepared from whole antibody
by a papain digestion using a 10:1 Wt:Wt ratio of
antibody:papain. After 2 hours incubation at $37^{\circ}$C
the reaction was terminated with 500mM of
iodoacetamide and the resulting digest diluted to
10mls using distilled water at $4^{\circ}$C. Contaminating
Fc chains were removed by Amicon filtration using
a Ym 30 filter. The buffering solution was
exchanged for 10mmol ammonium bicarbonate in the
filtration unit, and the preparation lyophilised
and stored in 100ug aliquots at $-20^{\circ}$C. SDS
polyacrylamide gel electrophoresis was performed
in an 8% gel, under reducing conditions, to check
the purity of the preparation.

Radiolabelling.

Both UJ13A and its Fab fragment were radiolabelled with $^{123}$I supplied by Harwell. During the eight months of the experiment, the form in which this was supplied was altered. The radioisotope was consistently supplied in dried form, prepared from a solution containing sodium hydroxide. A significant fluctuation in the level of sodium hydroxide was initially observed, and this resulted in a variable radiolabelled product. To overcome this problem, 123I was later supplied dried from a solution containing a low sodium hydroxide concentration.

Using a modified chloramine T technique, protein was radiolabelled to a specific activity of 5uCi/ug of protein. Free iodine was removed using a Sephadex G25 column equilibrated with phosphate buffered saline containing 1% human plasma protein fraction .(PBS/1% HPPF).

The biological activity of both preparations was determined before and after radiolabelling by an indirect immunofluoresence assay. Biological activity was defined by the lowest titre at which maximal fluoresence was observed. Free iodine in the radiolabelled product was measured by either trichloroacetic acid precipitation or thin layer chromatography in 85% methanol. Protein aggregation was determined by centrifugation of an aliquot of the preparation in PBS with 2% foetal calf serum at 10.000 x g.

Animal Studies.

Nine animals were entered into the study, 3 animals receiving whole UJ13A, 3 (Fab) monomer and a control group receiving free iodine. Prior to administration of the radiolabel, thyroid blockade was achieved by adding 3 drops of Lugol's iodine solution to a liquid feed. Under Halothane /Nitrous oxide and oxygen anaethesia, all animals had 0.5mls of blood withdrawn and stored as plasma. Experimental animals were then injected with 10ug/kg. 123-I/UJ13A (Ig) or 123-I/UJ13A (Fab) dissolved in 300ul of sterile PBS. Control animals received 0.3ml of a solution of free 123I. All administrations were followed by a further injection of 0.2mls of 0.9% saline to flush the syringe and needle. Repeat administration of Ig,

Fab or free 123I were performed on 3 further occasions 4 - 8 weeks apart.

Measurement of the injected dose was performed by counting the syringe and needle on the gamma counter before and after injection. The early biodistribution of the conjugate was studied using the gamma camera. A dynamic acquisition series was commenced at the moment of injection in 15 one minute frames. In order to estimate early organ uptake, measurements of counts in a standard region of interest were taken and expressed as a ratio of injected dose. Information on organ half life was obtained by sequential static scans from 1 hour to 48 hours after injection. The frequency and duration of counting was determined by the rapidity of fall of organ counts to background level.

To generate a time activity curve for blood, intermittent venous sampling was undertaken during the time period 30 minutes to 24 hours. In addition to plasma stored before each exposure to radiolabelled conjugate, plasma was also sampled and stored at approximately 4 weeks after injection. This was stored at $-70^{\circ}$C until assayed for presence of anti mouse Ig.

Preparation of Rabbit anti-Marmoset Ig and Measurement of an anti-mouse Ig in Marmoset sera.

Ig was purified from the sera of marmosets by ammonium sulphate precipitation. The Ig was emulsified in complete Freunds adjuvant. 2mg of the protein preparation was injected subcutaneously at multiple sites in rabbits. Injections were repeated at monthly intervals using Ig emulsified in incomplete Freunds (x5). Rabbit anti-marmoset Ig was affinity purified using an affinity column of marmoset Ig coupled to CNB activated Sephadex 4B. After dialysis and concentration to 1mg/ml the purified Ig was radiolabelled to a specific activity of 1ug protein/100uCi iodine.

For assay of an anti-mouse Ig response in marmosets, mouse Ig (monclonal antibody UJ13A) was coated onto 96 well vinyl plates (Dynatech). Serial dilutions of control and test sera were added to the wells. After a 30 minute incubation plates were washed using PBS/10% bovine serum

albumin and 100,000 cpm of rabbit anti- marmoset
Ig added. Following a further 30 minutes
incubation plates were washed and isotope bound
determined using a LKB Ultra- gamma counter.

**RESULTS.**

Fab Fragments and Radiolabelled Antibodies.
     A single band of approximately 50kd was
observed on SDS polyacrylamide gel electrophoresis
of the Fab preparation of UJ13A (Fig.1).

Fig.1. SDS polyacrylamide gel electrophoresis of
preparation.

Channel A, M,Wt. Markers
B, IgG1 - UJ13A
C, Fab - 2hr digest
D, Fab - 4hr digest
E, Fab - 6hr digest

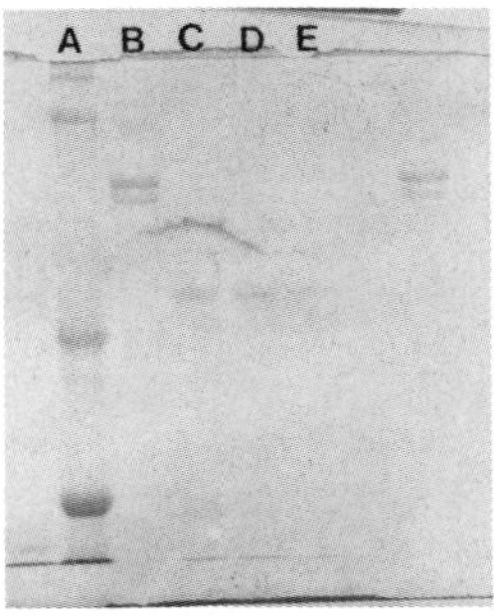

Whole Ig produced a single band of approximately
155,000 Mwt.  Both were shown to be biologically
active. Using standard neuroblastoma tissue a 1.0
mg/ml solution of whole UJ13A had a titre of
1/4,000  and an equivalent concentration of the
Fab preparation titred to 1/2,000.
     A reduction in biological activity was
generally observed after radiolabelling.  In
addition, the amount of aggregated protein and
free iodine contaminating the injected product,
varied significantly.  This was directly
attributable to the fluctuation in sodium
hydroxide content of the 123I over the period of
the experiment.

Direct Venous Sampling.
     On first administration of 123I UJ13A (Ig),
isotope was cleared relatively slowly from the
vascular compartment in a biexponential manner.
Direct venous sampling demonstrated a fast

clearance component with a mean biological half
life of 4.8 hours. The second component of the
curve had a half life of 19.6 hours. Isotope in
the blood remained attached to immunoglobulin as
in excess of 98% of the counts were precipitable
with 10% Trichloroacetic acid.

Coupling isotope to whole Ig dramatically
changed its biodistribution and pharmacokinetics
within the animal, as compared to the clearance of
unconjugated 123I. Although a biphasic clearance
curve for free iodine was suspected the first
component was so rapid that it could not be
accurately measured. Only 20% of the dose
remained in the blood thirty minutes after
injection. The second component of the clearance
curve of isotope showed a mean half life of 6
hours. No significant change in the rate of
clearance of unconjugated 123I was demonstrated at
the second, third or fourth administration. The
initial loss of 123I was estimated as 20% of
injected isotope at 30 minutes for each exposure.
Subsequent clearance had a biological half life of
5.5hrs, (range 5-5.8) 5.2hrs (range 4.4-5.7) and
5.7hrs (range 4.8-6.2) at sequential injections.

With each immunisation of 123I radiolabelled
Ig, isotope cleared from the blood in an
increasingly rapid fashion (Fig.2).

This was particularly marked for the first
half life where sequential changes of 5, 0.3, 0.2
and 0.1 hours were measured (injections 2,3,4).
This trend was similar for the second component
where changes from 19.6 to 17.3, 14.4 and 11 hours
were observed for successive administrations.
Variability within the group became more marked
with each injection of 123I UJ13A as indicated by
the dispersion of counts around the mean.

The kinetics of 123I Fab clearance from the
blood lay between those observed for whole Ig and
free isotope. An initial mean half life of 0.26
hours was observed (n=3) with the second clearance
component of 13 hours. With sequential
administration of the fragment there was little
change in the clearance kinetics. The scatter of
the points around the mean remained small and did
not change with increasing Fab exposure (Fig.3).

Figs. 2 and 3.

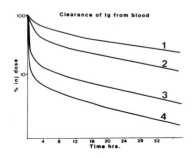

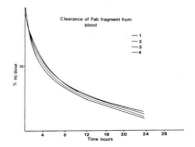

## Gamma Camera Scintigraphy.

Dynamic acquisition studies were undertaken
to provide information on organ uptake during the
early phase after 123I Ig administration. Liver
and heart were the only organs that were reliably
identified on the scans, the latter reflecting
conjugate in the vasculature. After
standardisation for injected dose it was apparent
that counts rapidly accrued in the liver during
the first 5 minutes of observation, with a slower
accumulation occuring during the next 8 minutes.
Towards the end of the observation period a
decline in activity was observed.

With succcessive exposures, dynamic
aquisition studies showed that uptake of the
radiolabel in liver increased with a quadrupling
of counts between the first and fourth
administrations. This increase in uptake was
consistent within the group and independent of
both the specific activity and degree of
aggregation of the injected protein (Fig.4).

Fig.4. Uptake of 123-I UJ13A into liver of
marmosets on sequential exposures.

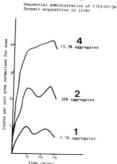

Sequential administration of I123-UJ13A
Dynamic acquisition in liver

Data on animals given the UJ13A was lost due to
computer failure. Observations on 2/3 animals are
also incomplete due to difficulties encountered on
repeated anaesthesia. However, static scans were
obtained on all animals. Loss of isotope from
liver was linear to 48 hours and was increasingly
rapid with successive administrations of antibody
(Table 1). Throughout the observation period
loss of the radiolabel from whole body was
monoexponential and became more rapid with each
exposure to Ig.

Table 1.

Half lives of blood and organs following successive
administration of 123-I/UJ13A - Marmosets.

| | Blood T 1 (h) | T 2 (h) | Liver (h) | Whole body (h) |
|---|---|---|---|---|
| 1 | 5 | 15.6 | 10.6 | 14.1 |
| 2 | 0.3 | 17.4 | 8.8 | 10.0 |
| 3 | 0.2 | 12.5 | 6.9 | 8.1 |
| 4 | 0.1 | 10.8 | 4.26 | 7.6 |

Early dynamic acquisition images of animals
given 123I Fab fragments of UJ13A showed uptake of
isotope in the kidney as well as in liver.
Maximal liver uptake occured within the first 2
minutes and then plateaued throughout the
observation period. Data was lost on one animal

due to cardiac arrest at anaesthesia and for one
time point on another animal due to computer
failure during the dynamic acquisition scans. The
level of peak uptake in the liver was calculated
to be approximately 75% of that seen on 1st
exposure to whole immunoglobulin. This did not
increase on successsive exposure of animals to
123I Fab (Fig.5). A similar pattern of uptake was
observed in the kidney. During the time period 1-
15 minutes, no activity was observed in the
bladder.

Fig.5. Uptake of 123-I UJ13A, Fab fragment into
liver and kidney of marmosets on sequential
exposures.

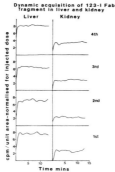

Static acquisition studies were performed up
to a time point of 6 hours. Scintigraphy was
discontinued after this time because of low count
rates, consequently late organ half lives could
not be obtained. The whole body clearance was
monoexponential and remained unchanged from
exposure to exposure. Mean effective half lives
of 6, 7.5, 5.3 and 5 hours were calculated for
injections 1-4 respectively.
The dynamic acquisition series on animals
receiving 123I alone support data obtained by
intravenous sampling showing a rapid loss of
isotope from the vascular compartment. Diffuse
homogenous activity was measured over the head,
thorax and abdomen. No organ could be identified
in the first 15 minutes of scanning with
distribution of isotope reflecting tissue mass
rather than specific organ uptake. By two hours a
region of activity was visible on the left upper

quadrant of the abdomen and a smaller amount
around the mouth. At later scans the activity
identified in the left upper quadrant was
diffusely distributed throughout the abdomen.
        Clearance of the isotope from whole body was
slightly longer than that observed for blood, with
a mean half life of 6 hours (Range 5.5 - 6.5
hours). This did not change on repeated exposure
of animals to isotope with mean body half lives of
6.5 (range 5.5-8) and 5 hours (range 4.8-5.2) for
the 3rd and 4th exposures. All data was lost for
the second exposure due to computer failure.

Screening of Sera for an Anti-Mouse Ig Response.
        An anti-mouse Ig response was only noted in
sera taken from animals receiving multiple
injections of 123I UJ13A. An illustration of the
change observed in sera are shown in Fig.6.

Fig.6. Rise in circulating marmoset anti-mouse Ig,
on multiple administrations of whole UJ13A.

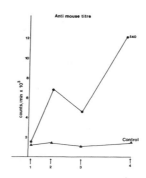

After the second injection of radiolabelled UJ13A,
a four fold increase in 125I rabbit anti-marmoset
Ig binding to plates preincubated with mouse Ig
(UJ13A) and marmoset sera was noted over
background levels (pre bleed scan). Levels of
anti-mouse Ig increased on subsequent exposure of
animals to UJ13A. In contrast no increase in
binding 125I rabbit anti-marmoset Ig was later
noted in sera from animals given multiple
injections of either 123I Fab or 123I alone
(control).

# DISCUSSION.

Investigation of the biodistribution of UJ13A in patients has suggested that several problems limit the use of the antibody. Significant hepato-splenic uptake of isotope occurs which limits the bioavailability of antibody for tumour targeting, as well as resulting in a significant radiation dose to these organs. Additional organ radiation dose delivery is derived from the relatively slow vascular clearance of conjugate.

This study, indicates that by utilising the Fab fragment of UJ13A the biodistribution of the conjugate is significantly changed. The initial rapid loss of conjugate from the vascular compartment suggests a more rapid equilibration of protein with the extravascular space. This feature coupled with more rapid clearance of isotope from whole body and other organs, lowers normal organ toxicity from equivalent levels of administered conjugate. In addition, the wider initial biodistribution of radiolabelled fragment may facilitate tumour uptake.

A similar therapeutic advantage may be seen with the Fab2 dimer of UJ13A. This was studied in the same model system, with results indicating a similar pattern of tissue distribution as documented for the Fab monomer. However it was not possible to obtain quantitative data on this fragment as preferential radiolabelling of a small molecular weight contaminant occurred. This contaminant was present in low amounts and was not detected in routine SDS gel electrophoresis.

The study also set out to determine whether the observed change in handling of UJ13A in patients at second exposure was the result of a circulating anti mouse Ig. It is clear from this study that repeat administrations of UJ13A produced increasingly rapid clearance of the conjugate from blood and organs. The initial vascular loss correlated with both hepatic sequestration and the strength of the anti-mouse Immunoglobulin. The magnitude of the immune response in influencing biodistribution appeared independent of other factors such as the degree of protein aggregation. Repeated injection of the

Fab fragment produced a stable biodistribution of conjugate and no anti mouse Ig activity. This data suggests that at this level of injected UJ13A, the generated anti mouse Ig is principally anti-Fc. It is likely that a stable bio-distribution of the Fab2 dimer would also be obtained.

These results indicate that the use of fragments will circumvent some of the problems experienced in our early work. Provided that tumour uptake of fragments is satisfactory, further progress in the use of monoclonal antibodies to target radiotherapy may be acheived.

## ACKNOWLEDGEMENTS.

Dr. Lashford is funded by the Neuroblastoma Society. This work has been supported by the Imperial Cancer Research Fund. Our thanks to patients, parents and staff at the Hospital for Sick Children, London.

## REFERENCES.

Goldman,A., Vivian,G., Gordon, I., Pritchard,J., Kemshead,J.T. Immunolocalisation of neuroblastoma using radiolabelled monoclonal antibody UJ13A. Journal of Paediatrics. 105:252-256. 1984.

Jones,D.H., Lashford,L.S., Dick-Mireaux,C., Kemshead,J.T. Comparison of pharmacokinetics of radiolabelled monoclonal antibody UJ13A in patients and animal models. NCI Monographs. 3:125-130. 1987.

Lashford,L.S., Evans,K.E., Jones,D.H., Gordon,I., Pritchard,J., Kemshead,J.T. The biodistribution of the monoclonal antibody UJ13A in children with stage IV neuroblastoma - implications for targeted radiation therapy. Submitted.

Lashford,L.S., Jones,D.H., Pritchard,J., Gordon,I., Breatnach,F., Kemshead,J.T. Therapeutic application of radiolabelled monoclonal antibody UJ13A in children with disseminated neuroblastoma. NCI Monographs. 3:53-59. 1987.

Schroff,R., Foon,K., Beally,S., Oldham,R.,
Morgan,R. Human anti-murine immunoglobulin
reponses in patients receiving monoclonal antibody
therapy. Cancer Res. 45:879. 1985.

Advances in Neuroblastoma Research 2, pages 619–632

# IMMUNOTHERAPY WITH $G_{D2}$ SPECIFIC MONOCLONAL ANTIBODIES

Nai-Kong V. Cheung, M. Edward Medof, and David Munn

Department of Pediatrics, Memorial Sloan Kettering
 Cancer Center, New York, NY 10021 and
Departments of Pediatrics and Pathology, Case Western
 Reserve University, Cleveland, OH 44106

## INTRODUCTION

In order to achieve durable disease free survival for children with metastatic neuroblastoma (NB), supralethal doses of chemoradiotherapy together with autologous bone marrow rescue have been utilized with some success in a number of clinical studies (Pritchard et al., 1982; August et al., 1984; Philip et al., 1985; Seeger et al., 1987). Patients treated at the time of complete clinical remission have benefited most from such approaches. Nevertheless, more than 50% will relapse and subsequently die (Seeger et al., 1987). In addition, more than one third of patients continue to have residual tumor after aggressive chemo- therapy and surgery and their disease progression is in- evitable. Although further escalation of drug dose or addition of more chemotherapeutic agents can be attempted, major organ toxicities and potential delayed side effects including second malignancies, are concerns. In addition, multi-drug resistance (Biedler et al., 1987) could emerge among these tumors that diminishes the efficacy of many cytotoxic agents. Like many childhood malignancies, an effective treatment of microscopic or residual tumor following maximal benefit from chemotherapy is needed.

Targeted immunotherapy focuses anti-tumor activity of antibodies and effector cells, which are actively developed by the host or adoptively transferred, onto tumor cells and into tumor sites. Such tumor selective therapy can be more specific and efficient. The value of such an approach is clearly evident in the classical interaction of antibodies and neutrophils directed to a focus of bacterial infection (Snyderman, 1985). Antibodies can diffuse into areas of infection to bind to the bacterial antigens whereupon the complement cascade is activated; vascular permeability is increased; chemotactic factors are released; so that the circulating neutrophils marginate and migrate into the infection site. Activated neutrophils then kill the organisms after binding through their Fc and complement receptors. Most infections can thus be eradicated. In order to develop a model system for targeted immunotherapy for human neuroblastoma, we have chosen the disialoganglioside $G_{D2}$ antigen system and murine monoclonal antibodies to $G_{D2}$.

The ganglioside $G_{D2}$ is an ideal antigen for specific tumor targeting because of (1) its relative lack of heterogeneity among human neuroblastoma, (2) its high density on tumor cells, (3) its lack of antigen modulation upon binding to antibody, and (4) its restricted distribution in normal tissues. We have previously reported murine monoclonal antibodies specific for $G_{D2}$ (Cheung et al., 1985). 3F8, an $IgG_3$, is suitable for targeted immunotherapy because (1) in vivo it distributes selectively to sites of metastatic disease in patients with NB without being intercepted by the reticuloendothelial system (liver, spleen) (Miraldi et al., 1986a; Miraldi et al., 1986b), (2) it activates human complement in tumor cytotoxicity (Saarinen et al., 1985), (3) it binds to IgG Fc receptors and thus mediates antibody dependent cell mediated cytotoxicity (ADCC), and (4) it can be safely administered intravenously in patients (Cheung et al., 1987).

## RELATIVE LACK OF $G_{D2}$ HETEROGENEITY AMONG HUMAN NEUROBLASTOMAS

In order to study $G_{D2}$ heterogeneity among human neuroblastomas, immunostaining of fresh human tumors were carried out. Specimens of NB were obtained at diagnosis, at debulking surgery and at autopsy. These included primary mediastinal and abdominal tumors, metastatic disease to liver, lymph nodes, subcutaneous and deep soft tissues. A total of 17 patient specimens were studied. 5 um sections were made and fixed in cold acetone. The sections were incubated for 1 hour at room temperature with 5 ug/ml of purified antibody 3F8 diluted in 1% normal goat serum. After rinsing in pH 7.4 Tris-HCl, the sections were reacted with FITC-conjugated goat anti-mouse antibody in Tris-normal saline pH 7.4. After another hour at room temperature, the sections were rinsed with Tris-HCl and mounted in 10% glycerol and studied using the fluorescent microscope. All 17/17 neuroblastoma specimens, irrespective of sites, previous chemotherapy, or disease status showed intense membrane (4+) and variable cytoplasmic staining. More than 95% of tumor cells were stained. Four ganglioneuromas were also studied. They showed fainter staining of neuropil in bands without discrete cell outlines. In tumors with nests of neuroblasts scattered among other benign elements, such clusters were obvious when stained with 3F8.

## ANTIGEN DENSITY OF GANGLIOSIDE $G_{D2}$ ON NEUROBLASTOMA CELLS

3F8 was labeled with $^{125}I$ using the chloramine T method as described (Cheung et al., 1986). Specific activity averaged $4 \times 10^5$ Ci per mole. Serial dilutions of the radiolabeled antibody was allowed to bind to a fixed number of tumor cells in microtiter polyvinylchloride wells for 2 hours at room temperature. Cells were separated from supernatant by centrifugation and counted in a gamma counter. The cpm bound and free were calculated. Dissociation constants (Kd) and number of antibody binding sites were computed. We observed nonlinear scatchard plots as well as nonsaturable binding of the antibody 3F8 onto neuroblastoma and melanoma cells. Estimates of Kd ranged from 1 nM to 17 nM depending on where on the curve the analysis was made. The higher dissociation constant probably represents non-specific interaction among $IgG_3$ molecules. Although the number of binding sites per neuroblastoma cell was calculated to be between $5 \times 10^6$ to $4 \times 10^7$, such estimations might not be accurate because of the nonsaturable binding characteristics. Using biochemical analysis, Wu et al. found an average of $10^7$ molecules per cell of $G_{D2}$ in human neuroblastoma (Wu et al., 1986). Such estimations might not take into account the extracellular $G_{D2}$ antigen in the stroma. Nevertheless, immunostaining of tumor sections suggested that most of the $G_{D2}$ resided on cell surfaces. Using a different $IgG_3$ anti-$G_{D2}$ antibody, Mujoo and colleagues estimated the density of $G_{D2}$ on neuroblastoma by Scatchard analysis to be around $2 \times 10^5$ (Mujoo et al., 1987). This lower estimate may be secondary to differences in fine specificities recognized by different $IgG_3$ mono-

clonals or to differences in the intermolecular interactions among $IgG_3$ molecules.

SENSITIVITY TO HUMAN COMPLEMENT MEDIATED CYTOTOXICITY

Previous observations from our laboratory using murine
monoclonal antibodies to $G_{D2}$ have shown that human neuroblastoma cells are very sensitive to human complement
mediated cytotoxicity (Saarinen et al., 1985). Both IgM
and $IgG_3$ antibodies were effective. As few as $10^4$ nano-
gram was adequate to achieve ca. 100% kill of $10^6$ tumor
cells. The ability of the monoclonal antibodies to effect
this cytotoxicity required the presence of surface $G_{D2}$
antigen, since normal marrow cells as well as other tumor
cell types that lack $G_{D2}$ were not damaged. However, a
number of $G_{D2}$ containing melanoma cell lines, despite their
ability to bind complement fixing antibodies, were resistant to in vitro complement killing (Panneerselvam et
al., 1986; Cheung et al., 1987). This finding suggests
that factors other than surface expression of target antigen must play a role in the susceptibility to complement
mediated cytotoxicity. Complement decay accelerating
factor (DAF) (Hoffman, 1969; Nicholson-Weller et al.,
1982; Pangburn et al., 1983; Medof et al., 1984) is a cell
membrane-associated inhibitor of complement activation
which protects blood cells from autologous complement
attack. By interfering with the assembly of C3 - (C4b2a
and C3bBb), and C5-convertases (C4b2a3b and C3bBb3b), DAF
blocks the amplification steps of both the classical and
alternative pathways. DAF is present on the membranes of
erythrocytes, platelets, neutrophils, monocytes, lymphocytes, vascular endothelium as well as epithelial cells
lining the extravascular compartments (Medof et al., 1987).

Utilizing monoclonal antibodies to DAF, the quantity
of surface and total cellular DAF protein can be measured.
Melanoma cell lines that are relatively resistant to human
complement mediated cytotoxicity have surface DAF (Cheung
et al., 1987). When the function of DAF is blocked by
anti-DAF monoclonal antibodies, the cells become sensitive
to antitumor antibody and human complement. Human neuroblastoma cell lines have no detectable DAF protein. In
contrast, human melanoma and breast carcinoma cell lines
are heterogeneous in DAF expression. In order to measure
the expression of DAF in fresh human tumors, fifteen

neuroblastoma tumors removed at surgery were studied with anti-DAF monoclonal antibodies by immunofluorescent staining as outlined above. 12/15 NB were negative while 3/15 showed faint surface staining. In comparison, melanoma and other sarcoma tissues showed positive but more heterogeneous staining. This consistent lack of, or low level expression of DAF may explain the susceptibility of NB tumors to in vitro killing by human complement and monoclonal antibody. Although the mechanisms by which cells regulate DAF expression are not understood, future experiments directed at the down regulation of DAF expression in tumors may yield sufficient activation of the complement cascade to impede tumor propagation. In addition to direct tumoricidal actions, complement activation can impact indirectly on tumor growth through effects on vessel permeability, cell trafficking, and improved adherence of tumors to effector cells via the complement receptors. Local formation of C3a can increase both blood flow and diffusion of proteins in the tumor-containing tissues. The generation of C5a will also increase the influx of phagocytes to tumor sites. The deposition of iC3b (or C3b) on target cell surfaces has been demonstrated to promote antibody dependent cell mediated cytotoxicity (ADCC) activity of lymphocytes (Perlmann et al., 1981).

SENSITIVITY OF NEUROBLASTOMA CELLS TO ADCC

Since neuroblastoma is not sensitive to major histo-compatibility complex (MHC) restricted T cell cytotoxicity, other means of targeting killer lymphocytes to this tumor is potentially of great interest (Lampson et al., 1985). In vitro studies have shown that neuroblastoma cell lines are sensitive to natural killer (NK) cells from human peripheral blood (Main et al., 1985). Recent studies clearly demonstrated that neuroblastoma cells are also sensitive to ADCC in the presence of murine monoclonal antibodies to ganglioside G$_{D2}$ (Mujoo et al., 1987; Munn and Cheung, 1987). Both peripheral blood mononuclear cells (PBMC) as well as granulocytes are effective.

Using $10^4$ target cells in a standard 4 hour chromium release assay, cytotoxicity by PBMC in the presence of 1 ug/ml of 3F8 was studied (Table 1). Cytotoxicity (>10%) in the absence of 3F8 observed in many of the neuroblastoma cell lines was secondary to their sensitivity to NK activity of PBMC. When cytotoxicity was compared in lytic units (Pross and Maroun, 1984), ADCC was consistently higher (300%) than NK killing of NB. ADCC was effective against cell lines which carried the $G_{D2}$ antigen. NK activity was minimal against the non-NB cell lines.

TABLE 1. % Lysis in ADCC of tumor cells by PBMC

| | | Effector to Target Ratio | | | | | |
| | | 100:1 | | 50:1 | | 25:1 | |
| TUMOR | CELL LINE | *+ | – | + | – | + | – |
| Neuroblastoma | NMB-7 | 68 | 29 | 55 | 22 | 41 | 14 |
| | IMR-6 | 73 | 25 | 50 | 21 | 40 | 15 |
| $(G_{D2}{}^{+})$ | IMR-32 | 67 | 26 | 56 | 20 | 38 | 9 |
| | LAN-5 | 43 | 5 | 33 | 5 | 14 | 3 |
| | LAN-2 | 43 | 14 | 40 | 12 | 17 | 8 |
| | LAN-1 | 62 | 4 | 44 | 2 | 33 | 2 |
| Melanoma | SKMEL-1 | 56 | 1 | 40 | 0 | 28 | 1 |
| $(G_{D2}{}^{+})$ | HT-144 | 54 | 5 | 48 | 3 | 34 | 2 |
| | SKMEL-5 | 23 | 2 | 17 | 1 | 3 | 0 |
| Breast | MCF-7 | 44 | 4 | 40 | 4 | 23 | 2 |
| $(G_{D2}{}^{+})$ | MDA-MB-175 | 50 | 9 | 48 | 5 | 25 | 1 |
| Melanoma | SKMEL-28 | 4 | 5 | 2 | 3 | 2 | 1 |
| | MALME-3A | 1 | 1 | 1 | 1 | 1 | 1 |
| $(G_{D2}{}^{-})$ | RPMI 7951 | 2 | 2 | 3 | 3 | 2 | 5 |
| Others | BT-20 | 3 | 3 | 4 | 3 | 3 | 1 |
| | U-373 | 9 | 4 | 6 | 4 | 6 | 4 |
| $(G_{D2}{}^{-})$ | A-204 | 6 | 4 | 5 | 4 | 4 | 2 |
| | SKCo-1 | 3 | 3 | 1 | 2 | 0 | 1 |

* + = with 3F8
  – = no 3F8

In order to separate the NK activity in PBMC from the overall ADCC phenomenon, neuroblastoma target cells were treated with pronase (1 mg/ml in Hank's buffer for 30

minutes at $37^{O}$). Since pronase would not digest $G_{D2}$, ADCC
target antigen was preserved. Thus, in the absence of 3F8,
no cytotoxicity of NMB-7 or IMR-6 was detected (Table 2).
The preservation of ADCC after pronase digestion of target
cells was consistently observed with other NB cell lines.
These observations suggest that if interaction molecules
other than 3F8 are essential for ADCC, they remain undam-
aged under these conditions by pronase. The data in
Table 2 indicates that the $IgG_3$ anti-$G_{D2}$ MoAb 3F8 was most
efficient in mediating ADCC, and without the Fc portion,
the $F(ab')_2$ fragment was ineffective. Figure 1-A summarizes the 3F8 dose dependence for ADCC using normal PBMC
against NMB-7. Half maximal lysis occurs at <0.01 ug/ml of
3F8.

TABLE 2. % Lysis in ADCC of pronased treated NB targets

| MoAb used | None | 3F8 | $F(ab')_2$ | 3G6 | 3E7 | N-S.7 |
|---|---|---|---|---|---|---|
| Antigen Specificity | - | $G_{D2}$ | $G_{D2}$ | $G_{D2}$ | NB | SRBC |
| Antibody Class | - | $IgG_3$ | $IgG_3$ | IgM | $IgG_{2b}$ | $IgG_3$ |
| **PBMC** | | | | | | |
| % lysis of NMB-7 | <1 | 60 | 5.3 | 5.2 | <1 | <1 |
| % lysis of IMR-6 | <1 | 63 | <1 | 6.5 | <1 | <1 |
| **Granulocytes** | | | | | | |
| % lysis of NMB-7 | <1 | 31 | 0.4 | 1.1 | <1 | <1 |
| % lysis of IMR-6 | <1 | 39 | <1 | <1 | <1 | <1 |

When the ADCC activity of PBMC was tested in normal
volunteers, 15/15 demonstrated efficient ADCC and NK activity against NB (Table 3). Moreover, repeated testing of
the same volunteers on separate days showed reproducible
lytic activity. In contrast, PBMC of 12 patients with
metastatic cancers (4 children, 8 adults: 9 of them had
recently recovered from chemotherapy) showed minimal spontaneous lytic activity against NB, with still appreciable
ADCC (50% of lytic activity of the PBMC from normal volunteers).

Interleukin-2 (IL-2) has recently been shown to

TABLE 3.  Mean ± SD of % lysis of NMB-7 cells by PBMC

| Donor | n | Effector to target ratio |  |  |  |  |  |
|---|---|---|---|---|---|---|---|
|  |  | 100:1 |  | 50:1 |  | 25:1 |  |
|  |  | 3F8 | no 3F8 | 3F8 | no 3F8 | 3F8 | no 3F8 |
| Volunteers | 15 | 68±14 | 29±11 | 55±13 | 22±8 | 41±14 | 14±7 |
| Patients | 12 | 47±16 | 7±3 | 31±12 | 6±3 | 20±9 | 4±2 |

Figure 1A                          Figure 1B

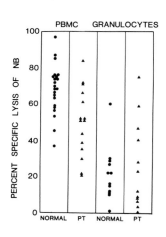

Figure 1A.  3F8 dose dependence of PBMC mediated ADCC
against NMB-7.  $10^4$ target cells were used per well in a
standard 4 hour $^{51}$Cr release assay.  Solid square=100:1 E/T
ratio, open square=50:1, solid circle=25:1, open circle=
12.5:1.    Figure 1B.  Cell mediated ADCC of NMB-7 at 100:1
effector to target ratio, with 1 ug/ml of 3F8 and $10^4$
target NB cells in a 4 hour $^{51}$Cr release assay.  PT=
Patients.  Normal= normal volunteers.


potentiate the NK activity of PBMC in vitro (Herberman et
al., 1985).  ADCC was also found to be enhanced (Honsik et
al., 1986; Munn and Cheung, 1987).  Since IL-2 could also
generate lymphokine activated killer (LAK) cells cytotoxic
for NK resistant cell lines and autologous tumors (Grimm et
al., 1982), an analysis of the relative role of each of

these cell mediated cytotoxicity components on neuroblastoma was carried out.

Effector cells were separated by adherence to immune complex (Munn and Cheung, 1987) before and after activation by IL-2. Fresh peripheral blood lymphocytes (PBL) nonadherent (Fc receptor negative, FcR$^-$) cells were unable to mediate ADCC or NK activities. After IL-2 activation of PBL, FcR$^-$ cells were cytotoxic to NK resistant cell lines. These cells constituted a subpopulation of the LAK cells able to kill NB efficiently in the absence of 3F8 (Table 4). In comparison, the FcR$^+$ cells mediated most of the ADCC, as well as showing lytic activity against NK-resistant cell lines. When each type of cytotoxicity was analysed in lytic units following interleukin-2 activation of PBL, the ability of FcR$^+$ cells to kill NMB-7 in the absence of 3F8 increased by >10 fold. Their ability to mediate ADCC was also enhanced by >10 times. In addition, the lytic activity of FcR$^-$ cells against NMB-7 was more than 10 times that of the unactivated NK activity of PBL.

TABLE 4. % Lysis of NB by IL-2 activated FcR$^-$ cells

| NB cell line | Effector to target ratio | | |
|---|---|---|---|
| | 4:1 | 2:1 | 1:1 |
| NMB-7 | 73 | 56 | 36 |
| IMR-6 | 56 | 44 | 31 |
| SKMEL-1 | 35 | 20 | 12 |
| K562 | 79 | 54 | 34 |

GRANULOCYTE MEDIATED ADCC OF HUMAN NEUROBLASTOMA

Granulocyte mediated ADCC of human NB is most efficient with the IgG$_3$ anti-G$_{D2}$ MoAb (Table 2). 3F8 dose titration studies showed that half maximal killing (E:T ratio of 12.5:1 to 100:1) occured at 0.04 ug/ml when NMB-7 was used as the target cell. In contrast to ADCC mediated by PBMC, where all targets with G$_{D2}$ tested so far have been sensitive, ADCC mediated by granulocytes were restricted to some tumor cell types (Table 5). The melanoma lines, HT-144 and SKMEL-31, both expressed the G$_{D2}$ antigens on their cell surface and although they were resistant to granulocytes, they were efficiently killed by PBMC (Table 1). In the experiments shown in Table 5, $10^4$ target cells and 1 ug/ml of 3F8 were used. No spontaneous killing was observed in the absence of 3F8.


TABLE 5. % Lysis of tumor cell lines in ADCC by granulocytes

| Cell line | Effector to target ratio | | |
| --- | --- | --- | --- |
| | 100:1 | 50:1 | 25:1 |
| NMB-7 | 64 | 50 | 37 |
| IMR-6 | 48 | 28 | 14 |
| IMR-32 | 60 | 49 | 32 |
| LAN-5 | 61 | 55 | 47 |
| LAN-1 | 43 | 28 | 16 |
| SKMEL-1 | 39 | 18 | 9 |
| HT-144 | 8 | 4 | 3 |
| SKMEL-31 | 5 | 4 | 4 |

When normal volunteers were studied, only 6/12 had appreciable ADCC activity (>20% lysis at 100:1 effector to target ratio) mediated by granulocytes. This same percentage was found in patients with metastatic cancer, with no clear correlation with prior chemotherapy (Figure 1B). These granulocyte preparations obtained by ficoll-hypaque gradient centrifugation and followed by dextran sedimentation had less than 1% contamination by PBMC. Thus, PBMC was unlikely to be directly responsible for the ADCC activity observed. When the number of eosinophils in the granulocyte preparations was counted, no correlation with the ability in ADCC was found by linear regression. Thus, it appears that the effector cell is most probably the neutrophils. Nevertheless, the mechanism of cytotoxicity will need to be clarified. The state of activation of the granulocytes can influence the degree of lysis of NB seen. The observation that granulocytes were unable yo kill certain $G_{D2}$ positive targets may suggest the presence of regulatory mechanisms on resistant tumor cells.


TOXICITIES AND ANTI-TUMOR EFFECTS OF 3F8 IN PATIENTS

Preliminary results from the Phase I clinical trial have shown that 3F8 had anti-tumor effects in patients with neuroblastoma and melanoma after they were injected with a single dose of the purified antibody 3F8 (Cheung et al., 1987). After antibody treatment, none of the patients received concurrent chemotherapy during the evaluation period. Although the side effects (pain, hypertension and urticaria) were severe, they were tolerable and had not led to any detectable long term neurological damage. The mechanisms of anti-tumor response were most likely due to both complement and cell mediated cytotoxicities. Immuno-staining of tissues after antibody treatment showed deposition of complement determinants as well as infil-tration of lymphocytes and a variety of other cell types. Phase II studies of the antibody 3F8 are in progress to further understand the immunological basis of these tumor responses as well as the observed side effects.

Given the sensitivity of neuroblastoma to human com-plement and ADCC, the targeting of complement fixing anti-body 3F8 can potentially activate a sequence of events that will lead to the selective influx of granulocytes and lymphocytes to the tumor. Methods developed to activate these effector cells will allow us to amplify the antitumor responses that will subsequently follow. Although G$_{D2}$ is present on most neuroblastomas with relative homogeneity, the identification of other antigen systems will be useful. The use of a panel of antibodies with different specific-ities for human neuroblastomas as well as the combined use of different targeted anti-tumor effector mechanisms, name-ly complement, ADCC, NK, LAK, toxins, and radioisotopes, will reduce potential problems of tumor heterogeneity in the final cleanup of microscopic disease.

ACKNOWLEDGEMENTS

This work was supported in part by grants from the American Cancer Society (CDA85-7, RD-226), NIH (CA-39320), and the Ireland Cancer Center, Cleveland, OH.
We want to thank Dr. P.F. Coccia, Dr. S. Strandjord, Dr. P. Warkentin, Dr. S. Susan, Dr. M. Gordon, Dr. B. Gordon, Dr. J. Stein, Ms. N. Albanese and nurses, and residents of Rainbow Babies and Childrens Hospital, Cleveland, OH for taking care of the patients in these studies.
We are grateful for the technical assistance of Ms. B. Landmeier, Mr. D. Donovan, and Mr. W. Smith-Mensah.

REFERENCES

August CS, Serota FT, Koch PA, Burkey E, Schlessinger H, Elkins WL, Evans AE, D'Angio GH (1984). Treatment of neuroblastoma with supralethal chemotherapy, radiation and allogeneic or autologous marrow reconstitution. J Clin Oncol 2:609-615.

Biedler JL, Meyers MB, Spengler BA (1987). Cellular concomitance of multi-drug resistance. Mechanism of Drug resistance in Neoplastic Cells. Bristol-Meyer Symposium. New York: Academic Press, in press.

Cheung N-KV, Saarinen UM, Neely JE, Landmeier B, Donovan D, Coccia PF (1985). Monoclonal antibodies to a glycolipid antigen on human neuroblastoma cells. Cancer Research 45:2642-2649.

Cheung N-KV, Landmeier B, Neely J, Nelson D, Abramowsky C, Ellery S, Adams RB, Miraldi FD (1986). Complete tumor ablation with iodine 131-radiolabeled disialoganglioside $G_{D2}$ specific monoclonal antibody against human neuroblastoma xenografted in nude mice. J Natl Can Inst 77: 739-745.

Cheung N-KV, Lazarus H, Miraldi F, Abramowsky C, Kallick S, Saarinen S, Spitzer T, Strandjord S, Coccia P, Berger N (1987). Ganglioside $G_{D2}$ specific monoclonal antibody 3F8: a phase I study in patients with neuroblastoma and malignant melanoma. J Clin Oncol (in press).

Cheung N-KV, Walter E, Smith-Mensah H, Tykocinski M, Medof ME (1987). Decay accelerating factor (DAF) protects tumor cells from complement mediated cytotoxicity. Proc. AACR.

Grimm EA, Mazumder A, Zhang HZ, Rosenberg SA (1982). Lymphokine-activated killer cell phenomenon. J Exp Med 155:1823-1841.

Herberman RB, Morgan AC, Reisfeld R, Cheresh DA, Ortaldo JR (1985). Antibody-dependent cellular cytotoxicity (ADCC) against human melanoma by human effector cells in cooperation with mouse monoclonal antibodies. In Reisfeld R, Sell S (eds): "Monoclonal Antibodies and Cancer Therapy", New York: Alan R. Liss, pp 193-203.

Hoffman EM (1969). Inhibition of complement by a substance isolated from human erythrocytes. I. Extraction from human erythrocyte stromata. Immunochemistry 6:391-404.

Honsik CJ, Jung G, Reisfeld RA (1986). Lymphokine-activated killer cells targeted by monoclonal antibodies to the disialogangliosides $G_{D2}$ and $G_{D3}$ specifically lyse human tumor cells of neuroectodermal origin. Proc Natl Acad Sci USA 83:7893-7897.

Main EK, Lampson LA, Hart MK, Kornbluth J, Wilson DB (1985). Human neuroblastoma cell lines are susceptible to lysis by natural killer cells but not by cytotoxic T lymphocytes. J Immunol 135:242-246.

Medof ME, Kinoshita T, Nussenzweig V (1984). Inhibition of complement activation on the surface of cells after incorporation of decay-accelerating factor (DAF) into their membranes. J Exp Med 160:1558-1578.

Medof ME, Walter EI, Rutgers JL, Knowles DM, Nussenzweig V (1987). Identification of the complement decay-accelerating factor (DAF) on epithelium and glandular cells and in body fluids. J Exp Med 165:848-864.

Miraldi FD, Nelson AD, Kraly C, Ellery S, Landmeier B, Coccia PF, Strandjord SE, Cheung N-KV (1986). Diagnostic imaging of human neuroblastoma with radiolabeled antibody. Radiology 161:413-418.

Miraldi FD, Nelson AD, Ellery S, Adams R, Landmeier B, Kallick S, Kraly C, Berger N, Cheung N-KV (1986). Imaging of melanoma, osteogenic sarcoma, and neuroblastoma using $G_{D2}$ specific I-131 labeled monoclonal antibody. J Nucl Med 27:881.

Mujoo K, Cheresh D, Yang HM, Reisfeld R (1987). Disialoganglioside $G_{D2}$ on human neuroblastoma cells: Target antigen for monoclonal antibody mediated cytolysis and suppression of tumor growth. Cancer Research 47:1098-1102.

Munn DH, Cheung N-KV (1987). Interleukin-2 (IL-2) enhances monoclonal antibody-mediated cellular cytotoxicity (ADCC) against human melanoma. Proc AACR.

Nicholson-Weller AJ, Burge DT, Fearon PF, Weller PF, Austen KF (1982). Isolation of a human erythrocyte membrane glycoprotein with decay-accelerating activity for C3 convertases of the complement system. J Immunol 129:184-187.

Pangburn MK, Schreiber RD, Muller-Eberhard HJ (1983). Deficiency of an erythrocyte membrane protein with complement regulatory activity in paroxysmal nocturnal hemoglobinuria. Proc Natl Acad Sci USA 80:5430-5434.

Panneerselvam M, Welt S, Old LJ, Vogel C (1986). A molecular mechanism of complement resistance of human melanoma cells. J Immunology 136:2534-2541.

Perlmann H, Perlmann P, Schreiber RD, Muller-Eberhard HJ (1981). Interaction of target cell-bound C3bi and C3d with human lymphocyte receptors. J Exp Med 153:1592-1595.

Perussia B, Trinchieri G, Jackson A, Warner NL, Faust J, Rumpold H, Kraft D, Lanier LL (1984). The Fc receptor for IgG on human natural killer cells: Phenotypic, functional, and comparative studies with monoclonal antibodies. J Immunol 133:180-189.

Philip T, Zucker JM, Favrot M, Bordigoni P, Plovier E, Robert A, Bernard JL, Souillet G, Philip I, Lute JP, Corton P, Kemshead J (1985). Purged autologous bone marrow transplantation in 25 cases of very poor prognosis neruoblastoma. Lancet 576-577.

Pritchard J, McElwain TJ, Graham-Pole J (1982). High dose melphalan with autologous marrow for treatment of advanced neuroblastoma. Brit J Cancer 45:86-94.

Pross HF, Maroun JA (1984). The standardization of NK cell assays for use in studies of biological response modifiers. J Immunol Methods 68:235-249.

Saarinen UM, Coccia PF, Gerson SL, Pelley R, Cheung N-KV (1985). Eradication of neuroblastoma cells in vitro by monoclonal antibody and human complement: method for purging autologous bone marrow. Cancer Research 45:5969-5975.

Seeger RC, Lenarsky C, Moss T, Feig S, Selch M, Ramsey N, Harris R, Reynolds P, Siegel S, Sather H, Hammond D, Wells J (1987). Bone marrow transplantation for poor prognosis neuroblastoma. Proc ASCO (abstract).

Snyderman R (ed) (1985). Contemporary Topics in Immunology: Regulation of leukocyte function. Vol. 14, Plenum Press, New York.

Wu ZL, Schwartz E, Seeger R, Ladisch S (1986). Expression of $G_{D2}$ ganglioside by untreated primary human neuroblastomas. Cancer Research 46:440-443.

Advances in Neuroblastoma Research 2, pages 633–639
© 1988 Alan R. Liss, Inc.

DISCUSSION

Chairman:      A.E. Evans and J. Kemshead

Discussants:   T. Philip, J.C. Genet,
               N.K.V. Cheung, L.S. Lashford

Seeger: Does the vancomycin-carboplatinum skin toxicity follow IV or po vancomycin for gut sterilization?

Philip: It follows IV vancomycin.


Kemshead: Please comment on the usefullness of animal models in experiments with radiolabelled monoclonal antibodies (MAb) and how they translate into the human situation.

Miraldi: We have looked at xenografts of NBL, Melanoma and Osteogenic Sarcoma which all gave excellent images with Nude mice. With NBL, we also get excellent images with the MoAb in the patient. With melanoma, the images are very variable and heterogenous, while in human osteosarcoma the images are good but not as good as in the mice model. There is not a direct correlation in image production between the mice and human model with the exception of NBL.

Lashford:. Animal models are limited and can only be used to address specific questions. With regard to the mouse NBL xenograft model. The disappointing finding in the mouse NBL xenograft modes is the excellent targeting with antibodies obtained in the animal is not seen in humans. For example, with UJ13A MAb, we obtain 20% of injected dose per gm of tissue in the mouse but in patients we obtain only $5 \times 10^{-3}$% per gm of NBL tissue. We can produce tumor ablation in the animal model with 150 microcuries of $I^{131}$ labelled UJ13A, but because of the poor concentration of the MAb in human NBL, this is unlikely to occur. The best use of animal models is to test an hypothesis and if encouraging to go onto other studies as applicable to humans. We have used primate animal models to give us useful information to make predictions of what may happen in humans.

Kemshead: The Imperial Cancer Research Foundation has done many animal model studies showing MAbs will target, image and ablate NBL xenograph tumors well. However, when you attempt to translate this effect into human NBL, you see the above figures quoted by Dr. Lashford. Instead of a $7\text{-}8\%$ injected dose/gm tissue one gets figures of $10^{-3}\%$ per gm tissue in humans. It shows the animal does not always behave in the same way as the human. I feel the biggest problem we face is getting the MAb through the capillary bed and onto the surface of the tumor. The mouse capillary supply to xenograft tumor allows this passage; hence one can deliver high percentages of injected dose to the tumor mass.

Cheung: I agree with previous panelists' comments. In mouse studies one can get 27-40% injected dose uptake. However, we do not take into account the size of the animal in these calculations which will influence the percentage uptake. Mouse models will be useful for qualitative data to compare MAbs but not for predicting quantitative data in humans.

Matthay: Can you share your knowledge and dosimetry data about the use of the positron emission scan? Did you correlate these data with actual tissue counts in your mice models?

Miraldi: We have just begun on the positron data. We have correlated with tissue samples in the other data presented with the standard scintillation camera. We were fortunate in obtaining surgical specimens enabling comparison of $I^{131}$ labelled MAb counts from these tissues with the data collected by the positron emission calculations. There was good correlation. Our interest in the positron is threefold: (1) It gives a twofold image with better definition of the tumor in relation to surrounding tissues; (2) Allows accurate dosimetry calculations anywhere in the body; (3) Can devise models which allow estimation of metabolic function in tissues. Standard camera techniques do not allow accurate dosimetry calculations with extensive calibration to allow for attenuation factors.

Pinkerton: I would like to comment on the kinetics of high dose CCPD. We need more toxicity data on the VP/Platinum protocols using infusions. In our experience very few patients got beyond three courses before significant glomerular filtration rates and hearing drops off. Rome data suggest that up to six courses of the high dose CPDD by infusion over five days can be given without demonstrable toxicity. The numbers, however, are small and we need prospective studies to confirm this lowered toxicity without compromising its therapeutic efficacy. The Italian group suggests the marrow and GI toxicity was higher in the five day infusion. Could you comment on that Dr. Genet?

Genet: I am not convinced that high dose CCPD increases marrow toxicity. However, high dose CCPD and VP16 is very hematotoxic. The Rome data are soft in supporting less toxicity with the infusion schedule. Other factors such as extent of bone marrow involvement at diagnosis play a role. We need more prospective studies to answer this question. In my patients there was not a real difference in toxicity between the pulse versus infusion CCPD schedules.

Lumbroso: I am very impressed with the quality of Dr. Miraldi's images. Others have suggested that the marrow toxicity following radiolabelled MAb targeting was due to gamma emissions. By using lower gamma emitters such as yttrium$^{90}$ or I$^{125}$ which has a short T1/2, the toxicity to bone marrow should be reduced. Is this so? The second question is why have you not used the FAB2' fragments in your studies which have been shown to have higher penetration and labelling of tumor tissues?

Cheung: In reply to the second question our unpublished studies showed a greater tumor to non-tumor concentration of the FAB prime 2 fragment but its half life was much shorter thereby decreasing the total exposure of the tumor to the radiolabelled MAb. I note Dr. Lashfords experience with FAB fragment and perhaps we should go back and look at FAB versus FAB prime 2 fragments.

Miraldi: The bone marrow toxicity in our patients was probably due to the fact that they had a lot of bone marrow disease leading to high bone marrow uptake of MAb and hence subsequent radiation. We have some data which shows that patients with little bone marrow tumor improvement showed much less bone marrow toxicity. We are looking at other radioisotopes and radiation particles in our program. The use of yttrium has its advantage with its emission but it may have a toxic effect on the bone marrow for other reasons.

Lashford: It is worth looking at the proportion of free iodine in the radiolabelled MAb preparations. In our preparations we have <3%. We only use 0.5 millicurie of isotope in our UJ13A preparations in patients we scan. In Cheung and Miraldi cases you use 3 millicurie and hence, one would expect better imaging of tumor uptake. With regard to $I^{125}$, in order for it to have a therapeutic effect (via electron emission), it needs to be close to the nucleus. UJ1BA MAb is membrane bound, and therefore, it would not get the $I^{125}$ close enough to the nucleus to be effective.

Seeger: Can you (Drs. Cheung/Miraldi) make any statement about bone marrow toxicity with radiolabelled MAbs in patients without bone marrow disease and about non-radiolabelled MAb effects or bone marrow stem cells?

Cheung: We have done three studies: (1) Purged marrow (with anti $GA_2$ ab) compared with non-purged marrow and did not see any difference; (2) Phase I study of IV injection with GD 2ab and saw no toxicity. In fact, the initial response was thrombocytosis or neutrophilia; (3) With radiolabelled isotopic MAb we did see bone marrow toxicity which we put down to bone marrow tumor uptake. However, there could have been a direct toxic effect of the isotope on stem cells.

Seeger: Since bone is a sanctuary for NBL will it prove difficult to deliver your $GD_2$ MoAbs to these sites?

Cheung: Many patients in the study with bone disease did respond to $GD_2$ MAb but there is a possibility that some bones may act as sanctuary sites due to poor vascularity. In addition, our study only used a single dose and hence, one may hypothesize that multiple doses of the MAb may reach these sanctuary zones.

Foster: Is there a role for radiolabelled MAb as initial therapy in patients without bulky disease, to attack micrometastases given its limitation in adequate tissue saturation in bulk disease? Will MAbs play a role in passive immunization and therapy for treatment of infection in patients with malignant disease who are immune suppressed secondarily to treatment?

Cheung: In any Phase I therapeutic trial we have to include patients with measurable hence bulky disease since they must be unresponsive to conventional treatment. In the future we would like to use this modality as adjuvant therapy. In our animal studies we have injected tumor cells then waited for disease establishment before injecting MAb. If you don't do this but inject MAb plus tumor cells simultaneously you may get an enormous therapeutic effect by preventing tumor establishment.

Lashford: I concur with Dr. Cheung. I believe if one can establish radiolabelled isotopic MAb at tumor site one will get a therapeutic oblative effect if one achieves a high enough concentration. We have been studying the use of labelled MAb intrathecally. This is seen in a "closed space" model with relapsed leptomeningeal disease and CSF injected isotopic MAbs giving a prolonged remission. However, I am less comfortable with delivery of MAb to tissue sites when given by IV route. Pharmacokinetics studies will help us to understand this better.

Kemshead: The quality of radiolabelled isotope received from the manufacturer can vary enormously and these are difficulties in labelling MAbs with the isotope guarantee as stable complex, free of aggregator and free isotopic iodine.

Voute: We are doing phase II studies with carboplatinum as a continuous infusion in varied relapsed pediatric solid tumors, with infusion 24 hours at 600 mg/m$^2$ of VM26 infused over 24 hours. We do not see toxicity and can repeat at three weekly intervals. Our curves for free carboplatinum are similar to Dr. Genet's. Could it be the peak levels of carboplatinum daily for five days that are responsible for the toxicity?

Genet: We have no information to date on peak levels of carboplatinum and bone marrow toxicity. There is however, a good correlation with peak levels and renal or ototoxicity.

Philip: I agree the best of delivery of carboplatinum is unclear at the moment. We like to deliver 800 mg/m$^2$ total dose in a four week period, perhaps 200 mg/m$^2$/week times four weeks will be better. Some of your patients have bone marrow disease, does this relate to marrow toxicity?

Voute: Our patient population was mixed and the study designed to address two questions only -- efficacy and toxicity. Some patients had invaded marrow and we used 600 mg/m$^2$ as a 24-hour induction every three weeks.

Philip (comment): It is easy to deliver carboplatinum q 4 weekly when patient has a normal marrow. With an abnormal marrow we find it impossible to deliver 800/m$^2$ carboplatinum every 4 weeks.

Greene: Our study reports CCPD as 40 mg/m$^2$/day times 5 days (200 mg/m$^2$ total) with VP16. Our initial pharmacokinetic data never correlated oto-, nephro- or hemopoetic toxicity with peak levels. However toxicity correlated with higher peaks on subsequent courses and longer T 1/2 lifes. These sequential studies identified a proportion of patients who would develop oto- and nephotoxicity.

Genet: Studies reported in Cancer 1985 showed relationships between peak CCPD levels and ototoxicity. Other studies have recently shown less fall off in GFR with infusions versus pulses. Our studies showed CCPD clearance, decreased when given in courses less than four weeks apart with no effect if courses spaced to six weeks.

Greene: My point was some patients showed sequential rises in peak CCPD levels in subsequent courses and these are the patients who manifested toxicity sooner and at lower cumulative doses than the other group, eg. ototoxicity is a dose related phenomenon. We have also seen retinal toxicity in a patient whose total CCPD cumulative dose was 2.4 gm (diminution in color vision and acuity -- down to 1:200).

Cornaglia: Can the granulocyte be activated against NBL cells without the use of MoAb by other means, eg. oxygen radicals?

Cheung: In our studies granulocytes were not activated unless MoAb was present. We are looking at activating granulocytes by other means but results will not be available for some time.

# [131]I-META-IODOBENZYLGUANIDINE THERAPY

Advances in Neuroblastoma Research 2, pages 643–654
© 1988 Alan R. Liss, Inc.

# A COMPARATIVE STUDY OF THE BIODISTRIBUTION OF META-IODOBENZYLGUANIDINE (mIBG) AND THE MONOCLONAL ANTIBODY UJ13A IN PATIENTS AND ANIMAL MODELS.

Lashford L.S.MRCP(1,2), Clarke J.MSc(1),
Gordon I.FRCR(2), Pritchard J,FRCP(2),
Kemshead J.T.PhD(1).

(1) Imperial Cancer Research Fund,Oncology
Laboratory, Institute of Child Health,
London.
(2) The Hospital for Sick Children, Great
Ormond Street, London.

## INTRODUCTION.

Two types of compound are available for
radiation targeting in neuroblastoma.  These are
the monoclonal antibodies exemplified by UJ13A,
and the small molecular weight radiopharmaceutical
meta-Iodobenzylguanidene (mIBG).

The monoclonal antibody UJ13A recognises a
cell surface antigen expressed on tissue of
neuroectodermal origin.  In 1984, Goldman et al.
demonstrated that radiolabelled UJ13A imaged both
primary neuroblastoma and secondary deposits.  In
subsequent studies the work was extended to
demonstrate that accumulation of UJ13A in human
neuroblastoma xenografts was a specific phenomena,
and that increasing the dose of radiolabelled 131-
I UJ13A produced a temporary ablation of the
xenografts (Jones D.H. et al.1985).

The radiopharmaceutical mIBG shares with
UJ13A the ability to accumulate at tumour sites.
mIBG is actively transported into neurosecretory
granules and unlike UJ13A is deposited intra-
cellularly (Buch J. et al.1985).  A number of
investigators have demonstrated that
administration of 100-200mCi of this radiolabelled
conjugate may produce a temporary response in

relapsed neuroblastoma (Hoefnagel C.& Voute T.1986).

The success of either delivery system in future clinical trials is dependent on the balance struck between radiation delivery to tumour and to normal organs.  To quantitate this latter aspect of radiation dose delivery, a comparative study of the biodistribution of both conjugates has been undertaken in non human primates (marmosets) and patients with stage IV neuroblastoma.

## METHODS.

UJ13A was prepared by the method of Jones et al.  The antibody was radiolabelled by the chloramine T technique, to a specific activity of between 8 and 16uCi/ug of protein.  Free iodine was separated from the radiolabelled product by column chromotography using Sephadex G25 equilibrated with phosphate buffered saline/1% human plasma protein fraction(PBS/1%HPPF).  Prior to injection into patients or marmosets the protein was passed through a 22um Millex filter to ensure sterility.  An aliquot of the solution was routinely checked for free iodine by precipitation with 10% trichloroacetic acid.  Protein aggregation was determined by either centri-fugation at 10,000 xg in PBS containing 2% HPPF or by high performance liquid chromotography.

The immunoreactivity of the radiolabelled antibody was confirmed before and after radio-labelling using an indirect immunofluorescence assay.

131-I mIBG was purchased from Amersham. 123-I mIBG was prepared in the laboratory by the method of Wieland et al.1980.  1-2mgs of mIBG were added to 10mCi of 123-I supplied in dried form from Harwell.  100ul of glacial acetic acid was added to this mixture followed by 3-5mgs of ammonium sulphate powder.  The bottle was sealed and heated for 45 minutes at 140-160$^{\circ}$C in a glycerol bath. 1.5mls of 0.005M acetate buffer was added (pH 4.1) and free iodine removed from the preparation by passage through a Cellex-D ion exchange column. Radiolabelled mIBG was sterilised by passage through a 0.22um Millex filter and collected in an evacuated vial.  The radiochemical purity was

determined by thin layer chromotography using a
3:1 mixture of propan-1 ol and 10% ammonia
solution.

Animal studies.
    To obtain a detailed understanding of the
pattern of clearance of the two compounds from
different organs, a quantitative assessment the
biodistribution of both compounds was undertaken
in marmosets.
    12 marmosets were injected with 10ug/kg of
131-I mIBG (S.A.2.5uCi/ug), and then sacrificed at
different time points.  Immediately prior to death
each animal was scanned using a Siemens gamma
camera fitted with a 410keV medium energy
collimator.  Blood and whole organs were then
removed and counted in a LKB ultragamma counter.
In this way a relationhip was established between
counts measured on the gamma camera and counts in
any organ.
    Six further marmosets received sequential
administrations of 131-I mIBG and 131-I UJ13A
in doses of 10ug/kg over a three week period.  The
pharmacokinetics of the radiolabelled conjugate
were studied by whole body scintigraphy at 1
minute, 20 minutes, 1,2,4,6,24 and 28 hours.
Using the tissue resection data from the initial
study, time activity curves were generated for
organs of interest.  Comparative organ radiation
dose estimates from the two compounds for each
animal, were undertaken by a comparison of the
accumulated activity in organs of interest.

Patient studies.
    Nine patients were entered into the study.
All patients had completed chemotherapy as defined
by Trial 1 of the European Neuroblastoma Study
Group.  Vincristine $1.5mg/m^2$, Cis platinum
$60mg/m^2$, VM26 $150mg/m^2$, cyclophosphamide $600mg/m^2$,
6-10 courses, randomised to high dose melphalan.
    To shorten the time period of the scanning
study, the first six patients with stage IV
neuroblastoma were sequentially injected with 123-
I mIBG (half-life of 123-I, 13.2hrs.) followed by
131-I UJ13A (half life of 131-I 8.04 days).  To
account for potential differences in isotope the
following 3 patients were injected with 131-I mIBG

and 123-I UJ13A. The early biodistribution of each
conjugate was followed in a dynamic acquisition
series of 30 x 1 minute frames of abdomen and
thorax. To define the later clearance of isotope,
sequential static images were obtained. These
studies comprised scans of right and left lateral
skull with the respective arm, anterior and
posterior thorax, anterior and posterior abdomen
and pelvis and posterior views of legs to include
feet. All scans were obtained on at least 3
occasions over the time period 4 hours to 48
hours. Time activity curves were generated for
the principle organs of uptake both for the time
period 1-30 minutes and for the later clearance 4-
48 hours.
    Radiation doseage was calculated using the
Medical Internal Radiation Dose formalism. The
assumption was made that the principle radiation
dose delivery to organs of interest came from a
single monoexponential clearance component, and
that this was adequately defined by estimates of
organ uptake over the three time points between 4
and 48 hours.

**RESULTS.**

Marmosets.
    Principle organs of uptake were defined as
kidney and liver for mIBG and liver for UJ13A.
The accumulation of mIBG in kidney was short
lived, and no significant activity over background
was detected in this organ by 1hour. From the
data provided by direct tissue resection,
accumulation of isotope in kidneys accounted for
10% of the injected dose at 20 minutes (Range 8-
11.6%,N=3). This fell to 0.52% by 4hrs (Range
0.36-0.64%,N=3). Loss of isotope through the
kidneys after 1 hour was monoexponential with an
effective half life of 7 hours. Examination of
urine by thin layer chromotography demonstrated
that the major excretory product was intact mIBG
in both the fast and slow phases of urinary
excretion (Fig 1).

Fig.1. Thin layer chrom-
atogram of administered
mIBG compared with
urinary excretion of mIBG
and contaminants over time
periods 0-20 minutes
and 20-60 minutes,
marmosets 1-free iodine,
2-mIBG, 3,4,5-larger
molecular weight bands.

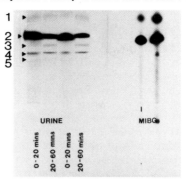

The impact of the initial urinary loss of mIBG was
to produce a fast and a slow component to the
clearance of mIBG from whole body.  The initial
rapid loss of isotope was sustained for a period
of 1 hour, and accounted for 17% of the injected
dose (Range 12-21%, N=6).  Subsequent loss was
monoexponential with an effective half life of
22.3hrs (Range 19-26.4hrs, N=6).
     No early period of renal excretion could be
identified for 131-I UJ13A.  Clearance of this
conjugate from whole body followed monoexponential
clearance kinetics.  The rate of clearance was
both variable between animals and prolonged (Mean
Teff:67.4hrs, Range 52-81, N=5).  Using these
results to derive the accumulated activity in
whole body from 1mCi of 131-I UJ13A and 1mCi of
131-I mIBG a mean of 3.8 times the whole body dose
is delivered from UJ13A as from mIBG.(Range 2.6-
5.3, N=5) (Fig.2).

Fig.2.  Comparison of
accumulated activity
(uCi hrs) in whole body
from 1mCi of 131-I UJ13A,
1mCi of 131-I low specific
activity mIBG and 1mCi of
131-I high specific
activity mIBG.

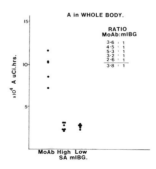

     Both mIBG and UJ13A were initially taken up
by liver before being cleared by this organ.  For

UJ13A, uptake was maximal at 1 hour and subsequent
clearance was monophasic.  A similar period of
isotope accumulation was demonstrated for mIBG,
with maximal uptake of isotope at 1 hour; however
subsequent clearance of the radiolabelled
conjugate isotope followed biphasic clearance
kinetics.

    The contribution of this initial period of
mIBG accumulation and loss to the total
accumulated isotope in liver was small (Teff 1st
component:Mean 2 hours, Range 1.2-3.6,N=6)
(Fig.3).  Estimates of accumulated activity in
liver were therefore based on information provided
by the influential second clearance component and
compared with the monophasic time activity curve
generated for UJ13A.  Both the proportion of
injected UJ13A removed by liver and its subsequent
rate of clearance  were significantly increased
over mIBG. This resulted in an estimated radiation
dose delivery from 1mCi of UJ13A to liver, of 6.4
times that delivered from 1mCi of 131-I mIBG
(Fig.4).

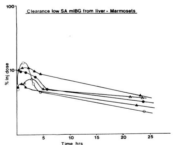

Fig.3. Time-activity
curves for low specific
activity mIBG in liver
of marmosets.

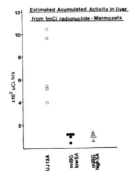

Fig.4. Estimated
accumulated activity
(uCi hrs) in liver of
marmosets, from 1mCi of
131-I UJ13A, 1mCi low
specific activity mIBG
and 1mCi of high
specific activity mIBG.

Patient studies.

The observations on the early biodistribution
of UJ13A and mIBG were confirmed in the patients.
Dynamic acquisition curves were generated for
heart, liver, kidney and bladder following
injection of mIBG. Similar curves were generated
for liver, spleen and heart following intravenous
administration of UJ13A. The heart curves suggest
that the initial rate of loss of radiolabel from
blood for both conjugates is similar (Fig 5).
This is not consistent with the values obtained by
blood sampling. By 1 hour, a mean of 95.6% of
administered mIBG is lost from the vascular
compartment (Range 90-98.5%,N=8). This compares
with a loss of 32% of injected UJ13A (Range 12-
44%,N=8) (Table 1).

Table 1.

CLEARANCE OF TARGETING AGENT FROM BLOOD
PATIENTS.

| Patient: | mIBG | | UJ13A | |
|---|---|---|---|---|
| | % inj dose (1 hr) | TBiol. (hrs) | % inj dose (1 hr) | TBiol. (hrs) |
| 1. | 4.6 | 19 | 76 | 64 |
| 2. | 6.8 | 130 | 76 | 64 |
| 3. | 2.7 | - | - | - |
| 4. | 2.4 | 19 | 64 | 39 |
| 5. | 1.5 | 18 | 60 | 18 |
| 6. | 10.0 | 10 | 88 | 19 |
| 7. | 2.3 | 23 | 56 | 68 |
| 8. | 5.0 | 43 | 61 | 38 |

The dynamic acquisition curves generated for UJ13A
over heart, reflect the measured rate of vascular
loss. The disparity between dynamic acquisition
data and vascular sampling for mIBG, indicates
that a period of myocardial uptake occured in all
patients studied.

This evidence of myocardial uptake of mIBG
was confirmed on the later static acquisition
scans.

Principle sites of isotope accumulation were
liver and salivary tissue for mIBG and liver and
spleen for UJ13A. The uptake and clearance of
isotope from liver was quantified for both
conjugates. The mean biological half life for
mIBG in liver was estimated as 27 hours (Range 8-
66 hours,N=8) (Table 2). This compared with 22
hours for UJ13A (Range 11-39 hours, N=8).

Table 2.  Clearance and Estimated Radiation
Doseage to Liver, of 1 mCi of Administered
Radionuclide.

|  | mIBG | | | UJ13A | | |
|---|---|---|---|---|---|---|
| Patient No. | Ao % | T(Biol) (hrs) | Dose rads | Ao % | T(Biol) (hrs) | Dose rads |
| 1. | 0.5 | 66 | 0.7 | 1.5 | 21 | 0.9 |
| 2. | 5.0 | 28 | 2.3 | 16.2 | 26 | 6.8 |
| 3. | NE | NE | NE | NE | NE | NE |
| 4. | 3.8 | 20 | 0.7 | 4.0 | 39 | 1.2 |
| 5. | NE | NE | NE | NE | NE | NE |
| 6. | 2.6 | 13 | 0.6 | 5.2 | 20 | 1.9 |
| 7. | 3.8 | 21 | 1.1 | 2.1 | 15 | 0.5 |
| 8. | 10.0 | 8 | 2.0 | 3.8 | 11 | 1.1 |
| 9. | NE | 27 | NE | NE | 22 | NE |
| 10. | 7.0 | 32 | NE | 11.0 | 23 | NE |
| Mean: | 4.6 | 27 | 1.2 | 6.2 | 22 | 2.1 |

Ao is the estimated % of injected dose present in
liver at time O.
T(Biol), is the biological half life of the
radionuclide in liver.
(hours), dose is the estimated radiation dose to
liver from 1mCi of injected conjugate.

Figure 5. Dynamic acquisition of isotope in various organs.

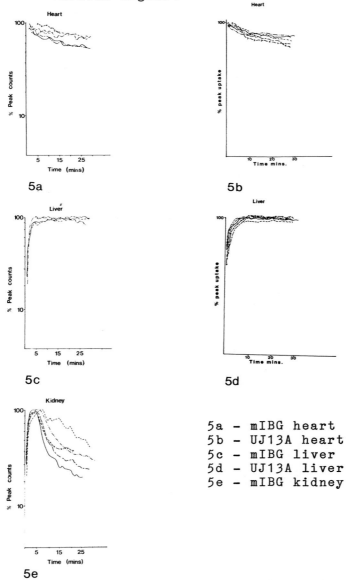

5a

5b

5c

5d

5e

5a – mIBG heart
5b – UJ13A heart
5c – mIBG liver
5d – UJ13A liver
5e – mIBG kidney

Estimates of maximal organ uptake were 4.7 for
mIBG (Range 0.5-10%) and 6.2% for UJ13A (Range
1.5-11%). The mean radiation dose delivered to
liver from these conjugates was estimated as 1.2
and 2.1 rads/mCi respectively (Table 2, see
separate sheet).

## DISCUSSION.

Whilst monoclonal antibodies and mIBG exploit
relatively specific mechanisms for localising
tumour deposits, additional specific and non
specific mechanisms operate in vivo which result
in the conjugate accumulating in a variety of
other tissues. The magnitude of these competing
mechanisms limit both the bioavailability of
conjugate for radiation targeting and set limits
on size of the administered dose.
Bone marrow is the tissue most likely to
limit escalation of the dose of radiolabelled
conjugate. In the absence of tumour infiltration,
this organ receives its principle dose delivery
from blood. The results clearly show that a
higher proportion of administered UJ13A remains in
blood at any time point. It is likely that on a
mCi for mCi basis UJ13A will be significantly more
marrow toxic than mIBG. This hypothesis is
supported by the whole body clearance data from
marmosets, which suggests that whole body
radiation dose is 3.8 times as great from 1mCi of
UJ13A as from 1mCi of mIBG. The data is in accord
with both our own observation of marrow toxicity
after administration of 55mCi of 131-I UJ13A
(Lashford L.S.et al.1987) and observations from
other investigators of marrow toxicity from 131-I
mIBG at between 150 and 200mCi of injected
conjugate (Hoefnagel C. & Voute T.1986).
Further dose escalation is possible provided
marrow rescue is available. It would seem likely
that the next dose limiting tissue might be liver.
The marmoset model demonstrates a clear advantage
of mIBG over UJ13A. This advantage appears to be
lost in our patients where no significant
difference is observed in dose delivery between
the two conjugates. Moreover in a larger series
of patients scanned with either mIBG or UJ13A the
trend is for mIBG to give a larger radiation dose

to liver (Lashford L.S.et al.manuscripts submitted).

The differences observed in marmosets are attributable to the higher uptake of UJ13A in liver and the more rapid clearance of mIBG. The difference in liver uptake is partly explained by the influence of splenic accumulation of UJ13A in patients, and the difficulty in making accurate measurements of total organ uptake in patients of varying sizes. Less easy to explain is the rapid clearance of mIBG from the liver of marmosets. Whilst it is possible that the difference between patients and animals reflects a physiological variation between lower and higher primates prior exposure to chemotherapy may also be an important factor.

Clearly, the factors that influence the metabolism of these compounds are complex. However, an understanding of the variables can only lead to a better appreciation of how to use these new delivery systems. At our current level of technology, mIBG is probably less likely to reach dose limiting toxicity than 131-I UJ13A. However, the potential to manipulate monoclonal antibodies by the preparation of fragments, and the possibility of using alternative isotopes, ensures that this technology remains an exciting possibility.

## ACKNOWLEDGEMENTS.

Dr. Lashford is funded by the Neuroblastoma Society. This work has been supported by the Imperial Cancer Research Fund. Our thanks to patients, parents and staff at the Hospital for Sick Children, London.

## REFERENCES.

Buch J., Bruchett G., Girgert,R. Specific uptake of 123-I meta-Iodobenzylguanidine in the neuroblastoma cell line SK-N-SH. Cancer Research. 45:6366-6370. 1985.

Goldman A., Vivian G., Gordon J., Pritchard J., Kemshead JT. Immunolocalisation of neuroblastoma using radiolabelled monoclonal antibody UJ13A. Journal of Paediatics. 105:252-256. 1984.

Hoefnagel C., Voute T. Radionuclide therapy of neural crest tumours. Nuclaire Geneestunde oud en niew. ed. REKJ.Pouwels. ISBN. 90-6767-120-7. 1986.

Jones DH., Goldman A., Gordon I., Pritchard J., Gregory BJ., Kemshead JT. Therapeutic application of a radiolabelled monoclonal antibody in nude mice xenografted with human neuroblastoma: tumouricidal effects and distribution studies. International Journal of Cancer. 35:715-720. 1986.

Lashford LS., Jones DH., Pritchard J., Gordon I., Breatnach F., Kemshead JT. Therapeutic application of radiolabelled monoclonal antibody UJ13A in children with disseminated neuroblastoma. NCI Monographs. 3:53-59. 1987.

Lashford LS., Moyes J., Ott R., Fielding S., Babich J., Mellors S., Gordon I., Evans K., Kemshead JT. The biodistribution and pharmackinetics of meta-Iodobenzylguanidine in childhood neuroblastoma. Submitted. 1987.

Lashford LS., Evans K., Jones DH., Gordon I., Pritchard J., Kemshead JT. The biodistribution of the monoclonal antibody UJ13A in children with stage IV neuroblastoma - implications for "targeted" radiation therapy. Submitted. 1987.

Wieland D., Wu J., Brown L., Manger T., Swanson D., Bierwaltes W. Radiolabelled adrenergic neuron blocking agents: Adrenomedullary imaging with (131) iodobenzylguanidine. J.Nucl.Med. 21:349. 1980.

Advances in Neuroblastoma Research 2, pages 655–667

THE THERAPEUTIC USE OF I-131 META-IODOBENZYLGUANIDINE (mIBG) IN NEUROBLASTOMA : A PHASE II STUDY IN 12 PATIENTS.

Olivier HARTMANN, Jean D. LUMBROSO, Jean LEMERLE, Martin SCHLUMBERGER, Marcel RICARD Bernard AUBERT, Sabine COORNAERT, Louis MERLIN, and Claude PARMENTIER.

Departments of Pediatry (O.H., J.L.), of Nuclear Medicine (J.D.L., M.S., C.P.), and of Physics, INSERM U66 (M.R., B.A.), Institut Gustave-Roussy, Rue Camille Desmoulins, 94805 Villejuif Cedex, France, ORIS-I-CEA (S.C., L.M.), Gif sur Yvette, 91190 FRANCE.

## INTRODUCTION

Despite the use of intensified conventional chemotherapy the complete response rate of advanced neuroblastoma remains low (Shafford et al.,1984). The use of high-dose chemo-radiotherapy followed by bone marrow transplantation (BMT) improved the duration of disease free survival (August et al.,1984, Hartmann et al. 1985) but, even after these high-dose regimens the relapse rate remains high. Metaiodobenzylguanidine (mIBG) (Wieland et al. 1980) labeled with I-131 or I-123 can be used for scintigraphic imaging of neuroblastoma (Treuner J. et al. 1984, Bousvaros A. et al 1986, Geatti O. et al. 1985, Munkner T. 1985, Voute P.A. et al. 1985, Hoefnagel CA. et al. 1985, Lumbroso J. et al. 1986). In order to evaluate the therapeutic role of I 131 mIBG in the treatment of neuroblastoma patients, a phase II study was performed in 12 patients.

### PATIENTS AND METHODS

Patient's characteristics
Twelve patients entered this study. Details are given in Table 1. According to Evans' classification (Evans et

TABLE 1 - PATIENTS CHARACTERISTICS

| N° OF PT | AGE AT DIAGNOSIS | SEX | PRIMARY TUMOR | STAGE | CONVENTIONAL CHEMOTHERAPY DURATION (MONTHS) | DRUGS | SURGERY | RADIATION THERAPY | HDC + ABMT |
|---|---|---|---|---|---|---|---|---|---|
| 1 | 13 | M | ABDO | 4 | 11 | C.V.A.E. | SUBTOTAL EXCISION | 30 Gy PRIMARY | HDM |
| 2 | 7 | M | ABDO | 4 | 21 | C.V.A.D.N.E.P. | COMPLETE EXCISION | 25Gy SKULL 35 Gy MEDIASTINUM | (BCNU + E + HDM) x 2 |
| 3 | 6 | M | ABDO | 4 | 9 | C.V.A.E.P. | SUBTOTAL EXCISION | - | BU.C |
| 4 | 8 | F | ABDO | 4 | 7 | C.V.A.D.E.P. | COMPLETE EXCISION | 20 Gy SKULL | V.HDM.TBI |
| 5 | 4 | M | ABDO | 4 | 10 | C.V.A.E.P.I. | COMPLETE EXCISION | - | (BCNU + E + HDM) x 2 |
| 6 | 5 | M | UNKNOWN | 4 | 6 | C.V.A.E.P. | - | 35 Gy PRIMARY | - |
| 7 | 3 | F | ABDO | 3 | 10 | C.V.A.E.P. | SUBTOTAL EXCISION | - | - |
| 8 | 2 | M | ABDO | 4 | 6 | C.V.A.E.P. | - | - | - |
| 9 | 4 | M | ABDO | 4 | 8 | C.V.A.E.P. | - | - | - |
| 10 | 5 | M | THORAX | 3 | 10 | C.V.A.E.P. | SUBTOTAL EXCISION | 35 Gy PRIMARY | - |
| 11 | 8 | M | ABDO | 4 | 6 | C.V.A.E.P. | SUBTOTAL EXCISION | 30 Gy PRIMARY | BCNU + E + HDM |
| 12 | 3 | M | ABDO | 4 | 9 | C.V.A.E.P. | COMPLETE EXCISION | - | (BCNU + E + HDM) x 2 |

Legends : ABDO = ABDOMEN ; A = DOXORUBICINE ; BU = BUSULFAN ; C = CYCLOPHOSPHAMIDE ; D = DITC ; E = VM26 ; HDC = HIGH DOSE CHEMOTHERAPY ; HDM = HIGH DOSE MELPHALAN ; I + IPHOSPHAMIDE ; P = CISPLATINUM ; TBI = TOTAL BODY IRRADIATION ; V = VINCRISTINE ; - = NOT DONE.

al., 1971) 10 patients had stage IV and 2 had stage III disease. Before entering this phase II study, all patients had been extensively treated. They had received, at least 2 different conventional polychemotherapy protocols, 4 to 7 different drugs (median 5) for a median duration of 9 months (range 6–21). Seven out of 12 patients (Nos 1 – 5,11,12) had also previously received high-dose chemora – diotherapy with autologous bone marrow transplantation. Surgical excision of the primary had been performed in 9/12 patients. Radiation therapy had been previously administred on tumoral bed volume and/or bone metastases in 6/12 patients (Nos 1,2,4,7,10,11).

Despite the use of such multimodal aggressive therapies, at the time of entering this phase II study, 4 patients had primarily resistant disease (Nos 3,6,8,9) ; 5 were in first refractory relapse (Nos 4,5,7,11,12) and 3 in second or third refractory relapse (Nos 1,2,10).

Prior to MIBG therapy, in addition to MIBG scan, all patients had measurable sites of the disease, details are given in Table 2.

### mIBG administration

mIBG was labeled according to Mangner's method (Mangner et al., 1982) with I-131, with a specific activity ranging from 0.74 to 1.5 GBq/mg (20 to 40 mCi/mg) and administered intravenously, using a shielded electric syringe. It was infused over 3 to 6 hours, in parallel with saline (NaCl 0.9 %) in a peripheral vein. During drug administration and for the 5 following days, patients were kept in an isolated room in order to avoid environmental contamination. Except in the case of pregnancy, the parents of the children after receiving the information on radioprotection pratices, were allowed to participate with the nurses in the care of their child.

Patients were to receive one course per month, treatment being stopped in case of disease progression under therapy and/or severe thrombopenia.

### Follow-up

During the five days of hospitalization, patients were monitored, several times a day, for blood pressure and clinical status. Whole body scans were performed every day from day 1 to day 6 using a rectilinear scanner with two opposite probes. Blood counts and hepatic tests were controlled every two days during the first week following

TABLE 2 – MEASURABLE DISEASE PRIOR TO MIBG THERAPY

| N° OF PT | PRIMARY | METASTASES | | | URINARY CATECHOLAMINES | MIBG SCAN | GENERAL CONDITIONS | PAIN | STATUS BEFORE MIBG THERAPY. |
|---|---|---|---|---|---|---|---|---|---|
| | | BONE | BM | OTHERS | | | | | |
| 1 | + | 0 | 0 | 0 | 0 | + | BAD | + | 3rd REFRACTORY RELAPSE |
| 2 | 0 | + | + | 0 | 0 | + | BAD | + | 3rd REFRACTORY RELAPSE |
| 3 | 0 | + | 0 | 0 | + | + | GOOD | 0 | PRIMARILY RESISTANT DISEASE |
| 4 | 0 | + | + | ORBITAL | 0 | + | GOOD | + | 1st REFRACTORY RELAPSE |
| 5 | 0 | + | + | 0 | + | + | BAD | + | 1st REFRACTORY RELAPSE |
| 6 | 0 | + | + | 0 | 0 | + | GOOD | 0 | PRIMARILY RESISTANT DISEASE |
| 7 | + | + | + | 0 | 0 | + | GOOD | 0 | 1st REFRACTORY RELAPSE |
| 8 | + | + | + | 0 | + | + | BAD | + | PRIMARILY RESISTANT DISEASE |
| 9 | + | 0 | + | 0 | 0 | + | GOOD | 0 | PRIMARILY RESISTANT DISEASE |
| 10 | + | 0 | 0 | SUBCUTANEOUS | 0 | + | GOOD | 0 | 2nd REFRACTORY RELAPSE |
| 11 | + | 0 | 0 | DISTANT L.H. | 0 | + | GOOD | + | 1st REFRACTORY RELAPSE |
| 12 | 0 | 0 | 0 | DISTANT L.H. | 0 | + | GOOD | 0 | 1st REFRACTORY RELAPSE |

the treatment. After discharge, blood counts were repeated at least once a week for the total duration of treatment and the month following the last mIBG administration.

In addition, biological hepatic tests, thyroid hormon assay and renal function tests were performed each month.

### Evaluation of response

Response was judged on serial evaluations of : a) urinary excretion of catecholamine metabolites ; b) changes of three dimensional measurements of primary and/or measurable metastases on ultrasonography and CT scan ; c) evolution of general condition and disease related pain ; d) changes of the number of lesions on mIBG scans.

Objective effect (OE) was considered when a < 50 % and > 20 % reduction of all measurable sites was obtained for at least 4 weeks. Stable disease (SD) defined a stable status of the disease without clinical manifestation of the disease for at least 8 weeks. All other situations were judged as no response (NR) or progressive disease (PD), wether progression was observed during or after the 4 weeks following injection.

## RESULTS

Five patients received one single course of mIBG, the seven remaining patients received 2 to 5 courses of treatment. Details are given in Table 3.

### mIBG biodistribution

All the post-therapeutic scans demontrated an intense uptake at the level of the tumor foci. In the case of patient n° 4 presenting a bone marrow relapse and an orbital metastasis, we could compute the radiation dose delivered to the orbital tumour. Its volume was estimated on CT and NMR to be of 50 $cm^3$ ; the uptake represented 11 % of the infused activity of I-131 mIBG and the biological half life was 9.3 days : the computed dose was 105 Gy. For the bone marrow tumor, the lack of volume measurement precluded any dosimetric estimate.

### Disease response

Details of response of each measurable site of the disease are given in Table 4. Overall, out of 7 patients with measurable primary, no shrinkage was observed. No measurable effect was observed on metastases in the 11

## TABLE 3 – MIBG THERAPY

| N° OF PT | N° OF COURSE | DOSE/COURSE (mCi) | INTERVALS BETWEEN COURSES (WEEKS) | CUMULATIVE DOSES (mCi) |
|---|---|---|---|---|
| 1 | 2 | 35, 49 | 12 | 84 |
| 2 | 1 | 42 | - | 42 |
| 3 | 5 | 49, 100, 104, 95, 108 | 4, 6, 6, 8 | 456 |
| 4 | 1 | 77.4 | - | 77.4 |
| 5 | 1 | 104 | - | 104 |
| 6 | 3 | 29, 3, 78, 6, 96 | 6, 8 | 204 |
| 7 | 4 | 65, 94, 95, 108 | 4, 4, 6 | 362 |
| 8 | 1 | 39.9 | - | 39.9 |
| 9 | 4 | 92, 95, 99, 5, 90 | 4, 5, 4 | 376.5 |
| 10 | 2 | 87, 101 | 4 | 188 |
| 11 | 2 | 98, 106.5 | 12 | 204.5 |
| 12 | 1 | 104 | - | 104 |

patients with these measurable sites. Out of 3 patients with elevated urinary catecholamine metabolites, one measurable improvement was observed. No improvement of general conditions but 4/6 dramatic relief of pain were observed. Overall, among the 12 patients, 2 OE, 2 SD, 5 NR, and 3 PD were observed.

### Duration of response
Duration of response observed in patients 3 and 9 was respectively 7 and 6 months. Disease remained stable in patients 6 and 7 respectively for 5 and 6 months until a new progression was observed (Table 4).

### Survival
In these very advanced patients, survival was short. As of May 1987, two patients (N° 9,10) are alive with disease at 7 and 10 months post mIBG, one patient (N°3) died of intercurrent complication 7 months post mIBG (measles encephalitis) ; 9 patients died of the disease 1.5 to 12 months post mIBG (median 3 months) (Table 4).

### Toxicity
### Early toxicity
In one patient (N° 3) a sudden elevation of blood pressure from 95/50 to 240/100 mm.Hg was observed following the third course of mIBG. It started 3 hours after the end of treatment (infusion over 3 hours) and recovered to normal values within 2 hours. No recurrence occurred for the two following courses in this patient. No elevation of blood pressure occured in any other patients.

A transient elevation of SGOT appeared within the week following drug administration in two patients (Nos 3,9). The values observed were between 2 and 3 times the normal values. These abnormalities remained clinically and biologicaly isolated and recovered spontaneously.

### Delayed toxicity
Delayed toxicity was exclusively marked by thrombopenia occurring in 7/12 patients. Profound thrombopenia was observed in four patients (Nos 2,5,11,12). One month after the first course of treatment the platelet numbers were under $40 \times 10^9/l$. clinical hemorrhagic complications were observed in one case. A moderate thrombopenia, maximum 4 weeks after the first course of treatment, occurred in one patient (N° 4). The lowest value

TABLE 4 : RESPONSE TO MIBG THERAPY

| N° OF PT | PRIMARY | METASTASES | | URINARY CATECHOLAMINES | MIBG SCAN CHANGES | PAIN | OVERALL RESPONSE | DURATION OF RESPONSE (MONTHS) | SURVIVAL FROM 1st COURSE (MONTHS) |
|---|---|---|---|---|---|---|---|---|---|
| | | BONE | BM | | | | | | |
| 1 | ↗ | NE | NE | NE | ↗ | ↗ | NR | - | 4 |
| 2 | NE | ↗↗ | ↗↗ | NE | 0 | ↗ | PD | - | 1,5 |
| 3 | NE | 0 | NE | ↗ | 0 | - | OE | 7 | 7 |
| 4 | NE | 0 | 0 | NE | 0 | ↗ | NR | - | 2 |
| 5 | NE | 0 | 0 | 0 | 0 | ↗ | PD | - | 3 |
| 6 | NE | 0 | 0 | NE | 0 | - | SD | 5 | 7 |
| 7 | 0 | ↗ | ↗ | NE | ↗ | - | SD | 6 | 12 |
| 8 | 0 | ↗↗ | ↗↗ | ↗ | ND | ↗ | PD | - | 1 |
| 9 | 0 | NE | 0 | NE | ↗ | - | OE | 6 | 10+ |
| 10 | ↗↗ | NE | NE | NE | ↗↗ | ↗ | NR | - | 7+ |
| 11 | ↗ | ↗ | ↗ | NE | ↗ | ↗ | NR | - | 5 |
| 12 | ↗ | NE | NE | NE | ↗ | - | NR | - | 4 |

LEGENDS :

↗ SLOW PROGRESSION  
↗↗ RAPID PROGRESSION  
↘ DECREASE  
0 = NO CHANGE  

NE = NOT EVALUABLE  
ND = NOT DONE  
NR = NO RESPONSE  
OE = OBJECTIVE EFFECT  
PD = PROGRESSIVE DISEASE  
SD = STABLE DISEASE

of the platelet counts was 51 x $10^9$/l. Mild thrombopenia was observed following 5/9 courses in two patients (N[os] 3,9). In patient 3, thrombopenia occurred after the third and the fourth course of mIBG therapy, the lowest value observed was 91 x $10^9$/l. In patient 9, thrombopenia followed the first, third and fourth course. The lowest platelet count was 80 x $10^9$/l. No change in RBC and WBC count was observed in any patient. No cardiac, pulmonary, renal or nervous complication was encountered.

### Radioprotection

The range of dose equivalent delivered to the parent, involved in the care of the child, by external irradiation and measured with a film dosimeter was from not detectable (threshold value : 0.2 mSv) to 2.9 mSv per treatment.

The internal contamination was estimated after counting an aliquot of urine : in one case, we found a urine activity of 7 Bq/l (100 pCi/l) which would lead to a thyroid dose equivalent less than 1 mSv assuming that the isotope was incorporated as free Iodine. In the other cases, no significant contamination was detected.

## DISCUSSION

mIBG uptake has been experimentally demonstrated in neuroblastoma cell line (Buck et al., 1985). Scintigraphic imaging with this drug, regularly shows a high uptake in neuroblastoma patients (Wieland et al., 1980, Voute et al., 1985). Therefore, the use of radioactive labeled mIBG for specific treatment of neuroblastoma appeared logical. Preliminary encouraging results have been published in the treatment of pheochromocytoma (Mc Dougall, 1984, Sisson et al., 1984, Thompson et al., 1984, Mac Ewan et al., 1985). In this group of heavily pretreated patients, the results observed were poor. The subjective effects of this treatment such as disappearance of pain in three patients and stabilization of the disease in two other patients were obvious. However, only 2/12 objective measurable effects were observed. Preliminary results have been published (Voute et al., 1986, Klingebiel et al. 1986) with higher response rate in neuroblastoma patients. Our patients were heavily pretreated and particularly resistant to any kind of chemotherapy. Although neuroblastoma is usually radiosensitive in vitro and in vivo (Deacon et al., 1985, Evans et al., 1986, Jacobson et al., 1984) is possible that chemoresistance increases resistance to radiotherapy. Following mIBG infusion, radiation dosimetry to the different tumor sites is always difficult to estimate. Precise measurement of the volume of the tumor was calculated for solid tumor from CT scan studies assuming spherical configuration but dosimetry estimates were impossible to calculate for diffuse bone marrow metastases. Hence the actual radiation dose administered to the different sites of the disease was often unknown. Moreover, the absence of tumor shrinkage with calculated doses up to 50 or 100 Gy suggests that the intra-tumoral distribution of the radiation dose is dramatically heterogeneous. Several parameters remain to be studied : duration of mIBG infusion (Buck et al., 1985), total dose necessary to obtain the best therapeutic effect, interval between each course of mIBG therapy.

Toxicity of this treatment was mild taking into account the endstage of these patients. The major side effect observed was thrombopenia. Platelets declined dramatically after the first course in 4 patients and successively after each course in two others. This complication has already been described with mIBG treatment (Sisson et al., 1984, Mac Ewan et al., 1985, Klingebielt et al., 1986). The presence of tumoral cells in the bone marrow, with a high uptake of rabiolabeled mIBG should play a role in this toxicity. However, it has to be emphasized that the greatest thrombopenia occurred in 4/7 patients previously treated with high-dose therapy and bone marrow transplantation. Similar toxicity in such patients has been described by Voute et al. (Voute et al., 1986).

The irradiation of the liver, always clearly seen on the post therapeutic scans, did not cause significant toxicity in our study. However, due to the short interval of follow-up of our patients, we cannot exclude the occurrence of delayed toxic effects after months or years. Despite Lugol administration, an image of the thyroid appeared on some post therapeutic scans, and the absence of late thyroid complications remains questionable.

For these treatments, the radiation dose to the staff has been lowered by the split of the exposure time between many persons and the involvement of the parents (Van der Steen et al., 1986). When helping the child with meals and toilet procedures, the parents were exposed to an acceptable dose for a single treatment.

Finally, as the contamination may multiply by a factor

2 the dose to the thyroid, Lugol administration to the parents should be discussed (Schlumberger, 1986), especially when the patients are young children requiring more care.

## CONCLUSION

With the doses and schedule used in this study, tolerance of this treatment was acceptable. However, the high hematological toxicity observed in previously bone marrow transplanted patients should represent an exclusion of this therapeutic approach for such patients. In these endstage patients, the effects observed, although transient, were encouraging. The absence of unpleasant side effects, usually encountered with chemotherapy, such as gastrointestinal toxicity and hair loss, rendered this therapy easy to manage in these heavily pretreated children.

## REFERENCES

August CS, Serota FT, Koch PA, Burkey E, Schlesinger H, Elkins WL, Evans AE, D'Angio GJ (1984). Treatment of advanced neuroblastoma with supralethal chemotherapy, radiation and allogeneic or autologous marrow reconstitution. J Clin Oncol 2:609–616.

Bousvaros A, Kirks DR, Grossman H (1986). Imaging of neuroblastoma : an overview. Pediatr Radiol 16:89–106.

Buck J, Bruchelt G, Girgert R, Treuner J, Niethammer D (1985). Specific uptake of m-($^{125}$I) iodobenzylguanidine in the human neuroblastoma cell line SK-N-SH. Cancer Res 45:6366–6370.

Deacon JM, Wilson P, Steel GG 1985). Radiosensitivity of neuroblastoma. Prog Clin Biol Res 175:525–531.

Evans AE, D'Angio GJ, Randolph J (1971). A proposed staging for children with neuroblastoma. Cancer 28:347–378.

Evans SM, Labs LM, Yuhas JM (1986). Response of human neuroblastoma and melanoma multicellular tumor spheroids (MTS) to single dose irradiation. Int J Radiation Oncology Biol Phys 12:969–973.

Geatti O, Shapiro B, Sisson JC, Hutchinson RJ, Mallette S, Eyre P, Beierwaltes WH (1985). Iodine 131 metaiodobenzylguanidine scintigraphy for the location of neuroblastoma : preliminary experience in ten cases. J Nucl Med 26:736–742.

Hartmann O, Zucker JM, Pinkerton R, Philip T, Beaujean F, Bernard JL, Soulliet G, Lutz P, Bordigoni P, Plouvier E (1985). Metastatic neuroblastoma in children older than one year old at diagnosis : treatment with intensive chemo-radiotherapy and autologous bone marrow transplantation. Blood Trans Immunohaematol 28:539-546.

Hoefnagel CA, Voute PA, De Kraker J, Marcuse HR (1985). Total-body scintigraphy with [131]I metaiodobenzyl - guanidine for detection of neuroblastoma. Diagn Imag Clin Med 54:21-27.

Jacobson GM, Sause NT, O'Brien RT (1984). Dose response analysis of pediatric neuroblastoma to megavoltage radiation. Am J Clin Oncol 7:693-697.

Klingebiel T, Feine U, Niethammer D, Müller-Schauenburg W, Schwabe O, Maul FD, Gerein V, Fischer M, Gahr M, Kraz K (1986). Initial experiences in the treatment of children with metastatic and recurrent neuroblastoma using meta-iodobenzylguanidine. Klin Padiatr 198:230-236.

Lumbroso J, Hartmann O, Guermazi F, Coornaert S, Rabarison Y, Leclere J, Lemerle J, Parmentier C (1986). The clinical contribution of I-123 and I-131 meta-iodobenzylguanidine (mIBG) scans in neuroblastoma. J Nucl Med 27:947 (Abstract).

McDougall IR (1984). Malignant pheochromocytoma treated by I-131 MIBG. J Nucl Med 25:249-251.

Mac Ewan AJ, Shapiro B, Sisson J, Beierwaltes WH, Ackery D (1985). Radio-iodobenzylguanidine for the scintigraphic location and therapy of adrenergic tumors. Semin Nucl Med 15:132-153.

Mangner TJ, Wu JL, Wieland DM (1982). Solid-phase exchange radioiodination of aryl iodide facilitation by ammonium sulfate. J. Org Chem 47:1484-1488.

Munkner T (1985). [131]I metaiodobenzylguanidine scintigraphy of neuroblastomas. Semin Nucl Med 15:154-160.

Schlumberger M (1986). L'iodure et la radioprotection de la thyroïde contre l'irradiation de la thyroïde par l'iode radiocatif. Radioprotection 21:277-300.

Shafford EA, Rogers DW, Pritchard J (1984). Advanced neuroblastoma : improved response rate using a multiagent regimen (OPEC) including cisplatin and VM26. J Clin Oncol 2:742-747.

Sisson JC, Shapiro B, Beierwaltes WH (1984). Radio-pharmaceutical treatment of malignant pheochromocytoma. J Nucl Med, 25:197:206.

Thompson NW, Allo DA, Shapiro B, Sisson J, Beierwaltes W (1984). Extraadrenal and metastatic pheochromocytoma in localization and management. World J Surg 3:605–611.

Treuner J, Feine U, Niethammer D, Müller–Schauenburg W, Meinke J, Eibach E, Dopfer R, Klingelbiel TH, Grumbach ST (1984). Scintigraphic imaging of neuroblastoma with ($^{131}$I) iodobenzylguanedine. Lancet 1:333–334.

Van der Steen J, Maessen HJ, Hoefnagel CA, Marcuse HR (1986). Radiation protection during treatment of children with $^{131}$I metaiodobenzylguanidine. Health Phys 50:515–522.

Voute PA, Hoefnagel CA, De Kraker J, Marcuse HR (1986). $^{131}$I MIBG as targeted radioisotope in treatment of children with neuroblastoma. Proceedings ASCO, Los Angeles, 836.

Voute PA, Hoefnagel CA, Marcuse HR, De Kraker J (1985). Detection of neuroblastoma with $^{131}$I metaiodobenzyl-guanidine. Prog Clin Biol Res 175:389–398.

Wieland DM, Wu J, Brown LE, Mangner TJ, Swanson DP, Beierwaltes WH (1980). Radiolabeled adrenergic neuron blocking agents : adrenomedullary imaging with ($^{131}$I) metaiodobenzylguanidine. J Nucl Med 21:349:353.

Advances in Neuroblastoma Research 2, pages 669–678
© 1988 Alan R. Liss, Inc.

MIBG-TREATMENT IN NEUROBLASTOMA; EXPERIENCES OF THE
TÜBINGEN/FRANKFURT GROUP

J.Treuner, V.Gerein, Th.Klingebiel, D.Schwabe,
U.Feine, J.Happ, D.Niethammer, F.Maul, R.Dopfer,
B.Kornhuber, F.Berthold, H.Jürgens, G.Hör

Department of Pediatrics (J.T., Th.K., D.N., R.D.) and
Department of Radiology (U.F.) of the University, D-
7400 Tübingen; Department of Pediatrics (V.G., D.S.,
B.K.) and Department of Radiology (J.H., F.M., G.H.)
of the University, D-6000 Frankfurt; Department of
Pediatrics of the University (F.B.), D-5000 Köln;
Department of Pediatrics of the University (H.J.), D-
4000 Düsseldorf

ABSTRACT

27 children with neuroblastoma were treated with
$^{131}$I-Metaiodobenzylguanidine (MBIG). They were
either refractory to conventional therapy or
experienced relapse after initially successful
treatment. 7 children revealed stage IV and 20 stage
III at the beginning of MIBG-treatment. MIBG was
administered by infusion lasting from 30 min to 30
hrs. In most children the dose was split    into two
portions each infused over a period of 4 hrs with a 24
hrs interval between. Courses were repeated up to 6
times and maximum activity given to one patient
cumulatively was 38,221 MBq. 24 patients were
evaluable for analysis of results. In 4 children (16.7
%) a CR was observed, in 10 (41.7 %) a PR, in 5 (20.8
%) a disease stabilization and 5 were nonresponders.
The 4 CR-patients were initially stage IV. 3 of them
were treated in addition by bone marrow
transplantation (bmt), one by further chemotherapy. 3
died of a relapse, 1 of complications from bmt. 5 of
the 10 PR-patients died of tumor progression, 3
achieved a CR by additional chemotherapy, 1 a PR by

bmt and 1 stays in PR without further measures. 2 of the 5 children with a disease stabilization were the first treated patients          to whom a fairly low dose was given.

In 3 of the 5 nonresponders no uptake of MIBG was observed; they died from tumor progression. 1 of the 2 nonresponders with uptake died of graft-versus-host disease after bmt, 1 other also of tumor progression. Duration of remission was between 1 and 12 months and depended upon uptake and dose of MIBG, interval between administrations and individual tumor behaviour. Side effects were seen as marked bone marrow depression; this was reversible in any case and we did not loose a patient due to MIBG-induced leuko- or thrombopenia. In cases of severely ill children we observed a very fast and dramatical amelioration in clinical conditions.

With this method even in neuroblastoma relapse and in nonresponders complete remissions are achievable. Important is the intensification of the therapeutical effect by additional chemotherapy or in combination with bmt. For a definitive evaluation further investigations are necessary to optimize therapeutic strategies.

INTRODUCTION

The substance benzylguanidine radiolabeled with [131]I or [125]I - Metaiodobenzylguanidine (MIBG) - was introduced by Beierwaltes and Sisson (Wieland et al., 1980; Sisson et al., 1981; Shapiro et al., 1983) more than 15 years ago for scintigraphic imaging of the adrenal gland and pheochromocytomas. We (Treuner et al., 1984) and another group in Germany (Kimmig et al., 1983) demonstrated that MIBG is also useful for scintigraphic imaging of neuroblastoma lesions. We undertook labaratory investigations to determine the cytotoxicity of highly labeled MIBG in neuroblastoma cell-lines and analyzed the uptake and storage mechanism (Buck et al., 1985). Using this background information we started treatment trials. Between 1985 and 1986 in two German centers - Frankfurt and Tübingen - 27 children with neuroblastoma were treated (Klingebiel et al., 1986). All of these children had relapsed after conventional

therapy or had shown no sufficient response to
cytostatic treatment.


PATIENTS AND METHODS

At initial diagnosis 7 children were at stage III and
20 at stage IV acccording to the Evans classification
(Evans et al., 1971); at the beginning of MIBG-
treatment 9 patients were assigned to stage III, 16 to
stage IV and in 2 cases MIBG was given for a suspected
minimal residual disease.
12 of 27 patients had relapsed after complete
remission (CR), the other 15 children showed signs of
tumor progression while still undergoing cytostatic
therapy. Thirteen children were boys and 14 girls, the
mean age at the beginning of MIBG-therapy was 4.9
years ranging from 1 to 21 years. Before start of MIBG-
treament the tumor burden was measured by CT-scan,
sonography and X-ray examinations. The expected uptake
of MIBG in the tumors was determined by a diagnostic
MIBG-scan. Liver, kidney, thyroid and adrenal function
were controlled before, during and after MIBG-
treatment. The thyroid gland was blocked with
potassium iodine 3 days prior MIBG treatment.
All of the 27 children had elevated catecholamine

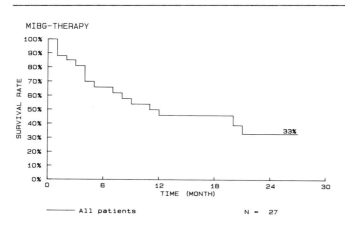

Figure 1: Survival time of all 27 treated patients
(Kaplan-Meier Plot)

levels at diagnosis. However, only 22 had increased
levels at onset of MIBG-treatment.
The radioactively labeled MIBG was administered in 1
to 6 therapy-cycles to the children, who were staying
on nuclear medicine ward. Altogether we gave 21 cycles
with a mean of 2.6 cycles per patient.
The administration was done by infusion lasting
between 30 minutes and 24 hours. Our definite approach
was to split the dosage into two portions, each
lasting 4 hours with 20 hours interval between.
Six of the children were transplanted after MIBG-
treatment by autologous or allogeneic bone marrow
transplantation (bmt).
Four of 27 patients did not show any uptake of MIBG,
none of these 4 patients had had elevated
catecholamine levels at the onset of therapy. Two of
these patients were stage at III.
The total radioactivity given ranged from 80 to 1033
mCi (2,960 - 38,221 MBq) with a mean dosage of 357 mCi
(13,209 Mbq).The radioactivity given per cycle ranged
from 35 to 450 mCi (1,295 - 16,650 MBq) with a mean
dosage of 134 mCi (4,958 MBq).

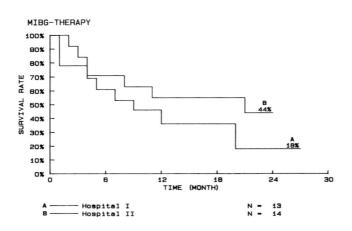

Figure 2a: Survival of patients treated in the two
hospitals.

The mean radioactivity related to body weigth per
cycle was 7.9 mCi/kg (292 MBq/kg) ranging from 1.4 to
21.4 mCi/kg (51.8 - 791,8 MBq/kg).


RESULTS

Twentyfour patients were available for the analysis.
In 4 patients (16.7%) a complete remission was
achieved, 10 (41,7%) achieved a partial remission, 5
(20.8%) a disease stabilization, and 5 did not respond
to MIBG treatment at all.
*The complete remission patients (CR) were at stage
IV, and 3 of them underwent a bmt after the MIBG-
induced remission. In spite of this additional
treatment 3 of the 4 patients died of tumor relapse
and the other one of transplantation complications.
* 5 of the 10 patients with partial remission (PR)
died of tumor progression, 3 achieved a CR by
additional chemotherapy , 1 achieved CR by bmt and 1
is still in PR without further measures.
*All of the 5 children with stable disease showed a
tumor progression later on and died of the disease.

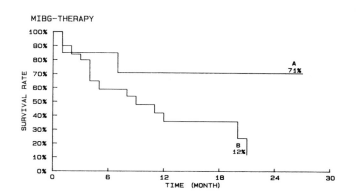

Figure 2b: Survival of patients according to their
stage at onset of MIBG-treatment. In hospital I more
patients with stage III disease were treated.

The first two of these patiens with stable disease
received a fairly low amount of MIBG.
*Three of the 5 <u>nonresponders</u> showed no uptake of
MIBG, they died from tumor progression. The other 2
nonresponders with uptake also died, one of graft-
versus-host disease after bmt the other of tumor
progression. The survival rate for the whole group was
33% with a mean survival time of 323 days ranging from
20 to 720 days (Fig. 1).
10 patients who are alive at present time show a
survival time between 120 and  720 days with a mean
value of 480 days after the start of MIBG-therapy.


DISCUSSION

The difference of the outcome (Fig. 2a) of the two
hospitals is not significant and could be explained by
the different pattern of patients in each group (stage
III and stage IV) (Fig. 2b).
There is the question what factors do influence the
effect of MIBG-treatment. We have looked at this point
and found some answers:

---

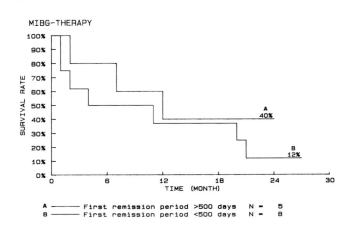

Figure 3: Survival of 13 patients with a CR before
MIBG-therapy according to the duration of this
remission.

*There is no correlation between the total
administered radioactivity and the survival rate.
*The expected tendency in favour of patients with a CR
prior to a relapse and subsequent MIBG-therapy could
not be observed.
*Duration of remission seems to influence the effect
of MIBG. The longer the duration of remission is, the
longer is the survival time (Fig. 3).
*It is not surprising that patients with additional
chemotherapy survive longer. There seems to be a
tendency in favour of additional chemotherapy but not
as expected in favour of bmt (Fig. 4).
*Patients with a higher dosage of radioactivity in the
first and second cycle of MIBG and patients with
higher uptake of activity in the tumor during the
first cycles have a longer survival period (Fig. 5).

However, it must be kept in mind that the number of
patients is too small to draw definitive conclusions.
The mentioned influencing factors of the MIBG-
treatment effect should be understood as tendency.
The limiting toxicity of MIBG-treatment is the bone
marrow depression, especially the effect on the
thrombocyte system. After 4 to 5 cycles of MIBG a

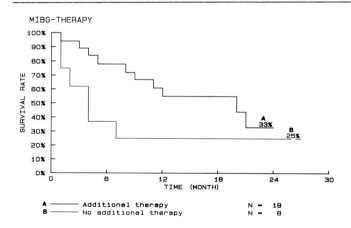

Figure 4: Survival of all patients according to an
additional therapy.

critical thrombopenia is achieved.


CONCLUSIONS

MIBG is a new therapeutic principle for the treatment
of neuroblastoma, which allows treating the tumor
specifically.
However, a breakthrough with this method in
neuroblastoma treatment does not seem to be possible
in the near future. The following factors seem to play
a role in the treatment efficacy:
*The specific activity as well as the dosage of the
first two cycles and perhaps in addition the infusion
time.
*The stage, the duration of a preexisting remission,
the radiation dose and an additional chemotherapy.
There are more questions left open by this pilot study
than answered at the present time:
*Why are some cases of neuroblastoma more sensitive
than others?

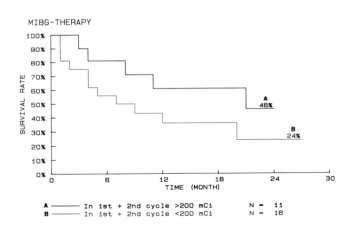

Figure 5: Survival of all patients according to the
administered MIBG-dose in the first two cycles.

*What minimal tumor volume can be killed by MIBG?
*What energy level is sufficient to destroy enough cells?
*What role does the state of cell differentiation play for the degree of response?
For the future there are three situations, where it seems to be feasable to test the use of MIBG:
*1) in cases with insufficient response to conventional therapy
*2) in patients with stage III and IV at diagnosis
*3) in combination with subsequent bone marrow transplantation.

REFERENCES

Buck J., Bruchelt G., Girgert R., Treuner J., Niethammer D.
Specific uptake of m-(125I)Iodobenzylguanidine in the human neuroblastoma cell line SK-N-SH
Cancer Res 46:6366-6370 (1985)

Evans A.E., D'Angio G.J., Randolph J.G.
A proposed staging for children with neuroblastoma
Cancer 27:374-378 (1971)

Kimmig B., Brandeis W.E., Eisenhut M., Bubeck B., Hermann H.J., Zum Winkel K.
Szintigraphische Darstellung eines Neuroblastoms
NucCompact 14:347-348 (1983)

Klingebiel Th., Feine U., Niethammer D., Müller-Schauenburg W., Schwabe D., Maul F.D., Gerein V., Fischer M., Gahr M., Kraz K., Wehinger H., Weinel P., Treuner J.
Erste Erfahrungen in der Behandlung von Kindern mit metastasiertem und rezidivierten Neuroblastom mit Metajodbenzylguanidin
Klin Päd. 198:230-236 (1986)

Shapiro B., Sisson J.C., Beierwaltes W.H.
Experience with the use of 131I-meta-Iodobenzylguanidine for locating pheochromocytomas.
In:Nuclear Medicine and Biology. Proc. 3rd World Congr. Nucl. Med. Biology Vol II p 1265; Pergamon Press Oxford 1983

Sisson J.C., Frager M.S., Valk T.W., Gross M.D.,
Swanson D.P., Wieland D.M., Tobes M.C., Beierwaltes
W.H., Thompson N.W.
Scintigraphic localization of pheochromocytoma
N Engl J Med 305:12-17 (1981)

Treuner J., Feine U., Niethammer D., Müller-
Schauenburg W., Meinke J., Eibach E., Dopfer R.,
Klingebiel Th., Grumbach St.
Scintigraphic imaging of neuroblastoma with
(131I)Iodobenzylguanidine
Lancet I,4:334-334 (1984)

Wieland D.M., Wu J.L., Brown L.E., Mangner T.J.,
Swanson D.P., Beierwaltes W.H.
Radiolabeled adrenergic neuron-blocking agents:
Adrenomedullary imaging with (131I)Iodobenzylguandine
J Nucl Med 21:349-353 (1980)

Advances in Neuroblastoma Research 2, pages 679–687
© 1988 Alan R. Liss, Inc.

# SIDE EFFECTS OF TREATMENT WITH I-131-META-IODOBENZYLGUANI-DINE (I-131-MIBG) IN NEUROBLASTOMA PATIENTS

P.A. Voûte, C.A. Hoefnagel, J.de Kraker and
M. Majoor
Werkgroep Kindertumoren, Emma Kinderziekenhuis
and Department of Nuclear Medicine, The Nether-
lands Cancer Institute, NL-1018 HJ Amsterdam,
The Netherlands

## INTRODUCTION

Meta-iodobenzylguanidine(MIBG), a guanethidine analogue,
coupled to Iodine-131(I-131), has been successfully used
for the diagnosis and treatment of pheochromocytoma(1).This
led to its use in other tumours, which are derived from the
neural crest and are capable of concentrating this radio-
pharmaceuticalin the neurosecretory granules of chromaffin
cells. In these chromaffin cells catecholamines are produced and stored. MIBG replaces the catecholamines in competi-
tion and is stored thereafter in these cells. In analogy
with the use of I-131 in thyroid cancer, I-131-MIBG-uptake
in tumours was found to be adequate for therapeutic use(2,3).

For treatment of neuroblastoma patients with I-131-MIBG
two patient groups can be distinguished: those with residual
disease in whom the treatment has a curative intention and
those with progressive, chemotherapy resistent disease in
whom the treatment is given for palliation.

22 children and 1 adult were selected upon the merits
of dosimetry and the availability of other treatment modalities to receive therapeutic doses of I-131-MIBG. All patients had recurrent disease and had been treated on different
chemotherapy protocols. 1.5-7.4 GBq(41-200 mCi) of I-131-
MIBG was administered intravenously over 1, 4 or 24 hours at
3-6 weeks intervals. The 23 patients received 74 therapeutic
doses of I-131-MIBG.

The patients were admitted to nuclear protected hospital isolation facilities for 4-5 days per treatment and used an iodide solution for 2 weeks to protect the thyroid. Whenever young patients had to be isolated, one of the parents or grandparents was asked to take care of the child. Continuous monitoring of the external radiation dose to these parents revealed cumulative doses of 0.3-1.25 mSv(30-125 mrem) per treatment dose; the calculated dose equivalent from internal contamination ranged 0.3-24 $\mu$Sv(0.03-2.4 mrem)(4). This was regarded to be acceptable. The advantage of having parents participating in this patient care can be obtained at essentially no increased radiation risk.


TREATMENT RESULTS

The first two patients, who received 1.85 GBq(50 mCi) doses of I-131-MIBG, showed a marked regression(50%) of the tumour mass together with good palliation in the form of relief of pain. However the initial response was followed by rapid progression. Subsequently higher doses of I-131-MIBG (3.7-7.4 GBq) were administered with shorter intervals (4 weeks). With this regimen the following overall results were obtained:
* 5 complete remissions: of these patients one had a relapse in the bone marrow 5 months after the start of therapy, two showed recurrent bone metastases respectively after 10 and 5 months, in one MRI revealed an intradural lesion after 23 months and the fifth patient died from a cerebral hemorrhage during a phase of thrombocytopenia: as at autopsy no tumour was found, this should be regarded as a toxic death;
* 10 partial remissions: i.e. more than 50% decrease in tumorvolume in 4 patients with measurable disease, and considerable scintigraphic improvement in 6 other patients;
* no change(stable disease) in 3 patients;
* progression in 2 patients;
* 2 patients are still on treatment and have not been evaluated yet, and 1 patient was lost to follow up.
In judging these results it should be kept in mind that all patients had metastatic disease and were only given I-131-MIBG treatment after all other treatment modalities had been exploited.

SIDE EFFECTS

Hematologic effects

Hematologic effects of I-131-MIBG treatment were observed in 19 patients, with particularly a predominance of the
occurrence of thrombocytopenia. As is shown in Figure 1, in
some patients the onset of thrombocytopenia is immediately
after the first dose, whereas other patients only develop a
decrease in platelet counts after successive therapy doses
(cumulative toxicity).

The bone marrow status was found to have an important
influence on the hematologic side effects(Table 1): in 2 of
3 patients who never had demonstrated any sign of bone marrow involvement no side effects occurred; 6 patients, who,at
the time of I-131-MIBG treatment,showed no bone marrow disease, but previously had been proven to have invaded bone
marrow, had thrombocytopenia only; however, 11 of 12 patients, who, during I-131-MIBG therapy, revealed bone marrow
involvement, developed severe bone marrow depressions.

In this respect it should be appreciated, that bone
marrow involvement occurs more frequently than can be demonstrated by bone marrow aspiration alone.

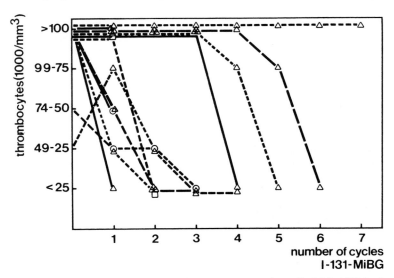

Figure 1. Platelet counts after successive I-131-MIBG doses.

TABLE 1.  Hematologic side effects of I-131-MIBG therapy
in 21 neuroblastoma patients

| bone marrow status (BMA/MIBG) | SIDE EFFECTS | | |
|---|---|---|---|
| | none | thrombocytopenia | BM-depression |
| negative | 2 | 1 | - |
| negative at therapy, previously positive | - | 6 | - |
| positive at therapy | - | 1 | 11 |

TABLE 2.  I-131-MIBG vs. Bone Marrow Aspiration(n=39) in
23 NBL patients treated with I-131-MIBG

| | BMA positive | BMA negative | total |
|---|---|---|---|
| MIBG positive | 13 | 7 | 20 |
| MIBG negative | 4 | 15 | 19 |
| total | 17 | 22 | 39 |

I-131-MIBG-scintigraphy, especially after administration of
therapeutic amounts, may reveal bone marrow involvement,
despite negative outcome of bone marrow aspirations. Table
2 shows a comparison of I-131-MIBG-scintigraphy and bone
marrow aspirations performed within 2 weeks, at 39 occasions
in the 23 treated patients. Although the majority of the
results are concordant, the 7 cases of bone marrow disease
only detected by I-131-MIBG-scintigraphy(and subsequently
confirmed) and the 4 cases only detected by bone marrow aspiration clearly demonstrate the complementary role of these
two procedures.

Figures 2 and 3 demonstrate cases, which, from the hematological point of view, are resp. ideal and not-ideal

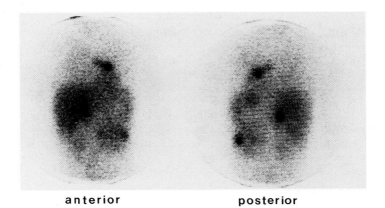

anterior                    posterior

Figure 2.   Posttherapeutic I-131-MIBG-scintigram in a 6 year old boy, showing intense concentration in a circumscript residual tumor mass behind the heart, as well as normal activity in a hyperplastic R-adrenal gland and in the bowel.

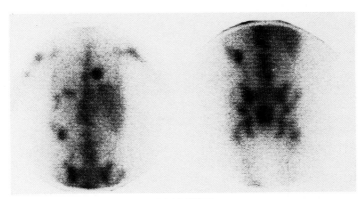

posterior

Figure 3.   Posttherapeutic I-131-MIBG-scintigram in a 5 year old girl treated for 3 small abdominal residual lesions after irradical resection of the primary tumour, which, despite negative bone marrow aspirations, shows intense concentration of the radiopharmaceutical throughout the bone marrow.

1<sup>st</sup> dose                3<sup>rd</sup> dose

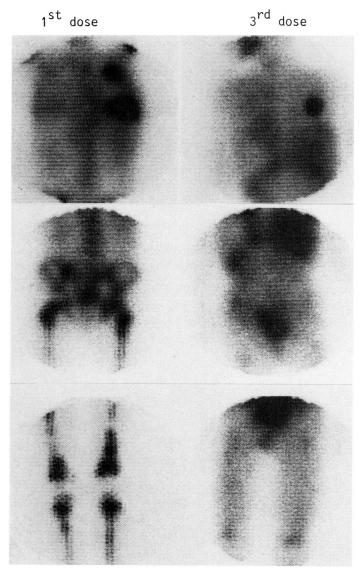

Figure 4.  Posttherapeutic scans of a 5 year old boy with
a neuroblastoma rib lesion and BM involvement(left); after
the 3rd dose(right) the bone marrow was cleared, but the boy
died due to a complication of severe bone marrow depression.

candidates for I-131-MIBG treatment: intense I-131-MIBG uptake with long retention in a circumscript lesion together
with a clear bone marrow may yield high absorbed radiation
doses to the tumour with relatively minor side effects.
As is shown by Figure 4, in patients with bone marrow involvement the bone marrow may be cleared by I-131-MIBG therapy,
but this practically always results in severe bone marrow
toxicity, and should only be anticipated when salvage methods are available.

## Nephrotoxicity

In 2 patients impairment of renal function(increase in serum
creatinine and decrease of creatinine clearance) was found
after treatment with I-131-MIBG. In most cases, however, no
detrimental effect to the kidneys was found(Figure 5). As
most of these patients had been treated with high dose Cisplatin before and some of them already had disturbances of
renal function at the start of I-131-MIBG treatment, it was
difficult to assess if any nephrotoxic effect can be attributed to  I-131-MIBG. However, in 1 patient, who had only
1 remaining kidney, we have observed that impairment of renal function, which had been induced by preceeding chemotherapy with Cisplatin, was enhanced after I-131-MIBG-therapy,
as is shown in Figure 6.

## Other side effects

Apart from occasional nausea on the day after the I-131
-MIBG-infusion, which may also be explained by the oral administration of Lugol's iodine, no gastrointestinal, hepatic
and cardiac side effects have been recorded.

## CONCLUSION

I-131-MIBG treatment is an effective treatment in neuroblastoma and can be used safely in patients with residual
disease without bone marrow involvement at any stage of
their disease.

Major toxicity can be expected when the bone marrow is
invaded, due to irreparable radiation damage to bone marrow
stem cells, especially to the megakaryocytes. In these patients I-131-MIBG can be used as a palliative treatment to re-
lieve pain, but with accepting hematologic toxicity.

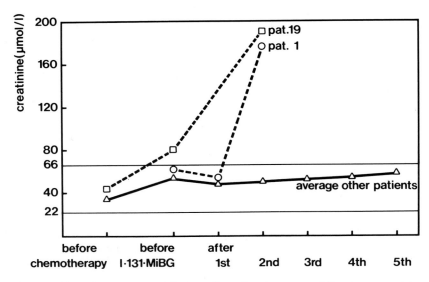

Figure 5.  Serum creatinine levels in neuroblastoma patients after successive therapeutic doses of I-131-MIBG.

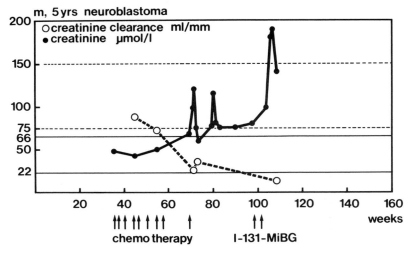

Figure 6.  Serum creatinine levels and creatinine clearance
in a 5 year old boy with neuroblastoma, during respective
treatment with Cisplatin and high dose(7.4 GBq= 200 mCi)
I-131-MIBG.

Using therapeutic doses of I-131-MIBG in patients who had bone marrow invasion at any stage of their disease can induce hematologic toxicity, which means that the use of I-131-MIBG has changed our concept of complete remission radically.

I-131-MIBG treatment can be used in the future in patients with invaded bone marrow, when methods to clean bone marrow in vitro for autologeous reinfusion, become available. It is a valuable method to destroy all neuroblastoma deposits in bone, bone marrow and other sites, but it will result in bone marrow aplasia.

In patients with impaired kidney function due to anatomical malformations, previous chemotherapy with platinum, or previous irradiation one might expect further impairment of the renal function. This may be due to a longer exposure of the kidney tissue to I-131 radiation or to a radiation effect enhancement by platinum deposits in the kidney. Patients with an impaired kidney function are also prone to more hematologic toxicity, probably due to a slower excretion of I-131-MIBG and a longer lasting body exposure to radiation.

No side effects of the gastrointestinal, hepatic and cardiac system were encountered.

Development of methods to access the absorbed radiation dose to tumours and normal tissues requires further research.

## REFERENCES

1) Sisson JC, Shapiro B, Beierwaltes WH, et al (1984). Radiopharmaceutical treatment of malignant pheochromocytoma. J Nucl Med 25: 197-206.
2) Voûte PA, Hoefnagel CA, Marcuse HR, et al (1985). Detection of neuroblastoma with I-131-meta-iodobenzylguanidine. In: Evans AE(ed): "Advances in neuroblastoma research", New York, Alan R Liss Inc, pp 389-398.
3) Hoefnagel CA, Voûte PA, de Kraker J, et al (1987). Radionuclide diagnosis and therapy of neural crest tumors using Iodine-131-meta-iodobenzylguanidine. J Nucl Med 28: 308-314.
4) Van der Steen J, Maessen HJM, Hoefnagel CA, et al (1986). Radiation protection during therapy with unsealed sources at young children. Health Physics 50: 515-522.

Advances in Neuroblastoma Research 2, pages 689–705
© 1988 Alan R. Liss, Inc.

META-IODOBENZYLGUANIDINE (mIBG) SCANS IN NEUROBLASTOMA :
SENSITIVITY AND SPECIFICITY,A REVIEW OF 115 SCANS

Jean D. Lumbroso,Fadhel Guermazi,Olivier Hartmann ,
Sabine Coornaert,Yvon Rabarison,Jérome G. Leclère ,
Dominique Couanet,Chantal Bayle,Jean M. Caillaud, '
Jean Lemerle and Claude Parmentier

Nuclear Medicine (J.D.L.,F.G.,J.G.L.,C.P.),Pedia-
tric Oncology (O.H.,J.L.), Radiology (D.C.),Hema-
tology (C.B.) and Pathology (J.M.C.) Dpts of Institut Gustave Roussy,Villejuif;U66-INSERM (J.D.L,
Y.R.,C.P.), Villejuif ; CEA-ORIS (S.C.),Gif-sur-
Yvette ; France.

INTRODUCTION

Neuroblastoma patients'survival and management with
often intensive therapy are strongly dependent on reliable staging and the detection of hidden tumor sites or
minimal residual disease. Radio-iodinated meta-iodobenzylguanidine (mIBG) is a new Nuclear Medicine tracer (Wieland et al., 1980) which has demonstrated an oxygen dependent uptake mechanism by adrenergic tissues resulting
in a high concentration contrast to other tissues. After
first successful imaging of pheochromocytoma in man (Sisson et al., 1981),this scanning agent was evaluated in
other neural crest tumours. The first positive results in
two neuroblastoma patients were probably reported by Baulieu et al. (1984); other case reports (Treuner et al.,
1984; Kimmig et al., 1984 ; Hattner et al., 1984) were
followed by preliminary results in series of patients
(Hoefnagel et al., 1985; Voute et al., 1985 ; Treuner,
1985; Munkner, 1985; Geatti et al., 1985 ; Hadley et al.,
1986 ; Kimmig et al., 1986; Muller-Gartner et al., 1986 ;
Hoefnagel et al., 1987). In vitro studies have already
demonstrated a specific and energy dependent mIBG uptake
in a human neuroblastoma cell line (Buck et al., 1985).

The aim of this paper is to present the practical
conclusions which can be drawn from the present status of

a work initiated in our Institution three years ago (Lumbroso et al.,1985,1986). We tried to evaluate the contribution of mIBG scans in the diagnosis and repeated staging of neuroblastoma patients as compared to the other
staging methods currently in use.


PATIENTS AND METHODS

Seventy children (3.7 ±3.3 y) with definitely confirmed diagnosis of neuroblastoma or ganglioneuroblastoma had 115 whole body scans carried out 24 hours after
slow intravenous injection of 3.7 MBq/kg of I-123 mIBG
(83 scans) or 0.7 MBq/kg of I-131 mIBG (17 scans) or 0.9
to 4.5 GBq of I-131 mIBG (15 post-therapeutic scans repeated daily for 5 days). The labelling of mIBG was done
according to Mangner's method (1982), using a convenient
kit for labelling with I-123. All the scans explored the
whole body and were performed using a large field gamma-
camera or a dual probe scanner, connected to a dedicated
computer. The total duration of each scan was in between
40 and 60 minutes in order to ensure a satisfactory image
quality.The scans were interpreted as positive in the
presence of any non-physiological uptake area (Nakajo et
al., 1983) or of any bone uptake of the tracer,even at
the level of the metaphyseal complex.
During the study, other well accepted diagnostic modalities including catecholamines assay in urine and conventional bone scans using 99m-technetium hydroxy-methy-
lene diphosphonate (HMDP) were executed as usual to obtain the stage of the disease (Evans et al., 1971). For
the primary tumour and for the detection of hepatic and
lymph node metastases, mIBG was compared to a standard
obtained by the combination of available results from ultrasonography, radiology, CT, NMR and surgery.The standard used for the detection of bone marrow metastases was
the cytological and histological examination (CHBMS), including, when 2 bone marrow aspirates were negative, 10
bone marrow aspirates (Bayle et al., 1985) and one or more trephine biopsies of the iliac bones.
The interpretation of mIBG scans was done prospecti-
vely after a training period of six months allowing two
independent observers (J.D.L.,F.G.) to be well used to
these new images; all the HMDP scans were re-evaluated
retrospectively; we do not consider in this paper the
possible demonstration of the primary tumour during a bo-

ne scan ( Martin-Simmerman et al., 1984).

RESULTS

Due to the rapidly changing nature of the disease,we did not find any significant difference between the results obtained in analysing only the first scan of each patient and the results obtained in analysing all the scans, which are listed below. For the same reason, when comparing mIBG to other modalities, the results were taken into account only if each study was done within 14 days of the other.

Normal and abnormal pattern

Negative scans are shown on figure 1 and 2, demonstrating the multiple physiological uptake areas, and the absence of any physiological bony uptake. Local disease is clearly seen on the scans of figure 3 and 4. Lymph node and bone marrow metastases are well recognized on figures 5 and 6. Tumour foci are significantly more intense than areas demonstrating a physiological uptake. The problem of urine radioactivity is shown on figure 5, where the image of the disposable nappy worn by the child reflects the important urinary excretion of the tracer.

Sensitivity and specificity

For the detection of the primary tumour, the sensitivity of mIBG scans was 73%. Ten false negative patients had an overlap of the tumour with the bladder or heart images (4 cases) or with positive metastatic images (6 cases:liver,spine). Three false negative patients had neuroblastomas which did not secrete catecholamines. The specificity of mIBG was 94%.

For the detection of hepatic and lymph nodes metastases,the sensitivity of mIBG was about 50% and the specificity was 100%.

For the detection of bone marrow metastases, the sensitivity of mIBG scans was 90%, and the specificity 68%, as compared to CHBMS, with in 2 cases additionnal bone marrow aspirates of the proximal femurs. However, reviewing the data from the 16 false positive scans, we

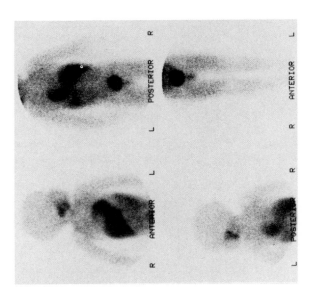

Figure 1

Normal I-123 mIBG scan of a 7y old male
child free of tumour. Left: anterior view,
with a clear image of the salivary glands,
the heart, the liver, a faint image of the
thyroid. Upper right: posterior view, the
spine appears as a photopenic region.
Lower right: no bony image on the limbs.

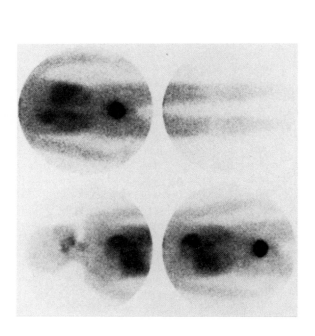
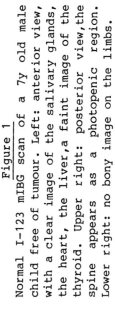

Figure 2

Normal I-123 mIBG scan of a 2.5y old male
child free of tumour. Upper left: demonstration of the salivary glands, the heart, the
liver and of an abdominal background. Other
views demonstrate no bony uptake of the tracer, with a muscular background at the level
of the lower limbs.

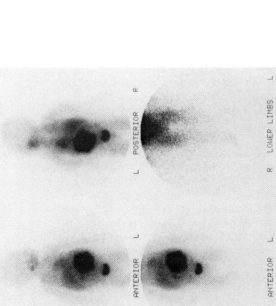

**Figure 3**

Abnormal I-123 mIBG scan of a 10m old female baby with an abdominal neuroblastoma. The tumour is clearly visualized on the left of the spine. A small uptake focus on the right was explained by CT images showing that the tumour was crossing the midline. No bony image and negative CHBMS.

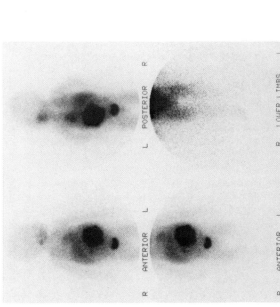

**Figure 4**

Abnormal I-123 mIBG scan of a 2.5y old female child with a thoracic neuroblastoma; tumour was seen on CT on the left of C7 to T7 vertebrae. Clear uptake of mIBG on this posterior view. Contrasting with no significant bony uptake, CHBMS showed rare metastatic cells in the bone marrow.

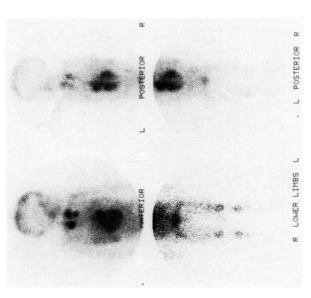

## Figure 5

Abnormal I-123 mIBG scan of a 2.5y old female child with an abdominal neuroblastoma. Clear uptake of the tumour (on the left of the lumbar spine) and of almost all the bones, consistent with a massively involved bone marrow on CHBMS. Notice the abnormal high uptake of the cranial base.

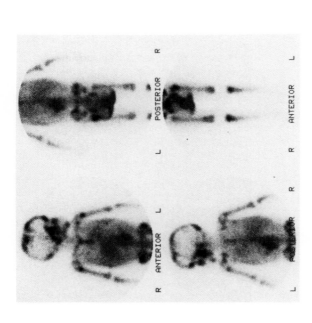

## Figure 6

Abnormal I-123 mIBG scan of a 3y old female child with a left suprarenal neuroblastoma, (5cm diameter on CT),with multiple abdominal and bilateral thoracic lymph node metastases. Clear demonstration of the cranial, pelvic and long bones was consistent with moderately positive CHBMS.

found 11 definitely proven bone metastases, 3 biological relapses without local disease, and 2 cases of delayed abnormal CHBMS supporting the positivity of the mIBG scans, raising the tumour specificity to 100%. Tc-99m HMDP bone scans had a sensitivity of 78% and a specificity of 51%, as compared to CHBMS.

The overall sensitivity of mIBG scans in patients with definitely proven tumour sites was 92% when the urinary excretion of VMA, HVA or dopamine was enhanced, and 45% when these catecholamine metabolites were normal.


DISCUSSION

Tolerance and dosimetry

We did not observe any clinically detectable side effect after injection of diagnostic amounts of mIBG, representing less than 1mg of this substance, intravenously infused over 5 to 30 minutes. Using mIBG labelled with the so-called "pure Iodine-123" (obtained by the p,5n nuclear reaction in cyclotrons), the radiation dose was about 1 cGy to the adrenal medulla and the thyroid if unblocked (Swanson et al.,1981), and less to other organs and the whole body. These doses compare favourably with those induced by Tc-99m HMDP conventional bone scans. The tolerance and the dosimetry of therapeutic doses of I-131 doses of mIBG are discussed in the paper of Hartmann et al., included in this book.


Detection of primary tumours and local disease

Since mIBG scans do not provide the anatomical data needed by the surgeon before tumour resection, their contribution is based on the functional information that can be obtained. In our opinion, their best application is to assess the activity of post-therapeutic remnants, after surgery, chemotherapy or radiotherapy. mIBG scans should be used in close relation with CT, providing functional information on questionable CT abnormalities; CT allows the precise anatomical identification of any mIBG uptake.

Another application could be the positive diagnosis of neuroblastoma when histological data are not available in a child presenting with an abdominal or thoracic tumour concentrating mIBG. We think that to date it is only possible to state that the child is bearing a neural crest tumour, among which neuroblastoma is the most frequent in children. We observed in a group of non-neuroblastoma children, excluded from this study, 1 positive uptake in a case of malignant pheochromocytoma and 1 positive uptake among 3 cases of benign ganglioneuroma.

## Detection of liver and lymph nodes metastases

The sensitivity of mIBG scans for detecting liver metastases is clearly lower than other methods, since there is a physiological uptake of mIBG producing a homogeneous image of the liver. Only in the case of focal metastases with increased uptake foci and a heterogeneous aspect of the liver, or massive liver involvement with a globally increased liver uptake as compared to other physiological uptake areas (especially the heart), will the scan be classified as definitely positive. For the same reasons, we believe that an abnormal hepatic mIBG image having changed into a normal one after therapy will never signify that there is definitely no residual tumour in the liver.

The results of lymph node metastases detection by mIBG scans demonstrate a low sensitivity probably due to the fact that in some cases the image of positive lymph nodes close to the primary tumour is hidden by the tumour image itself, and that in other cases lymph node metastases are small. However, we observed in at least 2 cases abnormal mIBG uptake foci at a distance from the tumour, out of the area primarily explored by CT ; subsequent CT images then confirmed the positive diagnosis of distant lymph node metastases.

## Factors limiting the sensitivity of mIBG scans

It is clear that even for large tumour sites, false negative mIBG scans may occur, due to the intrinsic lack of the tumour ability to concentrate mIBG. This may be observed primarily in patients whose tumour will never be demonstrated on mIBG scans, or after changes in the metabolic activity ( regarding the catecholamine storage or the oxygenation ) of the tumour and its recurrences or metastases later in the course of the disease. Other tumour sites may be hidden by physiological uptake areas, such as the heart, the liver, and especially the bladder for pelvic neuroblastomas ; some interesting results may be obtained in this situation by the use of delayed scans, lateral views, and single photon emission tomo-scintigraphy (Hoefnagel et al., 1987). Finally, there is obviously a threshold due to the signal to noise ratio, related to the tumour volume and the contrast, for the detection of small tumour masses surrounded by the background of normal tissues.

## False positive soft tissue images

Due to the important number of physiological uptake areas of mIBG in soft tissues, there is a risk of false positive interpretation of a normal mIBG scan. Of particular importance in children, we noticed in our study the frequence of the colonic uptake, the increased background in the right iliac fossa in contrast to the photopenic stomach area in babies, and the often intense uptake of a normal adrenal medulla after contralateral surgery of a supra-renal neuroblastoma.

On the other hand, even if CT is well recognized as the best tool for detecting soft tissue tumour sites in neuroblastoma (Couanet et al.,1981; Stark et al., 1983 ), it is impossible to state that its absolute sensitivity is 100% ; in one case of a metastatic neuroblastoma without identified primary, we believe that we found an abdominal tumour site concentrating mIBG and likely to correspond to the primary, without subsequent positive CT findings. In the present status of the study, such a result is classified as false positive mIBG scan.

## Bone and bone marrow metastases,comparison with CHBMS

We clearly demonstrate that mIBG scans are less sensitive than CHBMS, with a difference of about 10%. Two reasons may explain this difference : (i) some tumour cells, especially in non-secreting neuroblastoma, are basically unable to concentrate mIBG, and (ii) due to the signal to noise ratio, there is a volume and contrast threshold for the detection of a tumour site by any scintigraphic method, while histological and cytological methods, in their present status, are able to detect, if present in the sample, 1 metastatic cells clump per up to 1 million of normal bone marrow cells. The latter point was confirmed when we compared, versus CHBMS, the sensitivity of mIBG scans of the sternum and the pelvic bones, excluding any bony positivity elsewhere : this lowered again by 10% the sensitivity of mIBG scans. However, the fact that in 10% of the mIBG scans demonstrating bone marrow metastases, CHBMS was positive on samples from sternum and iliac bones with negative mIBG findings at their level, means that bone marrow metastases are often spread outside of commonly biopsied bones, and that any mIBG bony uptake should be considered as an evidence of a high probability of bone marrow or bone metastases, requiring further investigations. It is worthwhile to notice that in our study, in 2 cases, based on the result of mIBG scans, complementary bone marrow aspirates of the proximal femurs changed into positive false negative results of CHBMS.

False positive mIBG bony images

We never observed in any child of any age a physiological bony uptake of mIBG. The spine and the bones of the limbs always appeared as photopenic areas surrounded by muscular background. The pelvic bones cannot be identified on normal scans because they are superimposed to an important abdominal background. As described in our results, we do not have any data supporting the possibility of any false positive bony uptake. We obviously exclude technical artifacts such as urine contamination or residual Tc-99m bony activity if an interval of at least 3 days has not been observed when a conventional bone scan is followed by an I-123 mIBG scan.

Bone and bone marrow metastases, comparison with conventional Tc-99m HMDP bone scans

Using CHBMS as a standard, the overall sensitivity of mIBG scans is 10% higher than Tc-99m HMDP bone scans sensitivity. However, in patients with negative mIBG scans, the use of Tc-99m bone scans, which were previously considered as the most sensitive imaging modality for bone and bone marrow metastases in neuroblastoma (Howman-Giles et al., 1979 ; Baker et al., 1983 ; Heisel et al., 1983 ; Podrasky et al., 1983 ; Stark et al., 1983 ), is still recommended. The low specificity of Tc-99m HMDP bo-

ne scans and the discrepancies between observers we noticed retrospectively, are due (i) to the slight differences between normal aspect and scintigraphic signs of
bone marrow metastases with minimal changes in the structure and metabolism of normal bone, (ii) to the intense
physiological uptake of the tracer in many points of the
skeleton of a child, especially the metaphyseal complexes
(Kaufman et al., 1978), and (iii) to the difficulty in
ruling out a diffusely increased uptake at the level of
the spine or the pelvic bones, or on the contrary, to
identify areas of decreased uptake which have long been
described in some neuroblastoma osteolytic bone metastases.

## Differentiation between bone marrow and bone metastases

Detection of bone metastases has the same staging
significance as the detection of bone marrow metastases ;
however, the difference is of importance in delineating
the Stage IVs patients category.
Only high intensity bony uptake foci with an asyme-
trical distribution of the tracer will on mIBG scans be
an indication of possible bone metastases rather than
isolated bone marrow involvement. Conventional Tc-99m
HMDP bone scans demonstrating clear alteration from the
normal distribution of the tracer are indicative of bone
metastases, whereas subtle changes may only correspond to
the expression of bone metastases. However, on both scans, we believe that the differentiation between bone marrow and bone metastases may be inaccurate, and we usually
perform a radiological study of any area suspected to be
a bone metastasis on scans or on the presence of pain.
Total skeleton radiography is always performed before
classification of a child in the Stage IVs category in
our Institution.

## Positivity of mIBG scans and urine catecholamines

There is a clear relation between the sensitivity of
mIBG scans and the production of catecholamines (VMA, HVA
or dopamine) by tumour sites at the time of the scan. The
fact that the sensitivity of mIBG scans in the absence of
enhanced urinary catecholamine levels is 45% indicates
(i) that mIBG scans are more sensitive than urine cate-

cholamine assays in detecting a small tumour burden in a patient who had a secreting tumour, and (ii) that in some cases tumours which have never demonstrated their secretory activity in urine may demonstrate an mIBG uptake and therefore be detected by scintigraphy.

We have not to date a sufficient amount of data to correlate the mIBG scans results with the blood level of neurone specific enolase (NSE).

Aggressiveness of the disease and evolutionary potential

We have no data which could correlate on a single mIBG scan the scintigraphic aspect of a tumour site with the aggressiveness of the disease and the evolutionary potential of the so-demonstrated tumour foci. The intensity of the uptake is unlikely to answer this question, since well differentiated tumours like ganglioneuromas may demonstrate a high mIBG uptake. Worsening serial mIBG scans with an increasing number of uptake foci were always associated with a progressive disease.

mIBG scans for the follow up under therapy

Bone radiography and conventional bone scans explore the changes in normal bone structure and metabolism and do not visualize the tumoral process itself. Therefore, their positivity is delayed until the amount of tumour in the bone marrow reaches a threshold to produce detectable changes in normal bone. After a complete response to chemotherapy removing all the tumour cells, a delay of several weeks is necessary to allow the normal bone changes to disappear. It is accepted that residual weakly positive bone scans do not rule out the possibility of a complete remission. We observed after chemotherapy some dramatic changes in serial mIBG scans which may return to normal in an interval of six weeks. Although we have not yet quantitative data, it is likely that mIBG scans closely follow the course of the disease with "a low inertia", as do CHBMS and urine catecholamine assay, since these three modalities directly explore the tumour activity.

Iodine-123 or Iodine-131 for mIBG diagnostic use

For physical reasons, namely the energy of the principal gamma ray of each isotope, better images are provided by the use of I-123 rather than I-131 for gamma camera images.

Another reason which recommends the use of I-123 in children is the problem of environmental contamination and potential contamination of the parents or the nurses of Pediatric departments. Due to the radioactivity of the urine (see figure 5), the irradiation in the case of contamination of the skin or of the thyroid, which can occur if somebody taking care of the child does not respect the radioprotection recommendations, is lowered by a factor 100 using I-123 instead of I-131, and is therefore comparable to the risks induced by the use of Tc-99m HMDP.

When Iodine-131 mIBG is used for therapy, post-therapeutic scans, carried out 3 to 5 days after administration are of great value, since they are high activity scans therefore providing the highest sensitivity to the method.

CONCLUSION

A sufficient amount of data have been accumulated to accept mIBG scans as a major modality in neuroblastoma staging ,due to the tumour specificity of the tracer, playing the same role in neuroblastoma as has radioactive Iodide for four decades in differenciated thyroid cancer. The use of mIBG is simple and safe, especially when labelled with pure I-123.

Even if in most cases it is possible to stage correctly a neuroblastoma patient with a CT and bone marrow aspirates or biopsy, mIBG scans provide more accurate informations on the tumour burden in the whole body and may indicate additionnal CT images at a distance from the primary or additionnal bone marrow biopsies. When positive, mIBG scans replace conventionnal Tc-99m HMDP bone scans, and may reduce the frequency of CHBMS. When repeated during therapy, mIBG scans provide valuable information to quantitate a partial response and to confirm a complete response. Normal mIBG scans are progressively becoming an additional criteria of remission. As no data supports to date the possibility of false positive bony uptake of mIBG, a patient with such an image and negative findings from other staging methods should not be considered in complete remission, and should require further investigations.

As compared to CHBMS, mIBG scans are less sensitive for the detection of bone marrow metastases, but are not topographically limited since they explore the whole body: they provide a complementary approach to the problem of residual disease.

More clinical data are needed to correlate mIBG findings and the aggressiveness of the disease or the prediction of the outcome of intensive chemotherapy followed by a bone marrow transplantation.

## Aknowledgments:

We are indebted to the technologists' staff of the Nuclear Medicine Department and to the nurses of the Pediatric Department who took care of the children, and to Ingrid Kuchental who reviewed the manuscript.

## REFERENCES

Baker M, Siddiqui AR, Provisor A, Cohen MD (1983). Radiographic and scintigraphic skeletal imaging in patients with neuroblastoma: concise communication. J Nucl Med 24: 467-469.

Baulieu JL,Guilloteau D,Viel C,Valat C,Baulieu F,Chambon C,Iti R,Besnard JC,Pourcelot L (1984). Scintigraphie à la méta-iodobenzylguanidine:bilan d'une première année d'expérience. J Biophys et Med Nucl 8:27-33.

Bayle C, Allard T, Rodary C, Vanderplancke J, Hartmann O, Lemerle J (1985). Detection of bone marrow involvement by neuroblastoma:comparison of two cytological methods. Eur Paediatr Haematol Oncol 2: 123-128.

Buck J, Bruchelt G, Girgert R, Treuner J, Niethammer D (1985). Specific uptake of m-($^{125}$I)iodobenzylguanidine in the human neuroblastoma cell line SK-N-SH. Cancer Res 45: 6366-6370.

Couanet D, Hartmann O, Piekarski JD, Vanel D, Masselot J (1981). Apport de la tomodensitométrie dans le bilan d'extension des neuroblastomes de l'enfant. Arch Fr Pediatr 38: 315-318.

Evans AE, D'Angio GJ, Randolph J (1971). A proposed staging for children with neuroblastoma. Cancer 28: 347-378.

Geatti O, Shapiro B, Sisson J, Hutchinson RJ, Malette S, Eyre P, Beierwaltes WH (1985). Iodine-131 metaiodobenzylguanidine scintigraphy for the location of neuroblastoma: preliminary experience in ten cases. J Nucl Med 26: 736-742.

Hadley GP, Rabe E (1986). Scanning with iodine-131 MIBG in children with solid tumours: an initial appraisal. J Nucl Med 27: 620-626.

Hattner RS,HubertyJP,Engelstad BL,Gooding CA,Ablin AR (1984). Localization of m-Iodo($^{131}$I)benzylguanidine in neuroblastoma. AJR 143:373-374.

Heisel MA, Miller JH, Reid BS, Siegel SE (1983). Radionuclide bone scan in neuroblastoma. Pediatrics 71: 206-209.

Hoefnagel CA, Voute PA, de Kraker J, Marcuse HR (1985). Total-body scintigraphy with 131I-meta-iodobenzylguanidine for detection of neuroblastoma. Diag Imag Clin Med 54: 21-27.

Hoefnagel CA, Voute PA, de Kraker J, Marcuse HR (1987) Radionuclide diagnosis and therapy of neural crest tumors using Iodine-131 metaiodobenzylguanidine. J Nucl Med 28: 308-314.

Hoefnagel CA,Klumper A,Voute PA (1987). Single photon emission tomography using meta($^{131}$I)iodobenzylguanidine in malignant pheochromocytoma and neuroblastoma: case reports. Journal of Medical Imaging 1:57-60.

Howman-Giles RB, Gilday DL, Eng B, Ash JM (1979). Radionuclide skeletal survey in neuroblastma. Radiology 131: 497-502.

Kaufman RA, Thrall JH, Keyes JW, Brown ML, Zakem JF (1978). False negative bone scans in neuroblastoma metastatic to the ends of long bones. Am J Roentgenol 130: 131-135.

Kimmig B, Brandeis WE, Eisenhut M, Bubeck B, Hermann HJ, Zum Winkel K (1984). Scintigraphy of a neuroblastoma with I-131 meta-iodobenzylguanidine. J Nucl Med 25:773-775.

Kimmig B, Brandeis WE, Eisenhut M, Ludwig R, Adolph J (1986). Scintigraphic diagnosis of neuroblastoma using meta-iodobenzylguanidine. Klin Padiatr 198: 224-229.

Lumbroso J, Hartmann O, Lemerle J, Coornaert S, Desplanches G, Menard F, Gardet P, Schlumberger M, Parmentier C (1985). Scintigraphic detection of neuroblastoma using $^{131}$I and $^{123}$I labelled meta-iodobenzylguanidine.

Eur J Nucl Med 11 (number 2-3): A16 (Abstract).

Lumbroso J, Guermazi F, Coornaert S, Rabarison Y, Leclere J, Lemerle J, Parmentier C (1986). The clinical contribution of I-123 and I-131 meta-iodobenzylguanidine (mIBG) scans in neuroblastoma. J Nucl Med 27: 947 (Abstract).

Mangner TJ, Wu JL, Wieland DM (1982). Solid phase exchange radioiodination of aryl iodide facilitation by ammonium sulfate. J Org Chem 47: 1484-1488.

Martin-Simmerman P, Cohen MD, Siddiqui A, Mirkin D, Provisor A (1984). Calcification and uptake of Tc-99m diphosphonates in neuroblastomas: Concise communication. J Nucl Med 25: 656-660.

Muller-Gartner HW, Ertmann R, Helmke K (1986). Scintigraphy with radioiodinated meta-iodobenzylguanidine in the diagnosis of neuroblastoma. Nuklearmedizin 24: 222-226.

Munkner T (1985). 131I-meta-iodobenzylguanidine scintigraphy of neuroblastomas. Semin Nucl Med 15: 154-160.

Nakajo M, Shapiro B, Copp J, Kalff V, Gross MD, Sisson JC, Beierwaltes WH (1983). The normal and abnormal distribution of the adrenomedullary imaging agent m-(I-131)iodobenzylguanidine (I-131 MIBG) in man:evaluation by scintigraphy. J Nucl Med 24: 672-682.

Podrasky AE,Stark DD,Hattner RS,Gooding CA,Moss AA (1983) Radionuclide bone scanning in neuroblastoma:skeletal metastases and primary tumour localization of 99mTc-MDP AJR 141:469-472.

Sisson JC, Frager MS, Valk TW, Gross MD, Swanson DP, Wieland DW, Tobes MC, Beierwaltes WH (1981). Scintigraphic localization of pheochromocytoma. N Engl J Med 305: 12-17.

Stark DD, Moss AA, Brasch RC, De Lorimier AA, Albin AR, London DA, Gooding CA (1983). Neuroblastoma: diagnostic imaging and staging. Radiology 148: 101-105.

Swanson DP,Carey JE,Brown LE,Kline RC,Wieland DM,Thrall J H,Beierwaltes WH (1981). Human absorbed dose calculation for Iodine-131 and Iodine-123 labeled meta-iodobenzyl-guanidine (mIBG):a potential myocardial and adrenal medulla imaging agent. In:Proceedings of the third international symposium on radiopharmaceutical dosimetry, Oak Ridge,Tennessee. Oak Ridge Tenn:Oak Ridge Associated Universities,1981: 213-224.

Treuner J, Feine U, Niethammer D, Muller-Schaumberg W, Meinke J, Eibach E, Dopfer R, Klingebiel T, Grumbach S (1984). Scintigraphic imaging of neuroblastoma with ($^{131}$I)iodobenzylguanidine. Lancet 1:333-334.

Treuner J (1985). Use of 131I-meta-iodobenzylguanidine in pediatric oncology. Nuklearmedizin 24: 26–28.

Voute PA, Hoefnagel CA, Marcuse HR, de Kraker J (1985). Detection of neuroblastoma with 131I-meta-iodobenzyl-guanidine. Prog Clin Biol Res 175: 389–398.

Wieland DM, Wu J, Brown LE, Mangner TJ, Swanson DP, Beierwaltes WH (1980). Radiolabeled adrenergic neuron blocking agents: adrenomedullary imaging with ($^{131}$I) iodobenzylguanidine. J Nucl Med 21: 349–353.

Advances in Neuroblastoma Research 2, pages 707–720
© 1988 Alan R. Liss, Inc.

PITFALLS AND SOLUTIONS IN NEUROBLASTOMA DIAGNOSIS USING
RADIOIODINE MIBG: OUR EXPERIENCE ABOUT 50 CASES

Bouvier J.F.*, Philip T.**, Chauvot P.*, Brunat
Mentigny M.**, Ducrettet F.*, Maïassi N.*,
Lahneche B.E.*.
* Department of Nuclear Medicine ** Department
of Pediatrics, Centre Léon Bérard, 28 rue Laën-
nec, 69373 Lyon Cedex 08, France. Supported by
Grant INSERM 486022.

SUMMARY :
        We have been among the first authors to point out
that false negative cases could be observed with 131I-MIBG
scintigraphy for neuroblastoma. We have observed until now
ten of such false negative cases, 7 with primary tumor and
3 with bone metastases. Fifty 131I-MIBG scans were peformed
in 35 children with histologically proven neuroblastoma (24
grade IV) and compared to bone scans, CT and NMR images,
ultrasound and clinical results. The visualization of the
primary tumor shows a higher sensitivity with MIBG (79%)
than with bone scans (47%) and a 100% specificity with each
method. MIBG and bone scans, for bone metastases, are similar in the sensitivity (87.5%) but MIBG is much more specific (100%) than bone scan (81%). These results clearly
confirm the superiority of MIBG scan for detection of primary tumor as well as bone metastases. However, MIBG is not
always the most appropriate investigation, as shown by 11
observed pitfalls. Ten false negative cases have been observed and must be considered: in five out of 10 cases,
bone scans performed with 99m Tc-HMDP made the diagnosis
(3/7 cases of primary tumor and 2/3 cases of bone metastases). Moreover, one case was not usable due to a large
digestive uptake. Our aim is to understand the reasons of
the false negative by a meticulous analysis of every single
case. The optimal procedure for neuroblastoma diagnosis,
extent and follw up clearly seems to be the following strategy: MIBG scan must be firstly performed; in case of non-
demonstrative scan the bone scan, which is complementary,
will greatly contribute to the diagnosis.

The successful use of meta-iodo(131-I)benzylguanidine (131-I-MIBG) for the scintigraphic detection of pheochromocytoma (Wieland et al., 1981) led to its application in neuroblastoma, another neural crest tumor with fewer intracytoplasmic neurosecretory granules. The number of neurosecretory granules is a good indicator of the amount of hormone stored and not of the secretory status of the tumor (Bomanji et al., 1987). MIBG is structurally related to the neuron blocking agent guanethidine, an analog of norepinephrine, and is sequestered within norepinephrine storage granule. For storage of MIBG both an uptake system as well as storage vesicles have to be present (Buck et al., 1985; Guiloteau et al., 1984). MIBG $_+$ is taken up via the neuronal uptake system, the same Na$^+$-dependent, energy-requiring active transport mechanism as norepinephrine (Tobes et al., 1985). This specific uptake mechanism is the predominant uptake mechanism if MIBG concentrations are low, as is the case with bolus injections of radioiodine MIBG used for clinical diagnosis. MIBG is stored in vesicles through a poor specific H$^+$-dependent pathway (Gasnier et al., 1985). The first study (Nakojo et al., 1983) failed to demonstrate neuroblastoma by means of MIBG in two patients but several European centers (Kimmig et al., 1984; Treuner et al., 1984; Munkner et al., 1985) and other centers (Hattner et al., 1984) obtained excellent results confirmed later by the Ann Arbor group (Geatti et al., 1985). We pointed out that false negative cases could be observed with 131-I-MIBG scintigraphy for neuroblastoma and proposed a particular diagnostic strategy (Bouvier et al., 1986). Our experience is now based upon the results of fifty MIBG bone double scintigraphies.

MATERIALS AND METHODS

Since 1984, 35 children with histologically proven neuroblastomas have had fifty 131-I-MIBG and 99m-Tc-HMDP double scans. Twelve of our patients were girls, 23 were boys. The average age was 66 months. The average duration of the disease was 27 months at the time of the double scintigraphies. Three of our patients were in stage II, 8 in stage III and the majority had already reached stage IV (2 in stage IVs and 22 in stage IV). Seven scintigraphic examinations were performed before any therapy. Scans were performed after surgery alone in three cases and after treatment including cytostatics only in 12 cases or crytostatics associated with surgery in 27 cases. Fifteen out of these cases benefited in addition from bone marrow transplantation associated with radiotherapy in 6 cases. One scan was performed for a patient treated by cytostatics and bone marrow transplantation.

Radioiodine MIBG was supplied by CIS International (France). The synthesis of radioiodine MIBG was based on methods previously described by Wieland et al. (1981). We have chosen 131-I-MIBG because of its daily availability for our center. In addition, the alternative choice was MIBG radiolabeled with 123-I (p,2n), a radioisotope contaminated during its production by other compounds delivering appreciable doses of irradiation. The specific activity was about 45.25 MBq/mg. The thyroidal uptake was prevented by 200 mg perchlorate of potassium one hour before each injection and on the following day. The amounts injected intravenously ranged from 30 to 37 MBq. The studies were performed by means of a large-field-of-view gamma camera (Siemens) fitted with a high-energy, parallel-hole collimator and interfaced to a MDS computer (Philips). Multiple overlapping images were obtained at 24 hours after the injection. When necessary, supplementary studies were obtained after injections of 99m-Tc-phytate, DTPA, (Re) sulphide ... The resultant images (liver, kidneys, stomach, ...) were subtracted from 131-I-MIBG images using the computer, 99m-Tc-HMDP scans were systematically performed 3-5 days before 131-I-MIBG scintigraphies. The amounts injected intravenously ranged from 148 to 185 MBq. A dynamic study including sequential views, each view of 20 seconds, during 5 minutes after the injection was performed above the suspected primary tumor for each case without complete removal. In addition, anterior and posterior static images were obtained 5 minutes after the injection. In every case, multiple overlapping images were obtained 3 hours later and subtractions of liver and kidney imaged with 99m-Tc-phytate and DTPA were often realized using the computer.

RESULTS AND DISCUSSION

Normal distribution of 131-I-MIBG

The normal distribution of 131-I-MIBG includes clear portrayal of organs with adrenergic innervation, such as salivary glands and spleen, as well as in organs that process catecholamines for excretion, such as liver and urinary bladder. For the salivary glands the neuronal uptake one system prevails over the active accumulation of free 131-I as it seems to be demonstrated by the non-visualization of the stomach. The heart, lungs, colon, and kidneys can be visualized as the normal adrenal glands can be seldom seen.

## Criteria for positivity

We have the following criteria for MIBG scintigraphy: MIBG binding found in a primitive tumor but also a binding corresponding to any localization other than the normal sites of distribution of MIBG or to any increased intensity of an usual uptake site. Any bone binding is considered as positive as well any uptake by epiphyseal plates is considered. The actual number of metastases present at any particular time was not counted; in the clinical situation the first metastasis is by far the most important.

In addition to detecting skeletal metastases (Baker et al., 1983), bone scans also may image the primary neuroblastoma itself as it concentrates 99m-Tc-HMDP (Podrasky dt al., 1983; Heisel et al., 1983) without significant correlation between tumor uptake and calcification easily detectable by CT scan (Stark et al., 1983). Therefore in the case of an abdominal and/or thoracic mass by a child an uptake of 99m-Tc-HMDP indicates a very high probability of neuroblastoma and can eliminate a Wilms tumor.

Bone foci of 131-I-MIBG uptake can be due to bone involvement as well to bone marrow involvement while 99m-Tc-HMDP uptake can be seen only in case of bone involvement. For bone marrow metastases MIBG is well correlated with bone marrow biopsies (90%) and often confirmed by NMR results.

## Overall study

Each scan was compared with clinical and laboratory data, CT images, NMR or ultrasound results combined with results of biopsy and surgical findings and/or clinical follow-up. Each study was read as either positive or negative for primary disease and metastatic disease. Then true negative (TN), true positive (TP), false negative (FN) and false positive (FP) cases were obtained as indicated in the following table.

| | 131-I-MIBG | | 99m-Tc-HMDP | |
|---|---|---|---|---|
| | Primary tumor | Bone metastases | Primary tumor | Bone metastases |
| TN | 16 | 25 | 16 | 21 |
| TP | 26 | 21 | 16 | 21 |
| FN | 7 | 3 | 18 | 3 |
| FP | 0 | 0 | 0 | 5 |
| not usable | 1 | 1 | 0 | 0 |

Table 1 : Results obtained with 50 MIBG and bone double scintigraphies in 35 children with neuroblastoma

We can note the absence of false positive with 131-I-MIBG as well for primary tumor as for bone metastases. We must insist on the pitfalls observed with 131-I-MIBG. Its ability to diagnose primary tumor was absent in 8 cases (16%) because 7 false negative cases were observed and one case was not usable due to a large digestive uptake. The same problem and 3 false negative cases led to the absence of good diagnosis for bone metastases in four cases (8%). There is no significant correlation between the pitfalls observed with MIBG and urinary catecholamine levels.

Among the false positive cases observed with bone scans in bone metastases we have an interested case : a bone metastasis for which surgery revealed a sterilization by chemotherapy took up 99m-Tc-HMDP but not 131-I-MIBG.

Comparison between MIBG and bone scans

MIBG and bone scans are compared to see which is the more sensitive and specific for diagnosing primary tumor and bone metastases. The visualization of the primary tumor shows a higher sensitivity with MIBG (79%) than with bone scans (47%) and a 100% specificity with each method (Table 2). MIBG and bone scans, for bone metastases, are similar in the sensitivity (87.5%) but MIBG is much more specific (100%) than bone scan (81%)

| | Primary tumor | | Bone metastases | |
|---|---|---|---|---|
| | 131-I-MIBG | 99m-Tc-HMDP | 131-I-MIBG | 99m-Tc-HMDP |
| Sensitivity(%) | 79 | 47 | 87.5 | 87.5 |
| Specificity(%) | 100 | 100 | 100 | 81 |
| Accuracy(%) | 84 | 64 | 92 | 84 |
| PV + (%) | 100 | 100 | 100 | 81 |
| PV - (%) | 70 | 47 | 89 | 87.5 |

Table 2 : Comparison of results of MIBG and bone scans for the detection of primary tumor and for the diagnosis of bone metastases from neuroblastoma

For each study we compared the results obtained by 131-I-MIBG and 99m-Tc-HMDP scans. These results are similar in 24 studies. The superiority of MIBG is noted in 20 cases (7 detections of primary tumors and 13 diagnosis of bone metastases) for the positivity of detection or for the number of foci of uptake. On the other hand bone scan alone makes the diagnosis in 5 cases (3 primary tumors and 2 bone metastases) and one MIBG scan is not technically usable.

These results clearly confirm the superiority of MIBG scan for detection of primary tumor (Fig.1) as well as bone metastases , according to the literature data (Bouvaros et al.,1986;Lumbroso et al.,1986). MIBG scan presents a special interest to assess the tumor activity after treatment, especially in case of fibrosis after surgery and radiotherapy or in case of calcified tumors after chemotherapy.However 11 pitfalls are observed.Four reasons are possible : tumor can be too small to be detected, several organs can hid a tumor uptake, heterogeneousness of uptake can be observed sometimes and tumor tissue can not take up MIBG,especially because of pharmaceutical inhibition.

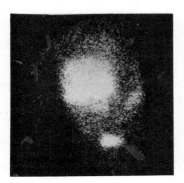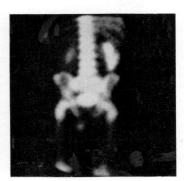

Fig. 1: Posterior MIBG scintigraphy (left) shows a large tumor above the left kidney while bone scan (right) does not reveal any uptake in this area but metastases of proximal femurs.

## Complementarity of MIBG and bone scans

In five out of the ten 131–I-MIBG false negative cases, bone scans performed with 99m–Tc–HMDP made the diagnosis, in 3/7 cases of primary tumor and in 2/3 cases of bone metastases.

For the detection of primary tumor the liver uptake can hide a neuroblastoma or its recurrence in the right upper abdomen. It is the case of a post–therapeutic remnant which was seen superimposed on the posterior end of the eleventh rib on the right side (Fig. 2). In such case Hoefnagel et al (1985) recommended the use of single photon emission tomography.

Accumulation of 131–I-MIBG in urinary tract can hide also abnormal uptakes. Hydronephrosis for instance could be considered as inducing a false negative with MIBG while the bone scan revealed a recurrence of neuroblastoma in the left upper lumber region (Fig. 3). In fact in this case new views were performed later to suppress hydronephrosis artefact. MIBG scan persisted in false negative (Fig. 4).

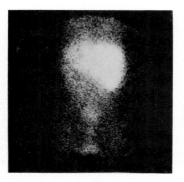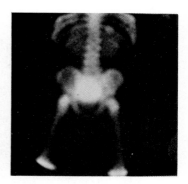

Fig. 2 : Posterior MIBG scintigraphy (left) considered as negative.Bone scan (right) shows a post-therapeutic remnant at the level of the posterior end of the right eleventh rib

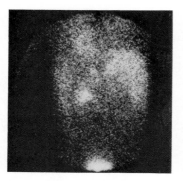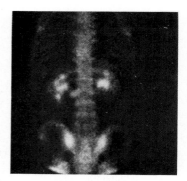

Fig. 3 : Left lumbar recurrence of neuroblastoma and hydro-nephrosis.Negative MIBG scan (left) and positive bone scan (right) (posterior views)

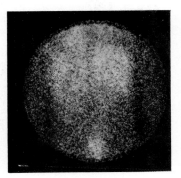 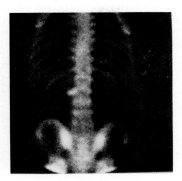

Fig. 4 : Later views of the lumbar region without hydronephrosis artefact.No MIBG abnormalities (left) while bone
scan (right) shows a left lumbar recurrence of neuroblastoma

    Bone scan revealed uptake in primary abdominal remnant
which was active while no abnormalities were demonstrated
by 131-I-MIBG (Fig.5).

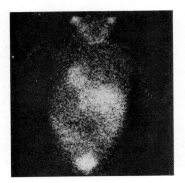 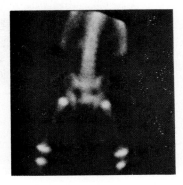

Fig. 5 : Active post-therapeutic remnant.99m-Tc-HMDP scan
(right) revealing uptake in left middle lumbar region.No
MIBG abnormalities (left)

For the diagnosis of bone metastases two false negatives with 131-I-MIBG were corrected by bone scans. 99m-Tc-HMDP scan revealed uptake in the left anterior vault of the skull while 131-I-MIBG scan did not show abnormalities. Two months later MIBG uptake was noted and bone metastasis was confirmed by biopsy (Fig.6).

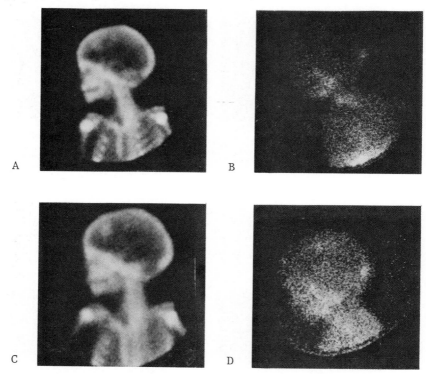

A    B
C    D

Fig. 6 : Left lateral scans of the skull.First bone scan (A) showed abnormal uptake in the anterior vault of the skull while MIBG (B) did not show abnormalities.Two months later MIBG (D) and bone (C) scans were positive

In a second case bone scan revealed a metastasis of the right acetabulum three months before MIBG (Fig.7).

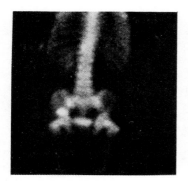

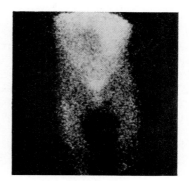

A                                    B

Fig. 7 : Right acetabulum metastasis of a neuroblastoma revealed by 99m-Tc-HMDP (A).First
MIBG scan (B) was negative and
three months later MIBG scan
(C) confirmed with other foci
of uptake

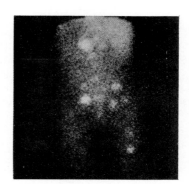

C

CONCLUSION

Our data show that the sensitivity of radioiodine MIBG
scan (79%) is much greater than that of 99m-Tc-HMDP scan
(47%) for detection of primary tumor in neuroblastoma, especially to assess the activity of post-therapeutic remnants.
MIBG scan appears more specific (100%) than bone scan for
diagnosis of bone metastases, in addition MIBG scan reveal
bone marrow metastases.

In our series a 16% false negative rate is found for
MIBG scans in primary tumor detection and 8% false negative
rate in bone metastases.Four reasons are possible : tumor
can be too small to be detected, several organs (liver, kidney with hydronephrosis, colon) can hide tumor uptake, heterogeneousness of uptake can be observed

sometimes and tumor tissue can not take up MIBG, especially because of pharmaceutical inhibition.

MIBG false negative diagnosis have a fifty chance of correction by complementary bone scans. Therefore the optimal procedure for neuroblastoma diagnosis, extent, therapeutic control and follow-up clearly seems to be the following strategy: MIBG scan must be performed first and in case of non demonstrative scan a complementary bone scan can greatly contribute to the diagnosis.

REFERENCES

Baker M, Siddiqui AR, Provisor A, Cohen MD (1983). Radiographic and scintigraphic skeletal imaging in patients with neuroblastoma: concise communication. J Nucl Med 24: 467–469.

Bomanji J, Levison DA, Britton KE (1987). Relationship between the number of chromaffin granules and 123-I-MIBG uptake in paraganglioma, nmeuroblastoma and carcinoid tumour cells. "MIBG and catecholamines. International Workshop", Tours France, pp. 14–16.

Bouvaros A, Kirks DR, Grossman H (1986). Imaging of neuroblastoma: an overview. Pediatr Radiol 16: 89–106.

Bouvier JF, Philip T, Mornex F, Brunat-Mentigny M, Chauvot P, Lahneche BE (1986). Requisite complementarity of 99m-Tc-HMDP and 131-I-MIBG in determining the extent of neuroblastoma. "MIBG in therapy, diagnosis and monitoring of neuroblastoma", Rome, p 1.

Buck J, Bruchelt G, Gigert R, Treuner J, Niethammer D (1985). Specific uptake of m-(125-I) iodobenzylguanidine in the human neuroblastoma cell line SK-N-SH. Cancer Res 45: 6366–6370.

Gasnier B, Roisin MP, Scherman D, Coornaert S, Desplanches G, Henry JP (1985). Uptake of meta-iodobenzylguanidine by bovine chromaffin granule membranes. Mol Pharmacol 29: 275–280.

Geatti O, Shapiro B, Sisson JC, Hutchinson RJ, Mallette S, Eyre P, Beierwaltes WH (1985). Iodine-131 metaiodobenzylguanidine scintigraphy for the location of neuroblastoma: preliminary experience in ten cases. J Nucl Med 26: 736-742.

Guilloteau D, Baulieu JL, Huguet F, Viel C, Chambon C, Vallat C, Baulieu F, Itti R, Pourcelot L, Narcisse G, Besnard JC (1984). Meta-iodobenzylguanidine adrenal medulla localization: autoradiographic and pharmacologic studies. Eur J Nucl Med 9: 278-281.

Hattner RS, Huberty JP, Englestad BL, Gooding CA, Albin AR (1984). Localization of m-iodo(131-I)benzylguanidine in neuroblastoma. AJR 143: 373-374.

Hoefnagel CA, Voute PA, DeKraker J, Marcuse HR (1985). Total-body scintigraphy with 131-I-metaiodbenzylguanidine for detection of neuroblastoma. Diagn Imag Clin Med 54: 21-27.

Kimmig B, Brandeis WE, Eisenhut M, Bubeck B, Hermann HJ, zum Winkel K (1984). Scintigraphy of a neuroblastoma with I-131 meta-iodobenzylguanidine. J Nucl Med 25: 773-775.

Lumbroso J, Hartmann O, Guermazi F, Coornaert S, Rabarison Y, Leclere J, Lemerle J, Parmentier C (1986). The clinical contribution of I-123 and I-131 meta-iodobenzylguanidine (mIBG) scans in neuroblastoma. J Nucl Med 27: 947.

Munkner T (1985). 131-I Metaiodobenzylguanidine scintigraphy of neuroblastomas. Semin Nucl Med 15: 154-160.

Nakajo M, Shapiro B, Copp J, Kalff V, Gross MD, Sisson JC, Beierwaltes WH (1983). The normal and anormal distribution of the adrenomedullary imaging agent m-(I-131) iodobenzylguanidine (I-131 MIBG) in man: evaluation by scintigraphy. J Nucl Med 24: 672-682.

Podrasky AE, Stark DD, Hattner RS, Gooding CA, Moss AA (1983). Radionuclide bone scanning in neuroblastoma: skeletal metastases and primary tumor. AJR 141: 469-472.

Stark DD, Moss AA, Brasch RC, de Lorimier AA, Albin AR, London DA, Gooding CA (1983). Neuroblastoma: diagnostic imaging and staging. Radiology 148: 101-105.

Stark DD, Brasch RC, Moss AA, de Lorimier AA, Albin AR, London DA, Gooding CA (1983). Recurrent neuroblastoma: the role of CT and alternative imaging tests. Radiology 148: 107-112.

Tobes MC, Jacques S, Wieland DM, Sisson JC (1985). Effect of uptake-one inhibitors on the uptake of norepinephrine and metaiodobenzylguanidine. J Nucl Med 26: 897-907.

Treuner J, Feine U, Niethammer D, Muller-Schauenburg W, Meinke J, Eibach E, Dopfer R, Klingelbiel TH, Grumbach ST (1984). Scintigraphic imaging of neuroblastoma with (131-I) iodobenzylguanidine. Lancet I: 333-334.

Wieland DM, Brown L, Tobes MC, Rogers WL, Marsh DD, Mangner TJ, Swanson DP, Beierwaltes WH (1981). Imaging the primate adrenal medulla with (123-I) and (131-I) meta-iodobenzylguanidine: concise communication. J Nucl Med 22: 358-364.

Advances in Neuroblastoma Research 2, pages 721–725
© 1988 Alan R. Liss, Inc.

DISCUSSION:

Chairman:      G.J. D'Angio and P.A. Voute

Discussants:   J. Lumbroso, J.F. Bouvier,
              L.S. Lashford, O. Hartmann,
              J. Treuner,

The discussion was opened by Matthay's request (San Francisco) for comments on the therapeutic effect of I-131 MIBG on bone marrow invasion. She reported her personal experience with a patient with neuroblastoma (NB) who had a positive response in a solid mass to I-131 MIBG but showed concurrent bone marrow progression. The different uptake in NB lesions have been confirmed by Dr. Treuner (Tubingen). In his experience, NB uptake of I-131 MIBG varied from one course to another in some cases. The presence of different clones of NB with different capabilities of MIBG uptake could explain this observation. In this regard, the status of tumor cell differentiation could be important. The need for more laboratory data on NB cell uptake of MIBG was emphasized. Dr. Treuner also pointed out that 1/4 of the complete responders in the study he reported had bone marrow involvement. His conclusion was that I-131 MIBG is effective for treating NB bone marrow involvement but the problem is the hematologic toxicity of the therapy under those conditions.

Dr. D'Angio (Philadelphia) asked whether extensive bone marrow involvement is a criterion for not treating a patient with I-131 MIBG. Dr. Treuner answered that according to their guidelines patients with more than 1/3 bone marrow involvement are not eligible so as to avoid excess toxicity.

In answer to the initial question regarding bone marrow progression during I-131 MIBG, Dr. Voute (Amsterdam) reported that he has never seen such an event. Obviously, he has seen bone marrow failures but never concurrent with I-131 MIBG response elsewhere. He went on to say that Stage III patients with post-surgical residual disease are ideal candidates for I-131 MIBG therapy in his opinion. In his institution, a trial of I-131 MIBG for such patients is now open. They still accept stage IV patients for I-131 MIBG therapy but only when this treatment represents the last chance for a long-term control. Dr. D'Angio asked Dr. Voute whether patients with extensive NB marrow infestation who have residual clumps of cells--or no residual cells visible--are accepted for treatment despite the known risks of severe bone marrow toxicity. Dr. Voute answered that the use of I-131 MIBG in these patients is always considered part of a Phase II trial, but emphasized that patients with known heavy bone marrow involvement are accepted. The role played by I-131 MIBG therepy in the treatment of Stage IV patients then was discussed by Dr. Hartmann (Villejuif). According to his experience, at the doses and at the schedules used, I-131 MIBG cannot be curative for Stage IV patients. Admitting them to I-131 MIBG studies is justified in order to collect Phase II data, not for definitive therapy. He also emphasized that the ideal patients for this treatment are those with Stage III disease. According to Dr. Lashford (London) I-131 MIBG from a theoretical point of view is not the correct isotope for treating a diffuse disease. Although its energy deposition extends about 1 mm around where it attaches to the cell, in fact, the major effect of I-131 MIBG is seen in bulky disease.

Dr. Philip (Lyon) noted that there were big differences in response rates recorded in the four studies presented. He concluded that a convincing Phase III study of I-131 MIBG is needed, but may still be premature because of uncertainty regarding best procedure.

Dr. Treuner commented that the results were not really so different except for that reported by Dr. Lumbroso (Villejuif) who did not have any positive responses. He went on to point out that another group of patients eligible for I-131 MIBG, i.e., Stage IV NB patients with an allogeneic bone marrow donor in whom the use of high dose MIBG could be tested. Dr. Voute advanced a possible explanation for the negative results in Villejuif namely, Dr. Lumbroso's compound was produced by a company different from the one used by the other European groups. He stressed that the same compound must be used to insure data comparability between centers.

Dr. Lumbroso believed this to be a pretty unlikely explanation for the negative results of their study. He explained that the activity of MIBG is always tested before the clinical use, and the same specific activity used by the other group is adopted in Villejuif.

Furthermore, with the same molecule they have achieved good results in pheochromocytoma. One possible reason for the failures registered is that the population of Dr. Lumbroso's study is represented mainly by end-stage patients, who actually in some instancess had some tumor shrinkage but always less than 50% of the initial tumor volume. Dr. Pinkerton (London) thought an explanation for the different results of the studies lay in the different schedules adopted. Dr. Voute commented saying that after having investigated many different possibilities, he has adopted a 4 hour infusion of 200 MCI of MIBG followed four weeks later by another 100. The tumor response is always assessed after the second course. According to Dr. Treuner, the best method has not been established yet; this problem is the object of a large controversy in German. For example, in Tubingen, they use a 24-hour infusion while in Frankfurt a split course is adopted consisting of two courses of four-hour infusions with a 20 hour interval between them. According to his laboratory data, long-term infusion of MIBG produces higher cytotoxicity in mice and in tissue cultures. Dr. Lashford introduced another variable: the time when I-131 MIBG is infused after defrosting. MIBG must be used no later than four hours after defrosting otherwise there is an excess of radiolytic breakdown products.

The problem of the dose of I-131 MIBG has been discussed. Dr. Matthay (San Francisco) asked if--when using doses of 20 mCi/Kg, as Dr. Treuner mentioned--an autologous bone marrow rescue is necessary. Dr. Treuner replayed that in each single patient, the dose of I-131 MIBG delivered is calculated according to the expected tumor uptake using the extent of bone marrow involvement, as limiting factor. The highest single dose used was 250 mCi and the highest cumulative dose was 450 mCi. Dr. Matthay gave her experience the highest single dose she administered (320 mCi), but it was used for an adult who thereafter experienced only a mild thrombocytopenia.

The next part of the discussion was focused on the diagnostic applications of I-131 MIBG. The first problem for discussion was proposed by Dr. Berthold (Cologne) who asked about the use of MIBG scans in patients with localized disease who did not excrete catecholamines. In

Dr. Lumbroso's experience, 98% of the patients secreting catecholamines had positive MIBG scans as did 50% of the non-secreting. In other words, it is possible to have a positive MIBG scan in the face of a negative catecholamine assay. That implies that the MIBG scan is more sensitive than is the biological assay for NB. Other than that, Dr. Hartmann added, it is pretty common in assessing the tumor response to initial chemotherapy in Stage IV children, to still have positive MIBG scans in patients who are no longer secreting catecholamines. The normalization of catecholamine secretion is not usually parallel to the normalization of MIBG scan.

Dr. D'Angio then asked the panel to provide their experience with discordant MIBG scan results in the same patient multiple lesions. According to Dr. Voute, this almost never happens. In his opinion, the MIBG scan is very sensitive and definitely superior to conventional Tc bone scans in diagnosing NB. In his institution they do not use Tc bone scans any more for the staging of NB patients because of the diagnostic effectiveness of MIBG scanning. The problem is that MIBG scans are not easy to do or to read. Dr. Treuner noted that MIBG can give false negative results in non-catechole secreting NB patients. In these cases, the conventional Tc bone scan was more sensitive. Anyhow, he also never had seen discordant MIBG scan results on the same patient. Dr. Lumbroso reported that the accuracy of the MIBG scan can be reduced in body regions with a high soft tissue background. Dr. Hartmann added that it is possible to have a positive Tc bone scan and negative MIBG scan. The possibility of using MIBG scan as a definitive diagnostic tool was also discussed. Dr. Lumbroso explained that many neural crest tumors can take up MIBG and thus the MIBG scan cannot be expected to provide an absolute, histologic diagnosis. He had experiences with MIBG positive abdominal masses in three children one of which turned out to be a pheochromocytoma and the other two were tumors with combined features of Wilms' tumor and neuroblastoma. MIBG can easily predict the diagnosis, but the basic diagnostic criteria are always necessary. He concluded emphasizing that the MIBG scan findings are difficult to interpret.

Dr. Voute stated that was not necessarily true. An MIBG positive large abdominal mass with high urinary levels of HVA and VMA is certainly a neuroblastoma. In this case, histologic proof is not necessary. Dr. Evans

commented briefly that she would also obtain a serum
ferritin assay to help clinch the diagnosis.

Dr. D'Angio believed there is a difference between
staging a NB patient in order to treat him or to study
him. In other words, if one has a positive conventional
Tc bone scan, what else is necessary to plan treatment?
Accurate identification of all involved sites is
important in studies of therapeutic efficacy, but is not
crucial in managing individual patients not enrolled in
such studies. A prolonged discussion ensued. According
to Dr. Hartmann, what Dr. D'Angio said is valid only for
planning a treatment but not for assessing a tumor
response. Dr. Voute disagreed with Dr. D'Angio. Not
performing an MIBG scan and utilizing only a conventional
Tc bone scan can result in a lot of lost information. In
fact, it may not be possible to judge if a newly
perceived lesion in a child under treatment represents a
real relapse or a persistant focus. The conventional Tc
bone scan gives information only related to calcium
metabolism and not directly related to the disease,
Dr. Lumbroso commented. But he also added that he has
had false positive MIBG scan. The importance of
performing MIBG scans for staging a NB patient also was
emphasized by Drs. Treuner and Philip.

The discussion was concluded by some notes regarding
the therapeutic use of MIBG. Dr. Carli (Padova)
requested a definitive comment on the possible use of
I-131 MIBG as front-line therapy for patients with
post-surgical residual disease and with microscopic
residues. Dr. Voute answered saying that in patients
with a good MIBG uptake after a dosimetric study, I-131
MIBG can be considered a possible primary therapy.
Anyhow, the superiority of I-131 MIBG versus local
radiotherapy has not been established yet. In
conclusion, as Dr. Philip also pointed out, in his
opinion the use of I-131 MIBG in Phase III trials is
probably still premature.

# Index

727